Introduction to Psychiatry

Introduction to Psychiatry

Preclinical Foundations and Clinical Essentials

Edited by

Audrey M. Walker

Albert Einstein College of Medicine

Steven C. Schlozman

Harvard Medical School

Jonathan E. Alpert

Albert Einstein College of Medicine

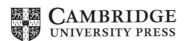

CAMBRIDGE
UNIVERSITY PRESS

CAMBRIDGE
UNIVERSITY PRESS

University Printing House, Cambridge CB2 8BS, United Kingdom

One Liberty Plaza, 20th Floor, New York, NY 10006, USA

477 Williamstown Road, Port Melbourne, VIC 3207, Australia

314–321, 3rd Floor, Plot 3, Splendor Forum, Jasola District Centre, New Delhi – 110025, India

103 Penang Road, #05–06/07, Visioncrest Commercial, Singapore 238467

Cambridge University Press is part of the University of Cambridge.

It furthers the University's mission by disseminating knowledge in the pursuit
of education, learning, and research at the highest international levels of excellence.

www.cambridge.org
Information on this title: www.cambridge.org/9780521279840
DOI: 10.1017/9780511846403

First published 2021

Printed in the United Kingdom by TJ Books Limited, Padstow Cornwall

A catalogue record for this publication is available from the British Library.

Library of Congress Cataloging-in-Publication Data
Names: Alpert, Jonathan Edward, editor. | Schlozman, Steven C., editor. | Walker, Audrey M., editor.
Title: Introduction to psychiatry: preclinical foundations and clinical essentials / edited by Jonathan Alpert, Steven Schlozman, Audrey Walker.
Description: Cambridge, United Kingdom; New York, NY: Cambridge University Press, 2021. | Includes bibliographical references and index.
Identifiers: LCCN 2020046956 (print) | LCCN 2020046957 (ebook) | ISBN 9780521279840 (paperback) | ISBN 9780511846403 (ebook)
Subjects: MESH: Mental Disorders | Psychiatry – methods
Classification: LCC RC454 (print) | LCC RC454 (ebook) | NLM WM 140 | DDC 616.89–dc23
LC record available at https://lccn.loc.gov/2020046956
LC ebook record available at https://lccn.loc.gov/2020046957

ISBN 978-0-521-27984-0 Paperback

Contents

List of Contributors   vii

1   Introduction   1
Audrey M. Walker, Steven C. Schlozman, and Jonathan E. Alpert

2   Clinical Neuroscience   9
Ayol Samuels, Matthew L. Baum, Joseph Luchsinger, Robert G. Mealer, and Rachel A. Ross

3   Introduction to the Patient Interview   38
Todd Griswold, Michael Kahn, Mark Schechter, Janet Yassen, Felicia Smith, and Rebecca Brendel

4   Mood Disorders   70
Scott R. Beach, Jeff C. Huffman, Ji Hyun Baek, Michael Treadway, Andrew A. Nierenberg, and Jonathan E. Alpert

5   Schizophrenia Spectrum and Other Psychotic Disorders   102
Dost Ongur, Francine Benes, Oliver Freudenreich, Matcheri Keshava, and Robert McCarley

6   Anxiety Disorders   128
Meredith Charney, Eric Bui, Elizabeth Goetter, Carl Salzman, John Worthington, Luana Marques, Jerrold Rosenbaum, and Naomi Simon

7   Obsessive-Compulsive and Related Disorders   146
Ryan J. Jacoby, Amanda W. Baker, Michael A. Jenike, Scott L. Rauch, and Sabine Wilhelm

8   Disorders Related to Stress and Trauma   166
Eric Bui, Meredith Charney, Mohammed R. Milad, Devon Hinton, Fredrick Stoddard, Terence Keane, Roger Pitman, and Naomi M. Simon

9   Substance Use Disorders   179
Hilary S. Connery, Mark J. Albanese, Jeffrey J. DeVido, Kevin P. Hill, R. Kathryn McHugh, Dana Sarvey, Joji Suzuki, and Roger D. Weiss

10   **Personality Disorders**   233
Lois W. Choi-Kain, Ana M. Rodriguez-Villa, Gabrielle S. Ilagan,
and Evan A. Iliakis

11   **Neurocognitive Disorders**   263
Brent P. Forester, Feyza Marouf, Ben Legesse, Olivia I. Okereke,
and Deborah Blacker

12   **Feeding and Eating Disorders**   289
Anne E. Becker, Kamryn T. Eddy, David C. Jimerson, and
Jennifer J. Thomas

13   **Child Psychiatry and Neurodevelopmental Disorders**   318
Scott Shaffer and Steven C. Schlozman

14   **Sleep Disorders**   329
Susan Chang and John Winkelman

15   **Psychopharmacology and Neurotherapeutics**   342
Steven Seiner, Ross Baldessarini, Joan Camprodon, Darin
Dougherty, Lior Givon, Jeffrey DeVido, and Jonathan E. Alpert

16   **Psychosocial Interventions**   389
Marshall Forstein, Alfred Marguiles, Robert Goisman, Elizabeth
Simpson, Eleanor Counselman, Miriam Tepper, Jennifer Greenwold,
Zev Schuman-Olivier, and Darshan Mehta

17   **Psychiatric Evaluation in the Medical Setting**   415
Fremonta Meyer, Oriana Vesga Lopez, Felicia Smith, Robert Joseph,
Ted Avi Gerstenblith, Theodore Stern, John Peteet, Donna Greenberg,
and David Gitlin

18   **Psychiatry of Gender and Sexuality**   448
Aaron S. Breslow

19   **Health Policy and Population Health in Behavioral Health Care in**
     the United States   473
Kirstin Beach and Bruce Schwartz

20   **Global Health and Mental Health Care Delivery in Low-Resource**
     Settings   486
Giuseppe Raviola

     Index   497

Contributors

AARON S. BRESLOW, PHD
Assistant Professor of Psychiatry and Behavioral Sciences, Albert Einstein College of Medicine

ALFRED MARGULIES, MD
Associate Professor of Psychiatry, Harvard Medical School, Cambridge Health Alliance/Cambridge Hospital

AMANDA W. BAKER, PHD
Assistant Professor of Psychology in the Department of Psychiatry, Harvard Medical School Massachusetts General Hospital

ANA M. RODRIGUEZ-VILLA, MD MBA
Psychiatry Resident, Harvard Medical School, Massachusetts General Hospital/McClean Hospital

ANDREW A. NIERENBERG, MD
Professor of Psychiatry, Harvard Medical School, Massachusetts General Hospital

ANNE E. BECKER, PHD, MD
Maude and Lillian Presley Professor of Global Health and Social Medicine, Harvard Medical School

AUDREY M. WALKER, MD
Associate Professor of Psychiatry and Behavioral Sciences, and Pediatrics, Albert Einstein College of Medicine, Montefiore Medical Center

AYOL SAMUELS, MD
Assistant Professor of Psychiatry and Behavioral Sciences, Albert Einstein College of Medicine, Montefiore Medical Center

BEN LEGESSE, MD
Cape Cod Healthcare Centers for Behavioral Health

BRENT P. FORESTER, MD, MSC
Associate Professor of Psychiatry, Harvard Medical School McLean Hospital

BRUCE SCHWARTZ, MD
Professor, Deputy Chair and Clinical Director, Psychiatry & Behavioral Sciences, Albert Einstein College of Medicine, Montefiore Medical Center

CARL SALZMAN, MD
Professor of Psychiatry, Harvard Medical School Beth Israel Deaconess Medical Center

DANA SARVEY, MD
Instructor in Psychiatry, Harvard Medical School, McLean Adolescent Partial Hospital Program

DARIN DOUGHERTY, MD
Associate Professor of Psychiatry, Harvard Medical School Massachusetts General Hospital

DARSHAN MEHTA, MD, MPH
Assistant Professor of Medicine, Harvard Medical School, Massachusetts General Hospital, Brigham & Women's Hospital

DAVID C. JIMERSON, MD
Professor of Psychiatry, Harvard Medical School, Beth Israel Deaconess Medical Center

DAVID GITLIN, MD
Assistant Professor of Psychiatry, Harvard Medical School, Brigham and Women's Hospital

DEBORAH BLACKER, SCD, MD
Professor of Psychiatry, Harvard Medical School, Massachusetts General Hospital

DEVON HINTON, MD
Associate Professor of Psychiatry, Part-time, Harvard Medical School, Massachusetts General Hospital

DONNA GREENBERG, MD
Associate Professor of Psychiatry, Harvard Medical School, Massachusetts General Hospital

DOST ONGUR, MD, PHD
William P. and Henry B. Test Professor of Psychiatry, Harvard Medical School,
McLean Hospital

ELEANOR COUNSELMAN, EDD
Private practice, Belmont, MA

ELIZABETH GOETTER, PHD
Assistant Professor of Psychology in the Department of Psychiatry, Harvard
Medical School, Massachusetts General Hospital

ELIZABETH SIMPSON, MD
Instructor in Psychiatry, Harvard Medical School, Beth Israel Deaconess Medical
Center-Mass Mental Health Center

ERIC BUI, PHD, MD
Assistant Professor of Psychiatry, Harvard Medical School, Massachusetts
General Hospital University of Caen Normandy & Caen University Hospital, Caen,
France

EVAN A. ILIAKIS, BA
McLean Hospital

FELICIA SMITH, MD
Assistant Professor of Psychiatry, Harvard Medical School, Massachusetts
General Hospital

FEYZA MAROUF, MD
Instructor in Psychiatry, Harvard Medical School, Massachusetts General Hospital

FRANCINE BENES, MD, PHD
William P. and Henry B. Test Professor of Psychiatry, Emerita, Harvard Medical
School, McLean Hospital

FREDERICK STODDARD, MD
Professor of Psychiatry, Part-time, Harvard Medical School, Massachusetts
General Hospital

FREMONTA MEYER, MD
Assistant Professor of Psychiatry, Harvard Medical School Brigham and Women's
Hospital

GABRIELLE S. ILAGAN, BA
McLean Hospital

GIUSEPPE RAVIOLA, MD, MPH
Assistant Professor of Psychiatry, Harvard Medical School, Massachusetts
General Hospital

HILARY S. CONNERY, MD, PHD
Assistant Professor of Psychiatry, Harvard Medical School, McLean Hospital

JANET YASSEN, MSW
Teaching Associate in Psychiatry, Harvard Medical School, Cambridge Health
Alliance

JEFFERY C. HUFFMAN, MD
Professor of Psychiatry, Harvard Medical School, Massachusetts General
Hospital

JEFFREY J. DEVIDO, MD
Assistant Clinical Professor of Psychiatry, UCSF Weill Institute for
Neurosciences

JENNIFER GREENWOLD, MD
Instructor in Psychiatry, Harvard Medical School, Cambridge Health Alliance

JENNIFER J. THOMAS, PHD
Associate Professor of Psychology in the Department of Psychiatry, Harvard
Medical School, Massachusetts General Hospital

JERROLD ROSENBAUM, MD
Stanley Cobb Professor of Psychiatry, Harvard Medical School, Massachusetts
General Hospital

JI HYUN BAEK, MD, PHD
Assistant Professor of Psychiatry, Sungkyunkwan University School of Medicine,
Samsung Medical Center

JOAN CAMPRODON, PHD, MD
Assistant Professor of Psychiatry, Harvard Medical School, Massachusetts
General Hospital

JOHN PETEET, MD
Associate Professor of Psychiatry, Harvard Medical School, Dana-Farber Cancer
Institute, Brigham and Women's Hospital

JOHN WINKELMAN, MD, PHD
Professor of Psychiatry, Harvard Medical School, Massachusetts General Hospital

JOHN WORTHINGTON III, MD
Assistant Professor of Psychiatry, Harvard Medical School, Massachusetts
General Hospital

JOJI SUZUKI, MD
Assistant Professor of Psychiatry, Harvard Medical School, Brigham and
Women's Hospital

JONATHAN E. ALPERT, MD, PHD
Professor of Psychiatry and Behavioral Sciences, Neuroscience, and Pediatrics,
Chair, Department of Psychiatry and Behavioral Sciences, Albert Einstein College
of Medicine, Montefiore Medical Center

JOSEPH LUCHSINGER
MSTP student, Vanderbilt University

KAMRYN T. EDDY, PHD
Associate Professor of Psychology in the Department of Psychiatry, Harvard
Medical School Massachusetts General Hospital

KEVIN P. HILL, MD
Associate Professor of Psychiatry, Harvard Medical School Beth Israel Deaconess
Medical Center

KIRSTIN BEACH, MPH
Vice President, Government Relations, Healthfirst

LIOR GIVON, MD, PHD
Assistant Professor of Psychiatry, Harvard Medical School, Cambridge Health
Alliance

LOIS W. CHOI-KAIN, MD MED
Assistant Professor of Psychiatry, Harvard Medical School, McLean Hospital

LUANA MARQUES, PHD
Associate Professor of Psychology in the Department of Psychiatry, Harvard Medical School, Massachusetts General Hospital

MARK J. ALBANESE, MD
Assistant Professor of Psychiatry, Harvard Medical School, Cambridge Health Alliance

MARK SCHECHTER, MD
Instructor in Psychiatry, Harvard Medical School, Massachusetts General Hospital
Chair, Department of Psychiatry, North Shore Medical Center

MARSHALL FORSTEIN, MD
Associate Professor of Psychiatry, Harvard Medical School, Cambridge Health Alliance

MATCHERI KESHAVA, MD
Stanley Cobb Professor of Psychiatry, Harvard Medical School, Beth Israel Deaconess Medical Center

MATTHEW L. BAUM, PHD
Clinical Fellow in Psychiatry, Harvard Medical School

MEREDITH CHARNEY, PHD
Psychologist/Director of Education, Psychology Specialists of Maine

MICHAEL A. JENIKE, MD
Professor of Psychiatry, Harvard Medical School, Massachusetts General Hospital

MICHAEL KAHN, MD
Assistant Professor of Psychiatry, Harvard Medical School, Beth Israel Deaconess Medical Center

MICHAEL TREADWAY, PHD
Associate Professor of Psychology, Emory College of Arts & Sciences

MIRIAM TEPPER, MD
Assistant Professor of Psychiatry, Harvard Medical School, Cambridge Health Alliance

MOHAMMED R. MILAD, PHD
Professor of Psychiatry, NYU Grossman School of Medicine, NYU Langone

NAOMI M. SIMON, MD, MSC
Professor of Psychiatry, NYU Grossman School of Medicine, Vice Chair, NYU
Langone Vice Chair NYU Langone/Psychiatry

OLIVER FREUDENREICH, MD
Associate Professor of Psychiatry, Harvard Medical School, Massachusetts
General Hospital

OLIVIA I. OKEREKE, MD, SM
Associate Professor of Psychiatry, Harvard Medical School, Massachusetts
General Hospital

ORIANA VESGA LOPEZ, MD
Monterey County Behavioral Health

R. KATHRYN MCHUGH, PHD
Assistant Professor of Psychology in the Department of Psychiatry, Harvard
Medical School, McLean Hospital

RACHEL A. ROSS, MD, PHD
Assistant Professor of Neuroscience, Psychiatry & Behavioral Sciences, and
Medicine, Albert Einstein College of Medicine

REBECCA BRENDEL, MD, JD
Assistant Professor of Psychiatry, Harvard Medical School, Massachusetts
General Hospital

ROBERT G. MEALER, MD
Instructor in Psychiatry, Harvard Medical School, Massachusetts General
Hospital

ROBERT GOISMAN, MD
Associate Professor of Psychiatry, Part-time, Harvard Medical School, Beth Israel
Deaconess Medical Center

ROBERT JOSEPH, MD
Assistant Professor of Psychiatry, Part-time, Harvard Medical School, Cambridge
Health Alliance

ROBERT MCCARLEY, MD
Professor and Chair of Psychiatry, Harvard Medical School (Deceased May 27,
2017)

ROGER D. WEISS, MD
Professor of Psychiatry, Harvard Medical School, McLean Hospital

ROGER PITMAN, MD
Professor of Psychiatry, Part-time, Harvard Medical School, Massachusetts General Hospital

ROSS BALDESSARINI, MD
Professor of Psychiatry (Neuroscience), Harvard Medical School, McLean Hospital

RYAN J. JACOBY, PHD
Assistant Professor of Psychology in the Department of Psychiatry, Harvard Medical School, Massachusetts General Hospital

SABINE WILHELM, PHD
Professor of Psychology in the Department of Psychiatry, Harvard Medical School, Massachusetts General Hospital

SCOTT L. RAUCH, MD
Professor of Psychiatry, Harvard Medical School; President & Psychiatrist in Chief, McLean Hospital

SCOTT R. BEACH, MD
Assistant Professor of Psychiatry, Harvard Medical School, Massachusetts General Hospital

SCOTT SHAFFER, MD
Assistant Professor of Psychiatry and Behavioral Sciences and Pediatrics, Albert Einstein College of Medicine Montefiore Medical Center

STEPHEN SEINER, MD
Assistant Professor of Psychiatry, Harvard Medical School, McLean Hospital

SUSAN CHANG, MD
Instructor in Medicine, Harvard Medical School, Brigham and Women's Hospital

STEVEN C. SCHLOZMAN, MD
Associate Professor of Psychiatry, Dartmouth Geisel School of Medicine

TED AVI GERSTENBLITH, MD
Assistant Professor of Psychiatry and Behavioral Sciences, Johns Hopkins University School of Medicine, The Johns Hopkins Hospital

TERENCE KEANE, PHD
Lecturer on Psychiatry, Part-time, Harvard Medical School, Veterans Affairs
Boston Healthcare System

THEODORE STERN, MD
Ned H. Cassem Professor of Psychiatry, Harvard Medical School, Massachusetts
General Hospital

TODD GRISWOLD, MD
Assistant Professor of Psychiatry, Harvard Medical School, Cambridge Health
Alliance

ZEV SCHUMAN-OLIVIER, MD
Instructor in Psychiatry, Harvard Medical School, Cambridge Health Alliance

1 | Introduction

AUDREY M. WALKER, STEVEN C. SCHLOZMAN, AND
JONATHAN E. ALPERT

Introduction

The essence of global health equity is the idea that something so precious as health might be viewed as a right.

Paul Farmer, Rx for Survival, Global Health Champions

Without mental health there can be no true physical health.

Brock Chisholm, first Director-General World Health Organization

The first edition of *Introduction to Psychiatry* is a textbook designed to reach medical students, house staff, primary care clinicians, and early-career mental health practitioners. It is the editors' hope that this text will enable its readers to understand the neuroscientific basis of psychiatry, best practices in the psychiatric assessment and treatment of the patient, the current understanding of core psychiatric diagnoses, and the important underlying issues of population health, public policy, and workforce recruitment and training that must be tackled to bring these advances to all.

Why create a textbook of psychiatry specifically for clinicians not trained for the mental health field? To answer this question, one must understand the troubling challenges facing the mental health workforce, the changing face of mental health care delivery, the enormous comorbidity between psychiatric illnesses and other health conditions, and the impact on non-psychiatric medical illnesses when a comorbid psychiatric disorder is present.

The Prevalence and Impact of Psychiatric Disorders

Across the globe, no category of human suffering equals that of mental illness. Mental disorders are highly prevalent, have their onset beginning in childhood through early adulthood, and are stubbornly chronic. One in five people annually have a diagnosable mental disorder, and a staggering one in two people will suffer from a mental illness during their lifetime. (Kessler, 2005; Steel et al., 2014). Though the prevalence of mental disorders is approximately equivalent among non-Hispanic whites, Hispanics, and non-Hispanic blacks, access to treatment and treatment intensity is lower among Hispanics and non-Hispanic blacks, leading to poorer outcomes (Alegria et al., 2008; US Dept of HHS, 2001).

Suicide is a frequent outcome of the more severe presentations of the most serious mental illnesses and is the second most common cause of death globally in young adults (Arensman, et al., 2020). Ninety percent of suicides are associated with a diagnosable psychiatric disorder. Substance abuse and death by drug overdose are a worldwide scourge.

Psychiatric disorders hit the child and adolescent population especially hard. Meta-analyses have found that the worldwide prevalence of mental disorders in children and adolescents is 13 percent (Polancyzk, 2015). Approximately half of all serious psychiatric disorders encountered in adults have their onset in childhood. Psychiatric disorders that have their onset in childhood and become chronic have a myriad of serious sequelae, following these young people through development and thus impacting their emerging identity, ability to learn, social development, and overall health and life expectancy.

Psychiatric disorders impede access to medical care and worsen clinical outcomes of medical illness. Virtually all medical problems have a poorer prognosis when accompanied by a comorbid mental illness. Individuals with mental illness in the United States and globally have a severely shortened life expectancy due to the mental illnesses as well as the poor overall health that accompanies them.

In spite of these staggering realities, the majority of individuals with psychiatric illness do not receive care.

Why Is This the Case?

The global population is growing. In 2021, the US population is projected to grow by 2,000,000 people from a combination of new births and immigration United Nations World Population Prospects U.S. Population Growth Rate 1950–2021. www.macrotrends.net. Retrieved 2021-03-29. Given this growing population, it can be predicted that the number of people needing mental health treatment will continue to increase.

Yet this growing demand for mental health care is not being met.

There is a severe workforce shortage in mental health globally, and indeed, in many cases that shortage may be expected to increase. For example, between 2003 and 2013, while the US population grew, the number of practicing psychiatrists declined (Bishop et al., 2016). A novel study analyzing data from the Association of American Medical Colleges (AAMC), American Board of Psychiatry & Neurology (ABPN), and US Census Bureau projected the psychiatrist workforce through 2050 (Satiani, et al., 2018). The study concluded that this workforce will continue to contract through 2024 if no interventions are implemented. In the United States, these shortfalls will continue to be felt most heavily in rural areas, among the poor and non-white population.

The shortfall of mental health clinicians who treat children and adolescents is especially severe. Most areas of the United States are in "severe shortage" for child and adolescent psychiatrists. Inequity worsens this lack of care and the shortfall is severe in the developing world (Shatkin, 2018; Bruckner et al. 2011).

What to Do

Integration of Primary Care and Behavioral Health

Traditionally, mental health and primary care have been isolated from one another, housed in separate clinical locations, often with no access to a shared medical record and with separate insurance and administrative/regulatory governance. A movement to integrate behavioral health care into primary care pediatric and internal medicine settings has gained momentum in recent years (Ramanuj, et al., 2019). The provision of behavioral health in these settings has a number of clear advantages over the current siloed approach, in which behavioral health care settings are institutionally separate from other medical settings. The evidence base for improved overall health outcomes when integrated mental health care is provided is growing. Integrated care allows for seamless transitions of care from the primary care provider (PCP) to the behavioral health provider (BHP); overall improvements in health care costs and the efficient leveraging of scarce psychiatric resources are additional benefits of this approach.

The significant global treatment gaps for mental health problems is another powerful rationale for the integration of mental health into the primary care setting. Integrated care improves access to care and overall health outcomes on both the individual and population scale.

The integrated care approach includes on-site collaborative models, as well as telepsychiatry. Telepsychiatry has been shown to be effective in settings where in-person access is limited, such as rural areas, high population urban areas, geographically difficult-to-reach areas, and in times of disaster when access is blocked.

Significant stigma accompanies a mental health diagnosis in most cultures. An advantage of the integration of mental health treatment into the primary care setting is the decreased isolation of patients being treated for mental health disorders. Eliminating this isolation will not only improve the care of the mentally ill, but also allow the larger medical community to increase their exposure to these patients, promoting greater understanding and, ideally, reducing stigma.

In addition to integrating behavioral health into primary care medical settings, integration of primary care medical services into mental health settings (sometimes referred to as "reverse integration") has also gained ground as an effective model, particularly for individuals with serious mental illness and substance use disorders whose closest and most frequent health care contacts may be with mental health clinicians. In addition, such individuals often have difficulty navigating general medical settings in which clinicians may have less familiarity with evaluating and treating general medical illness in individuals with significant psychiatric conditions and complex psychiatric treatment regimens. It is hoped that behavioral health integration into primary care as well as primary care into mental health settings will help address the substantial health disparities related to mental illness and substance use disorders.

Future Directions in the Scientific Basis of Psychiatry

Genetics

The field of psychiatric genetics has made extraordinary progress over the past twenty-five years. For a number of years, it had been firmly established through family studies that genes contribute significantly to the risk for psychiatric disorders. Indeed, for some disorders, such as bipolar disorder, schizophrenia, autism, and attention deficit disorder, the "hereditability" (i.e., amount of risk for the disorder attributable to genes) is as high as 80 percent. However, the search for single genes underlying specific psychiatric conditions utilizing linkage analysis and association studies with candidate genes for specific psychiatric disorders has been largely disappointing. An exception has been autism, in which about 20 percent of cases may be related to attributable to an identifiable genetic variant. This early research made it increasingly clear that most psychiatric disorders are likely to be polygenic "complex disorders" in which multiple genes interacted with epigenetic processes and environmental risk factors to determine the final outcome, in this respect resembling most other health conditions such as hypertension and diabetes

In recent decades, the sequencing of the entire human genome, the formation of large international collaborative consortia, and the availability of powerful computing abilities able to analyze data sets of genome-wide single nucleotide polymorphisms (SNPs) and copy number variants (CNVs) have revolutionized psychiatric genetic research. The International Genomics Consortium (PGC) is the largest of these centralized data banks (Sullivan et al., 2018). Progress has been made toward identifying risk loci for psychiatric disorders, including schizophrenia, bipolar disorder, autistic disorder, and ADHD (Cross-Disorder Group of the Psychiatric Genomics Consortium, 2013). The phenomenon of pleiotropy, in which many genes identified have been found to be shared across a number of disorders, is clearly a major genetic feature in psychiatric illness.

The emerging recognition that distinct psychiatric diagnoses may be associated with overlapping genetic risk has challenged the traditional categorical understanding of psychiatric diagnosis, which is the foundation of the Diagnostic and Statistical Manual (DSM) system of categorization (American Psychiatric Association, DSM-5, 2013). It also strengthens our understanding that many psychiatric disorders are "spectrum" disorders, captures the wide variations seen in individuals sharing a common diagnosis, and allows a data-driven approach to the variations so commonly seen in psychiatric presentations (Cross Disorder Group of the Psychiatric Genomics Consortium, 2019). These advances are sure to lead to a deep understanding of the biology of psychiatric disorders, transforming our diagnostic understanding and early screening of these illnesses and powerfully advancing our ability to treat these devastating disorders.

Neuroimaging and the Identification of Neural Circuits

Unlike common neurological disorders such as stroke, tumors, and multiple sclerosis, where gross pathological findings on brain imaging have allowed for accurate diagnosis and therapeutic intervention, psychiatric disorders, though often severe, are rarely accompanied by gross pathology on neuroimaging.

Advances in the field of non-invasive, in vivo functional neuroimaging over the past thirty years have begun to transform the field of psychiatry. These techniques have contributed to an understanding of the function of specific brain areas in psychiatric illness, along with how these areas communicate with one another and form interacting circuits. Knowledge of these circuits in normal development, health, and disease will aid in improving diagnosis, allowing for targeted therapies that do not currently exist in psychiatric practice.

Structural and functional MRI are increasingly refined and safer, with the capacity for longer and more detailed task observations, as well as better image resolution and processing. The structural and functional MRI work has been enhanced by PET studies that reveal metabolic and neurochemical processes in greater detail. Utilizing healthy controls and cohorts of patients with psychiatric symptoms, neural circuitry dysfunction has been localized and characterized in a number of psychiatric disorders, including major depressive disorder, schizophrenia, obsessive-compulsive disorder, and post-traumatic stress disorder. Though these approaches have not yet translated into concrete practical tools for psychiatric practice, such as establishing a psychiatric diagnosis or the probability of responding to a given treatment in an individual patient, they are helping to shed light on brain regions and circuits most likely to be relevant to psychiatric disorders. The promise is great that this will be forthcoming and transformative of psychiatric practice.

The Classification of Mental Disorders: The Diagnostic System of the Future

Various classification systems exist in psychiatry. Currently, the primary systems are DSM-5 (American Psychiatric Association) and the International Statistical Classification of Diseases and Related Health Problems-10 (ICD 10, The World Health

Organization). Both are based largely on differentiating psychiatric presentations into distinct disorders based on a constellation of symptoms, such as hallucinations, delusions, depressed or elevated mood, and disturbances in sleep, appetite, energy concentration, or memory. At the same time, the genetic and neuroimaging/neurocircuitry developments described here are providing the field with the much-needed scientific basis for understanding psychiatric symptoms and disorders. This, in turn, is fueling the paradigm shift from the DSM process of descriptive categorical diagnosis, which is related to symptoms but not necessarily to brain circuits or genes, to the more neuroscience-based, mechanistic Research Domain Criteria (RDoC) project proposed in 2008 by the National Institute of Mental Health. The RDoC approach is inherently translational. Rather than focusing on specific disorders such as major depressive disorder or generalized anxiety disorder, used in clinical psychiatry, it adopts the view that progress in research on the pathophysiology underlying these conditions may be greater if the focus is not on disorders as defined by DSM but rather upon particularly behavioral dimensions that may span multiple disorders. It further recommends assembling information from different levels of analysis – genes to behavior – in a matrix summarizing data about functional dimensions of behavior characterized by genes, molecules, cells, circuits, physiology, and behavior for each of the five domains that have been identified. The five current domains in the RDOc system are negative valence systems, positive valence systems, cognitive systems, systems for social processes, and arousal/regulatory systems. These domains of behavior were chosen not as comprehensive but as starting points to be built upon based on evolving knowledge. The RDoC matrix also includes a column that identifies paradigms which already exist and are well-validated – for example, Pavlovian conditioning in positive reward behavior.

While clinical psychiatry still relies heavily upon the symptom-based diagnoses reflected in the DSM (and similar ICD-10) classifications, the transdiagnostic approach reflected in RDoC has offered a promising roadmap to elucidate the neurobiological underpinnings of psychiatric conditions and potential new avenues to better understanding their etiology and to developing novel treatments.

The future of the field holds great promise that these breakthroughs will lead to early identification of risk factors, early diagnosis of psychiatric disorders and their subtyping, and precision therapeutics that will revolutionize the treatment of our patients.

Conclusion

With the recognition that individuals with serious mental illness die up to twenty-five years earlier than other individuals, often from general medical conditions; that most major medical conditions are associated with significantly worse outcome and higher health care costs when accompanied by untreated psychiatric conditions such as depression; and that major public health crises like the SARS-CoV-2 (COVID-19) pandemic are well known to have profound and enduring impacts on mental health, it is clear that mental health is an integral component of health and that a knowledge of psychiatry is a foundational aspect of health care. With steady advances in knowledge, the stigma associated with psychiatric conditions is gradually on the wane while the development of effective, evidence-based treatments with medications, psychotherapies, neuromodulation, and other approaches continues to expand. Worldwide, mental health is the most neglected aspect of health care.

Yet there is reason for optimism. The twenty-first century is witnessing explosive growth in the field of psychiatry and behavioral sciences. Paradigm-shifting scientific breakthroughs in the areas of psychiatric genetics, functional neuro-imaging, psychoimmunology, and cognitive sciences are upon us. The emerging fields of optogenetics and functional neural connectivity promise new advances in the future. The NIMH RDoC system classifies mental illness based on behavioral and neurobiological measures, thus bringing about a revolutionary dimensional understanding of mental disorders, as revealed by advances in neuroscience. The field of psychiatry is moving rapidly toward integration with the clinical neurosciences. The range of evidence-based treatments for psychiatric disorders is growing. In a powerful parallel development, due to breakthroughs in basic science and clinical applications, psychiatry is becoming more closely allied with its related fields of neurology, neurosurgery, and neuroradiology. Finally, the integration of psychiatric knowledge and clinicians into the primary care setting has begun to address the enormous problem of inadequate access to mental health care. This enhancement of shared knowledge is fueling hope for significantly greater access to mental health care for people across the globe. People with medical illnesses and co-occurring mental health disorders will benefit from the growth of this shared knowledge and integrated clinical care among their providers.

References and Selected Readings

- Alegría, M., Chatterji, P., Wells, K., Cao, Z., et al. (2008). Disparity in Depression Treatment among Racial and Ethnic Minority Populations in the United States. *Psychiatric Services*, 59, 1264–1272.
- American Psychiatric Association (2013). *Diagnostic and Statistical Manual of Mental Disorders*, 5th ed. Arlington: APA.
- Arensman, E., Scott, V., De Leo, D., and Pirkis, J. (2020). Suicide and Suicide Prevention from a Global Perspective. *Crisis*, 41(Suppl. 1), S3–S7.

- Bishop, T. F., Seirup, J. K., Pincus, H. A., and Ross, J. S. (2016). Population of US Practicing Psychiatrists Declined, 2003–13, Which May Help Explain Poor Access to Mental Health Care. *Health Affairs*, 35, 1271–1277.
- Bruckner, T. A., Scheffler, R. M., Shen, G., Yoon, J., et al. (2011). The Mental Health Workforce Gap in Low- and Middle-Income Countries: A Needs-Based Approach. *Bulletin of the World Health Organization*, 89, 184–194.
- Cross-Disorder Group of the Psychiatric Genomics Consortium (2019). Genomic Relationships, Novel Loci, and Pleiotropic Mechanisms across Eight Psychiatric Disorders. *CELL, 179*,1469.
- Cross-Disorder Group of the Psychiatric Genomics Consortium (2013). Identification of Risk Loci with Shared Effects on Five Major Psychiatric Disorders: A Genome-Wide Analysis. *Lancet*; 381, 1371–1379.
- Kessler, R. C., Demler, O., Frank, R. G., Olfson, M., Pincus, H. A., Walters, E. E., Wang, P., Wells, K. B., Zaslavsky, A. M. (2005). Prevalence and Treatment of Mental Disorders, 1990 to 2003. *New England Journal of Medicine*, 352(24), 2515–2523.
- Office of the Surgeon General (US); Center for Mental Health Services (US); National Institute of Mental Health (US) (August 2001). *Mental Health: Culture, Race, and Ethnicity: A Supplement to Mental Health: A Report of the Surgeon General.* Rockville, MD: Substance Abuse and Mental Health Services Administration. Available from www.ncbi.nlm.nih.gov/books/NBK44243/.
- Polanczyk, G. V., Salum, G. A., Sugaya, L. S., Caye, A., and Rohde, L. A. (2015). Annual Research Review: A Meta-Analysis of the Worldwide Prevalence of Mental Disorders in Children and Adolescents. *Journal of Child Psychology and Psychiatry*, 56, 345–365.
- Ramanuj, P., Ferenchik, E., Docherty, M., Spaeth-Rublee, B., Pincus, H. A. (2019). Evolving Models of Integrated Behavioral Health and Primary Care. *Current Psychiatry Reports*, 21, 4.
- Rx for Survival (2005). *Global Health Champions: Rise of the Superbugs*, Episode 2 (TV program), PBS. Available from www.pbs.org/wgbh/rxforsurvival/series/champions/paul_farmer.html.
- Satiani, A., Niedermier, J., Satiani, B., and Svendsen, D. P., (2018). Projected Workforce of Psychiatrists in the United States: A Population Analysis. *Psychiatric Services*, 69, 710–713.
- Shatkin, J. P. (2018). Mental Health Promotion and Disease Prevention: It's about Time. *Journal of the American Academy of Child & Adolescent Psychiatry*, 58, 474–477.
- World Health Organization (1954). *Outline for a Study Group on World Health and the Survival of the Human Race: Material Drawn from Articles and Speeches by Brock Chisholm.* Geneva: World Health Organization.
- United Nations World Population Prospects (2017). U.S. Population Growth Rate 1950–2021. www.macrotrends.net. Retrieved 2021-03-29.

2 Clinical Neuroscience

AYOL SAMUELS, MATTHEW L. BAUM, JOSEPH LUCHSINGER, ROBERT G. MEALER, AND RACHEL A. ROSS

Introduction

Psychiatry draws widely upon insights from many realms ranging from public health, the social sciences, and the humanities. As psychiatric disorders affect mood, cognition, perception, emotion, and behavior, brain science is recognized as foundational to understanding their pathophysiology. Along with the disciplines of neurology, neurosurgery, and neuroradiology, psychiatry is often regarded as one of the clinical neurosciences.

Although the clinical interview and observation of behavior continue to remain the mainstay for diagnosis of psychiatric disorders, growing insights about the pathophysiology of psychiatric conditions are likely to inform the assessment, treatment, and classification of psychiatric disorders in the coming years. A circuit-based understanding of brain function, the establishment of biomarkers for early identification and intervention, and genetic tools to stratify an individual's risk of disease and predict response to different treatment modalities promise to become increasingly integral to clinical psychiatry. As the field of psychiatry moves away from inefficient "trial-and-error" based approaches, toward precision medicine grounded in knowledge about individual variation in brain biology, fluency in neuroscience will be essential preparation for clinical practice.

This chapter will provide a general overview of neuroscience relevant to psychiatry. As progress is rapid, our focus is on neuroscientific concepts relevant to psychiatry, as well as on current efforts to identify clues about the underlying causes of psychiatric disorders, and discover promising targets for novel treatments.

Historical Context

In contemporary Western medicine, the impetus to link specific clinical syndromes to pathology in the brain dates to nineteenth-century Europe. The then-nascent field of neurology, led by notable physician-scientists, including Jean-Martin Charcot, Joseph Babinsky, Paul Broca, and Karl Wernicke, began to associate speech, motor, and cognitive abnormalities with lesions in particular brain regions. Preliminary attempts to explain emotional phenomena in terms of brain function were also made by Benjamin Rush in the United States and Wilhelm Griesinger in Germany.

One prominent clinician who believed that psychiatric symptoms could be explained neurologically was Sigmund Freud. Though best known for developing the field of psychoanalysis, focused on unconscious impulses and fears driving emotions and behavior, Freud was trained as a neurophysiologist and neurologist and was confident that psychological processes had neurophysiologic correlates yet to be discovered. As psychoanalysis was further elaborated between the late 1800s through the mid-1900s, becoming a leading force in psychiatry, the field increasingly diverged from brain science, though in recent years clinical practitioners and researchers of psychoanalytically based psychotherapies have shown renewed interest in neuroimaging and other methods for revisiting Freud's earlier vision.

In the latter part of the twentieth century, the discovery of effective pharmacological treatments for major psychiatric disorders, including antipsychotics and antidepressants, also brought renewed interest in the biology of psychiatric disease. These medications targeted neurochemical systems, particularly the so-called monoamines – dopamine, serotonin, and norepinephrine – which were being actively mapped in the brain during this same period. Their efficacy led to the *monoamine hypothesis of psychiatric illness*, the idea that alterations involving the levels or function of this group of neurotransmitters caused specific symptoms (e.g., depressed mood, anxiety, and psychosis). But without direct access to the brain in living individuals, more comprehensive approaches to understand the biology of mental illness were not yet possible. Scientists turned to animal models in order to probe the inner workings of individual cells and circuits in awake and behaving organisms, though their translational relevance to human psychiatric illness remains a considerable limitation. The development of functional brain imaging techniques in the 1990s enabled for the first time the study of altered brain function in vivo, and in conjunction with other advances in translational neuroscience, which will be discussed later, has revolutionized our understanding of mental illness as underlying brain and even whole-body disorders.

A New Neuroscience-Based Framework for Nosology

While the Diagnostic and Statistical Manual (DSM) remains the gold standard for clinical diagnosis in psychiatry, efforts to recategorize psychiatric disorders using neuroscience may ultimately reshape the way we think about psychiatric assessment. One such initiative is the Research Domain Criteria (RDoC) framework, championed in 2011 by Tom Insel, a psychiatrist, neuroscientist, and then-director of the National Institute of Mental Health (NIMH). Rather than using the DSM's distinct categories and checklists of symptoms and symptom duration for mental disorders, RDoC uses six domains of psychological processes that show

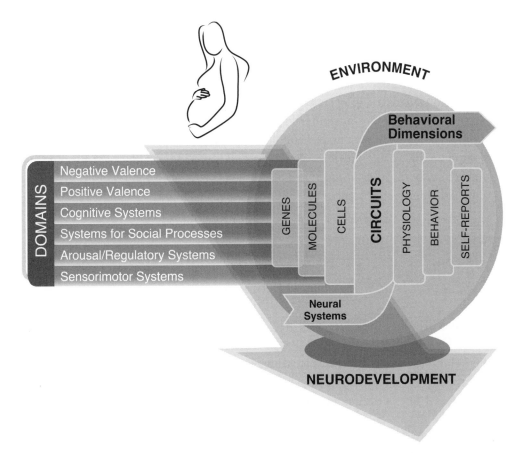

Figure 2.1 The Research Domain Criteria is a research framework developed by the National Institute of Mental Health (NIMH) to examine psychological processes based on seven levels of information. The image is reprinted from the NIMH website. www.nimh.nih.gov/research/research-funded-by-nimh/rdoc/.shtml

a continuous range of variation across the entire population (see Figure 2.1). These domains are not meant to be exclusive or finite but open to change with new research. They are also meant to be studied in multiple models from cells to human behavior. Extremes along these continua, perhaps in specific combinations, may underlie psychiatric symptoms that bridge across conventional diagnostic categories. Though RDoC was developed to help guide neuroscientific research into complex human behavior and mental disorders, it is hypothesized that these dimensions of psychopathology will more closely represent underlying variation in brain physiology compared to DSM-based diagnoses, and can be more directly mapped onto mechanistic models in both humans and other animals. It remains the work of clinicians and researchers to integrate RDoC and DSM categorization and determine if a more dimensional framework better advances meaningful research and clinical innovation.

In the RDoC framework, there are different hierarchical units of analysis used to investigate these constructs: genes, molecules, cells, circuits, physiology, behaviors, and self-reports. This chapter will take an analogous approach using the first five constructs to introduce the concepts and principles of neuroscience as related to psychiatric disorders. We will start with genetics and epigenetics; move on to receptors, neurotransmitters, and various immune and endocrinologic molecules; and conclude with neural circuits. We will discuss the studies within human, computational, and translational models and recommend Suggested Reading for further study of other promising model systems such as nonhuman primates and inducible pluripotent stem cells (iPSCs).

Psychiatric Genetics

Psychiatric Disorders Are Highly Heritable

"I have bipolar disorder. Will my son have it too?"
It has been known for centuries that psychiatric disorders run in families, and the heritability of mental illnesses is stronger than of most other medical conditions. Many patients diagnosed with a mental illness will worry about the chances of their loved ones developing the disease. Although we cannot say with certainty what will happen to any single individual, we can share with patients the "familial relative risk" for different disorders based on epidemiology and population studies. The familial relative risk tells us the increased likelihood that someone has of developing a particular illness compared to the general population given they have a family member with the disorder. For example, the risk of a first degree relative of someone with bipolar disorder of developing the illness is up to ten times the risk of the general population. Similarly, the risk of a first degree relative of someone with ADHD of developing ADHD is up to six times the risk in the general population. By knowing the incidence in the general population, clinicians can calculate the *absolute risk* of developing the illness in a relative. The incidence of bipolar disorder is about 1–3 percent in the general population, depending on how broadly it is defined, so the absolute risk for a first-degree relative developing the disorder is about 10–30 percent. The incidence of ADHD in the general population is 5 percent, so that the absolute risk for a first-degree relative is up to 30 percent.

Twin studies allow us to disentangle the relative contributions of genetic and environmental factors to mental illnesses on a population level. In these studies, large databases of monozygotic and dizygotic twins are analyzed. The question asked is, "If one twin develops a mental illness, what are the chances that the other twin will?" Dizygotic twins, like singleton siblings, share approximately 50 percent of their genetic information, whereas monozygotic twins share 100 percent.

Assuming that dizygotic twins share their environments as much as monozygotic twins do, any increased strength of correlation regarding mental illness in the monozygotic twins can be attributed solely to genetics. Indeed, monozygotic twins have a significantly higher rate of *concordance* for psychiatric disease than dizygotic twins; for example, the concordance of schizophrenia is nearly three times higher in monozygotic versus dizygotic twins (48 percent versus 17 percent, respectively). Information including differential concordance among family members is one way to calculate the *heritability* for a given disorder. The heritability tells us what percent of the variation in a given population (and a given environment) can be explained solely by genetics. Many psychiatric disorders have high heritability, including bipolar disorder (68 percent), schizophrenia (77 percent), autism (74 percent), and ADHD (79 percent). For context, the heritability of ovarian cancer is around 15–20 percent, and prostate cancer is around 5–10 percent. These numbers confirm a strong genetic component for psychiatric illness but do not tell us about an individual's risk or the specific genes involved. Can we identify specific genes involved in mental illness? Yes, but first, a brief genetics review is in order.

Organization of the Human Genome: Rare Variants Are Rare in Psychiatric Genetics

The human genome is composed of twenty-three pairs of chromosomes, each harboring millions of linearly arranged nucleotides, or *bases*. If a nucleotide sequence is in a region that codes for a protein, it is considered part of a *gene*, the functional unit of heredity. The physical location of a gene on a chromosome is termed a *locus*. Because chromosomes are inherited in pairs (one from each parent), most genetic loci have two copies that may be identical or different. The different loci that exist in a population are termed *alleles*, and the combination of alleles at a locus is referred to as a *genotype*.

Humans share 99.9 percent of their genome, with the remaining 0.1 percent accounting for all variation between individuals. To find genetic clues into why certain people develop mental illness and others do not, we need to understand the different types of variation that exist in our genomes, which can range from the duplication or deletion of an entire chromosome down to a change in a single letter of the DNA code.

Variation in the number of chromosomes present, termed *aneuploidy*, is relatively rare, but can be associated with profound effects in behavior and cognition as well as with substantial medical comorbidity. Down syndrome, for example, results from inheriting an extra copy of chromosome 21, and nearly all patients have some level of neuropsychiatric phenotype, namely intellectual disability. These chromosomal abnormalities can be detected by visualizing whole chromosomes using a simple light microscope to create what is called a *karyotype*.

Other large-scale variations can be caused by a deletion, duplication, or translocation of portions of the chromosome, which are large and easily detectable with current molecular techniques. A genetic variation with one of the largest effect sizes for developing mental illness is a large deletion of more than one million base pairs (nucleotides) encompassing several genes from the long arm of chromosome 22. This deletion can lead to a wide range of abnormalities including cardiac defects, immune deficiencies, and distinct facial features, and is most accurately referred to as 22q11.2 deletion syndrome, though other names have been used in the past (e.g., DiGeorge syndrome or velocardiofacial syndrome). Interestingly, 22q11.2 deletion syndrome carries an absolute risk of schizophrenia of approximately 30 percent, and patients already diagnosed with schizophrenia have a ten- to twenty-times higher prevalence of carrying this deletion. Despite the large effect size, 22q11.2 deletion still accounts for a very small portion of those diagnosed with schizophrenia due to the relative rarity of this variant (1 in 4,000). Large duplications have also been shown to increase the risk of psychiatric pathology. For example, duplications of a portion of chromosome 15 significantly increase the risk of developing autism and are found in 1–2 percent of cases. These large changes in DNA structure are often thought to have a causal effect on neuropsychiatric phenotypes; however, the deletion or addition of ten to a thousand genes only provides an incomplete glimpse into our understanding of the genetic basis of these disorders. Neuroscientists hope that by studying the mechanism by which 22q11.2 deletion influences schizophrenia-risk, or chromosome 15 duplication influences autism-risk, they will gain insights that will be helpful to a broader population.

Small variants with large effect can also cause substantial neuropsychiatric morbidity, with well-known examples, including Huntington disease (HD) and Fragile X. Both disorders are caused by an expansion of trinucleotide repeats (CAG, CCG) within a single gene; once the number of repeats crosses over a certain threshold, these small DNA variants have near 100 percent penetrance, meaning all carriers of the expansions express the disease. The genetic cause of these disorders was discovered in the last 30 years using the classic technique of linkage analysis, tracking increasingly smaller pieces of DNA that segregate in carriers of the disorder versus controls, eventually narrowing down to a single region or gene. More recently, a technique called *exome sequencing*, where the entire protein-coding sequence of DNA (exons) is determined, has been applied to psychiatric disorders and has started to find rare, novel mutations with large effects in single genes linked to disorders such as schizophrenia. While these inroads are exciting and important, it is equally important to recognize that even for disorders like HD and Fragile X linked to single genes the timeline for moving from genetics to clinical therapeutics has been much slower than most scientists and physicians originally anticipated.

Searching for Common Variants with Small Effects

Early genetic studies attempted to find "the gene" for a given mental illness. However, these monogenic investigations were largely unsuccessful in accounting for the strong heritability in developing these disorders. To address this so-called missing heritability, geneticists studying mental illness – as well as other common, complex human phenotypes such as diabetes and hypertension – have changed their focus from rare variation with large effect sizes toward common differences in the genome with subtle effects, and are generating promising results. These common variants, which include copy number variants (CNVs) and single nucleotide polymorphisms (SNPs), are present in large numbers in every individual. In general, common variants confer only minimal effects on most phenotypes in isolation; however, the aggregate effects of thousands can be substantial.

CNVs are duplications or deletions at the gene level, usually in the range of thousands of base pairs at a time. CNVs are common, making up an estimated 10 percent of the entire genome, and are thought to allow for additional genetic variation within a population. The cytochrome p450 system provides a good example of how these genetic variations can relate to psychiatry. The cytochrome P450 system contains enzymes that metabolize most psychiatric and other medications, and alterations in these enzymes can affect drug levels in the blood. CNVs in the gene encoding *CYP2D6* can increase or decrease the number of copies of this gene and change the amount of enzyme present, therefore affecting the ability of a patient to metabolize medications by this enzyme. Thus, if a patient has a CNV deletion at this site, they will have fewer enzymes. If this patient is prescribed a medication metabolized by this enzyme such as an antidepressant, they will be at higher risk for toxic side effects given higher medication levels. If, on the other hand, a patient has a CNV with additional copies of the gene, they will have more enzymes. If this patient is prescribed an antipsychotic metabolized by this enzyme, it is less likely to be effective at its usual doses due to lower levels. The field looking at how genetic variation influences medications is called pharmacogenomics while the field that studies how medications interact with receptors is called *pharmacodynamics*. Pharmacogenomic tests are already commercially available, although the field is nascent. Much remains to be learned about the genes most relevant for explaining the tolerability, safety, and effectiveness of most medications used in psychiatry.

The most common types of variation in the genome are single nucleotide polymorphisms, or *SNPs*. SNPs are single-base differences spread throughout the genome, with *low-frequency* variants occurring in less than 1 percent of the population and *high-frequency* variants occurring in more than 1 percent. Each individual has an estimated 4 million SNPs in their genome, and more than 100 million have been identified worldwide. The majority of SNPs occur outside of the coding region of genes and have no known functional relevance. The few SNPs with functional relevance are located in regulatory or protein-coding regions and likely can change the expression level of the gene or structure of the protein, respectively. In some cases, such as cystic fibrosis, SNPs can be devastating. It has become clear, though, that SNPs with this magnitude of an effect are infrequent in psychiatry;

however, their ubiquitous and variable nature makes them powerful markers to locate regions of a chromosome that are implicated in disease. How does this work?

During meiosis, before the paired chromosomes split apart, they swap some of their genetic material in a process called *recombination*. The closer genes or SNPs are to one another on a chromosome, the more likely they will undergo recombination together and remain together across multiple generations. These sections that stick together are called *haplotypes*. If a certain version (allele) of one of the genes in the haplotype is related to disease, the particular SNP on a different part of the same haplotype may be a marker for the disease allele as it is likely to be transmitted along with it. In addition, the locations where recombination takes place do not occur completely randomly: some SNPs are inherited together at a higher or lower frequency than expected by chance, which is referred to as SNPs existing in *linkage disequilibrium*. These factors allow geneticists to track down SNPs found with higher frequency in patients with schizophrenia compared to controls, and identify a nearby SNP or gene that may have a causal relationship to the disease. Thus SNPs can point to a region of the genome that confers risk for a disease, which can be a first step toward understanding the biology of an illness.

Genome-Wide Association Studies (GWAS) Deliver Promising Leads

The sequencing of the first human genome was completed in 2001 after more than a decade of work and a total project cost of $2.7 billion. Rapid breakthroughs in sequencing technologies now allow sequencing of a whole genome in a matter of days for around $1,000; similarly, a complete SNP analysis can cost as low as $50 per person. These technologies give geneticists the power to sequence a huge number of patients and controls at a relatively low cost to find both rare variants with large effects (whole genome and whole exome sequencing) and common variants with small effects (GWAS; genome-wide association studies).

In 2014, the Psychiatric Genomics Consortium published GWAS results from ~37,000 patients with schizophrenia and 110,000 controls, identifying 108 independent loci associated with the disorder. The findings of GWAS are commonly presented as a so-called Manhattan plot, given the resemblance to a city skyline (Figure 2.2). Each SNP is plotted on the x-axis and its corresponding p-value plotted on the y-axis – any SNP above the dotted line is significantly associated with the disorder. Though these results still only account for a fraction of the total heritability of schizophrenia (<10 percent), they provide an exciting and unprecedented avenue for exploration into the mechanism of disease. Evidence supporting the decades-old hypotheses of dysregulated neurotransmitter signaling was supported by the genetic associations of the dopamine D2 receptor (*DRD2*), the primary site of action for nearly all antipsychotic medications, and several glutamate receptors (*GRIA1*, *GRIN2A*, *GRM3*). Perhaps more interesting, novel clues of disease pathogenesis have started to emerge from the results. For example, the strongest GWAS association for schizophrenia was in the major histocompatibility complex (MHC)

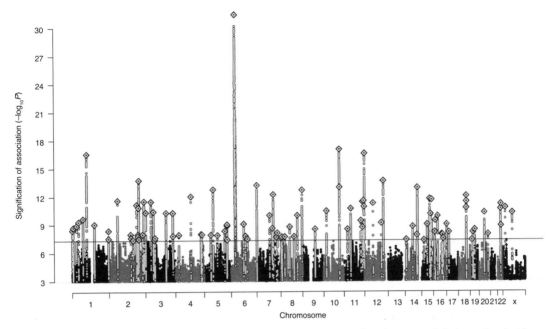

Figure 2.2 Manhattan plot from a large genome wide association study that found 108 genetic loci associated with schizophrenia. The *x* axis indicates the location of the SNP and the *y* axis indicates the significance of the association, where the red line shows the cutoff for genome-wide significance.
Reprinted from:
Schizophrenia Working Group of the Psychiatric Genomics Consortium., Ripke, S., Neale, B. *et al*. Biological insights from 108 schizophrenia-associated genetic loci. *Nature* **511**, 421–427 (2014)

locus and regulates the expression of a protein commonly used by the immune system, complement component 4 (C4). Changes in the expression of C4 were subsequently shown to effect synaptic pruning in the mouse brain, and for the first time, a disease-associated genetic variant was connected to a biological pathway implicated in schizophrenia. This finding has sparked interest in the potential immunologic etiology of mental illnesses including schizophrenia and will hopefully lead to new drug targets through pharmaceutical research.

Another powerful use of GWAS data is predicting an individual's risk for developing a phenotype by summing the effect size of every measured SNP in a single person, generating a *polygenic risk score (PRS)*. Though predictive validity has not yet been demonstrated, the hope is that PRSs can aid in screening and early detection, similar to the Framingham score predicting cardiac events, allowing for early and targeted interventions for those at highest risk. One current limitation to PRS is that GWAS are overwhelmingly performed in populations of European descent, limiting their applicability to only individuals of the same genetic background. However, as the Psychiatric Genomics Consortium continues to grow and analyze an increasing number of patients from diverse populations, additional disease-associated genes will be identified, and tools such as PRS will become more and more powerful.

Further studies in different mental illnesses have started to reveal shared genetic architecture and overlapping risk loci between certain psychiatric illnesses. For example, bipolar disorder and schizophrenia share considerable genetic overlap, as do autism spectrum disorder and ADHD, leading to new hypotheses about common biological bases of these disorders. Of note, the RDoC format accounts for some of this cross-disease relatedness. For example, these disorders all share phenotype dysregulation in the cognitive domain and genetic risk in genes encoding neurotransmitter receptors.

Epigenetics

Up to this point, we have only discussed variations among individuals that arise from the DNA sequence of the genome itself. We now know that gene expression ("turning a gene on") also plays a critical role in disease and depends on the external modification of genes, termed *epigenetics*, which has become another frontier in our endeavor to understand complex psychiatric illnesses. Genes are being expressed, enhanced, or repressed all the time and this external modification is influenced by environmental factors. The two most common ways in which gene expression is controlled are histone acetylation and DNA methylation. DNA is wrapped around proteins called histones, and this packaging, termed *nucleosomes*, can either be in an active state allowing transcription, or an inactive state where transcription is not possible. Acetylation, the enzymatic attachment of an acetyl group to lysine residues on histone proteins, relaxes the nucleosome complex and allows transcription, whereas deacetylation does the opposite. DNA methylation, which is also an enzymatic process, involves the addition of methyl groups directly onto cytosine and adenine nucleotides, which usually serves to repress gene transcription.

Several studies have shown that cocaine administration in mice induces histone acetylation, leading to increased expression of certain genes within the nucleus accumbens, a region in the basal ganglia that is related to motivation and reward. These epigenetic changes in this region are thought to be involved in propagating addiction behavior. One hurdle in these studies is they are often limited to animal models because these changes can be impermanent and difficult to track, unlike the DNA sequence, not to mention difficult to access in human brains. New collaborations with post-mortem brain repositories are allowing for larger-scale studies connecting epigenetic biology to lived history that can tell us about external and developmental-specific timing of gene expression, and potentially shed light on environmental modulation of neurobiological processes.

Key Take-aways on Psychiatric Genetics

Current clinical applications of genetics and epigenetics to psychiatric practice are limited. Still, the hope is that with a more sophisticated understanding and rapidly advancing technologies, we may be able to use genetics to predict and prevent the onset of disease, better understand and target distinct pathways of disease, and predict response to specific treatments. Given the complexity of genetic findings in mental illness, several points should be emphasized from this section:

1. Mental illnesses are highly polygenic, involving many different genetic pathways that arrive at the same final syndrome (which itself is highly heterogeneous).
2. Most genetic variants have a small effect size and are only present in a subset of patients; thus they are only found by studying large numbers of patients.
3. A single genetic variant may only show an effect in combination with other genetic variants, requiring a high level of computational analysis to determine.
4. In the majority of cases, genes are critical but alone not sufficient to cause mental illness (as suggested by a ~50 percent concordance of schizophrenia in monozygotic twins, who share 100 percent of their genes).
5. The environment plays an important role in developing mental illness through mechanisms including epigenetics, and looking at any single process in isolation may hinder our ability to find real effects.

Molecular Psychiatry

Neurotransmitters: Brain Signaling Molecules That Form Circuits

Our genetic code exerts its effects through *transcription* from DNA to RNA, followed by a *translation* of RNA into proteins which act as enzymes, transporters, receptors, neurotransmitters, hormones, and immune factors. The initial attention of biological psychiatry was focused primarily on neurotransmitters and receptors based on the fortuitous utility of medications initially intended for other use to treat other disorders. Shortly after chlorpromazine was developed as an anesthetic in 1950s France, Jean Delay and Pierre Deniker used it to treat psychosis in inpatients. Arvid Carlsson and Maria Lindqvist hypothesized that the effects were the result of the blockade of monoamine receptors. Similarly, the discovery of the antidepressants that appeared to share an effect on monoamines led to the hypothesis that the beneficial effects were secondary to increasing the amount of serotonin and norepinephrine in the *synaptic cleft,* the area between the presynaptic neuron and the postsynaptic neuron. It was extrapolated at that time that excess dopamine was at the root of schizophrenia, and serotonin and norepinephrine depletion is at the root of major depressive disorder (MDD). It is now understood that this explanation is overly simplistic; the mechanism of a treatment does not provide a clear window into the mechanism of the disease, even if the medication relieves symptoms. While neurotransmitters surely play a role in the development of these disorders, their role is quite nuanced, and we are only at the very beginning of understanding this complexity. In depression, for example, though serotonin specific reuptake inhibitors (SSRIs) quickly raise the level of serotonin at the synapse, this rise is often weeks before an antidepressant effect can be discerned.

Facility with how the different units of the nervous system work in concert and adapt over time is crucial to our understanding of both the biological basis of brain function (and dysfunction), as well as the rationale for how we treat mental illness. Neurons communicate by synthesizing and releasing different molecules, collectively called neurotransmitters, into the *synaptic cleft*. The postsynaptic neuron receives this transmission, or message, via receptors on its exterior. Through these receptors' actions, neurotransmitters alter the likelihood of the postsynaptic neuron firing an action potential. Because different receptors for the same neurotransmitter can have diverging actions, it is the receptor rather than the neurotransmitter that dictates the effect of the released neurotransmitter.

The action potential is an all-or-nothing signal that originates at the cell body and travels down a specialized outgrowth of a neuron, called an *axon*, causing the release of neurotransmitters at the next synapse. This continuity of neuronal transmission between cells and regions creates what is known as a *circuit*. Each "message" ends when the neurotransmitter is either degraded or transported back into the presynaptic neuron. Two of the most common neurotransmitters are glutamate and gamma-aminobutyric acid (GABA). They act by opening ion channels that raise or lower the voltage across the neuron's membrane by permitting the passage of positive or negative ions. If the neuron's voltage moves in the positive direction sufficiently, the neuron will fire an action potential. Glutamate binds to receptors that are usually excitatory, or increase the likelihood of an action potential. In contrast, GABA binds to receptors that are generally inhibitory, or decrease the likelihood of an action potential.

The expression of receptors, and synapse architecture more generally, is in constant flux. Dynamic modifications in the presynaptic and postsynaptic terminals, a process known as *synaptic plasticity*, can alter the efficiency of the synapse and can have lasting effects on the circuit. One example of this plasticity that is critical to lasting explicit memory formation is long term potentiation (LTP), a means by which repeated stimulation strengthens synapses. Signaling between neurons can be augmented in many ways: entirely new synapses can form, the presynaptic neuron can release more neurotransmitter, or the postsynaptic neuron can add receptors to enhance the effect of neurotransmitter in the synaptic cleft. Congruently, the reverse of these mechanisms is called long term depression (LTD) and can decrease interneuronal connectivity, a normal and essential part of neural homeostasis.

Beyond the ion-permeable receptors such as those mentioned previously, the brain has a plethora of modulatory receptors that adjust neuronal excitability through intracellular signals. These receptors act through intracellular second messengers that allow signals from the cell's surface (the neuromodulatory neurotransmitters) to change everything from protein phosphorylation to transcription to ion channel permeability. The family of dopamine receptors is a key example of modulatory receptors that act through a G-protein-coupled second messenger system. Importantly, some members of this family increase neuron excitability while others decrease it, further highlighting the flexibility of this messaging in the nervous system.

We will focus on the dopamine system to illustrate the clinical relevance of neurotransmitters. The effect of a neurotransmitter depends not only on the type of neurotransmitter and the receptor but also on the location of action. For example, the stronger an antipsychotic medication binds to the dopamine type 2 receptor in the striatum (thereby blocking dopaminergic transmission), the more likely it is to affect the positive symptoms of psychosis (e.g., hallucinations, delusions, and paranoia) and the more likely it is to cause dopamine-mediated side effects, as described later. There are four different major dopamine projections, each of whose name indicates from where it originates and to where it projects.

The mesocortical pathway originates in the ventral tegmental area of the brainstem and projects to the prefrontal cortex. The blockage of dopamine in this specific circuit is thought to account for the cognitive side effects of antipsychotic medications. The role of dopamine in executive functioning may also explain the use of medications that increase dopamine levels in the treatment of ADHD.

The location of action of a single neurotransmitter can be modulated further by the activity of other neurotransmitters/neuromodulators found in the same region, interacting either pre- or post-synaptically. For example, the tuberoinfundibular pathway projects from the hypothalamus to the stalk of the pituitary gland. The dopamine from this pathway inhibits prolactin, which is secreted from the post-synaptic cells of the pituitary gland. Thus, when dopamine is blocked in this pathway due to an antipsychotic medication, prolactin is increased and a patient may exhibit gynecomastia, galactorrhea, or amenorrhea. Risperidone has a particularly potent effect on this pathway more than other dopaminergic pathways, which accounts for these prolactin related side effects, even though the putative mechanism of action is merely dopamine blockade.

The nigrostriatal pathway projects from the substantia nigra to the striatum. When drugs or disease block dopamine transmission in this pathway, the patient will exhibit extrapyramidal symptoms, such as tremor, bradykinesia, and rigidity. These are similar to the symptoms described by and the mechanism of action of Parkinson's disease, which involves the degeneration of dopaminergic cell bodies in the substantia nigra. Remarkably, when secondary to the dopaminergic blockade, these symptoms can be improved by modulating acetylcholine levels in the region, which increases relative levels of dopamine within the synaptic cleft, again pointing to the interrelated relevance of multiple neurotransmitters from multiple pre-synaptic cell types interacting at the synapse.

As noted previously, dopamine has been central to hypotheses concerning piece the mechanisms underlying schizophrenia. The fourth major pathway, the mesolimbic pathway, has been the focus of attention here as well as in other psychiatric diseases, such as addiction and MDD. This pathway projects from the ventral tegmental area to the limbic and paralimbic structures, including the nucleus accumbens, amygdala, hippocampus, orbitofrontal cortex, and anterior cingulate cortex. These are all areas involved in various levels of emotional, motivational, and reward processing, and require multiple different neuromodulatory neurotransmitter systems working together to produce behavior and other psychological processes.

Much like the dopamine system, the serotonin system has been implicated in a broad swath of neuropsychiatric disorders that include MDD, generalized anxiety disorder, post-traumatic stress disorder, and obsessive-compulsive disorder. Serotonin, a biogenic amine that regulates complex cognitive processes and attention, is synthesized from tryptophan in midbrain neurons located in and near the raphe nuclei. These neurons project broadly throughout the nervous system and signal through the fourteen distinct types of serotonin receptors expressed across the brain. Each receptor subtype is unique and has a different affinity for serotonin, regional distribution, cellular localization, and downstream signaling. This variety of receptor attributes exemplifies the nuanced signaling that is possible using just one of the many neurotransmitters present in the mammalian brain. Though very intricate, this diversity of receptors also provides many potential inroads for treatment.

Similar to dopamine homeostasis, the reuptake transporter is a crucial regulator of the serotonin system's function, a property targeted by the first-line treatment of depression, the selective serotonin reuptake inhibitors (SSRIs). By blocking reuptake, SSRIs quickly increase serotonin at the synapse, yet weeks of treatment are typically required before antidepressant effects can be detected. Rather than direct action of serotonin, evidence suggests that relief from depression is due to increased plasticity and other "downstream" effects that occur at a much slower pace. Animal studies demonstrate that long-term treatment with SSRIs can increase a regulator of neural plasticity in the prefrontal cortex and hippocampus, brain-derived neurotrophic factor (BDNF). BDNF is a protein growth factor released from post-synaptic neurons and acts through its receptor TrkB on other cells. BDNF is critical for normal axon guidance, neuron development and survival, as well as the growth and maintenance of synapses and dendrites. Congruently, post-mortem brains from people with depression show decreased levels of BDNF, and the genetic knockout of BDNF in mice inhibits the antidepressant and pro-plasticity effects of SSRI treatment. These interesting findings highlight that much work remains to be done to more fully understand the functioning of neurotransmitters within circuits in order to more optimally target neural systems to treat disease.

Technologies to Study Neurotransmitters in Humans

All of the processes involved in neurotransmitter communication – synthesis, release, receptor binding, transport, reuptake, degradation – have been the focus of psychiatric research, with the ultimate goal of creating medications that can more precisely target these processes. Specialized non-invasive imaging techniques such as PET, SPECT, and MR spectroscopy are being used to quantify these processes, several examples of which are discussed in this section.

We mentioned previously that dopamine receptor DRD2 has been associated with schizophrenia by GWAS. In mice, overexpression of the DRD2 gene leads to hyperactivity in a novel environment, which can be related to human-illness behaviors seen in anxiety disorders and ADHD. The next step to understanding the biology that relates this polymorphism to disease is to examine the relative expression of the gene or the activity levels of the protein between populations. For example, a difference in expression levels of an SNP-associated gene between people with schizophrenia who have the risk SNP and those with schizophrenia without the SNP indicates a potential functional relevance of the SNP. There are a few techniques that allow us to do this with neurotransmitter genes and receptors, such as single-photon emission computed tomography (SPECT), a nuclear medicine imaging technique that uses a synthesized radioligand that binds to the receptor and can then be visualized and measured, thus estimating the concentration of those transporters. Another method of testing the impact of neurotransmitters on pathology is magnetic resonance spectroscopy (MRS). Functional MRS allows for the measurement of the levels of multiple neurochemicals in regions of the brain. Comparing signal at rest to signal during a task allows us to infer the activity of the receptors in different contexts. Positron emission tomography (PET) is another versatile neuroimaging approach that can provide regional measurements of brain physiology, including neurotransmission, metabolism, inflammation, and even histone modification. For example, there are numerous ways to canvass dopamine signaling using PET, including D1 and D2 receptor density, drug-induced dopamine release, and dopamine transport and turnover. The use of PET is limited by exposure to ionizing radiation, but its potential to measure activity at distinct receptor subtypes is virtually limitless.

Just as "one gene, one syndrome" does not work, so too "one neurotransmitter, one syndrome" does not work. Dopamine abnormalities have been documented in ADHD, addiction, and depressive disorders. For example, cocaine blocks reuptake at the dopamine transporter (DAT) and thus increases dopamine in the synaptic cleft. It is thought that through this excess dopamine, cocaine coopts the dopamine reward system, causing addiction; floods other areas of the mesolimbic system, causing psychosis; and can also lead to depression with the subsequent dopamine depletion. We continue the thread of tying research findings to clinical relevance through the lens of schizophrenia because this is the current lead-ing-edge – new information discovered in models of schizophrenia will likely be applied and lead to similar discoveries related to other presentations of mental illness as well.

Immune System: Molecules and Cells

In addition to neurotransmitters, recent research has begun to implicate immune factors in mental illness. One cause of chronic inflammation is past or present prolonged stress, which causes changes in cytokine signaling. Though it has been often taught that the brain is protected from the immune system (i.e., immune-priv-ileged), the field is rapidly correcting to recognize the connection between immune molecules and brain function. Several observations have led to this connection: (1) psychiatric disturbance during infections, (2) psychiatric symptoms arising in the context of known immune dysfunction, and (3) human genetics implicating immune molecules.

First, we have all experienced the feelings of malaise during a flu, sometimes called "sickness behavior." These feelings of fatigue, anhedonia, dysphoria, and social withdrawal are thought to often be an adaptive response to illness as the body recovers from illness. However, the symptoms also resemble those seen in depression and are thought to arise due to the cytokines released in response to infection that then affect the CNS. Those who have spent time on a general med-ical service have grown familiar with another example of psychiatric disturbance during an infection: a urinary tract infection in susceptible elderly patients can be a trigger of waxing and waning mental status, defects of working memory, agitation, and frank visual hallucinations called delirium. Patients seeing things like boats outside their windows or imaginary people come into their rooms are not uncommon. Though it is unclear exactly how an infection of the urinary tract can lead to these psychiatric symptoms, it is thought that centrally acting cytokines released in response to infection are involved, along with a range of age-related brain changes that may explain why some older individuals appear more susceptible. Delirium usually slowly resolves after the inciting UTI is treated. In the absence of acute infections, psychiatric symptoms can be produced by direct administration of cytokines, as seen when interferon-alpha, which is used to treat hepatitis C, induces symptoms of depression. Finally, depression is significantly more common among those with medical illnesses; patients with comorbid depres-sion have higher pro-inflammatory cytokines, and some depressed patients show increased levels of IL-6, TNF-alpha, and CRP. Neuropsychiatric manifestations of COVID-19 have been widely recognized during the recent pandemic. Preliminary suggestions relate to their association with pronounced inflammatory responses triggered in some individuals by the virus.

Second, immune cell dysfunction can produce psychiatric symptoms, as is the case when B-cells produce autoantibodies against neuronal antigens. The best-recognized example of this phenomenon is anti-NMDA-receptor encephalitis, the presentation of which can be indistinguishable from first-break psychoses of other causes. In the memoir *Brain on Fire*, for example, a young journalist for the *New York Post* describes how her own experience with anti-NMDA receptor encephalitis began with paranoid delusions of infidelity, the infestation of her apartment with insects, and progressed to full-fledged psychosis. Though the pathophysiology of the phenomenon is still emerging, there is evidence that autoantibodies to NMDA-receptors alter the function of those receptors in a way that leads to psychosis. Many, but not all, patients have relevant neurological signs, such as new-onset seizures, pointing to encephalitis. Once the underlying pathophysiology is diagnosed, different treatment options are available that provide better efficacy than symptom-managing antipsychotics. Sometimes, most commonly in young women, production of the autoantibodies is related to an ovarian teratoma, and surgical removal of the tumor is therapeutic. Without an obvious source of the antibodies, patients with suspected anti-NMDA encephalitis are treated with intravenous immunoglobulin or plasma exchange. The woman in *Brain on Fire*, for example, received these treatments and made a full recovery. Originally thought to be an ultra-rare disorder, recent studies suggest that as many as 3 percent of cases of first-episode psychosis involve anti-NMDA receptor antibodies. However, it is uncertain whether the antibodies are functionally active in all cases.

Third, human genetics has implicated several immune-related molecules in the pathophysiology of psychiatric illness. One prominent example of schizophrenia risk alluded to in the genetics section of this chapter is the genetic variation of complement component 4 (C4) within the MHC region of the genome. Individuals possess different copies of several versions of C4 genes, and the more copies of the C4A isoform an individual has, the higher the genetic risk of schizophrenia. The protein that encodes C4 is a member of the complement cascade, a set of innate immune molecules that cleave and activate each other in sequence, much like a set of dominoes, and deposit on the surface of invading microbes. The deposition of complement on microbes serves as an "eat me" signal to the phagocytes of the immune system, which eliminates the microbes through phagocytosis. Recent work in model systems has built a framework in which complement molecules are repurposed for normal development of the brain; they deposit not on microbes but on synapses, tag certain synapses for elimination by the brain's resident phagocytes, microglia, and thus mediate the sculpting of neural circuitry through synaptic pruning. The association of increased C4 with schizophrenia risk combined with the following observations has re-ignited a hypothesis that aberrant synaptic pruning may contribute to schizophrenia pathogenesis: (1) schizophrenia symptom onset occurs in late adolescence, a time of synaptic pruning; (2) correlates of synapse loss have been found post-mortem in the brains of people with schizophrenia; (3) youth identified with validated clinical tools to be at clinical high risk of developing psychosis, who then develop psychosis, have an accelerated rate of cortical thinning than high-risk youth who do not develop psychosis. What we know of the roles of immune molecules and cells in brain function is rapidly expanding – for example, brain astrocytes can also prune synapses and secrete cytokines like IL-33, which is also a regulator of synaptic pruning during development.

The study of immune factors provides another possible avenue toward precision medicine, combining this current cutting-edge science with practical use in clinical psychiatry through defining measurable biomarkers associated with illness. Unlike neurotransmitters, which are difficult to measure in humans without invasive procedures, immune molecules are blood-based and simple to test, if we know what test is relevant. As a first example, it is the subject of current research whether subgrouping patients with depression into those with elevated inflammatory markers and those without would be useful to guide treatment choices. As a second, we can detect anti-NMDA receptor antibodies in serum and CSF and use that information to guide further imaging (e.g., abdominal imaging for a teratoma) or treatment. Third, there is research underway to examine the usefulness of biomarkers of synaptic pruning, whether PET-imaging of microglia or fluid-phase biomarkers. This type of classification of illness would move away from DSM categories but potentially allow for improved diagnostic and treatment success for mental illness.

Hormones: Circulating Molecules Connecting the Brain and Body

Another group of molecules coded for by our genome and thought to contribute to the development of mental illness in some way is hormones. Like immune molecules, these are easily accessible in circulating blood, and an association between mental illness and hormonal changes has been long suspected, such that the field has the name: psychoneuroendocrinology. Circulating hormones released by the end organs of the endocrine system are directly associated with brain function and behavior. The entire system is coordinated by releasing hormones originating in the hypothalamus that respond to perturbations in the external or internal environment. These releasing hormones then directly activate subpopulations of pituitary neurons that secrete stimulating hormones into circulation to multiple end organs, such as the adrenal gland, the pancreas, or the thyroid. These circulating hormones provide regulatory feedback to the hypothalamus, so there is promise for simple treatments by manipulating the hormones themselves. For example, early connections were observed in people with low levels of circulating thyroid hormone and low mood, and a simple fix for this biological cause of depression is to replace thyroid hormone, though some individuals continue to experience depression requiring additional treatments. Conversely, hyperthyroidism is associated with elevated mood and mania, including occasional psychosis, which can be treated by reducing the thyroid hormone levels.

Two other major axes of the endocrine system have been linked to psychiatric illness. The first is the hypothalamic-pituitary-adrenal (HPA) axis, which coordinates the acute stress response in conjunction with the sympathetic nervous system (through which norepinephrine is a major signaling molecule). In response to an acute stressor, corticotropin-releasing hormone (CRH) from the hypothalamus stimulates adrenocorticotropin hormone (ACTH) release into circulation from the pituitary. The primary target organ for ACTH is the adrenal gland, which releases glucocorticoids like cortisol. Cortisol then circulates throughout the body to coordinate whole-body response; it is critical in mediating the body's physiological functions under acute stress. This can include the standard "fight-or-flight" response, arousal, energy utilization, and also immune cell response. Cortisol itself provides a signal back to the brain to downregulate the ongoing response, turning off further CRH production in the hypothalamus. It also tunes affective and cognitive functioning through effects in the hippocampus, amygdala, and prefrontal cortex to allow adaptive response to the stressor.

In the case of individual acute stressors, this system works well. However, the lifetime burden of stressors is correlated with a greater likelihood of developing depression. Furthermore, significant traumatic stressors are elemental to the diagnosis of PTSD, and acute stress frequently precedes the onset of a depressive episode, indicating there is an upset in the flexible function of the HPA system acutely when it has been taxed over time. In the setting of chronic stress, cortisol remains elevated, and this system, through the plasticity of the glucocorticoid receptors in various parts of the brain, adapts to ignore the feedback. The inability of this system to tone itself down is thought to underly the maladaptive hypervigilance response in PTSD, and an overly adaptive decrease in responsiveness is thought to relate to depression. This lack of adaptive plasticity is thought to be related to the expression and activity of the glucocorticoid receptor in different parts of the brain, which are epigenetically modified by stress. Genetic variants in regulators of the glucocorticoid response have also been associated with schizophrenia and MDD through GWAS. Because these changes are found primarily in the receptors (rather than circulating hormones themselves), they are not an easily accessible biomarker. Furthermore, as there is a wide range of normal baseline circulating levels of glucocorticoid hormones based on multiple factors (time of day, nutrient state, history of stress), such that it is hard to define levels that indicate a maladaptive HPA axis related to mood disorders or PTSD. But they remain a promising focus for further research to elucidate how to best target this axis for disease classification and precision treatment.

Another hormonal axis that has received attention, and has shown promise for new treatments for mood disorders, is the hypothalamic-pituitary-gonadal (HPG) axis. This interest followed robust observations regarding the higher incidence of MDD for females from adolescence to menopause. Furthermore, females experience acute periods of increased risk for psychiatric symptoms – premenstrual, postpartum, perimenopause – coinciding with fluctuations of sex hormones. Our understanding of the mechanism underlying this possible connection and why some women respond to these shifts and not others is in its infancy, but some progress is being made. In the 1980s, for example, it was discovered that metabolites of progesterone and deoxycorticosterone could stimulate certain neurotransmitter receptors like GABA receptors. Subsequent observation that one of these metabolites, allopregnanolone, increases during pregnancy and drops sharply in the post-partum period led to the development of a synthetic version of allopregnanolone called brexanolone, which was approved in 2019 by the FDA for the treatment of post-partum depression. These circuits show that the complexity of the nervous system extends to its effects on the whole body, and that the body's feedback mechanisms also play a role in driving altered brain function. If we can understand how these feedback circuits affect gene expression acutely, and behavior over time, we will find new biological targets for diagnosing and treating mental illness.

Neural Circuits in Psychiatry

Translation of Converging Circuits

Molecules such as neurotransmitters, hormones, and immune factors mediate the communication between two neurons at any given moment. Billions of these neurons work together in a *neural circuit* to respond to the environment and accomplish various complex behavioral, cognitive, and affective tasks. Unlike the field of neurology, in which many of the diagnoses lend themselves to gross anatomical localizations, in psychiatry, gross anatomical abnormalities have been few. Instead, it is the dysfunction of these microcircuits that is thought to occur in many mental disorders. These circuits may be a final common pathway for many of the various rare genetic (and resulting molecular) abnormalities in the development of certain mental illnesses. If this is the case, identifying these circuits could provide markers for predicting the development of the disorder and monitoring response to treatment. It would also be the first step toward finding methods to alter the pathways that could affect a large number of patients.

These neural circuits are pathways necessary for normal human function. To correlate these circuits with complex human psychology, though we need to break down our constructs into simpler forms. There is no "ADHD" neural circuit, and there is no one circuit that, when dysfunctional, results in ADHD. Instead, there are separate circuits involved in sustaining attention, shifting attention to a new and important stimulus, balancing internal and external attention, controlling motor function, and maintaining executive function – all functions that are affected in ADHD, as well as other psychiatric illnesses. Other examples of basic psychological constructs that have been used for correlation to the underlying biological networks are fear circuitry, reward circuitry, arousal circuitry, and circuitry underlying perception of self and others.

We will now take a deeper look at dopaminergic reward circuitry in the context of its relationship to addiction. The motivation to pursue such behaviors as eating, drinking, and sex is necessary for survival. Evolutionarily these behaviors are pleasurable in order to encourage and reinforce their continuation. In excess, though, these behaviors can interfere with normal functioning. Thus there also needs to be a regulatory mechanism. As mentioned earlier, dopamine is a key player in the reward pathway. Neurons at the top of the brainstem, in a region called the *ventral tegmental area*, synthesize dopamine. These neurons respond to one's behaviors or environmental stimuli that are deemed important for survival. In response, they send out a burst of dopamine to the nucleus accumbens, eliciting a positive, pleasurable feeling. These neurons interact with neurons in the orbitofrontal cortex, which is related to motivation and drive to continue the behavior. The prefrontal cortex, the most evolutionarily developed area of our brain, plays a modulatory and inhibitory role in behavior. Finally, the amygdala and hippocampus receive stimuli that allow the circuit to remember this behavior and how pleasurable it was. In cases of addiction, the addictive substance leads to a flood of dopamine release from the VTA, which overwhelms the regulatory pathways. In actuality, this is not a linear process. There is constant multidirectional communication and feedback within a circuit. Additionally, there is communication between circuits. For example, the amygdala plays a central role in the fear circuitry and stress-related disorders, and is commonly studied related to behaviors associated with PTSD. Stress and anxiety can be a trigger for the use of substances, and these stress-related disorders are known to be comorbid in a significant proportion of patients.

Technologies to study Neural Circuits

How are these circuits investigated in living humans? Magnetic resonance imaging (MRI) is a versatile tool that can evaluate structural and functional aspects of neural circuits and their relation to psychopathology. Task-based functional MRI (fMRI) is perhaps the best-known technique. In task-based fMRI, participants engage in a cognitive or emotional task while inside the MRI scanner. The instructions and task stimuli are presented in MR-compatible goggles or projected onto a small screen, and participants' performance can be measured through button presses. During task performance, changes are observed in both "task-positive" and "task-negative" networks. For example, during a test of working memory, an increase in the number of items that a participant must memorize associates with both a corresponding increase in activation of the frontoparietal control network (e.g., dorsolateral prefrontal cortex, inferior parietal lobe). However, it is also associated with increased *deactivation* of the default network (medial prefrontal cortex, posterior cingulate).

fMRI studies measure the blood oxygen level dependent (BOLD) signal, which is thought to index cerebral blood flow. The BOLD signal shows time-dependent oscillations that vary depending on where they are measured in the brain, and on task conditions (as noted previously). The BOLD signal is also present at rest, and regional correlations in the signal provide a way to measure the functional connectivity of those regions. Specifically, regions that are functionally interconnected show higher BOLD time-course correlations. These correlations have given rise to canonical brain networks, including the frontoparietal and default networks mentioned previously, but also those involved in sensorimotor, visual, attention, limbic, and salience processing. In 2013, an international collaboration called the Human Connectome Project (HCP) was established to create a baseline map of "normal" functional brain connectivity based on fMRI data from a growing database of subjects. In addition to showing differences in task-related activation (or deactivation), individuals with psychiatric syndromes have also been shown to have differences in intrinsic functional connectivity between and within these networks, relative to those observed in healthy HCP participants.

MRI scans also provide the opportunity to contrast measurements of brain structure within and between groups. For example, it is now well established that the thickness of the cerebral cortex diminishes linearly with age in longitudinal studies of healthy adolescents; this change is thought to reflect two processes, synaptic pruning and myelination, that are vital to cortical maturation. However, adolescents with psychotic symptoms (or who are at increased risk of such symptoms) demonstrate an early and accelerated pattern of cortical thinning, as mentioned in the context of immune molecules and synaptic pruning above. Another MRI technique, diffusion tensor imaging (DTI), indexes the structural integrity of white matter tracts. As with cortical thickness, DTI measurements change with age, and changes in these measures characterize psychiatric syndromes. In recent years, academic centers have begun combining PET and MRI machines, allowing for the combination of structural and functional data. The cost and risks associated with this combined technology have kept it in the realm of research at this time.

While researchers can use fMRI BOLD signal to determine the level of coordination between brain regions, complimentary techniques can map direct cellular connectivity. One new method that bridges the gap between brain-wide fMRI and the cellular resolution of fluorescent microscopy is light sheet microscopy. Unlike conventional microscopy, where thinly sliced samples are mounted on slides, light sheet microscopy scans large pieces of intact tissue. To permit researchers to image a sample on the scale of a whole mouse brain with its attached spinal cord, we make the brain completely transparent. This is accomplished by first removing the lipids from the brain and placing it in a solution with a matching refractive index. Light then passes through the sample without being refracted, and the sample appears clear. A sheet of light that is only a few micrometers thick then gently illuminates each plane, images of which are then reconstructed into a high-resolution model of the tissue. These data sets have the significant advantage of preserving the three-dimensional relationships within the large tissue sample. In this context, fluorescent neuronal tracers can identify inputs and outputs from regions across the brain. Likewise, genetically encoded reporters can show changes in the activity of neuronal subpopulations after experimental manipulation or drug exposure. This information can then be integrated with human imaging data and used to identify prospective target pathways for potential treatment.

Once structural and functional differences in brain circuits are discovered, how can we influence these aberrant pathways to improve the lives of patients with psychiatric illness? Several technologies are already available and in use. In deep brain stimulation (DBS), for example, electrical pulse generators are surgically placed in specific areas of the brain, and regular electrical pulses are sent at different frequencies to inhibit or activate the neuronal pathways in the area. In OCD, for example, electrodes are placed in an area of the basal ganglia called the striatum, presumably interrupting the pathways involved in this disorder. DBS is also under investigation at several medical centers for the treatment of MDD and anorexia nervosa. A less invasive tool, transcranial magnetic stimulation (TMS), uses magnetic fields to alter the functionality of certain circuits in the brain. It has shown particular efficacy in treatment-resistant depression, and research is ongoing in other areas. For both DBS and TMS, a better understanding of the circuits involved in the pathology will allow us to target these pathways more accurately.

Still, the macroscopic nature of both of these techniques limits their specificity. A new suite of tools may allow for more precise dissection and understanding of discrete neuron populations, currently used in animal models. The major advantage of these tools is their capacity to alter the function of specific neuron groups while leaving others largely undisturbed. The strategy is to use signals that do not normally induce a neuronal response. Perhaps the most well-known technology in this area is optogenetics. In optogenetics, scientists insert modified ion channels, which are sensitive to a particular wavelength of light, into the cell membrane. Because neurons are ordinarily insensitive to light, only those neurons expressing the light-sensitive proteins will respond when illuminated. Depending on the charge of the ions that the light-sensitive channel passes across the membrane, illumination may "turn on" or "turn off" those neurons. Genetic markers or cellular connectivity patterns can restrict the expression of these light-sensitive proteins to a desired subset of cells. For example, researchers use genetically modified mice to control which neuron types express the light-sensitive ion channels. We can then use fiberoptic implants to direct light to a particular brain region, giving researchers millisecond-level control over a precise set of neurons. In so doing, we can interrogate the role of those neurons during behavior and in models of disease. For example, if specific neurons in the ventromedial hypothalamus are stimulated with optogenetics, animals immediately become aggressive. While this may sound like science fiction, clinical trials using optogenetics are already underway.

The refined control of optogenetics has been a boon for our understanding of the brain; a growing capacity to "read" or detect signals in a similarly defined manner provides complementary information about neuronal function. New sensors based on fluorescent proteins make this possible by fluorescing when a specific ligand is present. GCaMP, a calcium indicator, is one of the most commonly used sensors today. When calcium concentrations increase in a cell, the calcium binds to and changes the conformation of GCaMP. The ensuing conformational shift permits the modified fluorescent protein in GCaMP to fluoresce. This is particularly useful because calcium increases are associated with neuronal activity. Miniaturized microscopes can be implanted in animal models to visualize the responses of individual cells during experiments. Other light-based sensors have been developed for a wide range of cellular signals, including glutamate, GABA, acetylcholine, dopamine, and protein kinase A (PKA). Much like optogenetic tools, these too can be targeted to discrete cell populations and pathways. Together, the "read and write" capabilities of these techniques have opened the door to questions about the brain and psychiatric illness that were never before possible. The ability to distinguish or control subpopulations of neurons in a molecularly specific, regionally defined, and time-locked manner allows us to dissect the workings of the behaving brain without reducing the layers of complexity of its function. That is to say, we believe we are starting to connect the language of the brain with the language of behavior.

Ethical Considerations and Translation Challenges

Ours is an exhilarating time because our understanding of the brain on multiple levels is rapidly expanding. Such an imminent explosion should ignite thoughtful discussion about how clinical practice *should* be affected – questions of what we *should* do compared to the range of what we *could* do is an ethical problem. For example, we highlighted here how our existing diagnostic categories do not map cleanly onto dysfunctions at the genetic, neurotransmitter, immunological, or neurocircuit level; rather, there is considerable pleiotropy (variations influencing the risk of multiple disorders) and heterogeneity (many different types of biological dysfunctions that lead to a similar "end state"). The messiness of remapping psychiatry onto clinical neuroscience is likely to expand, and with it, the field will have more pressure to decide how best to handle it. Answering questions like whether the psychological domains of RDoC are better than the DSM will involve the field deciding what makes a nosological framework valuable. If facilitating treatment is a value, for example, then would it be better to match nosology to the treatment approach. Should we use circuit conceptualizations when circuit interventions like DBS, or TMS might be useful? Should we use molecular conceptualizations when deciding whether to bathe the brain in small-molecules? We are starting to see this sort of reconceptualization in oncology: historically, anatomical diagnosis (lung, skin, or bowel cancer) has been useful when deciding on surgical treatment (an anatomical treatment), but the availability of small molecule targeting specific overactive pathways is leading to new categorization. Because the genetic driver mutations provide a potential pharmacologic target, and are shared between cancers of many different anatomical sites, new categorization drives new organization for medical treatment at the pathophysiologic root.

Because brain disorders often develop over time, efforts in clinical neuroscience will also expand our knowledge of earlier steps on these pathways and inform us more about individuals that have higher and lower likelihoods of developing symptoms. Although we are far from approaching the magnitude of predictive power that Mendelian genetics brought to Huntington's disease, risk estimation is rapidly entering the domain where it is clinically and morally relevant. We can already identify using clinical interviews a group of help-seeking young-people, 20–40 percent of whom will develop psychosis in the next two years, even though they have minimal current symptoms; whether to name this risk-state a "disorder" was hotly debated in the revision of the DSM-IV to DSM-V. These young people are often at crucial crossroads in life when they form their identities and make practical choices like whether and where to go to college. Already, imaging, laboratory, and data science are poised to refine these risk estimates further. At what risk threshold would a parent or clinician be justified in recommending for or against leaving for college, pursuing vocational training, joining the armed forces, or staying at home? Lowering or raising the teenager's expectations for future pursuits? Having a closer or more distant engagement with the health care system, should symptoms arise, especially if there was a financial cost of doing so? Disclosing this information to third parties, such as school counselors, current or potential employers, insurance companies? These questions of how to match psychiatric risk-magnitudes with actions are complicated. It is sobering to observe the precedent in other areas of medicine that small absolute-risks sometimes spur drastic measures. In vascular surgery, for example, a 1 percent per year risk of stroke from advanced carotid artery disease is often felt to be high enough to merit the risks of surgery.

Neuroscientific explanations of human behavior have already entered into the cultural zeitgeist. While many neuroscientists have a nuanced view of the complexity of the interaction between our biology and our actions, there is a danger of taking a more reductionistic and deterministic view. This view risks our patients' shifting to an external locus of control of their symptoms ("it is the dopamine, not me!") and not seeing the need to act to improve their lives. For example, though the campaign to emphasize addiction as a brain disease has had many proponents with a goal of decreasing blame and stigma, there have also been opponents who argue that the campaign exacerbates misconceptions around the ability of drug-related behaviors to be changeable. Another example, from forensics, has been the explosion of appeals to neuroscientific explanations of behavior in attempts to mitigate blameworthiness in courts.

In terms of translation, there are several overarching challenges that the field of neuroscience has faced in applying findings to psychiatric illness. While many of these challenges to successful translation are shared between psychiatry and other medical specialties, we try to highlight those that have particular salience in psychiatry.

1. *Definitions.* The DSM is based on distinct syndromes that have their origins in descriptive medicine. Categories based on descriptive medicine are present in many domains of medicine (e.g., fibromyalgia in rheumatology), but the fraction of entities of this sort in psychiatry is extreme compared to other medical specialties. Complicating things further, many patients have multiple diagnoses concurrently, the symptoms overlap between diagnoses, one presentation may morph into a different presentation, and the categories themselves are heterogeneous groups. Additionally, the definitions change with each new edition of the DSM. The starting point for understanding the biological underpinnings of an illness is first deciding what constitutes that illness, and thus uncertainty in nosology compounds challenges in clinical neuroscience.

2. *Causality.* When researchers find connections between psychiatric pathology and a neural network, gene, or neurotransmitter, they will often refer to it as a "correlate." Because disorder categories have been defined on clusters of symptoms as above, it has been a greater challenge than in other specialties for basic scientists to develop appropriate model systems that can aid in our understanding of causality. Though early efforts tried to model "symptoms of schizophrenia" in mice, or look at biological changes in an animal given an effective psychiatric medication, it is unclear if any of the biology studied in these systems was actually relevant to the cluster of symptoms in humans. Many of the basic and clinical neuroscience techniques described in this chapter are an effort to overcome this limitation.

3. *Effect size.* Many of our findings only account for the illness in a small portion of the population. Studies must use vast populations to find meaningful results, and the applications are then limited in scope. New techniques in math are helping to address this limitation.

4. *Reductionism.* We know that the disorders we treat have strong environmental influences that modulate and are modulated by our genetics. It is difficult, though, to quantify these environmental influences to better understand the interactions with our biology.

5. *History of stigma.* Though many diseases and disorders have carried a stigma and history of discrimination, psychiatric disorders have become surrounded by a unique legislative environment because of it. For example, because of the historical abuse of psychosurgery for social control, many states and countries have blanket prohibitions of any surgery for psychiatric indications; such regulations have meant that studies on the effectiveness of circuit-based treatments like DBS for psychiatric indications can only legally be pursued in certain legal jurisdictions.

These challenges to translation will become more surmountable with progress at each of the levels of investigations highlighted in this chapter: genomes, neurotransmitters, immune and hormonal molecules, and circuits. Some progress at one of these levels may enable the field to imagine different ways of categorizing and subgrouping disease, as it did in the development of the RDoC. Then this new subgrouping may open up new techniques for use in scientific investigation and translation into clinical diagnostics and treatment. Clinicians and patients can then provide further feedback as to whether the new categories, diagnostics, or treatments actually help them deal with their experience of mental illness. With each iteration of this process, slow as it may be, clinical neuroscience and psychiatric practice will move forward together to significantly advance both fields.

References and Selected Readings

- Charney, D. S., Nestler, E. J., Sklar, P., and Buxbaum, J. D., eds. (2018). *Neurobiology of Mental Illness.* 5th ed. New York: Oxford University Press.
- Cuthbert, B. N., and Insel, T. R. (2013). Toward the Future of Psychiatric Diagnosis: The Seven Pillars of RDoC. *BMC Medicine* 11, 126.
- Higgins, E. S., and George, M. J., eds. (2019). *The Neuroscience of Clinical Psychiatry: The Pathophysiology of Mental Illness.* 3rd ed. New York: Wolters Kluwer.
- Lieberman, J. A. (2015). *Shrinks: The Untold Story of Psychiatry.* New York: Little, Brown.
- Martin, A. R., Daly, M. J., Robinson, E. B., Hyman, S. E., and Neale, B. M. (2019). Predicting Polygenic Risk of Psychiatric Disorders. *Biological Psychiatry* 86, 97–109.

- McEwen, B. S., and Akil, H. (2020). Revisiting the Stress Concept: Implications for Affective Disorders. *Journal of Neuroscience* 40 (1), 12–21.
- Smoller, J. W. (2019). Psychiatric Genetics Beginning to Find Its Footing. *American Journal of Psychiatry* 176, 609–614.
- Stahl, S. M. (2013). *Stahl's Essential Psychopharmacology: Neuroscientific Basis and Practical Application*. 4th ed. Cambridge: Cambridge University Press.

Self-Assessment Questions

1. Which of the following is the most important difference between DSM-V and RDoC as frameworks for psychiatric disorders?
   A. RDoC places emphasis on broad domains of behavior that show a range of variation from normal to abnormal across populations and that can be studied across different levels of analysis from cells and circuits to observable behavior and subjective self-report.
   B. RDoC assess genetic variation in order to predict medication side effects and effectiveness in individual patients.
   C. DSM-V classifies disorders according to their symptoms and putative biological and environmental causes.
   D. DSM-V is more relevant to research than to clinical practice.
   E. Disorders may share symptom features in the RDoC framework but not in DSM-V.

2. Twin studies are most useful in which of the following ways:
   A. Predicting the severity of illness in affected individuals
   B. Explaining epigenetic mechanisms as in inter-generational adverse experiences
   C. Providing estimates of hereditability of psychiatric illnesses
   D. Highlighting specific risk genes underlying psychiatric illnesses
   E. Offering insights as to why genetic variants such as 22q11.2 deletion are associated with psychotic symptoms

3. Increased expression of certain genes in the nucleus accumbens related to histone acetylation induced by cocaine administration in mice is an example of:
   A. Pharmacogenomics
   B. Epigenetics
   C. Pharmacodynamics
   D. Reuptake inhibition
   E. Disinhibition

4. The most ubiquitous neurotransmitters in the brain are:
   A. GABA and glutamine
   B. Monoamines

    C. Opioids

    D. Cytokines

    E. Acetylcholine and histamine

5. Optogenetics is most closely associated with which of the following:

    A. The impact of light on cells in the retina thereby gaining influence on the central nervous system

    B. The use of genetic engineering to activate fibers along the optic nerve

    C. The insertion of modified ion channels that are sensitive to particular wavelengths of light into the nerve cell membrane

    D. The use of optical coherence tomography to detect genetic risk for certain neuropsychiatric conditions

    E. The application of light-emitting diodes to the scalp in order to stimulate superficial layers of cortical neurons

Answers to Self-Assessment Questions

1. (A)
2. (C)
3. (B)
4. (A)
5. (C)

3 Introduction to the Patient Interview

TODD GRISWOLD, MICHAEL KAHN, MARK SCHECHTER, JANET YASSEN,
FELICIA SMITH, AND REBECCA BRENDEL

Introduction

Interviewing patients is one of the most rewarding aspects of clinical psychiatry. It offers an opportunity to get to know someone, to find clues to diagnosis, and to relieve suffering. The psychiatric interview thus functions as an alliance-building process, diagnostic procedure, and therapeutic intervention. While this may sound complex, the interview process can be simplified by learning to approach it with the proper attitude. This can be considered analogous to helping a young musician learn how to have proper posture at the piano or to hold a violin and bow correctly. Without a good feel for the instrument, and without the appropriate perspective for learning what the music is about, the simple drilling of scales and fingerings will be misguided. Similarly, in the psychiatric interview, one must have a proper attitude toward the patient to be of the most help. The key qualities of this approach are curiosity, respect, and caring. If you notice obstacles to feeling interested in or caring about the patient, do not despair – such attitudes can be cultivated (see the section on empathy and compassion later in this chapter).

Effective psychiatric interviewing involves eliciting feelings as well as data, and in this way, it differs from the more typical "medical" interview. Data collection alone is often not as helpful with psychiatric patients, who suffer in highly personal ways that often involve feeling some combination of shame, fear, despair, or anger. People naturally want to protect themselves from such painful feelings, and of course, it takes time and tact for the clinician to approach sensitive matters. Furthermore, psychiatric symptoms can interfere with the cognitive functions required to answer questions in a straightforward manner. Disorganized thinking, inattention, suspiciousness, and cultural difference are just a few of the factors that can complicate the process of getting to know someone. Such challenges may be overcome not by asking more probing questions but instead by building rapport through respectful curiosity and conversational flexibility.

Trainees often mistakenly feel an inherent conflict between eliciting history and building rapport. In fact, rapport facilitates gathering history, and understanding history facilitates rapport. The quality of information one gathers is a direct function of the quality of connection the clinician establishes with the patient. The best and most meaningful interviews typically resemble a conversation more than an ordinary interview.

Context and Purpose of the Interview

The approach to a psychiatric interview, and the content covered, depend in large part on the clinical context – the setting and situation – and the purpose of the interview. An initial evaluation in a high-acuity setting – such as an emergency department or inpatient unit – will often prioritize eliciting symptoms and history to determine a provisional diagnosis and assess risk. Once rapport is established, more probing questions can easily follow. An initial evaluation in a low-acuity outpatient setting – particularly if the clinical risk is low and the patient will be seen again in ongoing treatment – may emphasize developing the alliance and facilitating an open-ended exploration of the patient's story. A teaching interview is unique in that its goal is educational as well as therapeutic. In this instance, patients must have the capacity to consent to such an interview, which generally avoids probing distressing issues unless the patient wishes to discuss them.

Therapeutic Alliance

Developing a therapeutic alliance is the first goal of an initial psychiatric interview. Establishing the alliance means joining with the patient in such a way that the two of you can work together toward the goals of understanding and relieving suffering. While there is no one correct way to establish an alliance, one should keep in mind the principle of "get the story first and the symptoms next."

Numerous studies of psychotherapy efficacy have identified the therapeutic alliance as the most robust predictor of treatment efficacy, regardless of the type of psychotherapy. A therapeutic alliance generally involves an emotional connection between the patient and the clinician, involving caring and trust. A clinician's benevolence and goodwill are not guaranteed to elicit a patient's trust. Many patients, perhaps especially psychiatric patients, have little reason to accept the assumed social contract of a cooperative suffering patient seeking help from a kind, more knowledgeable physician; trust must be earned rather than assumed.

Three actions help develop the therapeutic alliance:

1. Listen authentically, with curiosity and without judgment.
2. Protect the patient's self-esteem.
3. Show respect and compassion.

When seeking to accomplish these three tasks, it is helpful to remember Harry Stack Sullivan's observation that "we are all much more simply human than otherwise." Do not hesitate to consider responding in a more naturally human way. One can remain professional while still being authentic. Patients are remarkable, and their lives are astonishing – allow yourself to experience this. Clinicians can help protect patients' self-esteem by being aware of their own potential to judge or shame patients, even inadvertently. Patients coming to seek psychiatric care are vulnerable, often having been mistreated or abused by others, and so are acutely

sensitive to words or behavior that convey disrespect or disdain. Authentically acknowledging a patient's strengths is useful as well. Certain patients are fearful of
being coerced, so an authoritative stance may need to be softened. Finally, while
some patients with severe psychiatric illness may appear confusing to inexperi-
enced clinicians, it is important to recognize that they have the same feelings we
all have – loneliness, fear, anger, sadness, and the wish to be cared for.

A sound therapeutic alliance facilitates more accurate reporting by patients,
which fosters a clearer understanding of the problem. It engenders trust, which
allows the patient to more openly consider whether to accept any treatment recommendations. Most importantly, the connection itself can relieve suffering. By listening respectfully and expressing compassion for a patient in pain, a clinician can
benefit patients immensely. As an old saying posits, "A burden shared is a burden
halved." This is often hard for medical students to believe early in their training.

Confidentiality

Maintaining confidentiality is of the utmost importance in psychiatric care, given
the sensitivity of topics discussed, the importance of establishing trust, and the
stigma attached to psychiatric illness. Explicit exceptions to maintaining confidentiality include the so-called emergency exception and mandated reporting statutes.
The "emergency exception" primarily means that clinicians can disclose confidential information if the patient is in imminent danger of harming themselves or others. Clinicians should familiarize themselves with state-specific statutes regarding
mandated reporting of suspected neglect or abuse of children, elders, and disabled
persons. Finally, it is important to know that a typical signed "consent for treatment" will include the authorization to disclose some information to insurers,
including diagnoses and types of treatment. These data, generally entered into
the electronic medical record, are often submitted by insurance companies to a
national insurance exchange, which then shares this information among insurers.

Empathy and Compassion

Empathy has increasingly been the subject of research, and it now has multiple
and sometimes confusing definitions. Put simply, *empathy* means being attuned
to what another person is feeling, and being able to see and feel a situation from
another's perspective. Empathy involves affectively sharing some felt sense of the
patient's emotion and also cognitively understanding the patient's feelings and
perspective (Halpern, 2003). In this way, empathy is a part of deep understanding.

Compassion is related to empathy and involves recognizing that someone is
suffering and feeling emotionally moved to want to relieve their suffering. If empathy helps build a "being with" connection, compassion develops the "caring for"
response to suffering. Patients feel supported and less alone when they feel truly
understood, and they are soothed or even uplifted when they feel their clinician's

compassionate care for them. Skills for heightening empathy and compassion can be taught and cultivated.

Empathic connection can be facilitated in several ways. Just prior to an interview, clinicians may wish to take a moment to remind themselves that, as the ancient Roman playwright Terence put it, "nothing human is alien to me." More prosaically, one should assume a receptive, friendly demeanor and posture without an excessive focus on note-taking or an electronic device such as a computer or tablet. When a patient describes distress and difficulty, empathic validating comments can strengthen the connection. Tried-and-true responses such as "That sounds really difficult" or "I am so sorry that happened" can sound like clichés or genuine concern, depending on one's attitude.

Sometimes clinicians will find it hard to feel empathic, particularly if the interviewer perceives the patient as significantly different or upsetting. It may help to imagine how one has felt in an *emotionally* similar situation, aiming to connect with the common humanity of suffering. But it is also important to recognize the particularity of one's own emotional responses as well as the patient's. Regardless of how different or upsetting a patient may seem, the clinician can be certain that the patient would not be coming into contact with psychiatric treatment unless they were deeply struggling and suffering in some way. Caution must be used when considering whether one's own emotional responses accurately indicate something specific about the patient's psychopathology. "This patient makes me feel so angry she must be borderline" is the kind of formulation that should be questioned and ideally reviewed with a peer or supervisor before being assumed to be true.

When clinicians resonate deeply with a patient's painful feelings, it is important for this empathic resonance to be further developed into compassionate caring. Simply feeling a patient's suffering may lead to empathic distress, a self-related emotional state that is experienced as stressful (Singer & Klimecki, 2014) and can lead to withdrawal from patients and others. Compassion taps into kindness and generosity and has an other-directed focus. Undertaking an active treatment approach helps clinicians move from empathy to compassion, but medical students or other trainees in primarily learner roles may have more difficulty making this transition since they may be less actively involved in caring for the patient. Two ways to help students make this transition are (1) structuring the student role to be more active and (2) effectively conveying to students that listening and bearing witness to distress is in itself a caring intervention and a compassionate act to relieve suffering.

Boundaries

Understanding the nature and function of boundaries helps define the limits of the clinician-patient relationship. Basic boundaries in the psychiatric interview regulate physical contact, the extent of the clinician's questioning, and the extent of the clinician's self-disclosure. While many boundary issues are uncontroversial (we do not socialize with patients, use them as confidants, or ask them for financial guidance, for example), other issues are less clear. Should you shake hands with a patient when first meeting them? For many (probably most) patients, this is a powerful signal of acceptance and a wish for connection. For other patients (who usually appear guarded or make poor eye contact), this can pose a threatening intrusion. The clinician usually develops a sense of what he or she is comfortable with and learns to read the patient's body language. Some clinicians are overly fearful about any physical contact with any patient. The elderly patient who seeks a hug after revealing how vulnerable he or she feels is quite different from a patient who is about the same age as the therapist and asks "if we can end every session with a hug." A good rule of thumb for analyzing boundary dilemmas is to ask one's self "What is the meaning of this action, and is it good for the patient?" Asking these questions helps one analyze common boundary issues, such as physical contact, gift giving, and self-disclosure.

Safety and Respect

Fostering an atmosphere of safety is important for the patient and clinician alike. Two specific situations merit particular attention: interviewing a traumatized patient and interviewing an agitated patient.

We follow the "universal precautions" principle in assuming all patients may have experienced significant trauma. Practical approaches include respect for personal space, positioning oneself at eye level with the patient, and allowing the patient choice in the direction of the interview. Some patients will not be comfortable unless their back is to the wall and they can view the door to the room. If the clinician is unsure how far to probe, one can always "ask about asking." In effect, this is obtaining informed consent from the patient to continue a line of questioning that may lead to reactions (not necessarily unhelpful) such as crying, anger, or anxiety.

When a patient is agitated and angry, it is ideal (but not an absolute requirement) if the interview room can be set up so both the patient and the clinician have unimpeded access to the door. Patients in a state of high stress generally respond more to nonverbal cues than to verbal ones, and the clinician should make sure that body language, tone of voice, and eye contact convey calm reassurance. Even when firm limits need to be set on a patient's behavior, this can be done in a nonthreatening, nonshaming way.

Structuring and Directing the Interview

Some patients have difficulty organizing their thoughts and therefore struggle to coherently articulate their feelings. Other patients wish to conceal thoughts and feelings, often to guard against shame. Clinicians thus need to develop their clinical toolkit to tailor their approach to the particular style and needs of each patient. Following the "story first, symptoms next" principle, interviews will generally be more open-ended initially and will progress gradually to a closed-ended or structured format. If a patient starts to seem long-winded or disorganized during a diagnostic interview, it is useful to courteously let the patient know at the outset that, reluctantly, you may have to interrupt them and resort to more structured questions. If the clinician imposes structure prematurely or bluntly, the flow of the interview may become deadened and constrained, with the patient passively providing limited answers to a series of questions. Ideally, the clinician guides and structures the interview without sacrificing its conversational quality; the assessment is a conversation *augmented* with an inquiry. The clinician should take a stepwise approach to guiding the interview, gradually becoming more active in providing structure and monitoring the patient's response. If an interruption is required (such as with a hypomanic or obsessional patient), the clinician can apologize in a friendly manner and explain the need to interrupt (for example, due to time constraints or the importance of discussing certain topics).

Summary

Developing advanced interviewing skills is a long process, measured in years. Yet the beginner, even when feeling uncertain and awkward, can nevertheless be of enormous help to the patient, merely by showing interest and concern. Whenever students wonder "What am I supposed to be doing here?," it can help to imagine one's role as that of a "collaborative curious co-investigator."

Psychiatric Assessment and Write-Up

A careful psychiatric evaluation includes interviewing and data gathering, clinical reasoning, and documentation. This chapter focuses on the content and documentation of the evaluation, not the process of interviewing. There is broad agreement on the fundamental parts of a psychiatric assessment. Clerkships, residency training programs, and clinical services generally use similar templates. The American Psychiatric Association[1] has published guidelines for the psychiatric evaluation of adults.

This chapter includes a representative assessment outline. It is not meant to be an outline of the order in which questions should be asked in an interview, but rather the order in which data should be presented. The comments about specific sections do not comprehensively list everything to possibly include, but instead outline major points to help guide clinical thinking.

Goals of a Write-Up

Thoughtful documentation accomplishes many important goals, some of which can be undermined by forms, checklists, and a cumbersome electronic medical record (EMR).

---

[1] American Psychiatric Association, *The American Psychiatric Association Practice Guidelines for the Evaluation of Adults*, 3rd ed., 2016.

1. Organizing data and clinical reasoning to support diagnosis and treatment
2. Supporting treatment by communicating effectively with others, including current and future clinicians
3. Documenting evaluation and treatment planning for the patient and family
4. Including required regulatory content and demonstrating clinical thinking relevant to medicolegal issues

General Principles

- Do not let templates and the EMR diminish your observational skills and clinical thinking.
- Balance comprehensiveness with conciseness and clarity.
- Avoid objectifying language and personal judgments. Increasingly the medical record is shared by clinicians and patients, and patients may want to read their records.
- Choose clear, simple, and specific language over jargon to more accurately convey information.
- Visual clarity and organization support good patient care by allowing busy clinicians to quickly find relevant information by scanning for headings, subheadings, bullet points, bolded content, and so forth.

Outline of Representative Assessment

Identifying Data

- Capsule summary of current presentation with most relevant identifying details
- There is debate about how many descriptors to routinely list regarding – for example, age; sex/gender pronouns and sexual orientation; employment and housing status; self-identified race, ethnicity, or national origin. Some clinicians favor including a broad range of information with the intention of presenting the broadest picture of the patient, while others emphasize that listing identifiers at the start of a case presentation activates implicit and explicit bias. A general rule of thumb is to include a descriptor if it adds appreciably to the understanding of the patient's current clinical situation.

Chief Complaint

- In patient's words whenever possible
- *Chief concern* is a related term and may be less likely to foster implicit judgmental attitudes, but is not always considered synonymous to *chief complaint*.

Sources of Information

- For example, patient interview, medical records, collateral information from treating clinicians or friends/family

History of the Present Illness

Aim for an understandable narrative. Ask yourself, "Do I really understand what the patient is experiencing and how the patient arrived at this particular circumstance?"

- Recent symptoms/problems, impact on functioning, efforts at coping
- Recent context and circumstances leading to current evaluation
- Pertinent positives and negatives of common disorders for establishing differential diagnosis, including major psychiatric, neurological, and other medical conditions including substance use. One option is to use the mnemonic "follow the MAPS TO diagnosis":
  - M: Mood
    - depressive symptoms
    - manic symptoms
  - A: Anxiety
    - panic symptoms and somatic anxiety symptoms
    - worry
    - avoidance
  - P: Psychosis
    - hallucinations
    - paranoia and delusions
    - thought disorganization
  - S: Substances (see separate section for more detailed history)
    - recent use of substances
  - T: Trauma (see separate section for more detailed history)
    - recent trauma related to HPI
    - past trauma affecting current functioning (nightmares, flashbacks, hypervigilance/hyperarousal, dissociation, avoidance)
  - O: Other medical
    - current medical illnesses or treatments affecting current functioning, especially pain
- Precipitating or exacerbating factors
- Recent treatment including adherence or other changes in treatment
- Risk issues (i.e., suicidality, aggression, impulsivity)

Past Psychiatric History

- Pertinent diagnostic symptoms and diagnoses – for example, mood, anxiety and PTSD, psychosis, personality, somatic symptoms, eating disorder, and so forth
- Treatment history including duration, adherence, response (benefits and harms)
  - First psychiatric treatment

- ○ Prior diagnoses
- ○ Prior psychiatric medications
- ○ Previous psychotherapies, including type of therapy
- ○ Psychiatric outpatient treatment
- ○ Hospitalizations and/or emergency evaluations
  - ▪ precipitants
  - ▪ voluntary or non-voluntary
  - ▪ benefit/harm
- ○ Other treatments such as ECT, partial hospitalization, or residential treatment
- ○ Known barriers to treatment
- • Risk and safety: For risk issues such as suicidality or violence, it is crucial to include details of any instance such as a suicide attempt or episode of aggression. A lack of specificity can lead to underestimation or overestimation of risk and thereby adversely affect clinical care.
  - ○ Suicidality and self-harm
    - ▪ Prior thoughts of suicide or self-harm
    - ▪ Any suicide attempts including intent and estimated lethality
    - ▪ Self-injury/self-harm, such as cutting
  - ○ Aggression: gathering this history can often be done when asking about symptoms and coping related to anger.
    - ▪ Prior thoughts of aggression or violence
    - ▪ Aggressive behaviors, including assault, use of weapons, destruction of property
    - ▪ Threats to others; stalking
  - ○ Access to firearms

Substance Use History

This important area is sometimes integrated into the PPH, but it often benefits patients and clinicians to document separately. Separate documentation demonstrates the appropriate importance of this information and also supports more thorough evaluation. Substance use history should not be included in social history because substance use disorders are medical/psychiatric disorders – documenting substance use history as social history   should be considered an outdated practice reflective of historical ignorance but unfortunately is still widely taught and practiced.

- • Substance type, including alcohol and tobacco and misuse of prescription medication
  - ○ First use, mode of ingestion, quantity, frequency, last use
  - ○ Pattern of use over time

- Substance use disorder
  - Dose escalation, tolerance, withdrawal
  - Efforts to reduce, control or stop; periods of abstinence
  - Consequences, including psychiatric, medical, legal, financial, relationships
  - Relapse
  - Treatment: medications, peer-support, detoxification, residential
  - Recovery, supports for recovery

Trauma History

This important area generally merits careful separate documentation, but often trauma history is closely interwoven with HPI or social/developmental history, and in these situations, it may be integrated into those sections. Include direct and indirect exposure to violence such as witnessing violence.

- Emotional, physical and sexual abuse, and assault, in childhood and adulthood
- Bullying
- Intimate partner violence/domestic violence
- Military trauma, political trauma
- Traumatic events such as crime, accidents, serious medical illness, catastrophic loss of loved ones

Past Medical History

- Any significant medical or surgical conditions
- Special attention to neurologic/endocrine: head trauma, seizures, thyroid disorders
- Pain symptoms, especially chronic pain
- Sexual and reproductive history
- Current primary care provider and other medical providers

Current Medications

- Prescribed, unprescribed, OTC, supplements and herbal preparations, internet purchases

Allergies

- Drug allergies

Lifestyle

- Caffeine (not generally included in substance use history because of the relatively low rate of morbidity related to caffeine use)
- Exercise and physical activity

- Diet/nutrition, access and affordability of fresh groceries
- Wellness practices – wellness and stress management approaches, including mind/body practices such as meditation and yoga

Family History
- Psychiatric and substance history, especially first-degree relatives: diagnoses, symptoms, hospitalizations, completed suicide, violence
- Significant medical conditions

Social and Developmental History
- Brief description of early life, including childhood/adolescence, family life and home environment, behavioral problems, losses, adversities such as poverty or experiences of marginalization and oppression
- Educational history: learning or attentional problems, attainment
- Family relationships: family of origin, current family (including children)
- Social supports: friendships, intimate relationships, other supports within the community
- Financial: current income, disability income, poverty or difficulty covering expenses, insurance status
- Current housing situation and neighborhood/community, including sense of safety
- Occupational history: student status or job history; reasons for job changes or loss
- Typical daily activities – it can be illuminating to ask a patient to describe a typical day or a typical week
- Interests and leisure activities
- Legal history: including charges, convictions, time in prison, current status (e.g., probation), restraining orders
- Military service: nature of service, current status
- Identity and cultural factors (self-identified): emphasizing those that the patient identifies as important to them
  - Gender identity and use of pronouns, sexual orientation
  - Race, ethnicity, and/or cultural self-identification
  - Spirituality and religion
  - Connection or sense of belonging in a community
  - Cultural attitudes toward psychiatry and mental illness

Mental Status Exam
The EMR MSE checklist undermines the development of important clinical skills of observation and documentation here. Unless a checklist is required for important research or data gathering, writing free text with specificity and conveying the unique features of the patient is more clinically useful. The cognitive exam will differ based on clinical setting – in certain psychiatric settings with low medical

complexity, a relatively abbreviated cognitive exam is appropriate, focused primarily on brief screening questions for orientation, memory, and attention.

Here we include very brief descriptions of each section:

- Appearance – specific descriptive detail about clothing, grooming
- Behavior and motor activity – gait, posture, eye contact, movements, tremor, or abnormal movements
- Speech – rate, volume, articulation, pressure of speech
- Mood – in patient's own words
- Affect – emotion observed: quality (e.g., elevated, depressed, irritable/angry, or anxious/fearful), intensity, range, lability, congruence with stated mood and thought content
- Perceptions – particularly auditory and visual hallucinations
- Thought process – e.g. linear and goal directed, inclusive, circumstantial, tangential, or loose associations
- Thought content: including major themes, paranoia/delusions, suicidality, homicidality
- Insight – into symptoms and illness
- Judgment – plans for future management of health care and safety issues
- Brief cognitive exam:
  - Orientation – day, date, place
  - Fund of knowledge – based on interview, particularly relevant for knowledge about illness or treatment
  - Attention – digit span, days of the week backward, serial 7s or 3s
  - Memory: registration of 3 objects, recall in 5 minutes

Physical Exam

- May be omitted if not relevant to context (e.g., outpatient visit)

Laboratory/Testing Data

Toxicology screening for substance use can be crucial in determining diagnosis and treatment, and should be considered a standard part of psychiatric laboratory evaluation.

- Toxicology screen, TFTs, LFTs, therapeutic drug levels
- ECG, MRI, or CT

Assessment

Here the most important point is to demonstrate your thought process rather than simply summarize history.

- Summary of current presentation and history

- Differential diagnosis considerations
- Biopsychosocial formulation placing patient's presentation in the context of relevant biological, psychological and social, and cultural factors
- Risk assessment – including risk of harm to self and others, capacity to care for self, and risk of addiction
- Strengths assessment – including psychological and social resources, insight and motivation for treatment

Provisional DSM-V Diagnoses Listed

- Primary or working psychiatric diagnoses
- Secondary psychiatric diagnoses
- Relevant nonpsychiatric medical conditions

Treatment Plan

- Patient preference for treatment
- Consideration of type/level of care (e.g., inpatient, outpatient, partial hospitalization) and clinical rationale
- Relevant multimodal treatment plan including medication, psychotherapy, or other psychosocial treatment, device-based (e.g., ECT, TMS) treatments, and the clinical reasoning that supports their use
- Relevant further consultation or assessment (e.g., neurology, medicine, psychological testing)
- Additional input (e.g., case management)

Assessing Suicidality

Assessing suicidality is often poorly understood outside of the mental health field. People commonly think in terms of "prediction" of suicide, as though the astute clinician can use elements of the clinical interview or a set of signs and symptoms to know with some degree of certainty which patients will or will not kill themselves. The truth, however, is quite different: even the most experienced and expert clinician cannot "predict" with any degree of certainty whether a patient who is at risk will go on to complete suicide. Despite our best efforts, there are some patients assessed to be at low risk who may go on to complete suicide, and there may be many "high risk" patients who might never go on to do so. That being said, assessing suicidality is essential in guiding clinical interventions to work safely with patients who are at risk for suicide. We describe the elements of this assessment as follows.

Suicide Risk Factors

Suicide risk factors are things that one can learn about a patient that have been correlated with some degree of increased risk for suicide. These include demographic, historical, and psychosocial risk factors (see Box 1), as well as psychiatric diagnosis. Unfortunately, one cannot correlate the number of risk factors with degree of risk for suicide. Some patients with many risk factors will not go on to kill themselves or make an attempt; some with relatively few known risk factors may actually complete suicide. Knowledge that a patient has multiple risk factors, however, can serve to heighten a clinician's awareness. Some risk factors are "static" and cannot be changed (such as age or prior suicide attempt); however, there are some "modifiable risk factors" that have the potential to be improved with treatment and thus presumably lower a patient's risk for suicide.

A history of past suicide attempts is one of the strongest risk factors for later suicide. The higher the lethality and the stronger the suicidal intent of a past attempt, the more the patient is at risk for suicide in the future. Most people who make even the most lethal suicide attempts, however, do not go on to kill themselves. This suggests that if we can help a patient to safely get through a suicidal crisis there is a high likelihood that our interventions can be life-saving.

In addition to past suicide attempts, it is important to know about any past episodes of intentional self-harm such as cutting oneself, burning, and so forth. While these are generally of low lethality (and may be done without *any* intent to end one's life), this history still confers some degree of increased risk for future suicide attempts. Finally, it is important to ask about "aborted" or "interrupted" suicide attempts – times when a patient was in the act of making an attempt but stopped or was interrupted at the last minute. For example, if a patient went to a bridge with a plan to jump but was restrained by police and brought to the hospital, he or she might respond "no" when asked about any history of suicide attempts. However, this history is clearly a risk factor for suicide, in fact to the same degree as an actual suicide attempt.

While demographic and historical risk factors are clearly not amenable to change, some risk factors that are potentially modifiable and thus are important areas for clinical intervention. For example, optimizing pain management in a patient with severe chronic pain may decrease a suicidal patient's degree of risk. Helping a suicidal patient who has been socially isolated to develop greater supports and connections might similarly decrease risk. Finally, access to firearms in the home is an independent risk factor for suicide even in the absence of mental illness, and firearm suicides account for more than one-half of the completed suicides in the United States. Removal of a gun from the home can go a long way toward decreasing the risk of suicide for a patient at risk.

BOX 1 Demographic, Psychosocial, and Historical Risk Factors

- Gender: Male > female
  - Women more attempts, men more completions (4×)
  - Men more likely to use lethal means (firearms, hanging)
- Race: White, Native American > non-Hispanic Blacks, Asian, Hispanic
- FH of completed suicide or suicide attempts
- Increasing age (especially white men > 75)
- Recent losses/adverse events
- Physical illness, chronic pain
- Decrease in social support/connectedness
  - Marital status – widowed, divorced, single
  - Work status: unemployed, retired
  - Living situation: alone, social isolation
- Exposure to suicidal behavior in others – especially for adolescents
- Past history of suicide attempts or intentional self-harm
- Recent discharge from an inpatient psychiatric unit
- Firearms in the home

The majority of patients who complete suicides have been found retrospectively to have a psychiatric diagnosis. The highest risk diagnoses tend to be mood disorders, particularly depression. This includes unipolar depression, bipolar depression, and "mixed states" in which the patient has symptoms of depression as well as symptoms of hypomania or mania such as racing thoughts, severe anxiety, dysphoria, and agitation. It also includes depressed states in the context of other disorders such as PTSD, schizophrenia, schizoaffective disorder, substance use disorder, and personality disorders. When patients have psychotic symptoms such as delusions and auditory hallucinations in addition to depression (major depression with psychotic features, or "psychotic depression"), this greatly increases the risk for suicide. Some patients have "command hallucinations" to kill or hurt themselves; while this does not mean that the patient will act on these "commands," they should be taken seriously in the assessment of suicide risk. Alcohol use disorder and other substance use problems are themselves risk factors for suicide, and they especially increase risk when there is comorbid depression. Other clinical symptoms have been found to correlate with an increased risk for suicide, especially in the context of depression. A pervasive sense of hopelessness (i.e., feeling that things are bad and that there is little to no chance of ever making them any better) can predispose someone to suicidal thoughts and behavior. Similarly, depressed patients with severe anxiety (both panic attacks and generalized anxiety), as well as with severe insomnia may be at increased risk. These can be thought of as modifiable risk factors. Hopelessness may improve with treatment of depression, and can be targeted as a symptom for improvement in psychotherapy. Anxiety and sleep disturbance are often readily treatable both with both psychopharmacologic and non-pharmacologic interventions.

Experiential Aspects of Suicidality

Another important part of assessing suicide risk is to consider the patient's subjective experience. Patients who get to the point of feeling suicidal are generally suffering terribly, with an experience of anguish and desperation that has come to feel truly unbearable. Those who have made a suicide attempt often say that they did so because it was the only way they could come up with to escape this intolerable emotional state. Thus the risk of suicidal behavior increases if the patient feels that there is no alternative to escaping their suffering.

A focus on subjective experience also helps explain the subset of people who attempt suicide but lack a preexisting psychiatric illness. This often occurs in the context of a life crisis that the person perceives as catastrophic and unbearable, with no way out, which can lead a vulnerable person to impulsive action. The key here is to appreciate the degree to which the person's experience of his or her situation is one of feeling desperate and trapped, with suicide as the only escape. If he or she can be supported and helped to stay safe and not act on suicidal impulses, there is a high likelihood that the intense need to act on suicidal thoughts will pass.

When interviewing a suicidal patient, the clinician has the opportunity to allow the patient to talk about his or her subjective experience, which in and of itself is sometimes a tremendous relief. Suicidal patients often feel a high degree of shame, self-blame, and a sense that no one cares enough to try to understand what they are going through. The clinician's interest in the patient's experience can help the patient feel less isolated and alone. The goal is to come to a shared understanding of the patient's distress, how it was that he or she came to see suicide as the solution, and (when possible) begin to problem-solve alternatives. This is not only an aspect of the risk assessment but is the beginning of crisis intervention, and can enhance the patient's motivation to continue to seek help.

Assessment of Suicidal Thoughts

Suicidality is often thought of as a yes/no kind of phenomenon – that is, either someone is suicidal or they are not. In fact, people can have a wide range of suicidal thoughts, ranging from passive (e.g., "I sometimes wish I were dead; I wish I just would not wake up"); to more specific thoughts (e.g., "I think I would take an overdose"); to active suicidal thoughts (e.g., "I think about taking the pills in my medicine cabinet"); to active thoughts with plan/intent (e.g., "I feel like killing myself.... I have a stash of pills at home that I can take"). Some clinicians are concerned that asking about suicidal thoughts might make the patient feel uncomfortable; others worry that raising the topic might actually *suggest* suicide to the patient and make it more likely; still others feel that there is no point in asking, because if a patient wants to kill themselves they will not admit it to the clinician. There is no reason to believe that asking about suicide suggests or induces suicidal thoughts or behavior. In fact, patients generally experience this kind of open, non-judgmental discussion as more of a relief than an intrusion, and not asking risks inadvertently closing off this topic and increasing the patient's sense of isolation. While it is true that there are some patients who will conceal suicidal thoughts from the clinician, many are grateful to have been asked and will respond honestly.

If the patient has been having active suicidal thoughts it is important to explore how far he or she has gone with them (see Box 2). It is critically important that physicians and other health care providers feel comfortable enough in exploring the degree of a patient's suicidality in order to determine the proper course of action (e.g., support and outpatient referral versus potential need for hospitalization). Determining whether the patient actually has a plan and intent to kill themselves is the key goal, and also whether they have the means to carry out the plan. Often collateral information from family or friends can sometimes be enormously helpful in the assessment. For example, a patient may deny any suicidal thoughts, but if the family reports that he or she has written a suicide note and said good-bye to friends, there is clearly reason for acute concern. Making an effort to obtain collateral information is part of routine practice in emergency departments and crisis team evaluation settings.

"Mitigating" Factors

Just as there are risk factors that suggest a patient's potential increased risk for suicide, there are also "mitigating" factors that may decrease the degree of risk. We prefer this language to the commonly used term "protective factors," in that they do not actually "protect" against suicide but may serve to balance and mitigate a patient's suicidal thoughts and impulses. In general, mitigating factors are ways in which the patient actually experiences that he or she has *something to live for*, and that his or her life *matters* in some way. Examples include having positive relationships (including therapeutic relationships); caregiving responsibilities or other concerns about needing to be there for children, family, friends, and that one's death would be experienced as a genuine loss; engagement in and caring about work; belief in one's capacity to cope; active religious involvement and/or genuine engagement in some other group that one truly feels a part of; and moral/spiritual beliefs that suicide is wrong and an unacceptable option.

Summary

Assessing suicidality is not about "prediction" of suicide, but is about using what is known about the patient's risk factors, clinical symptoms, subjective experience, and protective factors to assess the degree of risk. This assessment can then guide clinical interventions for the safe care of the patient. Engaging with the patient in a way that allows the patient to feel understood by the clinician can help the patient to feel less alone, and can help alleviate distress and enhance motivation for further treatment.

BOX 2 Important Elements of an Interview for Suicidality

Asking about suicide:

- Have you felt so bad that you wished that you were not here anymore…that life is not worth living…that you would be better off if you were dead?
- Has it gotten to the point you have had thoughts of hurting or killing yourself?
- Do these thoughts come out of the blue, or are they only in specific situations?
- Have these thoughts gotten specific – have you thought about what you would do to hurt or kill yourself?
- What have you thought of doing? Has it gotten to the point of having a plan or an urge to do it?
- Have you taken any steps to act on or prepare to act on these thoughts (e.g., saving up medications for an overdose, going to a bridge, practicing taking a noose, practicing loading a gun)?
- Have you told other people that you are thinking about suicide, or written any kind of good-bye notes?
- Have you in any way started to plan for not being here (e.g., writing a good-bye note, writing a will, giving away possessions)?
- What has held you back from acting on these thoughts so far? How do you think your (*spouse/family/children/friends*) would feel if you were to kill yourself?

Asking about past attempts:

- Have you ever tried to hurt yourself or kill yourself in the past? What did you do?
- Do you think that you were trying to die? Did you think you would die?
- What happened? Did you call for help?
- Did you stop yourself, or were you interrupted in some way or rescued?
- How did you feel when you realized you were not going to die?

BOX 2 (cont.)

Asking about other relevant factors:

- Do you ever hear voices urging you to hurt or kill yourself?
- What is your pattern of using alcohol or drugs?
- Have you had problems sleeping at night?
- Have you been feeling very anxious or agitated?
- Are there people you feel you can turn to for support and help if you are feeling like hurting or killing yourself?
- Has anyone in your family or anyone close to you attempted to kill themselves or died by suicide?

Asking about current safety:

- How safe do you feel currently? Are you having thoughts about hurting or killing yourself? Are they specific?
- Do you feel that you would call someone to get help if they were to get worse or go to your local emergency department?
- Do you have a plan for what to do if you get into crisis? Are you familiar with how to page your treaters, with local emergency resources, with suicide hotline numbers?

Assessing Domestic Violence

Introduction

Physicians are encouraged to approach patients from a holistic perspective, which includes assessing psychosocial factors that impact health and well-being. With respect to domestic violence, physicians' skills can best be used to screen, assess, and refer (SAR) patients. In general, physicians cannot and should not be considered experts, unless they have received specialized training. As generalists, they can rely on the support of local domestic violence programs or state hotlines as the SAR process unfolds in a clinical encounter.

Definition

Domestic violence, or violation (DV), is defined as a pattern of actual or threatened coercive behaviors that are intended for power and control. These behaviors are perpetrated by someone who is or has been in an intimate partner relationship (intimate partner violence is known as IPV) or in a family relationship (parent, grandparent, child, sibling). Behaviors may include but are not limited to physical injury, forced sexual acts, social isolation, psychological abuse, intimidation, threats, financial/economic or basic needs deprivation, interference with medical care, threats to children or pets, violation of human rights, or even religious/spiritual abuse.

Prevalence and Impact

According to data published in the Annals of Internal Medicine (Moyer, 2013), it is estimated that nearly 31 percent of women and 26 percent of men report experiencing some form of IPV in their lifetime. Although domestic violence affects mostly women, there are also reports of heterosexual men who are abused in controlling relationships. Domestic violence affects people of all ages, backgrounds, socio-economic groups, ethnicities, gender identities, and sexual orientations. There are also certain risk factors that can be associated with IPV. Some of these include gender inequality and privilege, exposure to childhood maltreatment, cultural attitudes that condone violence, and women's access to paid employment (World Health Organization, 2017). Being either a witness to DV or a victim of DV has ongoing consequences that create an important medical and psychological public health concern.

Clinical Presentations

The effects of DV can be far reaching and are not always obvious. Physical manifestations include chronic medical conditions such as gastrointestinal disorders and somatic complaints (aches, pains, migraines). Mental health conditions include depression, anxiety, dissociative disorders, affect regulation difficulties, self-harming behaviors (e.g., excessive risk taking, substance abuse, eating disorders, suicide attempts, etc.), and post-traumatic stress disorder (PTSD). In addition, victims of DV are more vulnerable to being taken advantage of by others. Often these conditions combine to form a complex constellation of symptoms sometimes referred to as complex PTSD.

Patients may not fully describe the etiology of their injuries and may minimize the abuse because of shame, intimidation, or fear. While some injuries may be obvious, some may be inconsistent with the explanation. Some injuries may be hidden (e.g., pain from hair-pulling, arm twisting backward, etc.). Some often unrecognized indicators of DV include a history of unexplained injuries, a patient taking complete responsibility or blame for stress in the home life, undue anxiety about something that would not normally create anxiety (such as fears of being late or disclosing medical appointments), interruptive phone calls by their partner, an overly attentive or jealous partner, needing to ask partner permission to tend to daily activities, fear of having insurance bills sent to the house, or delay in seeking health care or prenatal care). It is therefore the recommendation of the American

Medical Association (1992), as well as the Joint Commission on Accreditation of Healthcare Organizations (2009), that universal screening be established in all settings.

Screening and Assessment

Guidelines

- Set the tone by letting patients know that you screen all patients for being hurt or experiencing violence. Avoid using the terms *domestic violence* or *abuse* when initially talking to patients.
- Screening must occur in a private setting away from partners, family members, or friends. If you are communicating with the patient using an interpreter, be sure the interpreter is not a family member.
- Assure confidentiality, unless there is evidence of serious danger to themselves or others. Most states have mandated reporting for child abuse, elder abuse, or disabled persons. Reporting requirements for DV vary from state to state and should be verified before you promise or compromise confidentiality.
- Convey patience, willingness to listen, and a nonjudgmental attitude.
- You do not have to be a trauma specialist, but you can be trauma-informed by treating the patient respectfully, understanding resources, trusting their knowledge of their own situation, and being collaborative in planning.
- Remember not to impose your own agenda for what is best or for what you hope for the patient. Patients are often more at risk when they take action. Helping the patient to decide what is best for him or her is an invaluable intervention in itself.

Screening Questions

The purpose of screening is to identify possible DV and to let the patient know your concern. This may set the stage for a disclosure at some later time and may facilitate accessing necessary services.

Here are some sample specific questions to ask:

- At any time has your partner or another family member hurt, or threatened you or someone you care about?
- Have you ever felt afraid of your partner/family member?
- Has anyone tried to control you (from seeing your family or friends, your finances, etc.)?
- Has anyone tried to hurt you or someone you care about physically, emotionally, or sexually?
- A more general question would be: "Every couple has conflicts; how do you and your partner resolve disagreements?"

Note: Many settings encourage clinicians to ask: "Are you safe at home?" This can be confusing since it can have many meanings: Do you have locks on your door? Or, for the elderly, are you at risk for falling? The more specific the inquiry, the better.

If a patient does disclose abuse or violence, then the next step is a further risk assessment.

Assessing Risk

If a patient discloses abuse, you then ascertain if there is a current risk to them or others in their care, and let them know that you are able to assist in safety planning. Safety planning involves gathering information: learning what they have already done to survive, assessing the dangerousness of their perpetrators, and collaborating with them to develop short term plans for their safety and help them access local resources.

It is important to assess the dangerousness of their perpetrator to determine the seriousness of the immediate risk. While it is difficult to accurately predict whether a perpetrator will seriously harm or murder a victim, understanding high risk can assist in planning. Some common warning signs of high-risk situations are:

- Severity of violence, injuries and if choking was used
- Use of or access to weapons
- Substance use
- Excessive jealousy, monitoring of patient's activities, stalking
- Mental illness, threats of suicide, or homicide
- History of violence
- Threatening children or pets
- Violence while the victim is pregnant
- Recent escalation
- Victim recently left or attempted to leave the relationship

If there is a high danger risk, safety planning must be more immediate. Essential elements of safety planning include identifying safe places to go and packing an emergency bag with important documents and other supplies, such as extra keys, medications, and money. The patient should identify a support person and know how to reach them in an emergency. This support person can help develop plans for safe escapes from home, work, or the street, and become knowledgeable about local resources and legal rights.

Safety planning is often ongoing and involves anticipating various scenarios. In order to build a collaborative alliance for safety planning, it is important to:

- Be collaborative, not directive.
- Provide supportive listening and encouragement.

- Communicate to patients that you will work with them at their own pace. Let the patient know that she/he can disclose at their own pace and that there is no pressure to leave a relationship.
- Be honest and transparent about concerns without blaming the survivor for the behaviors of her/his abuser.
- Encourage the patient to seek support for other areas of her life to build confidence and her own protective factors (e.g., medical care, building community, interests, going to school, etc.).
- Understanding the person's current life situation, as well as cultural context, can help you develop trust and plan treatment.

Referral

You are not expected to know everything about DV. It is important to let patients know that they are not alone and that there is help available. There are many community resources available to help guide you and your patient, both immediately or in follow-up care. If your setting has a social worker, involve them in assisting the patient. Community resources can be helpful for safety planning, decisions about criminal justice involvement, and counseling. Get to know your local providers. If there are none, use the Internet for education materials (e.g., Center for Disease Control, Department of Justice, Futures without Violence) and state-based domestic violence hotlines, which often have multiple language capabilities. If possible, arrange a safe/confidential space for contacting resources.

Restraining orders are available 24/7 but are not always the best choice. At the very least, you can convey that legal help is an option. Legal protections need to be safely accessed when appropriate.

Before discharge, be sure there is a follow-up care plan for medical or other needs.

Diagnosis and Documentation

As mentioned before, there may be many co-occurring conditions or multiple diagnostic considerations occurring in the DV patient. Sometimes abusers will try to access medical records and will use the records as a form of control, humiliation, or manipulation (e.g., in child custody cases). Patients who have a long history of trauma or current domestic abuse often develop physical or psychological symptoms in response to their abusive situations (Gondolf, 1998), so diagnoses should be made with caution. Initially, it is better to list something as a "rule-out" while getting to know the patient better. In addition, patients may also use substances and/or feel suicidal or homicidal as a survival strategy. These risks must be documented and addressed, while understanding that they are in the context of the DV. Mental status examinations can reference responses that are consistent with the disclosure of abuse.

Records should be written in a concise, descriptive, symptom-focused manner, with awareness of what it would be like if the patient were to read their own record. The interview and the record should include strengths and survival strategies. If a patient does not disclose DV, do not say that the patient 'denies' domestic abuse, but rather document that they did not discuss it. It is also recommended *not* to use the word "alleged" since it implies disbelief and is actually a legal term. Clinicians are not in a position to offer a legal opinion and should not consider it within their function to verify patients' narratives. Instead, it is recommended to use the word "reported" for describing what a patient has told you.

Helpful Interventions

Every encounter with a patient is a potentially therapeutic encounter, whether it is in an emergency room, inpatient unit, crisis intervention, or outpatient clinic (Yassen & Harvey, 1998). The following suggestions will help you achieve these mutual goals with the patient: completing an overall assessment including safety and psychiatric risk, and providing help for the patient in an empowering way. Keep the following in mind:

1. Prioritize physical and emotional safety, including self-care for basic coping such as safe living environment, eating, sleeping, and so forth.
2. Allow space for expression and validation of experience.
3. Provide psychoeducation and inform the patient about the impact of domestic abuse, the right not to be abused, and so forth.
4. Help mobilize the patient's internal resources (coping strategies, etc.) as well as external helping referrals.
5. Prepare and plan for the next steps in terms of getting therapeutic or medical help as part of closure.

Conclusion

Timely, sensitive, and comprehensive screening, assessment, treatment, and intervention can assist patients who have been exposed to domestic abuse achieve safe, healthy, and meaningful lives for themselves and their families. Medical providers in psychiatric settings have the potential to offer an important service to achieve these goals. In building coalitions with community providers, a comprehensive set of services can offer a holistic approach that can benefit patients and offer support for providers. While it may not be safe or possible for patients to make changes in their domestic situations, medical providers can offer information and a caring presence that may be a foundation for patients to use at some other time. Screening, assessing/treating, and referring patients exposed to domestic violence can be difficult for providers – so providers should be open to receiving good supervision and support.

Assessing Risk to Others

Introduction

"How dangerous is this patient?" is a question that raises significant concern among clinicians when there is suspicion that a person may be at risk of harming others. The relationship between violent behavior and mental illness is complex – people who commit violent acts do not necessarily suffer from mental illness, and the majority of people with mental illness are not violent. However, there are instances in which people with mental illness do become violent. Given that rates of severe mental illness are several times higher for incarcerated people than the general population, it is critical for mental health clinicians to be adept at assessing violence risk. Although this is not a perfect science, studies over the past couple of decades have elucidated numerous risk factors for violence among people with mental health disorders. This chapter outlines these risk factors as well as the key components of an approach to assessing violence risk in the mental health setting.

Risk Factors for Violence

Violence risk factors are aspects about a patient that have been correlated with an increased risk for violence. Just like suicide risk factors, these include demographic, historical, and psychosocial risk factors (see Box 1), as well as a psychiatric diagnosis. Broadly speaking, these risk factors fall into two categories: static and dynamic. Static risk factors are those that are not amenable to change (e.g., gender, age). Dynamic risk factors are able to be altered with treatment (e.g., psychosis, substance use). Although these risk factors can help us predict violent acts, some people with numerous risk factors may not go on to commit violence. Conversely, some with relatively few known risk factors may become violent. Although this ambiguity is challenging, the key point is that knowing a person has multiple risk factors should heighten awareness and prompt a more thorough assessment of violence risk. In addition, addressing dynamic or "modifiable" risk factors with treatment may lower the patient's risk for violence.

In general, a history of past violence or criminal behavior is the strongest risk factor for future violence. The more serious the past violence, the stronger the association with future episodes of violence. Moreover, those who commit first violent acts at a younger age have a higher likelihood of being violent in the future. It is, therefore, important to take a detailed history to develop an understanding of the exact nature of prior violent episodes. This can be a challenging endeavor given that there is often significant shame and avoidance of being forthcoming about a history of violence or aggression.

Men are more likely to be violent in the general population, though among mentally ill populations, men and women commit violent acts with similar fre-

---

BOX 3 Demographic, Psychosocial, and Historical Risk Factors

- Demographic factors
  - Men are more violent in the general population, though this is not necessarily true in the psychiatrically ill population, where rates of violence are similar in men and women
  - Age: younger > older (younger than 40)
  - Low socioeconomic status, low educational achievement
- Historical factors
  - History of prior violence is the most powerful indicator of future violence
  - Nature of past violence is important
  - Age of violence (younger is higher risk)
  - History of child abuse or witnessed domestic violence
  - Low IQ
- Psychosocial factors and environmental factors
  - Stress and lack of social support (financial, interpersonal, environmental)
  - Availability of weapons
  - Access to victim
  - Access to substances

---

quency. Other potential risk factors include low IQ and a history of child abuse or domestic violence. Psychosocial issues such as occupational, interpersonal, or environmental stress are also important in that these types of stressors may be the final straw that pushes a patient to commit a violent act. Finally, access to weapons and substances of misuse are key environmental risk factors that should be considered and that may be modified to lower the risk of violence. (See Box 1 for a list of non-clinical risk factors.)

Clinical Risk Factors

There are a number of clinical or psychopathological factors that may increase the risk of violence or aggression (see Box 2). Aside from a prior history of violence, substance use is perhaps the most significant predictor of assaultive behavior. The risk of violence while intoxicated is not only significantly higher than the general population, but the combination of intoxication and active psychosis magnifies the risk considerably. Interestingly, the age of onset of substance use is also important in that those who start using substances at any early age are more likely to become violent at some point.

Psychosis is also an important risk factor. Rather than a particular diagnosis (e.g., schizophrenia), it is the presence of active symptoms of psychosis that is most important. For example, delusions with a perception of threat or sense that one's actions are being controlled are particularly concerning. These patients often appear guarded, paranoid, or suspicious. They may avoid eye contact, appear fearful, or be excessively fidgety. Command auditory hallucinations (especially from a familiar voice) telling a patient to harm someone are also very worrisome symptoms. Finally, although stalking is a behavior rather than a diagnosis, those people who are psychotic and stalk the objects of their delusions are at higher risk of committing acts of violence.

Although the majority of people with mood disorders do not become violent, there are some relevant risk factors. Mania may be associated with aggression and impulsivity, though is rarely associated with intentional or targeted violence. Severe depression (especially when associated with hopelessness or guilt) occasionally leads to violent acts. An example of this would be a person who loses a job, becomes severely depressed and hopeless about the future, kills his/her family, and then commits suicide. Although these acts are rare, one should not overlook an assessment of thoughts of harming others in depressed patients. As discussed previously, the presence of psychotic symptoms or substance use disorder in this group increases risk even further.

Neurologic impairment may also increase the risk of violence. While patients with a history of brain injury from a variety of causes (e.g., traumatic, stroke, infection) may become aggressive, targeted violence is rare. However, those with a history of frontal lobe impairment resulting in impulsivity are at higher risk of becoming violent, especially when other comorbid risk factors as outlined above are present.

Finally, antisocial personality disorder is strongly associated with a risk of violent behavior. By definition, those with this disorder have a persistent disregard for others, are impulsive, lack empathy or remorse, and often break rules – all factors that may contribute to acts of aggression toward others. Antisocial personality disorder is highly comorbid with substance use disorder – this often compounds the problem.

For all of the clinical risk factors, treatment (reducing active symptomatology) is the mainstay of decreasing risk.

Assessment of Violence Risk

A key concept when assessing violence is that of chronically elevated risk versus imminent risk. Chronically elevated risk is present in a patient who has one or more of the above risk factors but is not having active thoughts of harming anyone and is not currently acting in an agitated or violent way. Imminent risk involves a patient who is either actively thinking about or planning to harm someone, or is acting in an aggressive or agitated manner. Although it is important to get as much history and violence assessment for both types of patients, treatment and intervention implications differ in that those who are at imminent risk require an immediate intervention. For a patient who is experiencing violent thoughts, it is also essential to discern whether these thoughts are directed toward a specific person (or persons) or whether these are more general impulses, as treatment and interventions differ depending on this context. It is, therefore, essential to make these key aspects of the clinical assessment.

In terms of approaching this evaluation, in most instances, the examiner would start with detailed questions to establish historical, psychosocial, demographic and clinical risk factors as outlined previously. Following this, the examiner would segue into a specific violence screening while maintaining as neutral a manner as possible. In general, the most effective way to begin a violence assessment is to begin with broad screening questions (e.g., "What makes you angry? What do you do when you get angry?"). Depending on the answers to the screening questions, more targeted questions should follow. For example, if the answer to a question such as "what is the most violent thing that you have ever done?" reveals that the patient assaulted someone, then a follow up question might be "What harm occurred to the other person?" (see Box 2 for more sample questions). A key concept during this examination is that safety is paramount. Although the majority of patients are not violent, any indication that someone is becoming agitated or aggressive during this examination should be taken very seriously and the examination should be aborted until safety can be assured. Some early signs of possible imminent aggression include staring, clenched fists or jaw, sweating, pacing, loud voice, angry, or threatening comments. Moving the patient to a safe setting (e.g., emergency department) or having a security guard or police officer standby are some of a few options to ensure a safe setting for continuing the examination.

BOX 4 Sample Violence Questions

- What makes you angry? What do you do when you get angry?
- Have you ever gotten in a physical altercation or been violent? How close have you come to getting into an altercation?
  - If so, did the other person sustain injuries? What type?
  - Were you under the influence of substances at the time?
  - Were you having psychotic symptoms (give examples) at the time?
  - What do you think caused you to become physically aggressive?
- Have you ever used a weapon to hurt someone?
  - If so, what type?
  - What was the extent of the injuries?
  - Do you own or have access to weapons now?
  - If so, where are the weapons? Are they secured?
- Have you ever been incarcerated?
  - If yes, what for? For how long?

BOX 4 (cont.)

- o Are you on probation?
- Do you experience any warning signs before becoming aggressive?
  - o If yes, can you stop yourself from becoming aggressive or violent?
  - o What helps?
  - o What makes the impulse worse?
- Are you having violent thoughts or impulses now?
  - o If yes, what are these thoughts?
  - o Are you thinking of hurting a specific person or group of people? If so, who?

Treatments and Interventions

Although a discussion of specific treatments for violence is beyond the scope of this chapter, some key concepts are worth outlining. The violence risk assessment most often involves chronic risk of violence, and interventions involve treating any modifiable risk factors and thereby reducing risk. This is why understanding and elucidating key risk factors are so important in terms of the violence assessment. When there is an imminent risk, an immediate intervention must be made. These may include psychiatric hospitalization, notification of intended victims, notification of police, and removing access to weapons or victims (among other possible interventions).

Conclusion

The violence risk assessment is not about "predicting" violence but rather is about using the patient's known risk factors and clinical symptoms to assess a degree of risk. This assessment will then help guide clinical care and interventions to ensure safety for the patient and others. While the assessment should be approached in a nonjudgmental and matter-of-fact way, special care should be taken to make sure that the assessment is done in a safe setting – any sign of agitation should result in aborting the examination until safety can be ensured. While most patients with mental illness do not become violent, it is critical to understand the risk factors for violence and how to complete a thorough violence assessment, as outlined previously.

Assessing Capacity

Every day, in the course of medical treatment, patients are asked to make decisions about their care. Through the process of informed consent, patients engage in a collaborative process with their providers in which the treater provides and the patient receives information and voluntarily agrees to or refuses care. Informed consent (or refusal) has been a central tenet of medical practice since the 1960s and recognizes the autonomy of patients to make decisions about what happens (or does not happen) to their bodies. In order to engage in the informed consent process, an individual must possess the requisite mental ability to make decisions. The clinical term for this threshold assessment of decision-making ability is *capacity*. The legal equivalent of capacity is competency, which the law presumes for all adults unless they are legally adjudicated otherwise.

Capacity may be global, as evidenced by the presumption that all adults are able to make decisions unless shown otherwise. Incapacity may also be global; for example, a patient in a coma has global incapacity. However, in the course of clinical treatment, it is more common for capacity to be delineated as specific to certain tasks. Examples of specific domains of capacity include medical decision-making, testamentary capacity (the ability to execute a will), contractual capacity (the ability to conduct business or enter into a contract), testimonial capacity (the ability to testify in court), and capacity to appoint a surrogate decision maker. In medical settings, psychiatrists are frequently asked to assist in determining patients' decisional capacity related to medical care due to psychiatrists' unique understanding of affect, behavior, and cognition. However, any physician can make a determination of capacity.

A practical approach to capacity assessment recognizes that different decisions require varying degrees of ability, knowledge, and understanding. Therefore, the first question in any capacity assessment should be, "Capacity for what?" Clear identification of the decision at hand (e.g., refusing some or all treatment or leaving against medical advice [AMA]) informs what information and reasoning capabilities are required to meet the capacity threshold. Once the medical decision before the patient is clarified, then the assessment of capacity involves an understanding of the illness, the proposed intervention(s), and the expected result of the treatment or lack thereof. The predominant framework for assessing medical decision-making capacity is a four-step model proposed by Appelbaum and Grisso. The four criteria include the following: (1) preference, (2) factual understanding, (3) appreciation, and (4) rational manipulation of information. All four elements must be met in order for the patient to possess capacity.

Preference refers to the patient's ability to express a consistent or stable position regarding a proposed treatment. A patient who is either unable (e.g., due to cognitive impairment) or unwilling to express a preference fails to meet this criterion. The second element, *factual understanding*, assesses whether the patient possesses the relevant information about his or her illness, treatment options, and prognosis. In assessing factual understanding, it is imperative that the evaluator consider the efforts that have been made to provide this information to the patient. If the patient has not been informed of the critical information, efforts must be made to inform the patient prior to a determination of incapacity.

The third prong of capacity is *appreciation*. This criterion requires that the patient go beyond the facts to appreciate how the facts specifically apply to the patient, including a broad view of the potential risks and benefits to the individual of his or her stated preference. Lastly, the patient must show the ability to rely on the information and rationally process the facts in coming to a decision. This element recognizes that some individuals may make decisions to refuse potentially life-saving care due to deeply held beliefs or religious practices, and therefore, the *assessment of rationality* must be contextualized in the individual's life history, culture, and belief system.

When a patient lacks capacity, an alternate decision maker must be identified. All 50 United States recognize the ability of a competent (capacitated) patient to appoint an alternate, or surrogate, decision maker to make decisions on the patient's behalf should the patient become incapacitated at a future time. These legal instruments are most commonly called *health care proxies* or *durable power of attorney for health care* but take different forms and have different legal requirements, depending on the jurisdiction in which they are executed. One important consideration is that because capacity is task-specific, an individual who lacks capacity to make a medical decision may nonetheless possess (retain) the ability to appoint an appropriate individual to make the decision on his or her behalf. Finally, because different jurisdictions have different provisions for the identification and implementation of a surrogate decision maker, it is critical for practitioners to be aware of prevailing requirements and consultative resources in the jurisdictions in which they practice.

References and Selected Readings

- American Medical Association (1992). Association Diagnostic and Treatment Guidelines on Domestic Violence. *Archives of Family Medicine*, 1, 39–47.
- Appelbaum, P. S., and Grisso, T. (1988). Assessing Patients' Capacities to Consent to Treatment. *New England Journal of Medicine*, 319, 1635–1638.
- Brendel, R. W., and Schouten, R. (2007). Legal Concerns in Psychosomatic Medicine. *Psychiatric Clinics of North America*, 30, 663–676.
- Gondolf, E. W. (1998). *Assessing Woman Battering in Mental Health Settings*. Thousand Oak: Sage.
- Halpern J. (2003). What Is Clinical Empathy? *Journal of General Internal Medicine*, 18, 670–674.
- Joint Commission on Accreditation of Healthcare Organizations (2009). *Joint Commission Standard PC.01.02.09. The Hospital Assesses the Patient Who May Be a Victim of Possible Abuse and Neglect* (Revised 2009).
- Moyer, V. A. (2013). Screening for Intimate Partner Violence and Abuse of Elderly and Vulnerable Adults: U.S. Preventive Services Task Force Recommendation Statement. *Annals of Internal Medicine*, 158, 478–486.

- Singer, T., and Klimecki, O. M. (2014). Empathy and Compassion. *Current Biology*, 24, R875–R878.
- World Health Organization (2017). Violence against Women. Who.int. Available at www.who.int/news-room/fact-sheets/detail/violence-against-women.
- Yassen, J., and Harvey, M. T. (1998). Crisis Assessment and Interventions with Victims of Violence. In *Emergencies in Mental Health Practice: Evaluation and Management*. New York: Guilford Press, pp. 117–144.

Self-Assessment Questions

1. Which of the following statements is true regarding the assessment of capacity?
    A. Only a board-certified psychiatrist is able to make a capacity determination.
    B. Competency is a clinical term, which signifies the global mental ability to make decisions.
    C. Any physician can make a determination of capacity.
    D. Because capacity is a global assessment, an individual who lacks the capacity for medical decision-making also lacks the capacity to appoint an alternate decision maker.

2. Which of the following is not an exception to the strict maintenance of confidentiality observed in the psychiatric assessment?
    A. Mandatory reporting of suspected child abuse
    B. The patient is deemed to be in imminent danger of harming another person.
    C. The patient discloses a chronic history of abuse of an illegal substance.
    D. There is suspicion that the patient is engaging in domestic abuse.

3. Which of the following patient characteristics do not represent a high-risk factor for completed suicide?
    A. Female gender
    B. Widower status
    C. Family history of suicide attempts
    D. Presence of firearms in the home

Answers to Self-Assessment Questions

1. (C)
2. (C)
3. (A)

4 Mood Disorders

SCOTT R. BEACH, JEFF C. HUFFMAN, JI HYUN BAEK, MICHAEL TREAD-
WAY, ANDREW A. NIERENBERG, AND JONATHAN E. ALPERT

Depressive Disorders

Classification

Over the years, attempts have been made to classify depressive syndromes based on various criteria. For several decades, the term *reactive depression* was used to describe cases involving an obvious precipitant, whereas *endogenous depression* lacked a recent stressor. Alternatively, the term *secondary depression* has been used in reference to cases related to a defined medical condition, as opposed to examples of *primary depression.* In the current classification scheme, the *Diagnostic and Statistics Manual of Mental Disorders,* 5th edition (DSM-V) lists fifteen distinct diagnoses related to disorders of mood, which are shown in Table 4.1. Eight of these disorders are considered depressive disorders, whereas seven categorize patients within the bipolar spectrum of illness.

Table 4.1 DSM-V Classification of mood disorders

Disruptive mood regulation disorder

Major depressive disorder

Persistent depressive disorder

Premenstrual dysphoric disorder

Substance/medication-induced depressive disorder

Depressive disorder due to another medical condition

Other specified depressive disorder

Unspecified depressive disorder

Bipolar I disorder

Bipolar II disorder

Cyclothymic disorder

Substance/medication-induced bipolar and related disorder

Bipolar and related disorder due to another medical condition

Other specified bipolar and related disorder

Unspecified bipolar and related disorder

Epidemiology and Impact of Illness

Prevalence

The prototypical depressive disorder is major depressive disorder (MDD). MDD is common, disabling, persistent, and deadly. Approximately fourteen million Americans (6.6 percent of adults) have a new or ongoing episode of MDD each year, and overall lifetime prevalence is 15 percent. The prevalence in women is thought to be approximately 25 percent, twice as high as that in men (12 percent). Prevalence of MDD in eighteen- to twenty-nine-year-old individuals is nearly three times that of those over age sixty.

Clinical Course

The onset of MDD follows a bimodal distribution, with most cases beginning in late adolescence or early adulthood, and a second peak occurring in middle-age. This latter peak approximates the onset of menopause in many women, leading to some speculation that hormonal factors may be involved. Overall, the average age of onset is in the late twenties, though more than half of cases first appear after age forty.

Though there is a common misconception that elderly patients are at higher risk for depression and many practitioners may attempt to "normalize" depression in this population, evidence suggests that the rate of clinical depression among the elderly is actually lower than that of the general population. Notably, however, rates of depression are elevated among residents of nursing homes. Further, the impact of depression may be greater in older populations, and the risk of suicide among depressed patients is thought to increase with age.

Risk factors for MDD include family history, adverse childhood experiences, stressful life events, neuroticism, chronic or disabling medical conditions, and comorbid mental illness.

Patients experiencing an episode of major depression tend to describe worsening of mood over a period of weeks. In the stress-diathesis model of depression, though some individuals have a vulnerability to developing depression related to genetics or to childhood events, the phenotype of depression may only manifest in the setting of a life stress. For others, a series of stressors culminates in an episode of depression even if no vulnerability exists. In both situations, there is an obvious precipitating stressor that contributes to early episodes of depression. Patients experiencing recurrent depressive episodes, however, may find that later episodes do not have a defined precipitant, and in fact, prior episodes of depression may represent additional life stressors that increase vulnerability. This phenomenon is referred to as *kindling*, similar to the phenomenon observed in epilepsy. The theory is supported by the observation that early depressive episodes are often separated by longer periods of remission that become shorter as the illness progresses.

From a neurobiological perspective, prior episodes of depression may induce brain changes at a cellular level, particularly in limbic areas of the brain, that convey a vulnerability to developing future depressive episodes even without provocation.

A typical episode of MDD lasts six months if untreated. Without treatment, approximately half of patients who experience a single episode of MDD will have a recurrence, including 15 percent who experience unremitting symptoms. After two episodes, the risk of recurrence increases to 70 percent, rising to 90 percent after three episodes. Subsequent episodes tend to occur more frequently and to last longer.

The course of MDD over the lifetime is quite variable, with some patients experiencing many years without symptoms and others experiencing an unremitting course. The presence of chronic symptoms may suggest an untreated comorbid personality, anxiety, or substance use disorder.

Morbidity and Mortality
MDD leads to major functional impairment and is the second leading cause of disability in the United States and worldwide.

Patients with MDD have greatly elevated general medical costs, and the total cost of MDD in the United States (health care costs + lost productivity) is a staggering $83 billion per year. MDD has been consistently and independently linked to elevated rates of death via suicide, heart disease, and all causes. Despite this, depression is the major illness with the least NIH funding proportional to the burden of disease in the United States.

Impact on Medical Illness
In addition to morbidity and mortality related to direct effects of depression, it also has a major impact on other medical illnesses. Depression following a variety of acute cardiac conditions has been consistently associated with cardiac and all-cause mortality over the following year, independent of sociodemographic variables and traditional risk factors. In patients with diabetes, depression has been linked to decreased adherence to diet and medication, higher levels of hemoglobin A1c, and worse outcomes. Similar effects have been shown for depressed patients with human immunodeficiency virus (HIV) and cancer. Depressed patients admitted to nursing homes have an increased risk of death in the subsequent year.

Cultural Factors
While some large epidemiologic studies have suggested higher rates of depression among Caucasians than among minority individuals in the United States, others have contended equal rates across racial groups.

Cross-cultural surveys suggest a significant (sevenfold) difference globally in twelve-month prevalence rates, though with the caveat that depression is underdiagnosed in many countries and that somatic symptoms may dominate the presentation in some cultures. Gender ratios and age of onset appear to be relatively consistent across cultures.

Clinical Features and Course

Major Depression

DSM-V diagnostic criteria for MDD are shown in Table 4.2. MDD is a persistent and pervasive condition, and diagnosis of MDD requires that depressive symptoms be present nearly every day throughout the duration of the episode. The hallmark of an episode of MDD is the presence of either depressed mood or anhedonia, a marked reduction in the ability to experience interest or pleasure. To meet the criteria for MDD, a total of five symptoms must be present. These include depressed mood, anhedonia, insomnia or hypersomnia, decrease or increase in appetite or weight, fatigue or loss of energy, psychomotor agitation or retardation, feelings of worthlessness or excessive guilt, decreased concentration, or recurrent thoughts of death or suicide; depressed mood or anhedonia must be one of the five symptoms. Symptoms (except for weight change and suicidal ideation) must be present nearly every day over a period of at least two weeks.

Table 4.2 DSM-V Criteria for major depressive disorder

A. Five (or more) of the following symptoms have been present during the same 2-week period and represent a change from previous functioning; at least one of the symptoms is either (1) depressed mood or (2) loss of interest or pleasure.

Note: Do not include symptoms that are clearly attributable to another medical condition

1. Depressed mood most of the day, nearly every day, as indicated by either subjective report (e.g., feels sad, empty, hopeless) or observation made by others (e.g., appears tearful). (Note: In children and adolescents can be irritable mood.)

2. Markedly diminished interest or pleasure in all, or almost all, activities most of the day, nearly every day (as indicated by either subjective account or observation).

3. Significant weight loss when not dieting or weight gain (e.g., a change of more than 5 percent of body weight in a month), or decrease or increase in appetite nearly every day. (Note: In children, consider failure to make expected weight gain.)

4. Insomnia or hypersomnia nearly every day.

5. Psychomotor agitation or retardation nearly every day (observable by others, not merely subjective feelings of restlessness or being slowed down).

6. Fatigue or loss of energy nearly every day.

7. Feelings of worthlessness or excessive or inappropriate guilt (which may be delusional) nearly every day (not merely self-reproach or guilt about being sick).

8. Diminished ability to think or concentrate, or indecisiveness, nearly every day (either by subjective account or as observed by others).

Table 4.2 (cont.)

   9. Recurrent thoughts of death (not just fear of dying), recurrent suicidal ideation without a specific plan, or a suicide attempt or a specific plan for committing suicide.
B. The symptoms cause clinically significant distress or impairment in social, occupational, or other important areas of functioning.
C. The episode is not attributable to the physiological effects of a substance or to another medical condition.
   Note: Criteria A–C represent a major depressive episode.
   Note: Responses to a significant loss (e.g., bereavement, financial ruin, losses from a natural disaster, a serious medical illness or disability) may include the feelings of intense sadness, rumination about the loss, insomnia, poor appetite, and weight loss noted in Criterion A, which may resemble a depressive episode. Although such symptoms may be understandable or considered appropriate to the loss, the presence of a major depressive episode, in addition to the normal response to a significant loss, should also be carefully considered. This decision inevitably requires the exercise of clinical judgment based on the individual's history and the cultural norms for the expression of distress in the context of loss.
D. The occurrence of the major depressive episode is not better explained by schizoaffective disorder, schizophrenia, schizophreniform disorder, delusional disorder, or other specified and unspecified schizophrenia spectrum and other psychotic disorders.
E. There has never been a manic episode or a hypomanic episode.
   Note: This exclusion does not apply if all of the manic-like or hypomanic-like episodes are substance-induced or are attributable to the physiological effects of another medical condition.

Together, the eight symptoms of depression (not including depressed mood) are frequently referred to as neurovegetative symptoms, and are recalled via the use of the pneumonic device "SIGECAPS," standing for "sleep, interest, guilt, energy, concentration, appetite, psychomotor activity, and suicidal ideation." The term "SIGECAPS" is meant to evoke the idea of prescribing a boost of energy for depressed patients, stemming from the Latin "Sig" for prescribe and "E Caps" for energy capsules.

Finally, it should be noted that patients may meet criteria for a major depressive *episode* (with all of the features listed previously) but have bipolar disorder, by virtue of having prior manic or hypomanic episodes; this has relevance for treatment and longitudinal course of illness.

A major depressive episode can be subclassified based on specific clinical features.

With Anxious Distress
Anxiety is a common feature of depressive episodes, and may convey a higher risk of suicide and treatment-resistance. The specifier "with anxious distress" is applied

to an episode of MDD if two of the following symptoms are present for the majority of the course: feeling keyed up or tense, feeling unusually restless, difficulty concentrating because of worry, fear that something awful might happen, feeling that the individual might lose control of himself. The severity of the anxious distress is rated from mild to severe on the basis of the number of symptoms present.

With Mixed Features

Though previous editions classified a mixed mood episode as one involving the simultaneous presence of both a depressive and a manic episode, the DSM-V allows for the specifier "with mixed features" to be applied to an episode of MDD. Patients with an episode of MDD involving mixed features have a higher likelihood of developing bipolar disorder. Criteria are met if three or more of the following symptoms of mania/hypomania are present for the majority of a depressive episode: elevated, expansive mood; inflated self-esteem or grandiosity; more talkative than usual or pressure to keep talking; flight of ideas or racing thoughts; increase in energy or goal-directed activity; increased or excessive involvement in activities with high potential for painful consequences; and decreased need for sleep. Activities considered to have a high potential for painful consequences include unrestrained buying sprees, sexual indiscretion, and foolish business investments. If the patient meets the full criteria for bipolar disorder but has prominent depressive symptoms in addition to mania or hypomania, they are considered to have a manic or hypomanic episode with mixed features in the setting of bipolar disorder, rather than MDD with mixed features.

With Psychotic Features

Major depression with psychotic features signifies the presence of either hallucinations or delusions accompanying mood symptoms. Psychotic features are subdivided into mood-congruent and mood-incongruent features. Commonly, psychotic symptoms in MDD are mood-congruent. Delusions in psychotic depression, for example, tend to be nihilistic, guilt-themed, or somatic. Patients may develop Cotard's syndrome, in which they believe themselves to be dead or dying, or believe that they have lost their internal vital organs. Other patients may believe that they are emitting toxic chemicals or that they are responsible for all of the bad events in the world. Hallucinations may involve olfactory sensations of decay or rotting, or voices commenting that the patient is evil or bad. Patients who develop a major depression with psychosis are at higher risk for developing psychosis during future mood episodes.

With Melancholic Features

A major depressive episode with melancholic features is heralded by the presence of either complete loss of pleasure in activities or loss of mood reactivity to pleasurable stimuli, in addition to three of the following: quality of depression characterized by despondency or despair, morning worsening of mood, early morning awakening, psychomotor retardation or agitation, decreased appetite, or excessive guilt. Patients with melancholic features are less likely to have a comorbid personality disorder, to have a clear precipitant for the depressive episode, or to respond to placebo. They may be more likely to respond to antidepressant medication or electroconvulsive therapy (ECT). Patients who develop melancholic features tend to be older and more often develop psychosis in conjunction with their depression. Melancholic features often do not persist across multiple episodes of depression.

With Atypical Features

The hallmark of major depression with atypical features is preserved mood reactivity. On exam, these patients are often capable of smiling or even laughing appropriately, and may not appear particularly depressed. Because of their mood reactivity, these patients occasionally may not engender as much empathy from the interviewer. Other atypical features include hypersomnia and hyperphagia rather than insomnia or decreased appetite, a feeling of heaviness in the arms and legs called "leaden paralysis," and heightened rejection sensitivity. Women more commonly exhibit atypical features of depression as compared to men. Patients with atypical features tend to have an earlier age of onset for their depression and may respond to different classes of medication. Atypical depression has been linked to higher rates of comorbidity with bipolar disorder, borderline personality disorder, and social phobia.

With Catatonia

Patients who develop a major depressive episode with catatonic features exhibit three or more signs of the syndrome of catatonia. These may include motoric immobility, excessive motor activity, peculiarities of voluntary movement (including grimacing or the maintenance of rigid positions known as posturing), negativism, mutism, or echophenomena. Negativism manifests most commonly as resistance to all instructions. Patients do not follow commands and may actively resist manipulation by the examiner, such as shutting their eyes during attempts to open them. Echophenomena may include mimicking of the examiner's speech (echolalia) or movements (echopraxia). Though patients with catatonia are classically thought of as being rigid and mute, the syndrome occurs on a spectrum, and many catatonic patients will be able to communicate with examiners and cooperate with the examination. Patients exhibiting catatonic symptoms can sometimes appear to be "playing possum," which may lead to doubts on the part of treaters regarding the validity of their symptoms. Indeed, one theory about catatonia is that it represents an evolutionary fear response and is similar to "playing dead" behavior in other species.

With Peripartum Onset

An episode of major depression with peripartum onset occurs during pregnancy or within four weeks of delivery and is estimated to occur in 3–6 percent of pregnancies. Women with prior episodes of depression are at the highest risk for peripartum depression, but some patients will experience the first episode of depression during the peripartum period. Peripartum depression can be distinguished from "baby blues," a normal, transient period of increased emotionality in the first three to seven days of the postpartum period, by both persistence and severity, though having the baby blues is a risk factor for developing peripartum MDD. Depression in the postpartum period often includes severe anxiety, spontaneous crying, disinterest in the infant and insomnia. Obsessional thoughts regarding violence to the child may be present and should be inquired after. Psychotic symptoms, such as delusions regarding the infant, occurring in 1 in 500 to 1 in 1,000 deliveries, are particularly worrisome and are a significant risk factor for infanticide. They tend to occur more in primiparous women and in those with personal or family histories of bipolar disorder. The risk of recurrence following an initial postpartum psychosis is up to 50 percent.

With Seasonal Pattern

Depression with seasonal variation refers to a pattern of depression in which the onset and remission of depressive episodes occur at characteristic times of the year. Most commonly, depressive episodes begin in the fall and resolve in the spring, though a minority of patients experience an opposite pattern. In order to meet criteria for the seasonal specifier, the pattern needs to have occurred for the past two years without any non-seasonal episodes. Further, over one's lifetime, the number of seasonal episodes must substantially outnumber non-seasonal episodes. Depressive episodes occurring with a seasonal pattern tend to have more atypical features, and there is some speculation that there is higher comorbidity with bipolar disorder. Prevalence appears to increase with higher latitudes and younger age. Though standard treatments for MDD may be effective in these patients, other treatments, such as bright light therapy, may be particularly useful in patients with a seasonal pattern of major depressive episodes.

Suicide

Patients with MDD are at increased risk for suicide. Among patients who die of suicide, depression is more common than any other psychiatric disorder. Suicidal thoughts and feelings of hopelessness are often key components of depression. Among depressed patients, symptoms that increase the risk of suicide include anxiety, panic attacks, desperation, and feeling burdensome. Additional risk factors for suicide among depressed patients are shown in Table 4.3. Suicide risk factors can be divided into static and dynamic factors. Static factors refer to elements of

Table 4.3 Risk factors for imminent serious self-harm in depressed patients

Static factors

Past self-injurious behavior or suicide attempts

Family history of attempted or completed suicide

Personality disorder

History of mood disorder or psychosis

History of abuse

Male gender

Older age

Dynamic factors

Current or recent suicidal ideation (including plan, intent)

Anxiety/panic

Substance use

Current mood symptoms

Current psychosis

Access to lethal means (firearms, etc.)

Impulsivity

Social stressors

Table 4.4 Protective factors for imminent serious self-harm in depressed patients

Lack of prior suicide attempts

Access to and engagement with psychiatric providers

Medication compliance

Social supports

Employment

Children and loved ones

Future orientation

patients' histories that are stable and cannot be changed or influenced, whereas dynamic risk factors represent those that are amenable to treatment or intervention. Factors that may mitigate the risk of suicide in depressed patients are shown in Table 4.4.

It appears that patients are particularly vulnerable to suicide during the early recovery from a depressive episode. One hypothesis is that energy and motivation tend to improve prior to the resolution of other symptoms, including low mood and suicidal ideation. Patients who have been experiencing suicidal ideation for weeks to months but who have not been motivated to act on these thoughts may suddenly find themselves with greater energy and impetus to act on these ongoing thoughts.

Depression Severity
Episodes of depression are rated as mild, moderate, or severe, based on symptom severity and degree of functional impairment. Mild depression is characterized by the presence of a minimal number of symptoms that result in only minor impairment in social or occupational functioning. Severe depression is characterized by the presence of several symptoms in excess of those needed for the diagnosis, as well as marked impairment in social or occupational functioning; patients requiring hospitalization for depression are in general thought to have a severe form. Under DSM-V, the presence of psychosis no longer by definition qualifies an episode as severe, though the majority of patients with psychotic depression will meet the criteria for a severe episode.

Remission
Full remission from depression is defined as a complete resolution of depressive symptoms for a minimum of two months. Though some patients with recurrent depression experience full remission, some will only achieve a partial reduction in symptoms, during which full MDD criteria are no longer met, or experience full remission for less than two months. Both of these latter patterns are classified as partial remission. Longitudinal course specifiers for depression differentiate between single episode and recurrent episodes of depression. In order to qualify as having a recurrent MDD, patients must experience a two-month period of at least partial remission followed by a return of a full syndromal episode.

The presence of residual symptoms between episodes conveys a worse overall prognosis. Unfortunately, trials of MDD treatments have found that remission of MDD is the exception rather than the rule, and millions of Americans have residual symptoms or ongoing syndromal depression with its attendant impairment, costs, and risks. Risk of recurrence declines as the length of remission increases. Factors conveying a higher risk of recurrence, aside from treatment, include symptom severity and younger age.

Persistent Depressive Disorder
Please see Table 4.5 for the DSM-V criteria for persistent depressive disorder. Persistent depressive disorder is a consolidation of two previous entities, chronic MDD and dysthymia. It is characterized by depressed mood more often than not for a period of at least two years. In addition to low mood, patients also exhibit at least two of the following: insomnia or hypersomnia, low self-esteem, low energy or fatigue, poor concentration, poor appetite or overeating, and feelings of hopelessness. In order to qualify for a diagnosis of persistent depressive disorder, patients

Table 4.5 DSM-V Criteria for persistent depressive disorder

A. Depressed mood for most of the day, for more days than not, as indicated by either subjective account or observation by others, for at least 2 years.
   Note: In children and adolescents, mood can be irritable and duration must be at least 1 year.
B. Presence, while depressed, of two (or more) of the following:
   1. Poor appetite or overeating
   2. Insomnia or hypersomnia
   3. Low energy or fatigue
   4. Low self-esteem
   5. Poor concentration or difficulty making decisions
   6. Feelings of hopelessness
C. During the 2-year period (1 year for children and adolescents) of the disturbance, the individual has never been without the symptoms in Criteria A or B for more than 2 months at a time.
D. Criteria for a major depressive disorder may be continuously present for 2 years.
E. There has never been a manic episode or a hypomanic episode, and criteria have never been met for cyclothymic disorder.
F. The disturbance is not better explained by a persistent schizoaffective disorder, schizophrenia, schizophreniform disorder, delusional disorder, or other specified and unspecified schizophrenia spectrum and other psychotic disorder.
G. The symptoms are not attributable to the physiological effects of a substance (e.g., a drug of abuse, a medication) or to another medical condition (e.g., hypothyroidism).
H. The symptoms cause clinically significant distress or impairment in social, occupational, or other important areas of functioning.
   Note: Because the criteria for a major depressive episode include four symptoms that are absent from the symptom list for persistent depressive disorder (dysthymia), a very limited number of individuals will have depressive symptoms that have persisted longer than 2 years but will not meet criteria for persistent depressive disorder. If full criteria for a major depressive episode has been met at some point during the current episode of illness, they should be given a diagnosis of major depressive disorder. Otherwise, a diagnosis of other specified depressive disorder or unspecified depressive disorder is warranted.

cannot be without symptoms for a greater than a two-month continuous period of time within the two years. Individuals who meet criteria for MDD consistently for two years should be given diagnoses of both MDD and persistent depressive disorder. Persistent depressive disorder occurs in approximately 2 percent of the population per year (75 percent of these patients have chronic MDD) and often has its onset in adolescence or young adulthood. Children and adolescents with persistent depressive disorder may experience irritable rather than depressed mood, and only require one year of mood and associated symptoms for the diagnosis. Earlier onset is associated with Cluster B and C personality disorders and substance use disorders. Risk factors include childhood parental loss or separation, and family history of MDD or persistent depressive disorder.

Patients with persistent depressive disorder have often grown so accustomed to their chronic mood state that they view their mood as a personality trait and do not report low mood unless specifically asked. This entity is sometimes called the "Eeyore phenomenon," after the character from *Winnie the Pooh* who frequently exhibits a pessimistic, gloomy attitude. Historically, an episode of MDD superimposed on the background of dysthymia has been referred to as "double depression." For many patients with persistent depressive disorder, as an acute episode of depression resolves, they return to their baseline dysthymia.

Premenstrual Dysphoric Disorder (PMDD)

Please see Table 4.6 for the DSM-V criteria for premenstrual dysphoric disorder. PMDD is a condition seen in women of childbearing age, marked by episodes of irritability or anger, anxiety, mood lability, and depressed mood, causing significant impairment in functioning and lasting several days surrounding menses. The typical pattern is one of dysfunction beginning

---

Table 4.6 DSM-V criteria for PMDD

A. In the majority of menstrual cycles, at least 5 symptoms must be present in the final weeks before the onset of menses, start to improve within a few days after the onset of menses, and become minimal or absent in the week postmenses.

B. One (or more) of the following symptoms must be present:
   1. Marked affective lability (e.g., mood swings; feeling suddenly sad or tearful, or increased sensitivity to rejection).
   2. Marked irritability or anger or increased interpersonal conflicts.
   3. Marked depressed mood, feelings of hopelessness, or self-deprecating thoughts.
   4. Marked anxiety, tension, and/or feelings of being keyed up or on edge.

C. One (or more) of the following symptoms must additionally be present, to reach a total of five symptoms when combined with symptoms from Criterion B above.
   1. Decreased interest in usual activities (e.g., work, school, friends, hobbies).
   2. Subjective difficulty in concentration.
   3. Lethargy, easy fatigability, or marked lack of energy.
   4. Marked change in appetite; overeating; or specific food cravings.
   5. Hypersomnia or insomnia.
   6. A sense of being overwhelmed or out of control.
   7. Physical symptoms such as breast tenderness or swelling, joint or muscle pain, a sensation of "bloating," or weight gain.

   Note: The symptoms in Criterion A–C must have been met for most menstrual cycles that occurred in the preceding year.

D. The symptoms are associated with clinically significant distress or interference with work, school, usual social activities, or relationships with others (e.g., avoidance of social activities; decreased productivity or efficiency at work, school, or home).

E. The disturbance is not merely an exacerbation of the symptoms of another disorder, such as major depressive disorder, panic disorder, persistent depressive disorder (dysthymia), or a personality disorder (although it may co-occur with any of these disorders).

F. Criterion A should be confirmed by prospective daily ratings during at least two symptomatic cycles (Note: The diagnosis may be made provisionally prior to this confirmation).

G. The symptoms are not attributable to the physiological effects of a substance (e.g., a drug of abuse, a medication) or to another medical condition (e.g., hyperthyroidism).

the week prior to menses with resolution mid-menses. Symptoms must be present in the final week before the onset of menses and must start to improve within a few days of the onset of menses, with minimal or absent symptoms in the week postmenses. Symptoms may be of comparable severity to those of MDD, but by definition are shorter-lasting and recur with the majority of cycles. Though symptoms of PMDD may be comorbid with dysmenorrhea, most females with PMDD do not have the latter condition. Brief periods of psychotic symptoms may occur, particularly in the late luteal phase, but are rare. Twelve-month prevalence appears to be about 2 percent of menstruating women. Onset can occur at any age, though symptoms may tend to worsen as women approach menopause. Symptoms resolve after menopause. Risk factors include psychosocial stress, trauma, and seasonal changes. Oral contraceptives may mitigate risk.

Disruptive Mood Regulation Disorder

Disruptive mood regulation disorder is a diagnosis applied to children and adolescents who exhibit severe, recurrent temper outbursts. These episodes are manifested either as verbal rages or physical aggression that is markedly out of proportion to the situation or precipitant. Episodes are inconsistent with developmental level, occur at least three times per week, persist for twelve or more months, and occur in at least two different settings. Further, the patient's mood between episodes is persistently irritable or angry most of the day, nearly every day. Symptoms must be present prior to age ten, and the diagnosis should not be given prior to age six or after age eighteen.

Differential Diagnosis

Depressive Disorder due to Another Medical Condition

Medical illnesses known to cause or contribute to symptoms of depression via a direct pathophysiologic mechanism are listed in Table 4.7. Classically, neurological illnesses associated with lesions in the left frontal lobe or left basal ganglia may be more associated with depression, though lesions in other brain areas may also be associated with mood symptoms. Among neoplasms, pancreatic cancer is most associated with depression, and symptoms of depression including fatigue and low mood are frequently the first signs of this illness. Endocrinologic disorders may mimic depression. Hypothyroidism is perhaps the best known of these, with prominent features of fatigue, low energy, weight gain, and amotivation, but hyperthyroidism, hyper- and hypocortisol states (Cushing's syndrome and Addison's disease, respectively), and hyperparathyroidism (and hypercalcemia in general) have also been associated with depression. Immune and inflammatory disorders, such as multiple sclerosis and systemic lupus erythematosus, may also be linked to

Table 4.7 Medical conditions associated with depression

Neurologic
  Degenerative diseases (Parkinson's, Huntington's, etc)
  Cerebrovascular disease
  Inflammatory Conditions (Multiple sclerosis, lupus cerebritis, etc)
  CNS lesions
Endocrinologic
  Thyroid disease (hypo- and hyperthyroidism)
  Cushing's disease
  Addison's disease
  Hypogonadism
  Hyperparathyroidism
Vitamin deficiencies
  Pellagra (Niacin)
  Vitamin B12 deficiency
Other
  Pancreatic cancer

depression. Among men, particularly those infected with HIV, low testosterone is a frequent cause of depressive symptoms.

Substance/Medication-Induced Depressive Disorder

Many prescribed and illicit substances may cause or contribute to symptoms of depression. Ideally, diagnoses of MDD should only be made in the setting of at least a two-month period of sobriety from mood-altering substances.

Among prescribed medications, systemic steroids are commonly associated with a wide variety of neuropsychiatric disturbances (e.g., psychosis, mania, delirium) that also include depressive episodes. Interferon, used for the treatment of hepatitis C or melanoma, is also highly associated with the development of depression. While older literature noted a propensity among beta-blockers to cause depression, more recent prospective studies suggest that this effect (with the possible exception of propranolol) is not typically seen. Other medications that have the potential to cause depression are listed in Table 4.8.

Alcohol is a known depressant, and patients with alcohol use disorders may exhibit a wide array of depressive symptoms in the setting of ongoing use. Sedatives, such as benzodiazepines and barbiturates, also act as depressants. Similarly, patients prescribed chronic opiates for pain, or those using illicit opiates such as heroin, may exhibit depressive syndromes. Other substances, including cocaine and amphetamines, have withdrawal phases that include intense dysphoria, typically lasting days to weeks.

Table 4.8 Medications associated with depression

Neurologic medications
    Barbiturates
    Vigabatrin
    Topiramate
    Flunarizine
Anti-infective agents
    Efavirenz
    Interferon-α
    Mefloquine
Other medications
    Corticosteroids

Dysphoria in Personality Disorders (Characterologic Dysphoria)

Patients with an underlying personality disorder are vulnerable to episodes of mood dysregulation. Sometimes there exists a comorbid mood disorder, such as MDD, but other times depressive symptoms occur in a subsyndromal pattern. This is particularly common in patients with Cluster B personality disorders, such as borderline and narcissistic personality disorders. These patients will frequently describe their depression as feeling like an emptiness, rather than the sadness commonly described by those suffering from MDD, and may lack prominent neurovegetative symptoms. Dysphoria in these patients is more transient, and tends to appear and disappear more suddenly, often in response to interpersonal relationships. Low mood in personality disorders has also been called a "mad-bad" depression, in which patients can experience significant periods of irritability while also viewing themselves as inherently bad people.

Adjustment Disorder with Depressed Mood

Adjustment disorders describe a group of syndromes in which patients develop clinically significant emotional or behavioral dysregulation in response to a specific stressor. Specific variants include adjustment disorder with depressed mood and adjustment disorder with mixed anxiety and depressed mood, both of which can mimic depression. By definition, adjustment disorders have their onset within three months of the stressor and resolve within six months of the stressor, except in cases in which the stressor is chronic or ongoing, such as relating to a general medical condition. An adjustment disorder is not diagnosed if the patient meets the criteria for another diagnosis, and MDD is thus said to trump adjustment disorders in the diagnostic hierarchy.

Demoralization

Demoralization stems from a persistent inability to cope with a particular ongoing stressor, combined with a sense of hopelessness and helplessness regarding the resolution of that stressor. It is most commonly seen in patients suffering from chronic medical or psychiatric illnesses. Patients most commonly describe a pervasive sense of powerlessness driven by a recognition that they cannot change or remove themselves from the situation. Unlike MDD, patients with demoralization rarely describe anhedonia and are often able to point to recent enjoyment or discuss upcoming events to which they are looking forward. Like patients with MDD, however, and particularly in the absence of being able to engage in pleasurable activities, those with demoralization may have a desire for hastened death and are at higher risk for suicide. They are also at high risk of developing a superimposed episode of MDD.

Bereavement

Bereavement describes the presence of depressive symptoms in the setting of the death of a loved one. Though bereavement previously represented an exclusion to MDD, patients who meet full criteria for MDD in the setting of a recent loss are now diagnosed as having MDD. Importantly, this new nosology does not suggest that sadness in the setting of loss or grieving is necessarily pathologic, and many patients experiencing normal bereavement in the context of a major loss have symptoms that overlap with MDD, including intense sadness crying spells, sleep/appetite disturbance, low energy, guilt, diminished interest, and wishes to join the deceased person.

However, several important features of normal bereavement can distinguish it from MDD in the context of grief. First, symptoms of bereavement tend to come in waves during and between days, with some "good days" and some "bad days." People with normal bereavement are often cheered by social support, able to access positive feelings and hope for the future, and also able to maintain some interest in activities. Guilt and impairment of self-esteem tend to be limited to feelings that one could have done more to support or engage the person while still alive, and thoughts of death typically are fleeting and related to wishes to join the deceased. In contrast, patients with MDD have persistent, pervasive symptoms most of the day, nearly every day. Such symptoms are less variable and less responsive to social support or other small positive life events. Guilt, hopelessness, loss of interest, and self-esteem are both more intense and go beyond feelings related to the death of the loved one; patients often feel that they are globally bad people and that they have much in their life about which to feel guilty. Finally, suicidal thoughts often come with intent and/or plan in MDD and, rather than focused on a wish to join the deceased, are more associated with ending their suffering.

Bereavement is not treated with medication, but may respond to supportive forms of therapy. Patients with bereavement remain at increased risk for developing MDD and should be closely monitored. The DSM-V also proposes the entity persistent complex bereavement disorder to describe the presence of ongoing depressive symptoms related to the loss more than twelve months after it occurs.

Normative Sadness

Many patients experience periods of sadness in response to life events. Though the term "depression" may colloquially be used by people to describe their mood state, it is important to keep in mind that only a very small percentage of those experiencing sadness actually meet the criteria for depression. As of yet, there is no treatment for sadness and no evidence that treating those with subsyndromal dysphoria is useful. Patients with situational sadness should be monitored for the development of depression, though no current evidence suggests that they are at higher risk than others.

Evaluation

Clinical Interview

Screening patients for MDD and other depressive disorders is straightforward and effective. Questions such as "Have you felt depressed much of the time in the past two weeks?" and "Have you experienced a loss of interest in pleasurable activities in the past two weeks?" that inquire about the cardinal symptoms of depressed mood and anhedonia can quickly identify patients who require further assessment. Such assessment will typically include assessment for neurovegetative symptoms of depression, associated symptoms of anxiety or psychosis, the presence of past or current manic/hypomanic symptoms, substance use, recent physical symptoms/illness, and medications.

Patients reporting low mood are often reserved in the interview setting and may offer little in the way of spontaneous speech. Open-ended questions can be a useful way to draw them out, as they may tend to give one- or two-word responses to more direct questions. Recent or ongoing stressors should also be asked about and their likelihood of resolution assessed.

To test for preserved mood reactivity, the interviewer may ask the patient to discuss an event that made them happy in the past or might attempt to inject humor into the interview in order to gauge the patient's reaction. In assessing for key symptoms of depression, the presence of low mood is sometimes denied but can be inferred from outward expressions and demeanor. Loss of interest may manifest as a report of not caring about things, being less interested in hobbies, or decreased libido. Sleep disturbances may present as difficulty falling asleep (initial insomnia), staying asleep (middle insomnia), or as early-morning awakening (terminal insomnia). Psychomotor changes may be observable as slowed movements, slowed speech, or increased latency in answering questions. Guilty thoughts may present as worthlessness, blaming oneself for failures, or as the misinterpretation of trivial events as evidence of personal defects. Decreased concentration may manifest as a decline in school or work performance, or in more severe cases as memory and executive functioning difficulties (pseudodementia).

On mental status exam, interviewers should be observant of signs of decreased attention to appearance, self-care, and hygiene, including disheveled appearance, unkempt hair, old or soiled clothing, or malodor. Psychomotor slowing may be readily apparent from observation of the patient's movements. Eye contact is often poor when patients are depressed. Speech may be slowed and is often low-volume or sometimes monotone. Affect may appear sad (with periods of tearfulness), irritable, or blunted to flat, with an absence of facial expressivity. Common thought content includes guilty ruminations, focusing on negative aspects of life, and lack of hope for the future. Thought processes may be slowed. Cognition may be impaired, with deficits particularly in attention, concentration, and executive functioning, leading to a picture of "pseudo-dementia."

Physical Exam and Laboratory Evaluation (to Rule Out a General Medical Condition)

Physical examination of depressed patients is focused on ruling out potential medical causes of depression. Stigmata of illnesses that may cause depression should be assessed. In particular, a good neurologic examination, including testing for reflexes, strength, movement abnormalities, and frontal release signs, is key to ruling out neurological causes of depression. Basic blood work may include thyroid studies, vitamin B12 and folate levels, and blood and urine toxicology screens. Further studies may be indicated if there is high suspicion for a specific medical condition.

Risk Assessment

Issues of risk and risk assessment are addressed in depth in Chapter 3. For patients who endorse thoughts that life is not worth living or otherwise appear to be at elevated suicidal risk, a more complete assessment of suicidal thoughts and urges is indicated. This will include thoughts about wishing to be dead, any suicidal plans, access to means of suicide (especially firearms), suicidal intent, protective features (e.g., "Who or what has kept you from doing it this far?"), and prior suicide attempts.

Treatment Approaches

In considering treatment options for patients with depression, the first decision involves the appropriate level of care for the patient. Many patients with depression can be treated on an outpatient basis using either pharmacotherapy or psychotherapy.

Patients who are experiencing depressive symptoms that are significantly impairing their ability to work or function at home, or those for whom significant medication changes are anticipated which may require closer monitoring, a higher level of care such as a day treatment program or a crisis stabilization unit may be warranted. For some depressed patients, particularly those exhibiting suicidal ideation with plan or intent, or those whose depression is affecting their ability to meet basic care needs, inpatient hospitalization on a locked unit may be warranted for safety and containment, medication initiation or adjustment, and aftercare planning. On an inpatient unit, where patients are monitored around the clock and typically kept for a minimum of three days, medications can be titrated more quickly, patients can benefit from being in a supportive and therapeutic milieu with others suffering from similar illnesses, and additional therapies that may not be readily available to outpatients, such as electroconvulsive therapy, may be offered.

After deciding on the appropriate level of care, the next key decision in the initial evaluation of the depressed patient is whether to institute pharmacotherapy or psychotherapy (or neither or both). Pharmacotherapy with an adequate dose of an antidepressant medication (e.g., a selective serotonin reuptake inhibitor [SSRI]) or treatment using evidence-based psychotherapy (e.g., cognitive-behavioral therapy [CBT] or interpersonal therapy [IPT]) is indicated for patients who meet the criteria for MDD or persistent depressive disorder. Patients with PMDD may benefit specifically from an SSRI.

Patients with more severe, prolonged, or refractory mood symptoms can benefit from combined treatment with both medications and psychotherapy; for patients with the most severe or refractory conditions, ECT can be very effective. For patients who have MDD with psychotic features, combination therapy using an antidepressant and antipsychotic is indicated; ECT can be effective in this condition as well. One important caveat is that patients with a major depressive episode who have bipolar disorder, or when the episode has mixed features, should in general not be treated with an antidepressant without also taking an adequate dose of a mood-stabilizing medication such as lithium, as antidepressants may induce hypomania or mania (or worsening of mixed features) in such patients.

With regard to the titration and duration of antidepressant treatment, it is often the case that dose adjustment (and potentially switching or augmenting treatment) is often required before response and remission can be attained. An adequate trial of an antidepressant can take at least six to eight weeks, and patients may have limited response to treatment within the first few weeks of treatment. Patients for whom antidepressants are prescribed should be able to adhere to a daily medication regimen, given the need to take such medications consistently for weeks prior to effect and their lack of efficacy until taken consistently. If depression limits the patient's ability to adhere, consideration may be given to the utilization of family members or home nursing services to ensure adherence.

There are no absolute medical contraindications to antidepressant treatment, though certain situations require caution. Patients taking other serotonergic agents should be closely monitored for the emergence of serotonin syndrome, and in rare cases (e.g., when patients are taking the antibiotic linezolid), serotonergic antidepressants are contraindicated and alternative agents may need to be used. Many antidepressants may affect blood levels of other medications, including warfarin and metoprolol.

Once a patient has remission of symptoms, it is generally recommended that patients continue the antidepressant at the effective dose for at least nine to twelve months of stability (with evidence for longer continuation treatment leading to lesser rates of relapse) for a first depressive episode and longer for a second episode. Most authorities recommend lifetime antidepressant treatment for patients with three or more lifetime major depressive episodes.

With regard to psychotherapy, such as CBT or IPT, therapy typically occurs on a weekly basis, for a period of at least two to three months. Other forms of psychotherapy, such as group therapy, psychodynamic therapy, or supportive therapy, may be helpful for patients who have less severe depression or comorbid illnesses that can make these interventions indicated. Finally, exercise has been found to be an effective antidepressant and should be recommended to those patients willing and able to perform moderate physical activity.

Bipolar Disorders

Classification

In contrast to unipolar major depressive disorder, in which individuals experience recurrent episodes of decreased mood, energy, motivation, and changes in sleep and eating patterns, those with bipolar spectrum disorders also experience episodes of mood elevation (i.e., manic, hypomanic, or mixed episodes).

There are several subtypes of bipolar disorders (see Table 4.1). They vary in terms of their severity and in the duration of manic symptoms. Those with bipolar I disorder show a lifetime history of major depressive episodes and manic episodes. On the other hand, bipolar II disorder is characterized by a lifetime history of major depressive episodes and hypomanic episodes. In hypomanic episodes, there are less severe manic symptoms compared to manic episodes (see the "Clinical Feature" section). Those with cyclothymia have alternating periods of hypomania and subsyndromal depression; however, they do not ever fully meet the criteria for manic episodes or major depressive episodes. All of these categorizations are consistent with the concept of a mood spectrum, with recurrent unipolar depression as an anchor on one end of the spectrum and with the full-blown manic episodes on the other end of the spectrum.

Additionally, the DSM-V lists other specified bipolar and related disorders that include a past history of a major depressive disorder either with hypomania lasting less than four days or with hypomania lasting more than four days but with fewer symptoms. The DSM-V also includes *substance/medication-induced bipolar and related disorder* and *bipolar and related disorder due to another medical condition*.

Epidemiology and Impact of Illness Prevalence

The prevalence of bipolar I disorder is approximately 1 percent of the general population. Bipolar II disorder is approximately twice as common as bipolar I disorder (0.3–4.8 percent). The prevalence of all bipolar spectrum illness, including mild forms, is approximately 4 percent of the general population (2.6–7.8 percent). Bipolar I disorder is equally prevalent in men and women, but the prevalence of bipolar II disorder is greater in women (3:2). The median age of onset is twenty-five years, with men having an earlier age of onset.

Clinical Course

Often patients with bipolar disorder experience depression first, with later episodes of mania/hypomania. Once patients experience a single manic episode, 90 percent have another mood episode. As the disorder progresses, the time interval between episodes generally decreases.

Manic episodes typically start abruptly and last about three months without treatment. The depressive episodes usually last longer than manic episodes, but bipolar depression tends to last for a shorter amount of time than does unipolar depression.

Overall, patients with bipolar I disorder will experience approximately nine mood episodes in their lifetime. When ill, most patients spend most of their time in depressive episodes, including both major depressive and subsyndromal depressive episodes. Patients with bipolar I disorder, for example, spent one-third of their time depressed and about one-tenth of their time manic or hypomanic. Those with bipolar II disorder spent over half of the time feeling depressed.

Morbidity and Mortality

Bipolar disorder is one of the world's 10 most disabling diseases. According to a report from 2009, the annual direct and indirect costs of bipolar disorder in the United States are about $151 billion; of this amount, $30.7 billion was direct costs. Annual insurance payments for patients with bipolar disorder are higher than those of patients with other behavioral health care diagnoses.

According to a recent national cohort study in Sweden, women and men with bipolar disorder died 9.0 and 8.5 years earlier (on average) than the rest of the population, respectively. In comparison with the rest of the population, there was a twofold increase in all-cause mortality in those with bipolar disorder compared to the rest of the population. Patients with bipolar disorder had increased mortality from cardiovascular diseases, diabetes mellitus, chronic obstructive pulmonary disease (COPD), influenza or pneumonia, unintentional injuries, and suicide. The suicide risk among women with bipolar disorder was increased tenfold, and an eightfold increase was found among men with bipolar disorder.

Impact on Medical Illness

Patients with bipolar disorder are often more vulnerable to medical illnesses; about half of patients have comorbid medical illnesses. Common medical illnesses that are frequently observed in bipolar disorder are cardiovascular, endocrine, and pulmonary conditions. The medical conditions of those with bipolar disorders tend to receive less clinical attention compared to the general population. For this reason, mortality rates due to medical illnesses are greater than in the general population. The increased rates of medical comorbidity are thought to be due to (i) medication side effects, (ii) shared pathophysiology, and (iii) negative health behaviors, including smoking, poor diet, overeating, and substance/alcohol use.

Clinical Features and Course

Major Depressive Episode

The diagnostic criteria for major depressive episodes are identical to the criteria used in major depressive disorder (MDD). This means that patients with bipolar disorder who have a depressive episode first cannot be initially distinguished from patients with MDD. Several studies suggest that there are some differentiating factors between unipolar and bipolar depression, including agitated depression, cyclical depression, episodic sleep dysregulation, refractory depression (failed antidepressants from three different classes), depression in someone with an extroverted personality or profession, depression with atypical features, postpartum onset, and depression with relatively earlier age at onset. However, no definite markers exist to distinguish unipolar and bipolar depression. The same course specifiers with MDD can be applied in major depressive episodes of bipolar disorder.

Manic Episode

The DSM-V criteria for a manic episode require the presence of a distinct period of abnormally elevated, expansive, or irritable mood and abnormally increased activity or energy (see Table 4.9). The episode must last at least one week without hospitalization; the duration is not relevant if hospitalization is necessary. In the DSM-V, changes in activity and energy are emphasized as well as mood; this is to enhance the accuracy of diagnosis and facilitate earlier detection. To meet the criteria for a manic episode, at least three (or four, if mood is only irritable) symptoms must be present. These include increased self-esteem or grandiosity, decreased need for sleep, talkativeness, flight of ideas or racing thoughts, distractibility, increased goal-directed activity or psychomotor agitation, and excessive involvement in pleasurable activities that have a high potential for painful consequences.

Manic episodes usually begin with an elevated, euphoric mood; they often evolve into irritability during the course of the episode. A variant of mania, known as *dysphoric mania*, involves a negative, sad, or angry mood. Increased self-esteem can vary from mildly inflated self-esteem to delusional and grandiose thoughts (e.g., "I'm a god. I'm Superman"). Some patients are psychotic during manic episodes, and the nature of psychotic symptoms often match the patient's mood (i.e., "mood-congruent" features). During the manic episode, patients usually feel rested with only a few hours of sleep and are excessively active and energetic. Spending sprees, irrational investments, increased sexual activity, and reckless driving are common examples of increased goal-directed, pleasurable activities that could cause painful consequences.

The DSM-IV-TR criteria included mixed episodes. In such episodes, patients would fully meet the criteria for both manic and depressive episodes simultaneously.

Table 4.9 DSM-V Diagnostic criteria for a manic episode

A. A distinct period of abnormally and persistently elevated, expansive or irritable mood and abnormally and persistently increased goal-directed activity or energy, lasting at least 1 week and present most of the day, nearly every day (or any duration if hospitalization is necessary).

B. During the period of mood disturbance and increased energy or activity, three (or more) of the following symptoms (four if the mood is only irritable) are present to a significant degree and represent a noticeable change from usual behavior:
  1. Inflated self-esteem or grandiosity
  2. Decreased need for sleep (e.g., feels rested after only 3 hours of sleep)
  3. More talkative than usual or pressure to keep talking
  4. Flight of ideas or subjective experience that thoughts are racing
  5. Distractability (i.e., attention to easily drawn to unimportant or irrelevant external stimuli), as reported or observed
  6. Increase in goal-directed activity (either socially, at work or school, or sexually) or psychomotor agitation (i.e., purposeless non-goal-directed activity)
  7. Excessive involvement in activities that have a high potential for painful consequences (e.g., engaging in unrestrained buying sprees, sexual indiscretions, or foolish business investments)

C. The mood disturbance is sufficiently severe to cause marked impairment in social or occupational functioning or to necessitate hospitalization to prevent harm to self or others, or there are psychotic features

D. The episode is not attributable to the physiologic effects of a substance (e.g., a drug of abuse, a medication, other treatment) or to another medical condition
Note: A full manic episode that emerges during antidepressant treatment (e.g., medication, electroconvulsive therapy) but persists at a fully syndromal level beyond the physiological effect of that treatment is sufficient evidence for a manic episode and, therefore, a bipolar I diagnosis
Note: Criteria A–D constitute a manic episode. At least one lifetime manic episode is required for the diagnosis of bipolar I disorder.

In DSM-V, a mixed specifier can be applied to both manic and depressive episodes, and involves the presence of at least three manic or depressive symptoms while simultaneously meeting full criteria for the opposite mood state.

Hypomanic Episode

The diagnostic criteria for a hypomanic episode are identical to those for a manic episode (see Table 4.10). However, the duration and severity are typically milder than a full-blown manic episode; hypomanic episodes need only last four days. The episode can cause changes in functioning, but are by definition not severe

Table 4.10 DSM-V diagnostic criteria for a hypomanic episode

A. A distinct period of abnormally and persistently elevated, expansive or irritable mood and abnormally and persistently increased activity or energy, lasting at least 4 consecutive days and present most of the day, nearly every day

B. During the period of mood disturbance and increased energy or activity, three (or more) of the following symptoms (four if the mood is only irritable) have persisted, represent a noticeable change from usual behavior, and have been present to a significant degree:
   1. Inflated self-esteem or grandiosity
   2. Decreased need for sleep (e.g., feels rested after only 3 hours of sleep)
   3. More talkative than usual or pressure to keep talking
   4. Flight of ideas or subjective experience that thoughts are racing
   5. Distractability (i.e., attention to easily drawn to unimportant or irrelevant external stimuli), as reported or observed
   6. Increase in goal-directed activity (either socially, at work or school, or sexually) or psychomotor agitation (i.e., purposeless non-goal-directed activity)
   7. Excessive involvement in activities that have a high potential for painful consequences (e.g., engaging in unrestrained buying sprees, sexual indiscretions, or foolish business investments)

C. The episode is associated with an unequivocal change in functioning that is uncharacteristic of the individual when not symptomatic.

D. The disturbance in mood and change in functioning are observable by others

E. The mood disturbance is not severe enough to cause marked impairment in social or occupational functioning or to necessitate hospitalization. If there are psychotic features, the episode is, by definition, manic.

F. The episode is not attributable to the physiologic effects of a substance (e.g., a drug of abuse, a medication, other treatment)

Note: A full hypomanic episode that emerges during antidepressant treatment (e.g., medication, electroconvulsive therapy) but persists at a fully syndromal level beyond the physiological effect of that treatment is sufficient evidence for a hypomanic episode diagnosis. However, caution is indicated so that one or two symptoms (particularly increased irritability, edginess, or agitation following antidepressant use) are not taken as sufficient for diagnosis of a hypomanic episode, nor necessarily indicative of a bipolar diathesis.

Note: Criteria A–F constitute a hypomanic episode. Hypomanic episodes are common in bipolar I disorder but are not required for the diagnosis of bipolar I disorder.

enough to cause marked impairment or hospitalization. Psychotic features, such as hallucinations or delusions, do not appear during hypomanic episodes.

Unlike manic episodes, which are destructive and easily noticed by others, hypomanic episodes can be hard to detect. Since they can be ego-syntonic or pleasurable for patients, it is also sometimes difficult to determine whether they have occurred previously. To complicate the issue further, hypomanic episodes are typically less frequent than depressive episodes and recall can be dependent on current mood.

Episode Specifiers

In depressive episodes, all of the specifiers used in MDD can be applied. In manic/hypomanic episodes, the following specifiers can also be applied: with anxious features, with mixed features, with psychotic features, with catatonia, and with peripartum onset. (see the "Depressive Disorders" section for a detailed explanation of each of these specifiers).

Course Specifiers Describing the Course of Recurrent Episodes

A seasonal pattern specifier can be applied to depressive episodes in bipolar disorder. It refers to having a regular temporal relationship between the onset of major depressive episodes and a particular time of the year recurrently. Full remissions (or a change from depression into mania or hypomania) also should occur at a characteristic time of the year (e.g., having a major depressive episode every winter with remission every spring).

Some patients are classified as having a bipolar illness with rapid cycling, implying that they experience mood episodes (including manic, hypomanic, and depressive) more than four times per year. Approximately 5–15 percent of patients with bipolar disorder are known to be rapid cyclers. Rapid cycling is generally thought to have a poor medication response and indicates a poor prognosis.

Suicide

Patients with bipolar disorder are at great risk for suicide compared to the general population and even compared to individuals with other mental health problems. During their lifetime, about half of patients with bipolar disorder attempt suicide. They attempt suicide not only when they are depressed but also during mixed affective states or dysphoric manic episodes. Controversies exist regarding whether those with bipolar disorder are at greater risk for suicide than those with unipolar depression.

Severity and Remission

The criteria for defining severity and remission are identical to those for MDD.

Differential Diagnosis

Bipolar Disorder Due to Another Medical Condition

Neurologic conditions such as brain tumors or multiple sclerosis are known causes of secondary mania. Classically, lesions in the right frontal lobe are associated with manic symptoms. Systemic illnesses have also been linked to manic symptoms. In particular, HIV has been associated with a secondary mania that may involve direct invasion of the CNS by the virus, though the pathophysiology remains unclear. Both hyper- and hypothyroid states have been shown to cause a secondary mania, with the latter being historically known as "myxedema madness."

Substance/Medication-Induced Bipolar and Related Disorders

Some pharmacological agents can also produce manic symptoms. In particular, intoxication with stimulants, such as cocaine or amphetamines, often mimics mania. Anabolic steroids may also cause maniform behavior. Prescribed medications such as corticosteroids, dopamine agonists, or isoniazid have also been associated with secondary mania, as have several classes of antibiotics, including macrolides.

When evaluating substance use patients present with mood symptoms, clinicians should consider the time course of symptom presentation. In some cases, patients might have taken medications due to the underlying manic symptoms. For example, a patient might have taken an amphetamine because of increased pleasure-seeking behaviors, which is part of manic symptoms. If the condition is a "secondary mood disorder" caused by a medical condition, theoretically, it could be corrected by resolving the current medical illness or discontinuation of the medication.

Major Depressive Disorder

When patients present with a current depressive episode, it is sometimes difficult to discover a previous history of a hypomanic/manic episode. The patient's history must be thoroughly taken; it is also important to get information from and about the individual's family. Often, patients may not have insight about past manic/hypomanic episodes.

As previously mentioned, some patients with MDD experience manic episodes after being diagnosed with MDD. Prior to the experience of a manic episode, it is impossible to differentiate unipolar from bipolar depression. Approximately 5–10 percent of patients with an initial diagnosis of MDD have a manic episode 6–10 years after the first depressive episode.

Schizophrenia

Psychotic mood episodes can be difficult to differentiate from schizophrenia. Inter-episodic functioning is relatively preserved and psychotic symptoms are observed only during the acute episode in bipolar disorder. Additionally, psychotic mood episodes tend to start abruptly, with psychotic symptoms concordant with mood symptoms (e.g., grandiose delusions in manic episodes; delusions of poverty in depressive episodes). Merriment, elation, and infectiousness of mood are also prominent in bipolar disorder. Half of patients with bipolar disorder have a family history of mood disorders, while schizophrenic patients are more likely to have a family history of schizophrenia. Catatonic features are more commonly seen in bipolar disorder than in schizophrenia. Sometimes long-term course evaluation is the best way to determine whether an individual is experiencing schizophrenia or bipolar disorder.

Schizoaffective Disorder

Schizoaffective disorder combines elements of schizophrenia and bipolar disorder. To meet the criteria for schizoaffective disorder, however, delusions or hallucinations must be present for at least two weeks in the absence of prominent mood symptoms.

Hyperthymic Personality

Hyperthymic temperament is a personality type characterized by an excessively positive disposition that is similar to hypomania. Individuals with hyperthymic temperament typically show increased energy and productivity compared with other people. They are also self-confident and enjoy risk-taking or sensation seeking. Sometimes they naturally do not need much sleep, feeling rested after only a few hours. Ostensibly, hyperthymic temperament can be thought of as hypomania, but the main difference is that hyperthymic temperament is a constant individual characteristic while hypomania is episodic. When individuals with hyperthymic temperament are depressed, some evaluate it as a variant of bipolar disorder.

Evaluation

Clinical Interview

When patients are in a manic or hypomanic state, they may have no insight about their current state. Along with questions about subjective mood, the behavioral patterns during the interview are important; manic patients are typically talkative and active, sometimes even restless. They can be irritable towards clinicians and speech may be rapid and difficult to interrupt ("pressured speech"). Reports on patients' premorbid personality and behavior are crucial, especially when evaluating possible hypomanic episodes, because changes and abnormalities can be subtle and sometimes difficult to distinguish from their natural characteristics. Reports from family and friends are also important. When an individual is manic, safety issues should be evaluated at the beginning.

Even if patients present with a depressive mood, concurrent manic symptoms should be evaluated since mixed features are quite common in bipolar disorder. Clinicians should look for symptoms such as irritability, talkativeness, inflated self-esteem, increased activity, and increased pleasurable activities. A family history of bipolar disorder makes a diagnosis of bipolar disorder more likely, but the most frequent disorder in first degree relatives of those with bipolar disorder is unipolar depression. Other psychiatric comorbid conditions also need to be evaluated. As described before, patients' alcohol or drug use history should be obtained.

Physical Exam and Laboratory Evaluation (to Rule Out a General Medical Condition)

To rule out neurologic conditions that present with mania-like symptoms, a thorough neurologic examination is necessary. If a patient presents with their first psychotic episode, neuroimaging is generally recommended to rule out a brain lesion. Additionally, blood examination including endocrinologic studies and toxicology should be ordered. Urine drug screening is also helpful to rule out substance use.

Risk Assessment

Suicide and violent behavior are the most important psychiatric emergencies related to bipolar disorder. When patients are highly agitated, psychotic, and paranoid, they might misperceive their surroundings and act out in self-defense. If any risk of self-harm or violence toward others is suspected, safety is the priority; clinicians need to protect themselves, patients, and patients' families. Risk assessment associated with suicidality and violence is further discussed in Chapter 3.

Treatment Approaches

The treatment strategy for bipolar disorder differs by phase: acute (hypo)manic, acute depressive, and maintenance phase. Across all phases, pharmacotherapy is the cornerstone of treatment for bipolar disorder, though adjunctive psychotherapy can reduce relapse and improve function. When preparing for treatment of an acute mood episode, an assessment for the most appropriate treatment setting should be completed. If patients are acutely at risk of self-harm or violence toward others, or if basic self-care has been neglected due to impaired judgment or severe symptoms, hospitalization is indicated. Otherwise, treatment of mood episodes in the outpatient setting can be pursued. As in depressive disorders, achieving remission of mood symptoms should be the primary goal for treatment, as patients with residual symptoms are more likely to experience a relapse or recurrence of mood episodes.

In the maintenance phase of treatment, the goal is to enhance function and prevent the recurrence of mood episodes. Mood stabilizing medications are used to achieve this goal. Lithium is the oldest and most well-known mood stabilizer, and it may have specific suicide-reducing properties. Other agents that are used in the maintenance phase of bipolar disorder include anticonvulsants, such as valproic acid, lamotrigine, and carbamazepine, and atypical antipsychotics, such as aripiprazole and olanzapine. Many patients require combination pharmacotherapy to achieve clinical stability. In addition, specific forms of psychotherapy, including CBT and interpersonal and social rhythm therapy (IPSRT), have been used to prevent relapse and improve function. Psychoeducation is also vital for patients with this illness to increase patients' understanding of the impact of sleep impairment, substances, stress, and other triggers for acute episodes.

Manic (and hypomanic) episodes can be effectively managed with a number of different agents. Lithium, anticonvulsants, and atypical antipsychotics (alone or in combination) are widely used to treat these elevated mood states, and typical antipsychotics and benzodiazepines may also be used adjunctively. In general, one or more of the agents used to treat mania should be an agent that is effective for the maintenance treatment of bipolar disorder, to allow a continuation of the agent following resolution of the acute episode as a means of preventing relapse.

Depressive episodes are more common, more prolonged, and more difficult to manage. Treatments for bipolar depression include lithium, lamotrigine, and atypical antipsychotics (e.g., quetiapine, lurasidone, and olanzapine in combination with fluoxetine). CBT and IPSRT have also been used in the treatment of bipolar depression, with some success. The use of standard antidepressants in the treatment of bipolar disorder is controversial. These agents should not be used as monotherapy in managing bipolar depression, as they can lead to a switch into mania/hypomania and may overall worsen the course of illness. Whether the use of these agents in combination with an established mood stabilizer provides benefit remains unclear. At this point, it appears that, for most patients, the addition of an antidepressant to mood stabilizer does not greatly increase the risk of mood destabilization/cycling but does not appear to consistently reduce depressive symptoms. For patients with refractory or severe depression, electroconvulsive therapy is effective, and it can be used as maintenance treatment as well as an acute intervention.

The duration of treatment in bipolar disorder differs from that of unipolar depressive episodes. Given the devastating impact that mood episodes can have and the data suggesting that 90 percent of patients with a single manic episode will have another mood episode, most practitioners recommend indefinite maintenance treatment for bipolar disorder with even a single episode and certainly for patients with multiple mood episodes. There may be circumstances under which closely supervised discontinuation of treatment may be attempted (e.g., a patient with a single manic episode with a clear precipitant and a period of prolonged stability), but these situations are the exceptions rather than the rule.

Neuroimaging of Mood Disorders

The neuroimaging literature of mood disorders has grown dramatically in recent decades. In unipolar depression, the most robust neuroimaging findings to date have been reductions of gray matter volume within corticostriatolimbic circuits, especially the hippocampus, basal ganglia, and medial prefrontal cortex. For bipolar disorder, findings from structural MRI scans are less consistent, with different studies and meta-analyses finding evidence for both increased and decreased greater volume associated with the disorder. In addition to alterations of gray matter, neuroimaging studies of both MDD and bipolar have repeatedly demonstrated the presence of enlarged ventricles and subcortical hyper-intensities, though the clinical significance of these findings remains poorly understood.

Functional imaging studies have also found that unipolar and bipolar depression is associated with altered neural responses during a wide range of tasks, including the processing of affective stimuli, cognitive control, attention, emotion regulation, reinforcement learning, and goal-directed behavior. In both bipolar and unipolar depression, meta-analyses have suggested an increase in responsivity of limbic regions, especially the amygdala.

References and Selected Readings

- Bauer, M., et al. (2013). World Federation of Societies of Biological Psychiatry(WFSBP) Guidelines for Biological Treatment of Unipolar Depressive Disorders, Part 1: Update 2013 on the Acute and Continuation Treatment of Unipolar Depressive Disorders. *World Journal of Biological Psychiatry*, 14, 334–385.
- Eisenberg, J. M., and the Center for Clinical Decisions and Communications Science (2007). Treatment for Depression after Unsatisfactory Response to SSRIs in Adults and Adolescents. AHRQ Comparative Effectiveness Reviews, 62. Rockville, MD: Agency for Health Care Research and Quality. Available from *Comparative Effectiveness Review Summary Guides for Clinicians*, www.ncbi.nlm.nih.gov/books/NBK158931/2013.
- Frye, M. A. (2011). Clinical Practice. Bipolar Disorder – A Focus on Depression. *New England Journal of Medicine*, 364(1), 51–59.
- Geddes, J. R., and Miklowitz, D. J. (2013). Treatment of Bipolar Disorder. *The Lancet*, 381(9878), 1672–1682.
- Joffres, M., Jaramillo, A., et al. (2013). Recommendations on Screening for Depression in Adults. *Canadian Medical Association Journal*, 185, 775–782.
- Kessler, R. C., Berglund, P., Demler, O., et al. (2003). The Epidemiology of Major Depressive Disorder: Results from the National Comorbidity Survey Replication (NCS-R). *Journal of the American Medical Association*, 289, 3095–3105.
- Lauder, S. D., Berk, M., Castle, D. J., et al. (2010). The Role of Psychotherapy in Bipolar Disorder. *Medical Journal of Australia*, 193(4 suppl.), S31–S35.

- McIntyre, R. S., et al. (2012). Managing Medical and Psychiatric Comorbidity in Individuals with Major Depressive Disorder and Bipolar Disorder. *Annals of Clinical Psychiatry*, 24, 163–169.
- Nierenberg, A. A., Akiskal, H. S., Angst, J., et al. (2010). Bipolar Disorder with Frequent Mood Episodes in the National Comorbidity Survey Replication (NCS-R). *Molecular Psychiatry*, 15, 1075–1087.
- Sachs, G. S., Nierenberg, A. A., Calabrese, J. R., et al. (2007). Effectiveness of Adjunctive Antidepressant Treatment for Bipolar Depression. *New England Journal of Medicine*, 356(17), 1711–1722.
- Savitz, J. B., Rauch, S. L., and Drevets, W. C. (2013). Clinical Application of Brain Imaging for the Diagnosis of Mood Disorders: The Current State of Play. *Molecular Psychiatry*, 18, 528–539.
- Villanueva, R. (2013). Neurobiology of Major Depressive Disorder. *Neural Plasticity*, article ID 873278, doi: 10.1155/2013/873278.

Self-Assessment Questions

1. All of the following are risk factors for major depressive disorder (MDD), except:
   A. Family history of MDD
   B. Adverse childhood experiences
   C. Stressful life events
   D. Age over 65 years
   E. Chronic medical illness

2. Which of the following medications are not usually associated with depressive symptoms?
   A. Beta-blockers such as propranolol
   B. Systemic steroids
   C. Interferon
   D. Opiates such as fentanyl
   E. Topiramate

3. In a patient with severe MDD with psychotic features, which of the following treatments is contraindicated?
   A. Electroconvulsive therapy (ECT)
   B. Antidepressant plus antipsychotic medication
   C. Antidepressant therapy alone
   D. Antidepressant plus antipsychotic medication combined with cognitive behavioral therapy (CBT)

4. Which of the following statements is true regarding MDD and psychosis with peripartum onset?
   A. Occurs during pregnancy or within 3 months of delivery

B. Occurs in <1 percent of deliveries

C. Obsessional violent thoughts regarding the child may be present

D. The risk of recurrence following an initial postpartum psychosis is 5 percent

5. Which of the following statements is false with regard to patients with a diagnosis of bipolar disorder?

A. Once a patient has experienced a manic episode, 90 percent will have another mood episode.

B. The first mood episode experienced by patients is usually a manic episode.

C. Patients with bipolar I disorder have more depressive than manic episodes.

D. Patients with bipolar disorder are at greater risk for suicide compared with individuals with other mental health problems.

Answers to Self-Assessment Questions

1. (D)
2. (A)
3. (C)
4. (C)
5. (B)

5 Schizophrenia Spectrum and Other Psychotic Disorders

DOST ONGUR, FRANCINE BENES, OLIVER FREUDENREICH, MATCHERI KESHAVA, AND ROBERT MCCARLEY

Introduction

Schizophrenia is the most common and important type of a primary psychotic disorder (i.e., not caused by drugs or a medical condition), representing more than half of all patients with a psychotic disorder. In this chapter, we will follow the DSM-5 framework and review schizophrenia and related disorders as schizophrenia spectrum disorders (i.e., schizoaffective disorder, delusional disorder, schizophreniform disorder, brief psychotic disorder). Schizotypal personality disorder, which is closely related (and often considered a schizophrenia spectrum disorder), is discussed elsewhere in this book.

Classification

All schizophrenia spectrum disorders are diagnoses of exclusion – that is, the physician needs to obtain a clinical history and carry out the mental status and physical examination in order to rule out other (secondary) causes of psychotic symptoms to make the diagnosis of a primary psychiatric condition as the cause for the psychosis. A distinction between the various psychotic disorders themselves is made based on presenting symptom patterns and illness course.

Schizophrenia

Schizophrenia is one of the most devastating psychiatric disorders and most important public health problems in the world. It strikes just as individuals are preparing to enter adulthood and often follows a relapsing-remitting lifelong pattern. It affects not only the patients but also their families and friends.

The term "schizophrenia" is derived from the Greek "schizo" (split, fragmented) and "phrenia" (mind) to describe the disjointed experience of people with the disorder (e.g., contradictory thought content and affect). This term was not meant to convey the idea of split or multiple personality, as many assume. Although the term "schizophrenia" is relatively new, schizophrenia-like psychosis has been recognized since at least the second millennium BC. In 1893, Emil Kraepelin coined the term "dementia praecox" for this condition, which was renamed "schizophrenia" by Eugen Bleuler in 1911.

Table 5.1 Diagnostic criteria for schizophrenia (DSM-5)

A. *Characteristic symptoms:* Two (or more) of the following, each present for a significant portion of time during a 1-month period (or less if successfully treated). At least one of these must be (1), (2), or (3):

    (1) delusions

    (2) hallucinations

    (3) disorganized speech (e.g., frequent derailment or incoherence)

    (4) grossly disorganized or catatonic behavior

    (5) negative symptoms, i.e., diminished emotional expression or avolition

B. For a significant portion of the time since the onset of the disturbance, level of functioning in one or more major areas such as work, interpersonal relations, or self-care, is markedly below the level achieved prior to the onset (or when the onset is in childhood or adolescence, there is failure to achieve expected level of interpersonal, academic, or occupational functioning).

C. Continuous signs of the disturbance persist for at least 6 months. This 6-month period must include at least 1 month of symptoms (or less if successfully treated) that meet Criterion A (i.e., active-phase symptoms) and may include periods of prodromal or residual symptoms. During these prodromal or residual periods, the signs of the disturbance may be manifested by only negative symptoms or two or more symptoms listed in Criterion A present in an attenuated form (e.g., odd beliefs, unusual perceptual experiences).

D. Schizoaffective Disorder and Mood Disorder with Psychotic Features have been ruled out because either (1) no Major Depressive, Manic, or Mixed Episodes have occurred concurrently with the active-phase symptoms; or (2) if mood episodes have occurred during active-phase symptoms, they have been present for a minority of the total duration of the active and residual periods.

E. The disturbance is not due to the direct physiological effects of a substance (e.g., a drug of abuse, a medication) or a general medical condition.

F. If there is a history of autism spectrum disorder or a communication disorder of childhood onset, the additional diagnosis of Schizophrenia is made only if prominent delusions or hallucinations, in addition to the other required symptoms of schizophrenia are also present for at least a month (or less if successfully treated).

The following course specifiers are to be applied only after a 1-year duration of the disorder:

First episode, currently in acute episode; First episode, currently in partial remission; First episode, currently in full remission

Multiple episodes, currently in acute episode; Multiple episodes, currently in partial remission; Multiple episodes, currently in full remission

Continuous

Unspecified Pattern

Specify if: With catatonia (note that catatonia is not specific to schizophrenia and can be seen in other conditions)

Specify current severity: Severity is rated by a quantitative assessment of the primary symptoms of psychosis on a scale of 0 (not present) to 4 (severe). The diagnosis can be made without using this severity specifier.

In DSM-5, schizophrenia is defined by a group of characteristic symptoms, such as delusions, hallucinations, negative symptoms; deterioration in social, occupational, or interpersonal relationships; and continuous signs of the disturbance for at least six months (Table 5.1). The tenth edition of the International Classifications of Disease (ICD-10) system, which is used in many countries, is broadly comparable to the DSM classification, although it differs in some details. For example, schizophrenia can already be diagnosed after thirty days of typical symptoms, and no deterioration in function is required.

Schizoaffective Disorder

Schizoaffective disorder is characterized by a combination of symptoms found in patients with schizophrenia and in patients with mood disorders. In order to consider schizoaffective disorder, hallucinations or delusions must be present for two weeks or more in the absence of prominent mood symptoms, but mood symptoms must be present for a majority of the total duration of illness. The correct application of the criteria for schizoaffective disorder requires knowledge about the longitudinal illness course and cannot be made based on a cross-sectional symptom review alone. DSM-5 diagnostic criteria for schizoaffective disorder are presented in Table 5.2.

Schizoaffective disorder shares many features with schizophrenia. The key distinction is the prominent role played by mood episodes (depression and mania) in this condition. Note that patients with schizophrenia often experience mood symptoms as well. But the diagnosis is not converted to schizoaffective disorder unless mood symptoms are prominent and present for a majority of the total

---

Table 5.2 Diagnostic criteria for schizoaffective disorder (DSM-5)

A. An uninterrupted period of illness during which there is a major mood episode (major depressive or concurrent with Criterion A of Schizophrenia).

Note: The Major Depressive Episode must include Criterion A1: depressed mood.

B. Delusions or hallucinations for 2 or more weeks in the absence of a major mood episode (depressive or manic) during the lifetime duration of the illness.

C. Symptoms that meet criteria for a major mood episode are present for the majority of the total duration of the active and residual periods of the illness.

D. The disturbance is not due to the direct physiological effects of a substance (e.g., a drug of abuse, a medication) or a general medical condition.

Specify type

Bipolar Type: if a manic episode is part of the presentation. Major depressive episode may also occur.

Depressive Type: if only major depressive episodes are part of the presentation.

duration of illness. Symptoms usually begin in early adulthood. The lifetime prevalence of the disorder is somewhat less than 1 percent (i.e., comparable to that of schizophrenia). Therefore, this is a common clinical problem for clinicians treating psychotic disorders. It may occur more often in women. The most important psychiatric differential diagnosis for schizoaffective disorder consists of schizophrenia and psychotic mood disorders such as bipolar disorder. However, psychotic disorders induced by medical illness (e.g., HIV, neurosyphilis, epilepsy) or drugs (amphetamine) can mimic the course and symptom psychiatric symptom mixture seen in schizoaffective disorder. As a group, patients with schizoaffective disorder have a more favorable prognosis than those with schizophrenia, and a worse prognosis than those with psychotic mood disorders. The mainstay of treatment are antipsychotic medications, just as in schizophrenia, but in this case, antipsychotics may need to be combined with a mood stabilizer, or an antidepressant, or both.

Delusional Disorder

Delusional disorder is a psychotic disorder in which patients experience persistent delusions as the main psychiatric symptom (i.e., there are no accompanying prominent hallucinations or a formal thought disorder or negative symptoms). The delusions are typically not bizarre (clearly implausible such as violating laws of physics), but the distinction between bizarre and non-bizarre can be difficult to draw in specific cases. Delusions need to last for at least one month for this disorder to be considered.

Table 5.3 Diagnostic criteria for delusional disorder (DSM-5)

A. The presence of one (or more) delusions with a duration of 1 month or longer.

B. Criterion A for Schizophrenia has never been met. Note: Hallucinations, if present, are not prominent and are related to the delusional theme.

C. Apart from the impact of the delusion(s) or its ramifications, functioning is not markedly impaired and behavior is not obviously odd or bizarre.

D. If manic or major depressive episodes have occurred, these have been brief relative to the duration of the delusional periods.

E. The disturbance is not due to the direct physiological effects of a **substance** (e.g., a drug of abuse, a medication) or a general medical condition.

Specify type:

  Erotomanic Type: This subtype applies when the central theme of the delusion is that another person is in love with the individual

  Grandiose Type: This subtype applies when the central theme of the delusion is the conviction of having some great (but unrecognized) talent or insight or having made some important discovery

Table 5.3 (cont.)

Jealous Type: This subtype applies when the central theme of the delusion is that the individual's spouse or lover is unfaithful

Persecutory Type: This subtype applies when the central theme of the delusion involves the individual's belief that he or she is being conspired against, cheated, spied on, followed, poisoned or drugged, maliciously maligned, harassed, or obstructed in the pursuit of long term goals

Somatic Type: This subtype applies when the central theme of the delusion bodily functions or sensations

Mixed Type: This subtype applies when no one theme predominates

Unspecified Type

Delusional disorder is not common, and when it does occur, individuals come to treatment infrequently because functioning is preserved in all areas other than the delusional beliefs. It affects more women than men. Some studies suggest that men are more likely to develop paranoid delusions while women are more likely to develop erotomanic ones. Associated factors include being married, being employed, recent immigration, and low socioeconomic status. This disorder has its onset much more commonly in the middle decades of life, unlike other psychotic disorders, which have typical ages at onset of eighteen through twenty-five.

Differential diagnosis includes other causes of psychosis such as drug-induced conditions, dementia, and other psychiatric disorders. In delusional disorder, mood symptoms tend to be brief or absent; delusions are almost always non-bizarre and hallucinations are minimal or absent. Antipsychotic medication may be useful, particularly for accompanying anxiety and agitation if not for dissolving the core delusional belief.

Schizophreniform Disorder

In schizophreniform disorder, typical schizophrenia symptoms are present for a significant portion of the time within a one-month period, but signs of disruption are not present for the full six months required for the diagnosis of schizophrenia. In this condition, full criteria for schizophrenia would have been met with the exception of the six-month overall duration. As a corollary, most individuals who receive this diagnosis are simply in the early stages of schizophrenia and the diagnosis will convert to schizophrenia (or schizoaffective disorder) once the duration criterion has been met.

Brief Psychotic Disorder

In this condition, patients have psychotic symptoms that generally last at least a day, but not more than a month, and there is an eventual return to full baseline functioning.

Signs and symptoms are similar to those seen in schizophrenia, and other etiologies have been ruled out as causing the symptoms. In the DSM-5, three specifiers for brief psychotic disorder can be assigned: with marked stressor(s) (i.e., brief reactive psychosis); without marked stressor(s); and with postpartum onset (during pregnancy or within four weeks postpartum). In other nomenclatures, this condition is accordingly referred to as brief reactive psychosis or acute and transient psychotic disorder (ATPD).

Since brief psychotic disorder is by definition associated with a full return to premorbid level of functioning, it is a condition with a good prognosis. As such, it appears to represent a different kind of psychotic disorder than the other schizophrenia spectrum disorders. Its prevalence is unknown. It occurs at least twice as often in women than in men. Hospitalization may be necessary for acute stabilization as well as for the protection of the individual and others. During the symptomatic phase, antipsychotic medications are uniformly used but long-term pharmacotherapy is not indicated if the diagnosis is well-established. However, the relapse risk can be high, and patients might opt for maintenance treatment (antipsychotic or lithium) to prevent another episode once it has become clear that a patient has a remitting-relapsing form of the illness.

Shared Psychotic Disorder

Shared psychotic disorder (folie à deux), is a rare and peculiar form of psychosis that is not listed in the DSM-5. Since its recognition can lead to effective treatment, we discuss it here. This is a delusional disorder in which an otherwise healthy person shares the delusional beliefs of a person with a psychotic disorder. This disorder usually occurs in long-term relationships in which one person is dominant and the other is submissive. Most cases involve two members of the same family, most commonly siblings or a parent and child. The treatment is to separate the two individuals, as this results in rapid improvement of the person who does not have a chronic psychotic illness.

Attenuated Psychosis Syndrome

DSM-5 includes the attenuated psychosis syndrome as a "condition for further study" – that is, a condition where further research is encouraged with consideration of placement in the official diagnostic system in future editions. This syndrome requires the presence of attenuated psychotic symptoms sufficient to warrant clinical attention but criteria for any psychotic disorder have never been met. Attenuated psychotic are, as the name implies, milder forms of psychotic symptoms. Typically and in contradistinction to severe psychosis, patients retain insight into the abnormal nature of their experiences. Some individuals who meet criteria for this syndrome progress to be diagnosed with psychotic disorders in the future; therefore the concept is related (but not identical) to the prodrome described under the "Clinical Course" later in this chapter.

Epidemiology and Burden of Illness

Schizophrenia is among the more common disorders in medicine and is the most common psychotic condition. In population-based studies, the prevalence of schizophrenia worldwide is typically found to be in the range of 0.5–1.5 percent of the general population. According to the National Institute of Mental Health (NIMH), about 1.1 percent of the population over the age of 18 in the United States has schizophrenia, which amounts to about 2.5 million people. The World Health Organization (WHO) estimates that schizophrenia affects about 24 million people across the world.

In addition to being common, schizophrenia is also costly to both the afflicted individual and to the society. According to the Global Burden of Disease study of the cost of illness worldwide, schizophrenia is among the ten leading causes of disability among people in the fifteen to forty-four age range. The financial cost of schizophrenia in the United States is estimated to be $130 billion annually, including direct health care costs but also disability income and community services. Nationwide in the United States, individuals with schizophrenia account for approximately 20 percent of all social security disability days, and 25 percent of psychiatric hospital bed days are devoted to individuals with schizophrenia. In terms of the average cost per patient, schizophrenia is the second most costly disease, at more than $16,000 patient/ year (Figure 5.1). This makes the average cost per patient greater than that for cancer, stroke, and diabetes mellitus (DM) because the condition is chronic and relapsing-remitting.

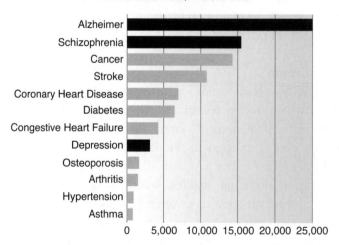

Figure 5.1 Yearly cost per patient of selected medical conditions: United States US$/patient/year

Source: WHO, 2003

Suicide, Violence, and Mortality

The World Health Organization calculates the lifetime global risk of suicide globally for people with schizophrenia as 10–13 percent, twelve times the general population risk. However, recent studies indicate that this figure represents risk in early stages of illness because the highest risk of suicide is usually within a year or two of symptom onset. Total lifetime risk of suicide is probably closer to 5 percent in schizophrenia. More than 40 percent of people with schizophrenia will attempt suicide at least once (60 percent of males and 20 percent of females), and twice that rate will develop suicidal ideation. Completed suicide is more common in males.

Although many in society believe that people with schizophrenia are likely to be violent, violence is not a core and characteristic symptom of schizophrenia, although some acutely psychotic patients can be violent, with drug use and antisocial personality traits being risk factors. Individuals with schizophrenia are in fact at higher risk of being victims of violence than perpetrating it. In addition, people with schizophrenia are far more likely to harm themselves than harm anyone else. Mortality rates are eight times higher in this condition than in the general population, due to suicide, accidents, and violence, as well as medical causes. As a result, patients with schizophrenia have on average a reduced life-expectancy that is a decade and a half shorter than their peers without schizophrenia. Cardiovascular and cerebrovascular diseases and cancer are the main medical causes of death in these patients. Contributing factors include fragmentation of care, smoking, and iatrogenic morbidity. While mortality rates are falling in the general population, they are still rising among people with schizophrenia. Advances in modern medicine generally and improved treatments for the condition itself have not made the desired impact for this patient population of patients with serious mental illness.

Risk Factors

Risk factors for schizophrenia have been the subject of much debate. The most widely accepted risk factors include the following.

Family History

Twin, adoption, and family studies show that schizophrenia has a strong genetic component. Family history of schizophrenia is the best-established risk factor for the disorder. A child whose parent has schizophrenia has about a 10 percent chance of developing schizophrenia. The risk is even higher, as high as 50 percent, among monozygotic twins who share their entire DNA.

Insults to Early Brain Development

People who are born during times of famine are more than twice as likely to develop schizophrenia as those born in previous or subsequent years in the same part of the world. This relationship has been demonstrated in Holland during the famine of 1944 and in parts of China during the Cultural Revolution. Likewise, people who were exposed in utero during a particularly severe flu epidemic in Helsinki, Finland, had a threefold higher risk of schizophrenia as adults than the general population. Finally, people with schizophrenia are more likely to have had difficult births, particularly perinatal hypoxia. Perhaps related to this literature on early brain development are the studies suggesting that individuals who experience abuse in early childhood are at higher risk of being diagnosed with schizophrenia in the future.

Socioeconomic Status

Schizophrenia is much more prevalent in the lower socioeconomic groups, perhaps in part as a result of increased stress and poor nutrition. Equally important, however, is "downward drift" into poverty after the onset of disease because many people suffering from schizophrenia are unable to earn a living and rely on public assistance. Schizophrenia occurs twice as often in unmarried and divorced people as in married or widowed individuals, also likely due to the influence of the disease itself.

Advanced Paternal Age

A subset of patients with schizophrenia has older fathers and advanced paternal age has been established as a risk factor for schizophrenia. The leading explanation for this phenomenon is the accumulation with age of genetic mutations, such as copy number variations, in sperm. These deletions or duplications in the genome may set up the offspring for abnormal brain development and function. More than 10 percent of schizophrenia cases may be accounted for by these non-inherited de novo mutations. This mechanism is not specific to schizophrenia but has been described in other neuropsychiatric conditions like autism.

Sex

Although the overall sex ratio is almost equal, males tend to have an earlier onset than females. Schizophrenia symptoms are more severe during the follicular phase of the menstrual cycle when estrogen levels are low. Such findings have suggested that estrogen has antipsychotic properties. Higher estrogen levels in female patients with schizophrenia are associated with better outcomes and estrogen receptor agonists are being explored as antipsychotics.

Cannabis Use

Cannabis use is associated with a future diagnosis of schizophrenia. Prospective studies have suggested that there is a dose-response, with daily smoking conferring a greater risk than less frequent use; in addition, the risk is most pronounced for use in teenage years.

Clinical Features and Course

It is possible for schizophrenia to develop at almost any age, but it tends to first develop between adolescence and young adulthood, especially in the eighteen to twenty-five age range. Schizophrenia that has its onset in children is likely to be severe. Although the incidence of new cases of schizophrenia declines with age, there is a small peak at about age fifty.

The symptoms of schizophrenia fall into three broad categories: positive symptoms (hallucinations, delusions, and formal thought disorder), negative symptoms (avolition, flat affect, impoverished thought and speech), and cognitive symptoms. These will be discussed in more detail later.

Several studies suggest that individuals who are later diagnosed with schizophrenia already have subtle cognitive, social, and neuromotor impairments in a premorbid phase. Following this clinically asymptomatic premorbid phase, three typical illness phases of schizophrenia can often be delineated. It usually begins with a prodromal phase before the onset of frank psychotic symptoms. Approximately 80–90 percent of patients with schizophrenia report a variety of unspecific symptoms, including changes in perception and beliefs (attenuated psychotic symptoms), cognition, mood, affect, and behavior that typically begin late adolescence or early adulthood and precede frank psychosis by some months or even years. The patient may not disclose these symptoms to others, and many patients go without treatment during this time. Those who do come to medical attention are often diagnosed with mood or anxiety disorders and treated for such. This phase is important because, as we will discuss in more detail later, intervention in the early phases of illness carries great promise for improving outcomes for patients with schizophrenia.

The prodromal phase is followed by an active illness phase characterized by delusions, hallucinations, disorganized speech, and behavior. Most patients come to medical attention during this phase and antipsychotic therapy is initiated. Hospitalizations are common during the active phase. The active phase is followed by the "post-psychotic phase" (or transitional phase, characterized by a tendency to relapse and remit) which evolves into a residual phase where frankly psychotic symptoms are absent or no longer prominent. During this phase, patients often experience role impairment, negative symptoms, and/or attenuated positive symptoms. For many patients, acute exacerbation or relapse may reemerge periodically during the residual phase. There is good evidence that active phases of illness take a cumulative toll on cognition as well as community functioning in patients. After several such cycles, most patients settle into a stable but lower-than-expected level of functioning without further progression.

What makes schizophrenia a major challenge for patients, places a significant burden on families, and turns the disorder into a public health problem is the loss of functioning in the community experienced by many patients. This disorder leads most patients to lower levels of educational and professional attainment than they would otherwise have, lowers marriage and fertility rates, and even makes independent living a challenge. The best predictor of community functioning appears to be cognitive deficits and not positive symptoms. Antipsychotics have limited if any benefit for cognition, and accordingly effective treatment for cognitive symptoms of schizophrenia is a major unmet need in the field. However, not all patients with schizophrenia have a poor prognosis. In fact, most people with schizophrenia can live independently with community support. Even among patients experiencing a severe first episode of psychosis, one-third of patients will have a good long-term outcome (working and living independently), one-third will have an intermediate outcome, and one-third will have a poor outcome. A small minority of patients (fewer than 5 percent) have very good outcomes and lead fully satisfying lives, even with active positive symptoms. Understanding the biological and psychological characteristics of these patients may offer an opportunity for more effective intervention for the remaining group of patients. An interesting literature suggests that community outcomes for schizophrenia appear better in the developing world than in the West. The reasons for this phenomenon are not clear but may have to do with the support provided to such patients in the community and expectations placed on them. An important feature of care is the family atmosphere to which a patient may return after a hospitalization. Families with a high degree of expressed emotions (e.g., a family very critical of a patient) have a higher relapse rate than those with lower expressed emotions, and working with families becomes an important aspect of treatment. Here the social worker dealing with the family is an important team member of the treatment team.

Clinicians who care for patients with schizophrenia need to be skilled at treating all major domains of psychopathology, not just psychosis. Mood episodes (major depression and mania), anxiety disorders (especially panic attacks and obsessive compulsive disorder), and substance use are all highly comorbid with schizophrenia and need to be adequately addressed. In addition, impulsivity and anger can be significant components of the clinical presentation. Finally, partial or poor treatment adherence is common in this condition and this is associated with poor outcomes.

Another important clinical aspect of schizophrenia is its heterogeneity. Patients with this condition present with a variety of clinical pictures. Some have a classic paranoid psychosis with hallucinations and delusions but preserved cognition; others have poorly formed delusions but pronounced negative and cognitive symptoms; others still evolve in their presentation over time. Note that the symptomatic criteria for schizophrenia can be satisfied equally well by totally non-overlapping presentations (e.g., in Table 5.1 criterion A, items (1+4) by one patient but (2+5) by another). Previous classification schemes had described schizophrenia subtypes based on this heterogeneity. DSM-5 no longer recognizes the historical subtypes of schizophrenia (i.e., paranoid, hebephrenic, and catatonic), as they are unstable and as they do not adequately capture the diversity among patients with the condition. Instead, clinicians are asked to capture dimensions of psychopathology to describe individual patients.

Description of Symptoms

Positive symptoms include delusions, hallucinations, (formal) thought disorder, and disorganized motor and social behavior. Delusions are false beliefs that cannot be attributed to the patient's culture or background and are resistant to change. The person continues to believe delusions even in the face of overwhelming evidence to the contrary. Delusions are the most common psychotic symptoms and are extremely variable in content. *Persecutory delusions* are the most common type and involve the theme of being persecuted or harassed by spouse, friends, and neighbors; or being followed, attacked, monitored, or spied on by the government (e.g., FBI, CIA, NSA). *Somatic delusions* involve the belief that the body is somehow diseased, abnormal, or changed (e.g., that the body is infested with parasites or the heart is not beating). People with grandiose delusions have an exaggerated sense of self-importance and are convinced that they have special powers, talents, or abilities, or are an important figure (e.g., a rock star or Christ). In nihilistic delusions, one believes that a part of the body, other persons, or the whole world have ceased or will cease to exist. *Religious delusions* involve beliefs that the affected person is a God, has a special relationship to God, or is part of a larger struggle between good and evil. *Erotomania* is a special case of a delusion where the person believes that another person, usually someone of higher status, is in love with him or her. This may lead to stalking behaviors in an effort to communicate to the object of the delusion that the patient is also romantically interested in them.

Hallucinations are sensory perceptions experienced without an external stimulus, with a compelling sense of their reality, and without control over the sensation by the subject. Patients with schizophrenia commonly report hallucinations in the auditory modality but visual, tactile, gustatory, or olfactory hallucinations or their combination can all be seen. Most typical of schizophrenia are auditory verbal hallucinations (i.e., hearing voices). These voices are often derogatory or persecutory, and sometimes command patients to carry out certain acts. Command auditory hallucinations are an established risk factor for completed suicide in psychosis patients. In his search for pathognomonic symptoms of schizophrenia, the German psychiatrist Kurt Schneider identified a series of "first rank" symptoms which included voices running commentary on the patient's actions and voices conversing with one another. Subsequent research has shown that even though these symptoms are indeed typical of schizophrenia, they are also seen in other conditions (i.e., they are not pathognomonic). Accordingly, Schneiderian first-rank symptoms have been de-emphasized in DSM-5 where they are no longer specifically listed.

(Formal) thought disorders are unusual ways of speaking that can make communication difficult. The most common types of thought disorder include tangentiality (oblique, digressive, or irrelevant replies to questions; the responses never address the point of the question), derailment, or disorganization (lack of a logical connection between one thought and the next). If disorganization is severe, the patient can be incoherent and produce word salad. Circumstantiality (delay in getting to the point due to interpolation of unnecessary details and parenthetical remarks) is another thought disorder that is not necessarily pathological. Other features of abnormal speech in a patient include the use of neologisms (use of words that have meaning only to the patient) or and illogicality.

Disorganized motor and social behavior include markedly unusual appearance, style, or general character as well as catatonic stupor (marked decrease in response to the environment with a reduction in spontaneous movement), catatonic excitement (characterized by extreme agitation), stereotypy (repetition of meaningless gestures or movements), mannerisms (exaggerated or affected style or habit, as in dress or speech), and echolalia/echopraxia (involuntary imitation of speech or movements made by others). Catatonic symptoms may also be seen in other mental illnesses such as affective disorders and may be due to other medical conditions.

Negative symptoms are disruptions of normal emotions and emotion-related behaviors. These symptoms are harder to recognize as part of the disorder and can be mistaken for depression or other conditions such as apathy. Family members can mistake those symptoms for willfully not participating (e.g., "being lazy"). They include flattening affect, alogia, avolition, and anhedonia. Flattening or blunting of affect refers to the complete or nearly complete absence of emotional expression and response. It is manifested by unchanging facial expression, decreased spontaneous movements, poverty of expressive gestures, poor eye contact, and slowed speech. Alogia is impoverished thinking evidenced by poverty of speech and by poverty of content of speech. Avolition is the absence of initiative or motivation to begin and maintain behavior in pursuit of a goal, and it is comparable to the apathy of neurology. Anhedonia is the inability to experience pleasure from usually enjoyable activities.

Finally, cognitive symptoms in schizophrenia involve multiple domains of information processing and problem solving. It is well established in prospective studies that individuals who will later develop schizophrenia display cognitive deficits prior to the prodromal phase and subsequent diagnosis of schizophrenia. This finding is consistent with the evidence that neurodevelopmental abnormalities sustained long before diagnosis are a key feature of the disorder. Like negative symptoms, cognitive symptoms may be difficult to recognize as part of schizophrenia but they are among the most disabling symptoms because they interfere with psychosocial adjustment and in extreme cases with the ability to even perform routine daily tasks (i.e., can reach the level of dementia, hence the old term for schizophrenia, "dementia praecox"). There appears to be a general cognitive problem in this disorder as well as superimposed abnormalities in specific domains of cognition. Specific cognitive symptoms include problems with attention, processing speed, episodic and working memory, social cognition (e.g., ability to perceive or infer others' emotions and thinking), and executive functions that impair the ability to order multilevel tasks, make plans for the future, and flexibly guide behavior in the face of changing contingencies.

One specific kind of cognitive symptom is the inability to recognize that there is any form of brain dysfunction (lack of insight or anosognosia), which is seen in about 60 percent of patients with schizophrenia. Individuals with anosognosia are unaware of having a disease and will deny it. Logically from their perspective, they will often reject treatment and nonadherence with resulting stuttering and poorly effective treatment can result. In other contexts (e.g., certain neurological conditions), anosognosia has been associated with abnormalities in parietal and frontal circuit functions, and this may also be the case in schizophrenia.

Differential Diagnosis

The causes of psychosis are legion and can broadly be divided into primary (psychiatric) and secondary (medical-neurological and toxic) causes. The determination of primary versus secondary causes of psychosis is made complicated by the frequent presence of comorbidity (e.g., drug use or delirium in patients with schizophrenia). Unfortunately, psychotic symptoms are nonspecific with regards to etiology, and no single psychotic symptom is pathognomonic for a psychiatric disorder. The aforementioned Schneiderian first-rank symptoms, for example, while typical for patients with schizophrenia, can be found in a wide variety of "organic" diseases. Conversely, no constellation of psychiatric symptoms unequivocally points toward the presence of an "organic" syndrome or one specific medical disorder as the cause of psychosis.

A delirium that is accompanied by psychosis (i.e., hallucinations and delusions) in almost half of all cases is an important and potentially reversible cause of psychosis and needs to be excluded first. Time course of symptoms (rapid development of psychosis over hours or days) with a waxing and waning course in the right setting (e.g., an elderly patient in an ICU) makes a diagnosis of delirium very likely. Similarly, illicit substance use intoxication or iatrogenic medication intoxication are reversible causes of psychosis that need to be excluded before attributing psychosis to a lifelong psychiatric illness like schizophrenia. Most drugs of abuse cause psychosis during intoxication but alcohol and sedatives can cause psychosis also during withdrawal states. Drugs often associated with psychosis are stimulants, PCP, and hallucinogens. Designer drugs, including synthetic cannabis sold over the Internet, are rapidly becoming important causes of psychosis. Many prescription medications have been associated with psychosis as a side effect.

Steroids are an important class where psychosis is relatively common. However, for other medications (e.g., malaria drugs, INH) psychosis would be considered very unusual but possible. While the list of medical conditions that can potentially present with psychosis is lengthy, a careful history and follow-up will generally provide enough clues to diagnose the medical condition (see Table 5.4 for a partial list of more common medical illnesses associated with psychosis).

Once secondary causes of psychosis have been ruled out, the main distinction is between schizophrenia spectrum disorders as discussed in the DSM-5 (e.g.,

Table 5.4 Medical conditions associated with psychosis (partial list)
Epilepsy
History of head trauma
Dementias
Parkinson's disease
Stroke
Space-occupying lesions: tumors, vascular malformations
Demyelinating diseases: leukodystrophies, MS (rare)
Neuropsychiatric diseases: Huntington's disease, Wilson's disease
Narcolepsy
Autoimmune disorders
Systemic lupus erythematosus (SLE)
Paraneoplastic syndromes
NMDA receptor encephalitis
Infections
Viral encephalitis: herpes simplex
Neurosyphilis
Neuroborreliosis (Lyme disease) (?)
HIV
CNS-invasive parasitic infections: cerebral malaria, toxoplasmosis
Endocrinopathies
Hypoglycemia
Hyper- and hypothyroidism
Hyperparathyroidism
Nutritional deficiencies
Vitamin B12 deficiency (pernicious anemia)
Niacin deficiency (pellagra)
Chromosomal abnormalities
Velo-cardio-facial syndrome (VCFS)

schizophrenia, schizoaffective disorder, and delusional disorder) and episodic mood disorders with psychosis (i.e., bipolar disorder and recurrent psychotic depression). The specific psychiatric diagnosis is made based on the specific symptom pattern over time. While the longitudinal course allows a diagnosis in many cases, atypical cases pose nosological and clinical problems. A category of rapid-onset and recurrent psychosis with good inter-episode functioning (varying terminology depending on local tradition include acute and transient psychotic disorder, Bouffée délirante, reactive psychosis, or cycloid psychosis) is a third important category of primary psychotic illness. Some personality disorders are characterized by temperaments similar to attenuated positive symptoms (paranoid and schizotypal personality disorder) or are associated with stress-associated short-lived psychosis (borderline personality disorder).

Evaluation

A diagnosis of a DSM-5 defined schizophrenia spectrum or other primary psychotic disorder is made on the basis of history and physical exam, supplemented by laboratory testing to exclude secondary causes of psychosis. The initial diagnostic evaluation of psychotic patients has the goal of excluding treatable "organic" causes of psychosis while collecting information supporting a diagnosis of schizophrenia: while schizophrenia is a diagnosis of exclusion, it is still diagnosed based on typical illness course and symptoms. Establishing a diagnosis of schizophrenia can be complicated if the evaluation leads to the discovery of toxins and drugs or medical conditions that could explain the presence of psychosis. The relevance of such "organic" factors with regards to the causation of psychosis can be judged based on biological plausibility, temporality, and typicality of presentation. However, often the distinction between etiological relevant factors (e.g., cannabis use) and incidental findings (e.g., brain imaging abnormality) requires longitudinal follow-up.

Clinical Examination

The history of present illness attempts to delineate the time course of psychotic symptoms prior to presentation and the acuity of onset as well as premorbid functioning; in many patients, a typical prodromal period with nonspecific symptoms (depression, anxiety, cognitive complaints) can be ascertained before psychotic symptoms emerge. The physical examination with emphasis on the neurological examination and mental status examination comprehensively assesses the main symptom clusters that characterize psychotic illnesses (i.e., motor symptoms; psychosis in the form of disorganization, delusions, and hallucinations; negative symptoms; cognition problems; and mood symptoms). Patients with schizophrenia can display a variety of neurological findings including catatonic symptoms; soft motor signs; or antipsychotic-induced problems (i.e., tardive dyskinesia and extrapyramidal symptoms). The mental status exam might be dominated by psychotic symptoms so care must be taken to not overlook a delirium. A basic screening for cognition that includes an assessment of attention and memory is therefore important to exclude delirium or dementia, respectively. The clinical examination can be difficult in uncooperative patients or in patients who have limited insight into the nature of their illness; obtaining collateral information can be the most critical component of the evaluation of psychotic patients. A family history is helpful if positive for schizophrenia or bipolar disorder in first-degree relatives, or if positive for movement disorders or rare syndromes that are genetically transmitted.

Laboratory Investigation

The extent of the medical work-up for a patient presenting with psychosis needs to be guided by the clinical history and cross-sectional symptom picture. More tests are not necessarily better as false-positive findings are likely if screening is done indiscriminately for diseases with a low index of suspicion. See Table 5.5 for a suggested work-up for patients presenting with psychosis.

In most cases, it will be sufficient to obtain routine blood work to exclude an acute illness supplemented by laboratory tests to specifically exclude disorders that should not be missed because they are treatable (i.e., thyroid disease, HIV infection, neurosyphilis). A urine drug screen (UDS) should be routinely included as part of the initial work-up. However, many drugs of abuse (e.g., designer drugs) are not detected by routine UDS batteries: a negative UDS does not necessarily mean that drug use was not present. Conversely, a positive drug test does not exclude a diagnosis of a primary psychotic disorder as drug use is commonly comorbid with schizophrenia. Broadly screening for infections and inflammations with sensitive albeit unspecific tests (i.e., ESR, ANA) is often done but remains of questionable value.

More extensive testing including a lumbar puncture is indicated in patients where the diagnosis remains unclear, particularly if a central nervous system infection or inflammation is suspected. Specific laboratory tests should only be ordered if the clinical picture suggests the presence of a specific syndrome (e.g., NMDA autoantibodies for NMDA receptor encephalitis). Currently, genetic testing is only pursued in cases where there is clinical suspicion of a neurodevelopmental disorder based on the presence of premorbid difficulties like learning disabilities and examination findings suggestive of a genetic syndrome (e.g., velo-cardio-facial syndrome).

Brain neuroimaging is not routinely recommended for young patients presenting with typical first-episode schizophrenia and a normal neurological exam. However, given the lifelong morbidity of schizophrenia a one-time (normal) structural MRI to support a clinical diagnosis of schizophrenia is reassuring and should be considered. In some patients, nonspecific cortical thinning will be visible. A routine electroencephalogram is similarly not recommended as a screening test as its yield is very low. Complicating this issue, more than 50 percent of first-episode patients have nonspecific EEG abnormalities. An EEG is best reserved for patients

Table 5.5 Initial medical psychosis work-up

Laboratory studies
Basic (all patients)
CBC
Electrolytes, BUN, creatinine
Glucose
Liver function tests
TSH
ESR
Urine drug screen
Urinalysis
Extended (consider for screening)
ANA
Ceruloplasmin
Vitamin B12 and folate
HIV*
FTA-Abs for neurosyphilis
Extensive (only if high-index of suspicion)
Chest x-ray
Arterial blood gases
Lumbar puncture
Genetic testing
EEG**
Neuropsychological testing**
Brain imaging studies**
MRI (preferred over CT unless bleeding suspected)
*HIV testing is recommended as a routine part of medical care
**Low yield if used for screening

with a history of head injury or in cases where a delirium or seizures are clinically suspected. If a seizure disorder is suspected, a routine, random EEG is not sufficient, and serial sleep-deprived EEGs or EEGs with special lead placements might be necessary to make a diagnosis of epilepsy.

Neurocognitive Testing

The majority of patients with schizophrenia have cognitive deficits that can reach the level of dementia in a subgroup of severely affected patients. However, the degree of cognitive difficulties is not necessarily obvious on bedside exams of cognition, particularly if only higher-order cognitive functions such as executive functions are impaired. Therefore, patients should undergo formal neurocognitive testing to better delineate the nature of their specific deficits. Key domains to examine include verbal memory, attention, working memory, problem solving, processing speed, and social cognition. This part of the assessment will help with treatment planning but not usually diagnostically.

Treatment Approaches

The treatment of patients with psychotic disorders can be divided into four overlapping phases: the prodromal phase, the acute psychosis and post-psychotic phase, and the maintenance phase. Each of these phases has its own goals and poses its own challenges, which are summarized in Table 5.6. Overarching goals of treatment not tied to any specific phase are optimal treatment to prevent disability and social exclusion and to prevent psychiatric and medical morbidity and mortality.

Table 5.6 Phase-specific treatment goals and challenges

Phase	Goals	Challenges
Prodrome	Prevention of psychosis	Early identification of true cases
		False-positive cases
		Unclear optimal treatment
Acute psychosis	Prevention of social toxicity	Lack of insight
	Keeping DUP short	Early treatment resistance
	Prevention of suicide/self-injury	
	Prevention of violence	
	Achieving initial symptomatic response	
Post-psychotic phase	Achieving early remission	Residual symptoms
	Ensuring treatment compliance	
	Lack of insight and early medication discontinuation	
	Psychoeducation	
Maintenance phase	Achieving sustained remission	Residual symptoms
		Recurrent illness course
	Achieving functional recovery	Poor function and disability
	Prevention of medical morbidity	Antipsychotic-related morbidity

Prodromal Phase

Intervening during an early stage of disease as a form of secondary prevention (screening for cancer as an example) is desirable if the intervention prevents the development of a more-severe disease. By analogy, trying to identify incipient schizophrenia when psychosis is only present in attenuated form holds the promise of preventing late-stages of schizophrenia with ongoing symptoms and severe disability. The importance of this approach is underscored by brain imaging studies which show progressive gray matter loss in the first few years after a diagnosis of schizophrenia – whether as a result or cause of the emerging disability. If we can arrest this biological progression through early detection and treatment, we will be in a position to improve long-term clinical outcomes as well. The challenge lies in that recognizing such cases of incipient psychosis prospectively as a prodrome by definition can only be achieved in retrospect. To complicate matters, several cohort studies have shown that a majority of patients (60–85 percent) presenting for help and who are considered at high risk for psychosis do not go on to develop schizophrenia. Nonetheless, the risk for psychosis is much higher in individuals with certain clinical features (clinical high risk, attenuated positive and negative symptoms), as well as those with risk because of affected family members (familial high risk), than in the general population. These features must thus be considered when an individual presents for treatment. Current treatment recommendations propose cognitive-behavioral treatment and supportive treatment as the mainstay of treatment. If clinical syndromes like depression are present they should be treated with the standard approach in so-called putatively prodromal patients. Antipsychotics are reserved for patients with serious concerns for a psychotic illness (e.g., rapidly worsening psychosocial functioning). There are early, unreplicated, reports of both pharmacological (e.g., omega-3 fatty acids) and psychological interventions being effective in preventing a transition from prodromal symptoms to frank psychosis. It remains to be seen if early intervention can prevent schizophrenia itself or merely delay its onset.

Acute Psychosis and Post-psychotic Phase

Once a patient has developed clear-cut psychosis, treatment with an antipsychotic is indicated. In first-episode patients, the choice of the antipsychotics is guided more by side effect profile and patient preference than by efficacy considerations as all antipsychotics (with the exception of clozapine) are similarly effective in treating psychosis (see Chapter 15 for a discussion of various antipsychotic medications). Unfortunately, in many instances, psychosis goes unrecognized for lengthy periods (one to two years on average of so-called duration of untreated psychosis [DUP]) until treatment is initiated. Keeping the DUP short is critical to avoid social toxicities that can result from being in a prolonged state of psychosis. Examples of such social toxicities are loss of a job and relationships, legal problems due to psychotic behavior, or stigmatization in one's community and among peers from being clearly psychiatrically ill and untreated. Treatment might have to be instituted involuntarily and in the hospital to allow for the protection of the patient and the community. While a full response can take several weeks, improvement in overall symptomatology is usually seen more quickly (e.g., sleep and agitation already improve after a few doses). The post-psychotic phase is characterized by unspecific symptoms and complaints about poor energy and motivation, depression, as well as cognitive difficulties. The resolution of negative, affective, and cognitive symptoms takes several weeks or months, and in some patients marks the beginning of lifelong disability. Since psychosis often responds to antipsychotics, many patients stop the antipsychotic during this phase of recovery prematurely, greatly increasing the risk for early relapse and incomplete recovery. About 20 percent of patients who had an episode of psychosis will never have a second episode. Unfortunately, it is currently not possible to predict who will relapse and who will not.

Some patients will be refractory to standard antipsychotics but show a good response to the atypical antipsychotic clozapine. Clozapine should not be reserved for chronic patients after years of illness but be considered early in the course of schizophrenia as soon as the refractory nature of the illness has become clinically apparent. Other indications for clozapine are sensitivity to extrapyramidal symptoms and chronic suicidality in the setting of a schizophrenia spectrum disorder. Some patients with severe psychosis and aggression can also greatly benefit from clozapine. Due to its more difficult use (e.g., need for regular blood monitoring because of an increased risk for agranulocytosis), this potentially life-saving and life-course-altering treatment remains underused.

Maintenance Phase

Once a patient has recovered from an illness episode to the extent possible, prevention of a chronic course with frequent relapses and incomplete remissions leading to accrued disability over time becomes paramount. The mainstay of treatment during this phase is maintenance treatment with an antipsychotic as these greatly reduce the risk of relapse. It is very difficult to recover psychosocially if the process of rehabilitation and reintegration into society is interrupted by psychotic relapses and hospitalizations. Lack of insight and drug use but also side effects from antipsychotics (e.g., antipsychotic-induced weight gain and tardive dyskinesia) are important threats to optimal long-term adherence. Unfortunately, even optimal and comprehensive treatment does not guarantee full resolution of symptoms, and many patients have to adapt to residual symptoms and to functional limitations.

Antipsychotics alone do not constitute a comprehensive treatment of schizophrenia. Most importantly, while antipsychotics are effective for positive symptoms, their benefit for negative symptoms and cognition is limited at best. Ancillary psychosocial treatments are needed for a more full recovery from illness beyond simply staying out of the hospital and not experiencing psychosis. Cognitive-behavioral therapy is effective to address residual positive and negative symptoms. Cognitive remediation and rehabilitation might be effective in improving cognitive deficits and helping regain lost function.

During all phases of illness, prevention of suicide and prevention of medical morbidity are critical goals. The risk of suicide is increased in all phases of illness but is highest in the early years of illness, particularly around the time of the first episode of psychosis. High premorbid functioning, depression, and partial insight are risk factors for suicide. In addition, treatment programs for patients with psychotic disorders should focus in particular on smoking cessation and prevention of weight gain and its metabolic consequences. This requires close attention to metabolic screening in all patients treated with antipsychotics, but particularly if antipsychotics with high liability for metabolic problems are used (e.g., olanzapine and clozapine). It needs to be stressed that not treating psychotic illness with antipsychotics when clinically indicated for fear of iatrogenic morbidities is not a strategy that leads to better long-term outcomes. Untreated psychiatric illness often prevents good treatment of medical illness, and in many cohort studies, the overall death rate is highest in untreated patients with schizophrenia.

Etiological and Pathophysiologic Insights

The etiology and pathophysiology of schizophrenia remain poorly understood. Although much progress has been made in delineating risk factors and brain abnormalities in this condition in over a century of research, we still lack an understanding of how pathophysiological brain changes arise from risk factors and antecedents leading to the formation of symptoms seen in the clinic. In many ways, this issue is the major unsolved problem at the intersection of neuroscience and medicine.

Nonetheless, several statements can be made about the etiology of schizophrenia as follows. There are likely multiple causal pathways to developing the condition. For any given patient, no one cause can be identified for their disorder. Abnormalities in genes having to do with brain development and plasticity increase the risk for schizophrenia. Risk genes are likely to interact with environmental risk factors such as trauma, hypoxic injury, and exposure to substances like cannabis and predispose to schizophrenia. Genetics is an area of active investigation and there are now very large genome-wide association studies (e.g., with > 25,000 patients and a similar number of controls) showing allelic variation in single nucleotide polymorphisms (SNPs) associated with disease risk at the population level. Each SNP confers a very small amount of additional risk, but there appears to be a hundred or more such SNPs. It is believed they may interact in their effects on key intracellular biochemical pathways to predispose individuals to risk for the condition. Additional recent research suggests rare copy number variants (CNV – deletions or duplications of larger portions of the genome) can also be associated with schizophrenia. CNVs are associated with greatly elevated risk (tenfold or greater) for schizophrenia when they are found in individual patients.

The pathophysiology of schizophrenia is thought to have both neurodevelopmental and neurodegenerative components. This means that insults during brain development increase the morbid risk for the condition, but once an active disorder is triggered, additional loss of functioning ensues. This hypothesis is supported by the finding that a longer DUP is associated with worse biological measures such as gray matter volume as well as with worse clinical outcomes. Note that neurodegeneration in this context does not refer to neuropathologically defined changes, as in Alzheimer's disease, but rather to progressive dysfunction in neural circuitry and grey matter volume loss.

Some theories of biological abnormality in the brains of individuals with schizophrenia focus on the dopamine system. This is because substances of abuse that enhance dopamine signaling are psychotomimetic, whereas drugs that block dopamine neurotransmission are antipsychotic. The latter were discovered through serendipity, as there was no a priori reason to suspect dopaminergic dysfunction in schizophrenia. Although dopamine no doubt plays a role, it is only one of multiple neurochemical systems where abnormalities are found. Research has identified significant abnormalities in GABAergic interneurons in the cerebral cortex and limbic system of people with schizophrenia. This is significant because these neurons may function as inhibitory filters, allowing information signals to be transmitted while silencing inappropriate background activity. In addition, multiple lines of convergent evidence suggest that the ionotropic glutamate NMDA receptor is hypofunctioning in schizophrenia. This would lead to abnormalities in learning and memory, as well as moment to moment information processing in the human brain. Several small molecules (e.g., glycine and D-serine) that enhance NMDA receptor function have shown modest therapeutic effects in schizophrenia.

Extensive postmortem and brain imaging research has shown that there are widespread but subtle cellular, structural, and functional abnormalities in the brains of people with schizophrenia. Thus there is no unique site for the lesion in this condition, and there is no one region that if lesioned can reliably cause psychosis. In fact, this pattern has led some to suggest that it is not dysfunction in any one brain region that characterizes the brain in schizophrenia but rather the integration of activity across distant brain regions. One recent line of work has focused on brain region communication, which is synchronized at particular brain frequencies, especially those in the gamma band range, at about 40 Hz. Although not specific to this disorder, abnormalities of gamma-band oscillations are a consistent feature of the disorder.

The search for the etiology of schizophrenia is motivated by the desire to find effective treatments and ultimately a cure for this often devastating condition. Based on what has been discovered so far, we can safely say that no single biological mechanism will transform the clinical practice of treating patients. Rather, it is likely that multiple interventions will be required, some of which will be at the level of normalizing cognition and behavior. For example, plasticity-based cognitive remediation approaches have shown recent promise. These interventions improve cognition and consequently community functioning. They do not require sophisticated knowledge of biological abnormalities in schizophrenia, but nonetheless they likely have a positive impact on exactly these abnormalities. They also have the additional benefit that patients often desire help with their cognition and therefore accept this intervention willingly – unlike the situation with antipsychotic medications. Last, stigma remains a major barrier for patients who would benefit from currently available, evidence-based treatments. Inadequate funding of mental health services and the resulting lack of access to high-quality care is not an intrinsic feature of the "natural" course of schizophrenia but a societal decision.

Future Directions

What does the future hold for patients with schizophrenia, their families, and clinicians who work with them? Over a century of research since Kraepelin's seminal initial description of "dementia praexoc" has given us a deeper understanding of the complexity of the biological and psychological mechanisms active in this condition. We now know many important facts about the disorder and have treatments that are broadly as effective as treatments for many other medical conditions (e.g., non-insulin-dependent diabetes mellitus). However, we continue to be dogged by the lack of pathophysiology that can explain symptom formation, and by the related absence of mechanistic treatments.

For future directions, we focus on two emerging phenomena: one related to advances in neuroscience and the other to our disease management strategies. Modern neuroscience has already provided us with multiple important insights regarding brain function, especially about how complex systems function and respond to changing environments. Similar to developments in cancer research and clinical oncology, our growing biological sophistication may take away the hope of a quick cure for schizophrenia, but also provide ever more numerous targets for refined interventions.

Clinical researchers are increasingly applying ideas borrowed from other branches of medicine to improve outcomes for patients with schizophrenia. Foremost among them is the concept of disease staging and the superiority of primary over secondary intervention. We know that most medical conditions are easier to treat in earlier stages, and in some cases, arrest of disease progression is possible with early intervention. This suggests that attention focused in early stages of schizophrenia may be particularly salutary in improving outcomes and reducing morbidity. Evidence to support this notion is coming in from studies conducted around the world. But most recently researchers are asking whether we should wait for schizophrenia to be diagnosed at all before intervening. Just as cardiologists identify individuals at high risk of developing coronary artery disease and engage in risk factor modification long before a myocardial infarct takes place, perhaps psychiatrists should identify individuals at high risk of developing schizophrenia and attempt to reduce this risk. This sort of primary prevention, if successful, would constitute the most hopeful intervention.

Finally, our notions of disease management as they apply to schizophrenia continue to evolve in other ways. Throughout history, clinicians have often seen people with psychotic disorders as passive subjects in their own treatment, partly as a result of the patients' cognitive deficits and partly due to societal attitudes toward individuals at the margins of society. There is now a growing movement of individuals with psychosis taking part in medical decision making (in the spirit of patient-centered medicine), and even in providing mental health care as "peer-counselors." This recovery movement can be seen as a natural progression of the de-institutionalization movement, which advocated moving the care of mentally ill people away from asylums where people were warehoused in often terrible conditions to the community. It should be noted that changes in societal attitudes and expectations alone (reducing stigma, involving patients actively in managing their disease) have vastly improved the quality of life for many people with schizophrenia without any neuroscientific advances or new treatments.

The suffering caused by schizophrenia is incalculable. Our ability to relieve this suffering is little but quickly growing. Future clinicians caring for patients with schizophrenia will have an unparalleled opportunity to make a positive impact in the lives of people afflicted with one of the most feared conditions known to humankind.

Self-Assessment Questions

1. Which of the following is not an established risk factor for the development of schizophrenia?
   A. Perinatal hypoxia
   B. Married or widowed status
   C. Family history of schizophrenia
   D. Advanced paternal age
   E. Cannabis use in adolescence

2. Which of the following is the peak age of onset of schizophrenia:
    A. 8–12 years
    B. 18–25 years
    C. 25–30 years
    D. Over age 50

3   Which of the following symptoms seen in schizophrenia is least responsive to treatment with antipsychotic medications?
    A. Auditory hallucinations
    B. Delusions
    C. Cognitive deficits
    D. Grossly disorganized behavior and agitation

4. Which of the following would not be helpful in distinguishing delirium from symptoms of schizophreniform disorder?
    A. Time course
    B. Presence of hallucinations
    C. Waxing and waning course
    D. Disorientation

5. D. F. is a 20-year-old male with a 2-year history of schizophrenia. He has had 4 hospitalizations during this time and has had 3 trials of medication (Risperdal, olanzapine, and haloperidol), which have not improved his symptoms. He had significant extrapyramidal side effects during the haloperidol trial. What would be the best next treatment for this patient?
    A. Chlorpromazine
    B. Clozapine
    C. Ziprasidone
    D. Electroconvulsive therapy (ECT)

Answers to Self-Assessment Questions

1. (B)
2. (B)
3. (C)
4. (B)
5. (B)

6 Anxiety Disorders

MEREDITH CHARNEY, ERIC BUI, ELIZABETH GOETTER, CARL SALZMAN, JOHN WORTHINGTON, LUANA MARQUES, JERROLD ROSENBAUM, AND NAOMI SIMON

The Spectrum of Anxiety Disorders

Classification

Anxiety is a common human emotion and is experienced by all people at some point in life. It is characterized by a state of apprehension about a perceived threat or potentially dangerous situation. In addition, fear is a negative emotion caused by the belief that someone or something is dangerous, likely to cause pain, or a threat. At mild to moderate levels, anxiety can be adaptive, motivating, and can help improve performance and attention. For example, prior to a significant life event such as an important test or presentation, some individuals may experience anxiety, which could serve as a motivator to work harder and perform better. Similarly, fear can be an adaptive response when one is confronted with a life-threatening situation, and a fight or flight response to danger is present and adaptive across many animal species. However, for some, anxiety or fear may be overwhelming, distressing, and interfere with functioning. This may require a person to seek treatment depending on the level of interference and could also result in the development of a psychiatric condition.

According to the fifth edition of the *Diagnostic and Statistical Manual of Mental Disorders* (DSM-V), anxiety becomes a disorder when it reaches a level at which it interferes with social, occupational, or familial functioning or causes significant distress. When anxiety interferes with normal function, it can interfere with quality of life and contribute to other disorders. For example, someone who is persistently concerned about having a panic attack may avoid leaving their home to reduce the risk of having a panic attack in public. Avoiding going out could then result in job loss and isolation from friends and family, which could further worsen anxiety and other mood sequelae.

The symptoms of anxiety are both psychological and physical in nature. Psychological symptoms may include worry, nervousness, panic, and fear. Physical symptoms may include a racing heart, sweating, trouble breathing, and physical tension. The psychological and physical health symptoms almost always co-occur and can be severely disabling.

Conceptualizing anxiety-related symptoms as unique disorders is a relatively recent phenomenon in the field of medicine. Historically, anxiety was discussed in terms of "neuroses" or "nervous disorders." In early editions of DSM, anxiety disorders were defined broadly under "psychoneurotic disorders" and included such diagnostic labels as "anxiety reaction," "phobic reaction," and "obsessive-compulsive reaction." Incidentally, "depression reaction" and "conversion reaction" were conceptualized similarly (i.e., as a psychoneurotic disorder). In DSM-II, the term *reaction* was replaced with *neurosis*, as it was becoming increasingly understood that mental illness was not a mere reaction to life circumstance. The publication of the DSM-III in 1980 brought about further change. Phobic neurosis was divided into specific diagnoses, including agoraphobia with and without panic attacks, social phobia, and simple phobia. Anxiety neurosis was eliminated in favor of generalized anxiety disorder and panic disorder. Obsessive-compulsive disorder (OCD) replaced obsessive-compulsive neurosis, and posttraumatic stress disorder (PTSD) was formally introduced.

Anxiety classification has remained largely the same since the publication of DSM-III. With the publication of DSM-IV, there was a movement toward empiricism in understanding and defining mental illness and the standard for evidentiary support was raised. With the publication of the fifth edition of DSM, our classification of anxiety disorders underwent its largest shift since 1980. Most notably, PTSD and OCD were be removed from anxiety disorders to "trauma and stressor-related disorders" and "obsessive-compulsive and related disorders," respectively, while agoraphobia became a diagnosis of its own (independent from panic disorder).

Epidemiology and Impact

Epidemiology and Course
Anxiety disorders are the most prevalent category of mental health disorders. According to the National Comorbidity Survey Replication (NCS-R), specific phobia is the most common lifetime anxiety disorder (12.5 percent), followed by social anxiety disorder (SAD; 12 percent), panic disorder (PD; 5 percent), and generalized anxiety disorder (GAD; 6 percent). Agoraphobia without a history of PD is somewhat rare, with a prevalence of 2 percent.

Compared to mood and psychotic disorders, the age of onset is often earlier in life, and the course of illness is more chronic. SAD has a bimodal age of onset, typically occurring in adolescence or early adulthood, while PD, agoraphobia, and GAD have more variable ages of onset, with a median age of onset in the early to mid-twenties.

Comorbidities
Both psychological and medical comorbidities are common among individuals with anxiety disorders. Approximately half of individuals with a lifetime anxiety disorder meet the criteria for two or more *distinct* anxiety or traumatic stress disorders.

Mood and anxiety disorder comorbidity is also well documented. Results from the NCS-R indicate that compared to those without anxiety disorders, individuals with an anxiety disorder are approximately three to five times more likely to have a lifetime diagnosis of major depression, three to six times more likely to have a lifetime diagnosis of dysthymia, and four to six times more likely to have a lifetime diagnosis of bipolar disorder. For twelve-month prevalence rates, the strongest association between mood and anxiety disorders is found among PD, GAD, and SAD. Additionally, SAD, GAD, and PD have been found to be uniquely associated with a lifetime history of suicidal ideation and behaviors, highlighting the significant impact of these disorders on public health, with analyses by gender indicating that all three disorders are associated with suicidality in women, while only PD is uniquely associated with suicidality among men.

Individuals with anxiety disorders are also at higher risk for comorbid substance use disorders. Individuals with anxiety disorders in the past twelve months are shown to be three to four times more likely to have met criteria for alcohol dependence and three to nine times more likely to suffer from drug dependence in the last year, suggesting screening all patients with anxiety disorders for these issues is indicated. While alcohol dependence is strongly correlated with most anxiety disorders (with the exception of GAD), drug dependence tends to be most strongly associated with social and specific phobias.

Finally, anxiety disorders often co-occur with medical illnesses. Anxiety disorders have been shown to be associated with a number of somatic diseases such as respiratory conditions, gastrointestinal problems, allergies, atopic conditions, or migraine, even after controlling for the effect of depression. Although the direction of the causality varies and may not be well understood, patients presenting with anxiety disorders and somatic symptoms should undergo a review of systems and concurrent medical conditions should be considered in the differential diagnosis.

Impact

The social and economic burden of anxiety disorders is high. On an individual level, the presence of an anxiety disorder is associated with school dropout, marital discord, reduced educational attainment, and job dissatisfaction. All anxiety disorders, except specific phobia, are associated with lost economic productivity and reduced work efficiency. Furthermore, the cost of anxiety disorders in the United States during the 1990s was estimated to exceed $40 billion.

Clinical Features and Course

Evaluation of anxiety disorders may be challenging as patients present with feelings of distress and concern about disease in the absence of objective evidence. Suffering no less from the subjective nature of their ailment, individuals with anxiety disorders may fear something is amiss with their bodies and persistently seek an acceptable explanation and relief. The autonomic arousal accompanying anxiety may affect many organ systems and imitate physical disease. Anxiety disorders are also associated with marked impairments in quality of life and function. For example, panic disorder is associated with higher rates of alcohol abuse, along with marital and vocational problems. Panic and phobic anxiety are also associated with increased rates of death by cardiovascular events.

While most patients with anxiety disorders improve with treatment, some do not achieve full and sustained remission with current evidence-based interventions. Further, relapse after discontinuation of pharmacotherapy is frequent, supporting the benefit of years of maintenance therapy for many patients.

Panic Disorder

Panic disorder is a syndrome characterized by recurrent unexpected *panic attacks* about which there is persistent concern, or that are accompanied by significant behavioral changes such as extensive avoidance, for one month or more. Per DSM-V, *panic attacks* are discrete episodes of intense anxiety that develop abruptly, reaching a peak within minutes and associated with at least *four* symptoms across different domains including psychological (e.g., derealization, depersonalization, a fear of losing control or going crazy, or a fear of dying) and autonomic arousal (e.g., sweating, chills, or hot flashes), as well as cardiac (e.g., tachycardia, palpitations, chest pain, or discomfort), pulmonary (e.g., feeling of choking or shortness of breath), gastrointestinal (e.g., nausea or abdominal distress), and neurological symptoms (e.g., dizziness, lightheadedness, faintness, trembling and shaking, or paresthesias). Additional diagnostic criteria include persistent concern about having another attack or their consequences (e.g., losing control) and maladaptive behavior changes related to the attacks. In addition, the panic attacks are not accounted for by any other mental disorder (for example, panic attacks only during exposure to social situations in social anxiety disorder).

Whereas the initial panic attack is, by definition, unprovoked and spontaneous, panic attacks may also become linked to typical triggers, and apprehension frequently develops about future attacks (anticipatory anxiety). The age of onset is typically between late adolescence and the thirties, but many patients experience anxiety dating from childhood, often in the form of inhibited, anxious temperament or childhood anxiety disorders. In addition, many patients have *limited symptom attacks* (only 3 or fewer of the panic symptoms experienced); however, these subsyndromal symptoms are also associated with significant morbidity.

Panic disorder is often a chronic disease, with rates of relapse after discontinuation of treatment as high as 60 percent. Untreated panic disorder is often complicated by persistent anxiety and avoidant behavior, social dysfunction, marital problems, alcohol and drug abuse, as well as by increased utilization of medical services, and an increased mortality rate (from cardiovascular complications and suicide). Avoidant behavior often leads to a progressive constriction of a patient's social interactions. Patients may experience chronic distress and demoralization which can trigger depression. Although alcohol can temporarily alleviate symptoms of anxiety, patients who abuse it may experience rebound anxiety, tolerance, and withdrawal, which may all exacerbate anxiety.

Agoraphobia

While Agoraphobia was associated with panic disorder in DSM-IV, it is no longer the case in DSM-V. Agoraphobia involves fear or anxiety in two or more of these situations from which ready escape might be difficult (or embarrassing), or where help may be unavailable in the event of a panic attack or in case of incapacitation: (1) outside home alone; (2) public transportation; (3) open spaces, including large parking lots or markets; (4) enclosed spaces (stores, theaters, or cinemas); and (5) standing in line or a crowd. The clinical significance criterion includes either avoidance of agoraphobic situations, or the need of a companion to face these situations, or intense worry and alarm in the situations. To meet the diagnosis, the fear or anxiety also needs to be out of proportion to the danger posed and typically persist for more than 6 months. Agoraphobia therefore significantly restricts a patient's daily activities, with individuals occasionally becoming homebound.

Generalized Anxiety Disorder (GAD)

GAD was introduced in 1980 as a "catch-all diagnosis" for disorders not fitting in another category. Patients with GAD suffer from *excessive anxiety or worry that is out of proportion to situational factors*. As per DSM-V, the worry over a variety of concerns, must occur on more days than not for longer than six months and be associated with three associated symptoms including: muscle tension, restlessness, insomnia, difficulty concentrating, easy fatigability, and irritability. The anxiety must cause significant distress or impairment in function. Finally, the worry must not be related to features of other disorders, and the anxiety is not attributed to an organic cause (e.g., substance use, medical condition). Typically, people with GAD have been worrying excessively for years with the level of severity of anxiety, ruminations and other symptoms waxing and waning over time.

Specific Phobia

A phobia is an irrational fear related to a specific stimulus. On exposure to that stimulus, the individual reliably manifests an anxiety response. A patient may suffer from a specific phobia of any specific stimulus. Although specific phobias commonly generate circumscribed symptoms, they may interfere with some aspect of a patient's functioning due to avoidance of the phobic stimulus or perseverance in the face of great discomfort (e.g., fear of flying leading to difficulty with travel). To meet the diagnosis, the fear or anxiety also needs to be out of proportion to the danger posed, typically persist for more than 6 months, and interfere with the person's normal routine or cause marked distress.

When making the diagnosis, specific subtypes (e.g., animal, natural environment, blood-injection-injury, situational) should be specified.

Social Anxiety Disorder (SAD) or Social Phobia

Patients with SAD exhibit marked fear or anxiety about social situation(s) in which they are the focus of attention or might be scrutinized publicly. The patient fears that he or she will act in a way (or show anxiety symptoms) that will be negatively evaluated (e.g., leading to humiliation or embarrassment). This perception leads to persistent fear and ultimately to avoidance or endurance with intense distress of the social situation. To meet the diagnosis, the fear or anxiety also needs to be out of proportion to the danger posed, typically persist for more than six months, and interfere with the person's normal routine or cause marked distress. The anxiety can be limited to circumscribed performance situations, like "performance anxiety" (e.g., public speaking); although discomfort related to public speaking is relatively frequent, significant distress or impairment is still required to warrant the diagnosis of the performance only subtype of SAD.

Patients frequently report early onset during childhood. The course of the disease is chronic but may fluctuate as symptoms may be worsened by stress as well as the level of exposure to social and performance activities. Finally, the symptoms should not be better accounted by an organic condition or by another mental disorder (e.g., trembling in Parkinson's disease, stuttering); however, if the fear due to such condition is excessive, SAD may be diagnosed.

Differential Diagnosis

There are distinct differences across anxiety disorders. Both social anxiety disorder and specific phobias are specific fear-based conditions; social phobia includes fear of social or performance situations, while specific phobia includes fear of a specific object or situation such as flying, needles, or blood. In DSM-V, agoraphobia (fear of a situation where one may have a panic attack or pass out) is included in this group of fear-based conditions. Panic disorder and generalized anxiety disorder are not associated with fear of a specific cue, although they may be exacerbated by a range of situations and stressors that may become triggers of heightened symptoms. Panic disorder includes the presence of panic attacks and persistent concern about having future attacks. Generalized anxiety consists of worry and nervousness about an array of day to day issues, rather than any specific concerns, and while somatic symptoms such as muscle tension and gastrointestinal distress are common, it does not require the presence of panic attacks.

Due to anxiety's nonspecific nature, it can also be due to a variety of other psychiatric or medical issues. Anxiety symptoms including panic, worry, and rumination can be present in other psychiatric illnesses including mood disorders, psychotic disorders, adjustment disorder with anxious mood, somatoform disorders, drug withdrawal, and personality disorders. It is important to gather a detailed psychiatric and medical history when assessing for anxiety disorders to best determine the nature of the anxiety as well as determine the primary disorder to optimize selection of the most appropriate treatment. Further, comorbid anxiety has been linked to greater severity for mood disorders and may be associated with greater initial side effects with some medications, such as antidepressants, which can impact treatment selection.

Anxiety symptoms may also be present in certain medical conditions, and clinicians should make sure that symptoms of anxiety are not reflecting an underlying somatic condition that would need specific medical attention. Neurological differential diagnoses include migraine headaches, temporal lobe epilepsy, post-concussive syndrome, multiple sclerosis, stroke, brain tumor, and limbic encephalitis. Cardiovascular differential diagnoses include myocardial infarction and pulmonary embolism. Furthermore, hypoglycemia, hyperthyroidism, and pheochromocytoma are endocrine diseases that may mimic anxiety disorders or panic attacks.

Evaluation

Completing a detailed clinical interview to assess for the presence of anxiety as well as psychiatric and medical issues is vital to making an accurate clinical diagnosis (see the "Sample Interview Questions" later in this chapter). Anxiety disorders can develop from a range of life experiences. From early childhood difficulties to adult life stressors, a variety of situations and circumstances can trigger anxiety. Some people report being unable to remember a time when they were not anxious; some in this childhood-onset group may not realize these symptoms are part of a treatable condition. It is important to understand how a patient has made sense of and responded to the situations that are related to their anxiety. Have they generalized their beliefs about their anxiety to other situations? Do they avoid situations that make them anxious? When they experience anxiety, do they try to avoid the anxious feelings? Understanding their response to their anxiety helps determine why their anxiety is still present and whether it has worsened over time. It is also important to identify the course and onset of the anxiety as well as search for potential accompanying somatic symptoms (headaches, chest pain, etc.) in order to rule out a somatic (e.g., myocardial infarction) or toxic (e.g., caffeine) etiology that would need further investigation and a targeted etiological treatment.

In addition to the clinical interview, structured assessment tools may be used to evaluate for the presence of anxiety disorders. One of the most optimal methods for evaluating anxiety disorders is through the use of clinician-administered diagnostic interviews. Two of the most widely used diagnostic assessments are the Structured Clinical Interview for DSM Axis I Disorders (SCID) and the Anxiety Disorders Interview Schedule (ADIS). Both interviews are designed to be administered by a clinician with knowledge of the diagnostic criteria and phenomenology of mental health disorders. Shorter, clinician-administered symptom scales for specific anxiety disorders, including the Liebowitz Social Anxiety Scale (LSAS) and the Panic Disorder Severity Scale (PDSS), are also available. In clinical practice, self-report measures can be used to assess the severity of a diagnosed anxiety disorder and to help monitor change with treatment over time. For instance, the LSAS and PDSS both have corresponding self-report forms, and the Generalized Anxiety Disorder 7-Item Scale (GAD-7) is a common self-report measure of generalized anxiety disorder. Additionally, there are a variety of other self-report measures of anxiety symptoms, such as the Beck Anxiety Inventory, Anxiety Sensitivity Index, and State-Trait Anxiety Inventory.

Furthermore, when evaluating patients with anxiety disorders, it is important to screen for depression and substance use disorders, given their high comorbidity rates. These disorders can be assessed through the SCID, as well as through screening tools such as the AUDIT-C for alcohol.

Treatment Approaches

Pharmacological Treatment of Anxiety

Pharmacological agents are among the most common and safest treatments for both acute and chronic states of anxiety. Four categories of drugs are in current use for treating anxiety and the anxiety that may be associated with other psychiatric and/or medical disorders: benzodiazepines, antidepressants, antipsychotics, and beta-blockers. Other drugs may also be used, either by prescription or over the counter: hydroxyzine, buspirone, and antihistamines.

Benzodiazepines

These drugs, members of the general class of sedative hypnotics, are rapidly effective and safe when medically prescribed in usual therapeutic doses. Time-limited but distressing anxiety symptoms, such as those associated with an acute medical illness or procedure, are commonly treated with as-needed agents to manage anxiety symptoms, rather than being disorder based. For example, in an acute setting or for specific phobias such as fear of flying, short-term benzodiazepines are among the most commonly prescribed anxiolytics and have high acceptability by patients. The use of short-term benzodiazepines in these situations is effective, has a rapid onset of action, and is generally safe. Benzodiazepines enhance inhibitory neurotransmission in the mood regulatory centers of the central nervous system. Their pharmacology and safety profile is well understood: the drugs may have short or long half-lives and may be low or high potency. The most common side effects are sedation, unsteadiness, and mild cognitive impairment; thus benzodiazepines should be initiated at low doses and titrated slowly, with extra caution in the elderly. Perhaps of greatest concern, benzodiazepines may cause physiological and psychological dependence and withdrawal and thus require careful monitoring. Because benzodiazepines do carry some risk of abuse and interact with alcohol, clinicians are advised to carefully assess for alcohol and substance abuse prior to prescribing.

For the major anxiety disorders with daily symptoms that are more chronic, the risk/benefit profile for benzodiazepines and the manner in which they are dosed should be considered in treatment selection. Paradoxically, monotherapy with as-needed benzodiazepines may reinforce dependence on the agents while simultaneously under-treating a significant and impairing anxiety disorder; thus as-needed use is not recommended as the only treatment for these types of anxiety disorders. Further, such use may interfere with exposure-based psychotherapies for some patients with these conditions. Patients prescribed benzodiazepines as the primary treatment for an anxiety disorder other than specific phobias should thus receive scheduled daily doses sufficiently titrated up as tolerated to achieve symptom resolution. Finally, patients with anxiety disorders should be assessed for the commonly occurring comorbid mood disorders, as benzodiazepine pharmaco-therapy alone would not address these conditions.

Antidepressants

This class of drugs, long known to have anti-anxiety properties, has become broadly recommended for the long-term treatment of anxiety disorders such as social anxiety, panic, OCD, and PTSD. Due to their relatively favorable risk-benefit profile without the same risks for abuse as benzodiazepines, selective serotonin reuptake inhibitors (SSRIs) and serotonin-norepinephrine reuptake inhibitors (SNRIs) have become popular and are commonly recommended for the long-term treatment of anxiety disorders. See Table 6.1 for the United States Food and Drug Administration's approved SSRIs/SNRIs for anxiety disorders and the typical daily dose ranges. Antidepressants are still associated with some side effects that can impair quality of life. With the exception of associated sexual dysfunction, these are generally greatest with treatment initiation and include headaches, insomnia, and gastrointestinal dysfunction. Because side effects may occur prior to initiation of effects, slow titration with careful monitoring and education about the expected time course of side effects and response, as well as the need for daily dosing, are needed to enhance treatment compliance. Documented risks that need to be monitored are the relatively rare serotonin syndrome and a potential increase in suicidal ideation, especially in young adults. Sexual dysfunction might also be a significantly impairing side effect that should be assessed and addressed. Typical therapeutic doses are often higher for anxiety than for depression. To reduce increased anxiety with treatment initiation, antidepressants should be titrated more slowly,

Table 6.1 Food and Drug Administration approved SSRIs/SNRIs for anxiety disorders, typical daily dose ranges, and common side effects

	Class	Indications			Initiation dose	Typical doses	Common side effects
		GAD	SAD	PD			
Escitalopram	SSRI	✓			5 mg	10–20 mg	Nausea/loss of appetite/ diarrhea, anxiety/ irritability, insomnia/ drowsiness, decreased libido, headaches, serotoninergic syndrome
Fluoxetine	SSRI			✓	10 mg	20–60 mg	
Paroxetine	SSRI	✓	✓	✓	10 mg	20–60 mg	
Paroxetine CR	SSRI		✓	✓	12.5 mg	12.5–62.5 mg	
Sertraline	SSRI		✓	✓	25 mg	25–200 mg	
Duloxetine	SNRI	✓			30 mg	60–120 mg	Same as above + Hypertension
Venlafaxine XR	SNRI	✓	✓	✓	37.5 mg	75–225 mg	

Notes: GAD, generalized anxiety disorder; PD, panic disorder; SAD, social anxiety disorder; SNRI, serotonin-norepinephrine reuptake inhibitor; SSRI, selective serotonin reuptake inhibitor

and time-limited co-prescription of a benzodiazepine may be helpful. While tricyclic antidepressants and monoamine oxidase inhibitors were the earliest antidepressants to have demonstrated efficacy for some anxiety disorders, their use has become less common as first-line agents due to their greater risk profiles.

Antipsychotics
While atypical antipsychotics have a lower risk profile than older antipsychotics and can significantly reduce anxiety, agitation, and insomnia with a rapid onset of action at doses lower than those used for psychosis, they still carry significant risks, such as a metabolic syndrome including weight gain, hypercholesterolemia, and diabetes. Thus, despite demonstrated efficacy for some agents, these drugs are not commonly used as first-line treatments for anxiety and are reserved for use as needed for more severe states or in daily dosing for refractory disorders that have not responded to other interventions or for anxiety comorbid with other conditions for which antipsychotics are indicated.

Beta-blockers
Because the peripheral effects of beta-blockers can rapidly block some of the somatic experience of acute anxiety, such as sweating, tachycardia, and tremulousness, they are sometimes used as needed prior to public performance for those with fear of public speaking, a limited form of social anxiety disorder, or adjunctively to manage refractory somatic symptoms. Because of their effects on blood pressure, they should be initiated at a low dose and tested at home prior to

use in important performance settings. These medications do not, however, have demonstrated efficacy for other anxiety disorders.

Miscellaneous Drugs

Buspirone is often prescribed by family physicians and some psychiatrists for chronic states of anxiety but has demonstrated efficacy as monotherapy only for generalized anxiety disorder. Because its clinical effect can take days to weeks to occur, buspirone is rarely used for acute states. Buspirone may be utilized as an augmentation strategy for disorders refractory to an antidepressant. Antihistamine drugs such as diphenhydramine and hydroxyzine, a sedating medication that is often used for states of itching, may also be used for milder states of subthreshold anxiety. They lack demonstrated efficacy, however, for adults with anxiety disorders. Similarly, gabapentin, pregabalin, or other anticonvulsants are sometimes useful, especially in the setting of bipolar disorder, pain, or as an adjunctive strategy, weighing risks and benefits for each individual agent and type of anxiety disorder.

Psychotherapy

Research studies strongly support the efficacy of cognitive-behavioral therapy (CBT) approaches for the treatment of anxiety disorders. CBT targets maladaptive chains of thoughts, feelings, and behaviors. CBT is used across all anxiety disorders with some modifications made based on the disorder. The common elements of CBT include psychoeducation, cognitive restructuring, and exposure. Psychoeducation involves providing information to the patient on their specific anxiety disorder and how the treatment will help address their difficulties. This is an important component of the treatment, as it provides the rationale for the active parts of the treatment. Having a sound understanding of their disorder can increase treatment engagement. Cognitive restructuring involves identifying maladaptive thoughts, observing how these thoughts escalate anxiety, and then helping patients modify them to be more balanced. For instance, a patient with panic may say, "I can't go to the store; I will have a panic attack." Cognitive restructuring would involve evaluating the reality of that situation (e.g., Have they had a panic attack every time they have gone to the market?) and helping the patient think in a more balanced way (e.g., "The odds suggest I won't have a panic attack if I go to the market."). Techniques used in cognitive restructuring include the completion of thought records (i.e., records to track how situations make a person think and feel), labeling cognitive distortions, and Socratic questioning to help a patient challenge their cognitions. Exposure, arguably the most crucial component of CBT for anxiety disorders, involves patients repeatedly confronting the anxiety-provoking situation until their fear subsides. The goal of exposure is for the patient to habituate to the feared stimulus and gain confidence in their ability to approach rather than avoid feared situations. Exposure therapy includes constructing a hierarchy of feared and avoided situations and having the patient work their way up the hierarchy (starting at moderate levels of anxiety and building to more severe). For example, an exposure hierarchy for a patient with SAD includes speaking in a small group (moderate anxiety) to a formal presentation in a larger group (severe anxiety).

A range of psychotherapy approaches may be useful for subsyndromal or situational anxiety, while a number of other targeted psychotherapy approaches that address anxiety disorders such as psychodynamic psychotherapy for panic, and mindfulness-based strategies for GAD, may also be quite useful in practice, although fewer research studies are available to support the efficacy of other psychotherapy approaches for each of the anxiety disorders.

Etiological Insights

Earlier etiological formulations of anxiety disorders were proposed by psychodynamic theorists. In the psychodynamic framework, anxiety is produced by a superego (moral part of the unconscious mind) that overly restricts the id (unconscious part of the mind fueling basic urges), resulting in the ego (the conscious part of the mind) experiencing neurotic anxiety.

From a cognitive-behavioral standpoint, anxiety disorders can be understood as a problem in information processing and behavioral reactions. Distorted cognitions and behaviors such as avoidance serve to activate anxiety and maintain fear responses. These faulty cognitions are often characterized by overprediction of the likelihood, or impact, of negative events. Attempts to neutralize anxiety with avoidance or compulsive behavior serve to "lock in" anxiety reactions and contribute to the chronic arousal and anticipatory anxiety that mark anxiety disorders. For example, distorted beliefs for a person with social phobia include "I will embarrass myself if I speak up," resulting in avoiding public speaking.

Although well beyond the scope of this chapter, much progress has been made in understanding the neurobiology of anxiety disorders with tools such as neuroimaging and genetics. For example, several central nervous system structures, including the amygdala, and neurotransmitter systems, including serotonin pathways, have been clearly implicated in the pathophysiology of anxiety. Acute (normal) alarm states have been tied to central noradrenergic systems, including the locus coeruleus. Thus stimulation of this system provokes panic attacks while its blockade decreases them. Anxiety, worry, and vigilance have also been shown to be mediated by the gamma aminobutyric acid (GABA) neurons from the limbic system, helping explain why GABA receptor binding with benzodiazepines reduces a heightened state of vigilance.

Future Directions

With the introduction of DSM-V, the classification of anxiety disorders will undergo major changes. Notably, anxiety disorders will no longer include OCD and PTSD that have been shown to significantly differ in terms of neurobiological substrate.

While advances in the field over the past two decades have provided strong support for the efficacy of both pharmacological (SSRI) and cognitive-behavioral (CBT) approaches, anxiety disorders remain to date the most prevalent psychiatric disorders in the United States, in part due to a lack of availability of these treatments. Further effort should be directed toward the dissemination of these evidence-based treatments in the community, to address these unmet needs.

In addition, recent advances in the understanding of the underlying neurobiology of these conditions have introduced the possibility of using pharmacological manipulations of fear acquisition and extinction as potential novel treatment avenues. In particular, the use of enhancers of NMDA transmission to potentiate learning processes during CBT sessions has yielded some promising results that warrant further investigation.

Sample Interview Questions

General Screening Questions to Explore for the Presence of an Anxiety Disorder

- Do you notice yourself becoming fearful, anxious, or uncomfortable in situations where other people might not feel as nervous?
- Have you ever been nervous or uncomfortable in situations involving other people, like speaking to others, public speaking, going to parties, eating, or writing?
- Have you ever had a panic attack, when you suddenly developed several physical symptoms, such as heart racing, breathlessness, sweating, hot flashes, or chills?
- Have you ever been uncomfortable or afraid when confronted with specific situations, like getting your blood drawn, seeing blood, flying, heights, tight spaces, animals, or insects?
- Do you feel like you worry excessively or feel nervous/on edge most of the time?

Follow-Up Questions

- When do you experience this fear/discomfort/anxiety?
- What are you afraid will happen (*if confronted with the feared stimulus*)?

- Do you avoid doing anything, going anywhere, or being in certain situations because of a fear that (*consequence*) will occur?
- What (if any) physical sensations of anxiety do you experience when confronted with (*feared stimulus*)?
- Have you experienced panic attacks as a result of your fear?
- Do these panic attacks ever happen out of the blue, or only in situations where you were expecting to feel uncomfortable?
- Has this fear interfered with your ability to socialize or take care of (work, family) responsibilities?
- How much has this fear or anxiety bothered you?
- When did this fear or anxiety begin? Was anything going on at the time?
- Have there been periods in your life when this fear or anxiety was more/less distressing to you?
- How have you traditionally coped with your anxiety/fear?

Case Examples

Generalized Anxiety Disorder

Ricardo was jittery, anxious, and very talkative during the first session. He sought help because he "just could not stop his brain from worrying." When prompted about his worries, Ricardo noted that he worried about everything and anything. He worried about his finances, his children's health, his job stability, his wife's job, his elderly parents, and more. In Ricardo's own words, "The real question doctor is: What don't I worry about?" Ricardo described himself as a "worrier" from an earlier age, which was different from his laid-back parents, who were Latin and abided by the cultural beliefs that "life should be relaxed and fun."

Ricardo had only decided to seek treatment at his wife's request. Andrea and Ricardo had been married for ten years and currently had two young children at home. Andrea noticed that Ricardo's worries had increased since the birth of their second child. She believed that it was because as dual working parents they were more stressed than ever and spread thin with childcare and work regardless of the reason, Ricardo's worry patterns had started to interfere in their relationship and, according to Andrea, the worries were also interfering with Ricardo's work.

Upon further investigation, it was clear that Ricardo's worries were severe enough to warrant a diagnosis of generalized anxiety disorder (GAD) for a number of reasons. First, Ricardo reported worrying more days than not for the past year, consistent with the six-month requirement for GAD. Second, as observed during our initial assessment, Ricardo's worries were associated with increased irritability and being keyed up and on edge, which led to exhaustion and muscle tension by the end of the day. Additionally, Ricardo would often have trouble falling asleep because he was lying in bed worrying, or would fall asleep immediately due to the day's exhaustion only to find himself awake midway through the night worrying. Ricardo described significant difficulties concentrating at work, reducing his work function, which was generating additional stress and worry for Ricardo. In fact, Ricardo reported that he was two months behind on some of the editing he was supposed to have done at his newspaper job. Finally, in addition to the work-related interference, Ricardo also reported significant relational interference, mostly related to arguments with Andrea, in addition to being quite distressed by his worries and associated symptoms, confirming that Ricardo's anxiety symptoms were at a clinical level that warranted a diagnosis of GAD.

Panic Disorder without Agoraphobia

Angelina was in her mid-twenties when she first saw a psychologist at the request of her primary care physician. Angelina had recently gone to the emergency room after feeling she might be having an acute heart-related problem but was told her heart was normal. Angelina was a young, vibrant, active college student, who prided herself on her good grades, a strong group of friends, and a very active life. However, Angelina's life had become restricted after her ER visit as she had begun to avoid anything that reminded her of what she believed was an "almost heart attack."

Angelina had out-of-the-blue, meaning uncued by any explicit stimulus, panic attacks that happened during one of her weekly runs. She could not pinpoint what had happened; all she recalled was a strong sense of intense anxiety, being out of her body, dizziness, difficulty breathing with a sense of chest tightness, shakiness, blurry vision, palpitations, and much-increased sweating. Angelina felt she was certain she was having a heart attack or that something was wrong with her. Angelina took herself to a nearby ER where many tests were done to ensure she did not have a medical condition, such as asthma or a heart condition. The test results were negative, suggesting it was likely that Angelina had experienced a panic attack. Angelina had had occasional panic attacks in high school but reported it was nothing like this panic attack.

In the past three months, since this very intense uncued attack, Angelina denied any attacks as intense as the first and had only a few attacks when she was hot or sweaty, but after that, she had significantly changed her life to ensure she would not have another attack. Angelina had given up all physical activities, as the associated physical sensations were too frighteningly similar to what she experienced during the attack. Furthermore, she restricted substances that could be associated with increased anxiety or related physical symptoms, such as caffeine or chocolate. Because Angelina was so scared of what would happen if she were to have another attack (i.e., that she would have a heart attack, not be able to escape or get help), she also avoided being alone and going to places where it was too crowded and rapid escape might be difficult (i.e., movie theaters and concerts). Angelina had gone as far as to avoid any intimacy with her fiancé, as the "excitement" and physical sensations associated with sexual activity were also now linked to fear.

Despite her phobic avoidance, Angelina managed to get out of the house and still attend classes, but she was only able to do that because she had friends in most of her classes, which allowed her to feel safe. Angelina was very bothered by her symptoms, she felt that they had started to guide her life, and had significantly changed the way she engaged in activities. As such, these symptoms were severe enough to warrant a diagnosis of panic disorder without agoraphobia.

Social Anxiety Disorder (SAD)

Bob was a single man in his late forties who had been a "loner" most of his life when he first sought treatment. Bob came in after reading a newspaper article about shyness and began wondering if he was not a "loner" but instead suffered from SAD, or extreme shyness. Bob was always shy; from an early age, he recalled blushing or feeling embarrassed when talking to other people, especially if they were authority figures (i.e., his teachers). Bob reported that, when he was in social situations, he would get very nervous and feel mild to moderate panic-like sensations (e.g., heart racing, sweaty hands, flushed face), which in turn would impact his concentration. During these interactions, he would worry that other people would think poorly of him and was fearful of "stumbling" over words or saying something "offensive." As a result, Bob kept to himself, often avoiding people especially if they were strangers or authority figures (e.g., his boss). Bob also avoided most social situations where he would be evaluated due to the fear that he might either be judged negatively or that he would accidently hurt other people's feelings. Such avoidance had significantly hampered Bob's career trajectory. Originally, he was passionate about the law and wanted to pursue a career as an attorney. However, when Bob realized that he would have to be in the "public eye," he gave up and instead became a computer scientist, and took a position where he did not have to interact with anyone.

In addition to work interference, Bob also reported interpersonal distress related to his social anxiety symptoms. He had rarely dated in his youth and only recently had attempted to try electronic dating sites, but with no success. He would chat with women online and ask for their phone numbers, but he could never call them or set up a date. Bob remained single and had never married. This was in sharp contrast to Bob's desire to be in a loving relationship and eventually become a father.

Bob was accurate when he sought assessment for his social fears; he indeed suffered had been suffering from social anxiety disorder, a treatable condition, for decades.

References and Selected Readings

- American Psychiatric Association (2000). *Diagnostic and Statistical Manual of Mental Disorders*, DSM-IV-TR, 4th edition (text revision). Washington, DC: American Psychiatric Publishing.
- American Psychiatric Association (2013). *Diagnostic and Statistical Manual of Mental Disorders*, 5th edition. Arlington, VA: American Psychiatric Publishing.
- Borkovec, T. D., Newman, M. G., Pincus, A. L., and Lytle, R. (2002). A Component Analysis of Cognitive-Behavioral Therapy for Generalized Anxiety Disorder and the Role of Interpersonal Problems. *Journal of Consulting and Clinical Psychology*, 70, 288–298.
- Heimberg, R. G., Salzman, D. G., Holt, C. G., and Blendell, K. A. (1993). Cognitive-Behavioral Group Treatment for Social Phobia: Effectiveness at Five-Year Followup. *Cognitive Therapy and Research*, 17, 325–339.
- Kessler, R. C., Berglund, P., et al. (2005). Lifetime Prevalence and Age-of-Onset Distributions of DSM-IV Disorders in the National Comorbidity Survey Replication. *Archives of General Psychiatry*, 62, 593–602.
- McHugh, R. K., Smits, J. A., and Otto, M. W. (2009). Empirically Supported Treatments for Panic Disorder. *Psychiatric Clinics of North America*, 32, 593–610.
- Pollack, M. H., Otto, M. W., Roy-Byrne P. P., et al. (2008). Novel Treatment Approaches for Refractory Anxiety Disorders. *Depression and Anxiety*, 25, 467–476.
- Stein, M. B., and Steckler, T. (2010). *Behavioral Neurobiology of Anxiety and Its Treatment*. New York: Springer.

Self-Assessment Questions

1. Which of the following statements regarding anxiety disorders is false?
   A. Anxiety disorders are the most prevalent category of mental health disorders.
   B. Half of the individuals with anxiety disorders meet the criteria for two or more distinct anxiety or traumatic stress disorders.
   C. Patients diagnosed with social and specific phobias are at high risk to develop substance abuse disorders (SUDs).
   D. Age of onset of anxiety disorders is later than mood and psychotic disorders.

2. S is a 25-year-old woman who recently began a doctoral program in a new city. The patient comes to the medical emergency room in acute distress with a 1-year history of episodes of severe tachycardia, palpitations, chest pain, and dizziness. During these episodes, which are abrupt in onset and last 10 minutes, the patient is certain she is dying. She has had a dozen such episodes in the preceding month. A full medical work-up reveals no abnormalities. Family history is significant for a father who died 1 year ago from an acute myocardial infarction and a mother with a diagnosis of major depressive disorder. Which of the following is the most likely diagnosis?

A. Agoraphobia

B. Major depressive disorder

C. Generalized anxiety disorder

D. Panic disorder

E. Post-traumatic stress disorder

3. A phobia is:

A. A persistent and recurrent involuntary thought that cannot be eliminated from consciousness by logic

B. An irrational fear related to a specific stimulus

C. A false belief based on an incorrect inference about external reality despite objective, contradictory proof, or evidence

D. An acute, intense attack of anxiety associated with feelings of impending doom, somatic sensations, and personality disorganization

4. Which of the following is not included in the differential diagnosis of an anxiety disorder?

A. Post-concussive disorder

B. Temporal lobe epilepsy

C. Hypothyroidism

D. Limbic encephalitis

E. Hyperthyroidism

5. Which of the following medications have not been demonstrated to have efficacy in the treatment of adults with anxiety disorders?

A. Clonazepam

B. Paroxetine

C. Venlafaxine

D. Hydroxyzine

E. Duloxetine

Answers to Self-Assessment Questions

1. (D)
2. (C)
3. (B)
4. (C)
5. (D)

7 | Obsessive-Compulsive and Related Disorders

RYAN J. JACOBY, AMANDA W. BAKER, MICHAEL A. JENIKE, SCOTT L. RAUCH, AND SABINE WILHELM

Introduction

This chapter presents an overview of the nature, assessment, and treatment of obsessive-compulsive and related disorders (OCRDs), including obsessive-compulsive disorder (OCD), body dysmorphic disorder (BDD), hoarding disorder (HD), hair-pulling disorder (HPD), and skin-picking disorder (SPD). Specifically, we review the DSM-V diagnostic criteria, epidemiology and impact, clinical features and course, and etiological insights for each of these disorders in turn. Next, we discuss key points to consider when making a differential diagnosis with disorders outside the OCRD category. From there, we turn to a discussion of the assessment and treatment of these disorders using pharmacological, cognitive-behavioral, and neuromodulation interventions. Future directions in the research on OCRDs then follows.

The Spectrum of Obsessive-Compulsive and Related Disorders

Diagnostic Criteria

The fifth edition of the *Diagnostic and Statistical Manual of Mental Disorders* (DSM-V) was the first version of the DSM to classify obsessive-compulsive and related disorders (OCRDs) in a newly created category, including obsessive-compulsive disorder (OCD), body dysmorphic disorder (BDD), hoarding disorder (HD), hair-pulling disorder (HPD; i.e., trichotillomania), and skin-picking disorder (SPD; i.e., excoriation). The core symptoms of OCRDs include preoccupation/obsessional thinking patterns and repetitive behaviors/compulsions (American Psychiatric Association, 2013). Across disorders, difficulties inhibiting behavioral responses may result in the manifestation of a variety of clinical symptoms such as repeated checking, acquisition of items, hair pulling, skin picking, or repetitive mental rituals. The rationale for grouping the OCRDs together was based upon common symptoms (i.e., repetitive thoughts and/or behaviors), associated features (e.g., age of onset, comorbidity patterns, heredity), etiology (i.e., neurobiological and neurotransmitter abnormalities), and similar treatment response profiles. (For comprehensive reviews on the development of this diagnostic class, see Abramowitz & Jacoby, 2015; Phillips et al., 2010).

Obsessive-Compulsive Disorder

Previously included within the anxiety disorders category in DSM-IV, OCD is the flagship disorder of the OCRDs in DSM-V. OCD is characterized by unwanted intrusive thoughts, images, or impulses (i.e., *obsessions*) that cause significant distress and anxiety. The content of patients' obsessions can be very heterogeneous, including fears of contamination, doubts about making a mistake, unwanted aggressive or sexual impulses, or a need for symmetry. Moreover, the content of obsessions is typically incongruent with the person's belief system and not in line with how the individual sees him/herself (i.e., ego-dystonic). In response to obsessions, individuals with OCD engage in ritualistic *compulsions* (both covert mental rituals and overt behaviors) in order to reduce the anxiety triggered by the obsessional thoughts. Such compulsions may include checking for signs of harm, repeating/arranging rituals, washing/cleaning, and/or praying. Additionally, patients often rely on avoidance in order to escape distressing obsessions and time-consuming compulsions. In order to receive a diagnosis of OCD, the level of obsessions and/or compulsions must be severe enough to cause marked distress or interferences in functioning (American Psychiatric Association, 2013).

Body Dysmorphic Disorder

BDD is a distressing preoccupation with one or more perceived flaws in physical appearance that are slight or unobservable. BDD is also associated with repetitive behaviors (e.g., mirror checking, excessive grooming or make-up use, skin picking in response to appearance concerns, touching/measuring body parts, and reassurance seeking) or mental acts (e.g., comparing one's appearance with that of others) in response to the body image concerns. These behaviors take up significant time and interfere with other social/work/school/role obligations (American Psychiatric Association, 2013). BDD was moved from the somatoform disorders in DSM-IV to the OCRD section in DSM-V; however, the diagnostic criteria were essentially unchanged.

Hoarding Disorder

HD is characterized by persistent difficulty discarding or parting with possessions (regardless of their actual value), which often results in the amassing of possessions that fill up and clutter living areas of the home, car, or workplace to the extent that their intended use is no longer possible. If living areas are uncluttered, to meet criteria for HD, this must be due to interventions of a third party (e.g., family member or authority; American Psychiatric Association, 2013). Hoarding is also associated with distress or impairment in social, occupational, or other important areas of functioning (including maintaining a safe environment for self and others). Hoarding was previously listed as a symptom of obsessive-compulsive personality disorder (OCPD) and often considered as a symptom of OCD, although research strongly suggests it is distinct from OCD (e.g., Mataix-Cols et al., 2010), supporting its separation as a new diagnosis included in DSM-V.

Hair Pulling and Skin-Picking Disorders

Finally, HPD and SPD both involve repetitive grooming behaviors. Research suggests that these problems frequently co-occur, have substantial similarities in symptom presentation and course of illness, and may have common risk factors (e.g., genetic vulnerabilities; Snorrason, Belleau, & Woods, 2012). HPD was previously classified as an impulse control disorder in DSM-IV and is characterized by the recurrent pulling out of one's hair (e.g., using fingernails and tweezers to pull hairs from their head, face, and pubic or other areas), with repeated attempts to stop hair pulling, resulting in measurable hair loss. While not a criterion for DSM-V, patients sometimes report feeling tension prior to or during pulling (i.e., a premonitory urge) and experiencing pleasure, relief, or gratification while pulling. In order to meet diagnostic criteria for HPD, the pulling behavior and/or the significant loss of hair must lead to significant distress or impairment in social, work, or role functioning.

Similarly, SPD is a new diagnosis in DSM-V and is characterized by recurrent skin picking (e.g., using fingernails or other implements to pick at the face, arms, legs, or other areas) that results in visible tissue damage and at times scarring. As a result of the skin picking and damage, patients with SPD also experience significant distress and/or functional impairment due to problems socially, at work/school, or at home.

Epidemiology and Impact

Each of the OCRDs has a significant public health impact. First, OCD is a substantial impairing and burdensome psychiatric condition, with a lifetime prevalence of approximately 2 percent in the population. It is identified as one of the top ten causes of health-related disability worldwide among all medical and psychiatric conditions due to the extreme distress patients experience, the amount of time the disorder consumes, as well as its relatively early onset and chronic course. Next, large population-based surveys have found the current prevalence rates for BDD to be approximately 1.7 to 2.4 percent (e.g., Buhlmann et al., 2010). Increased rates of cosmetic surgery, hospitalization, suicidal ideation, and suicide attempts due to appearance concerns are reported by these patients (e.g., Buhlmann et al., 2010). Thus, BDD is not only a commonly occurring disorder but also one that is associated with significant morbidity and mortality.

Although there have been only a few studies to date investigating the prevalence rates of HD by DSM-V criteria, preliminary estimates indicate that HD occurs at a prevalence of approximately 4–5 percent in the general population (Steketee & Frost, 2014). HD is associated with a considerable public health burden, especially in regard to the commonly hazardous living conditions that result. In extreme cases, the hoarded material has endangered the lives of not only the individual with HD but also neighbors (e.g., been a cause of fires).

Finally, large epidemiological studies of HPD and SPD have not been conducted; however, in the general population, SPD has reported prevalence rates ranging from 1.4 percent to 5.4 percent and HPD around 0.6 percent (Grant & Chamberlain, 2016; Grant et al., 2012). Patients with HPD and SPD report social, occupational, and academic impairment, financial burdens, as well as additional medical or mental health concerns (such as depression and anxiety), which they attribute to hair pulling and skin picking (Grant & Chamberlain, 2016). Additionally, HPD has the potential for mortality from trichobezoars (i.e., a buildup of ingested hair in the gastrointestinal system, often requiring surgical intervention), whereas severe skin picking can lead to infections which also may require surgery.

Clinical Features and Course

OCD is a heterogeneous disorder in which symptom expression may include a broad array of obsessions/compulsions that tend to vary within and across the following four types of symptom clusters or dimensions: (1) contamination/decontamination-related obsessions and washing/cleaning rituals, (2) responsibility for harm/doubting obsessions and checking rituals, (3) need for symmetry and ordering/arranging rituals, and (4) autogenous/unacceptable/"taboo" thoughts (e.g., related to violence, religion, sex, immorality, etc.) and covert mental neutralizing.

DSM-V also includes two clinical specifiers of OCD, including (a) the degree of insight patients have into their obsessive beliefs (ranging from good/fair insight to absent insight/delusional beliefs), and (b) whether the OCD is tic-related (i.e., whether the individual has a history of a tic disorder). The majority of patients with OCD have good insight regarding their obsessions (Phillips et al., 2012); in other words, they acknowledge that the obsessions and/or compulsions are unreasonable or excessive (e.g., "I know that I most likely won't contract AIDS if I use this public restroom, but the thought of having the disease is so horrible that I think it's better to be safe than sorry"). Poor insight is correlated with worse symptom severity and treatment outcomes.

Like all OCRDs, OCD tends to be chronic in nature without treatment and has a waxing and waning course that tends to correspond with general life stressors. Approximately half of OCD cases begin in childhood (ages 8–12); however, symptoms may also onset in late teens and early adulthood. The male to female ratio of OCD is approximately 1:1 in adults; however, girls have a later mean age of onset, resulting in more boys with pediatric OCD.

BDD is typified by a preoccupation with perceived appearance defects, with patients reporting that their appearance is ugly, abnormal, or deformed. Perceived defects can involve any area of the body, and hair preoccupations are the most common areas of concern (Bjornsson, Didie, & Phillips, 2010). Patients with BDD often attempt to hide or camouflage their perceived defects and frequently compare their appearance to others. Many will seek consultation or request clinical procedures from dermatologists and/or cosmetic surgeons. DSM-V specifiers for BDD include whether there is muscle dysmorphia (i.e., the preoccupation with the idea that one's body build lacks muscular tone) and/or limited insight. The degree of insight is often compromised in BDD, and patients may be quite delusional regarding their body image (Phillips et al., 2012). In comparing patients with BDD and delusional insight to nondelusional patients with BDD, research has shown that when controlling for symptom severity, the two groups differ only in terms of educational attainment, suggesting that BDD's delusional and nondelusional forms have many more similarities than differences and constitute the same disorder. BDD typically onsets during early adolescence, has a waxing and waning symptom course, and estimates of the male to female gender ratio range from 1:1 to 2:3 (Bjornsson et al., 2010).

For HD, DSM-V also includes two clinical specifiers to provide additional information about the hoarding diagnosis, including whether there is excessive acquisition (i.e., collecting of items) and/or limited insight. Patients with hoarding may or may not have issues with severe domestic squalor (i.e., unsanitary conditions in the home) due to their hoarding symptoms (e.g., accumulating spoiled food). Hoarding disorder most commonly onsets in adolescence and, in the majority of patients, before age twenty. HD has a chronic course with very little waxing and waning of symptoms (Steketee & Frost, 2014). Stressful and traumatic events are common in patients with HD, and relationship changes and interpersonal violence are temporally associated with symptom onset or exacerbation. The gender ratio of HD is inconsistently reported in the literature but appears to occur in an approximately 1:1 male: female ratio or be slightly more prevalent in men.

Patients with HPD and SPD often pull hair/pick skin from primarily one site on the body, but this site can change over time. Individuals with both disorders tend to pull hair and pick skin with imperfections; specifically, patients with HPD often seek to pull hairs that are "different" from other hairs (e.g., coarse, curly, or gray hairs), and patients with SPD target bumps/blemishes on the skin. Of note, HPD and SPD are similar to the other OCRDs (i.e., OCD, BDD) in the shared difficulty resisting or inhibiting repetitive maladaptive behaviors. However, the repetitive behaviors in HPD/SPD are not solely performed with the desire to reduce or avoid distress/anxiety (i.e., negative reinforcement; although individuals do at times report the urge to pull/pick in order to regulate emotions), but these behaviors are also associated with positive reinforcement (e.g., gratification).

Hair pulling and skin picking behavior can occur within the context of a BDD diagnosis, with approximately one-third of patients with BDD reporting skin-picking or hair-pulling symptoms. Thus, it is important to conduct a functional assessment to determine whether the picking/pulling is only performed in order to improve the appearance of a perceived defect (vs. to regulate emotions, derive pleasure, etc.). HPD and SPD tend to onset in adolescence, with an average age of onset of 11.8 years old, but these conditions have been seen in patients as young as 1-year-old. While longitudinal data is lacking, cross-sectional studies suggest that both disorders are chronic, with waxing and waning symptom severity (Grant & Chamberlain, 2016).

Etiological Insights

In general, research supports the idea that OCRDs run in families and there is likely a genetic component in the development of each of the disorders. Several genes have been implicated as potentially conferring risk for OCD and/or related disorders in human studies, or in the context of animal models (e.g., SLC1A1, OLIG2, SAPAP have been studied as candidate genes in OCRD genetic studies; e.g., Stewart et al., 2013). Still, there is no single gene or genetic make-up that has been shown to cause any of the OCRDs, indicating that psychosocial variables (cognitive processes or temperamental antecedents such as perfectionism) and life stressors also play a developmental role (Phillips et al., 2010).

Findings from functional brain imaging studies support a neurobiological model for the pathophysiology of OCD, which involves hyperactivity in the frontostriatal system (Dougherty et al., 2018). Specifically, the orbitofrontal and anterior cingulate cortex, caudate nucleus, and the thalamus have all been implicated as nodes in this hyperactive circuit; activity within these regions has been observed to be elevated during resting or neutral states, increased during symptom provocation, and attenuated following successful treatment. Moreover, OCD has been characterized by fear extinction abnormalities (evidenced by elevated psychophysiological responding during extinction recall relative to healthy controls), with identifiable neurobiological correlates as measured by functional brain imaging (e.g., reduced activation in the ventromedial prefrontal cortex; Milad et al., 2013). Additional neurobiological research implicates dysfunctional serotonergic and dopaminergic systems in OCRDs.

Differential Diagnosis

OCRDs share similarities with many other diagnoses and diagnostic groups in the DSM-V. Thus, several important differential diagnoses are discussed in this section. Specifically, important similarities and distinctions in symptom functionality to consider when making a diagnosis will be briefly reviewed. A number of the differences between the OCRDs and the differential diagnoses discussed as follows have to do with the ego-dystonic versus ego-syntonic nature of the disorder. In general, the OCRDs tend to be ego-dystonic disorders, indicating that the obsessional beliefs are incompatible with the patient's self-identity or image.

Tic Disorders

OCRDs and tic disorders (e.g., Tourette's disorder) both exhibit repetitive behaviors in response to a trigger and OCRDs commonly co-occur with tic disorders. However, in tic disorders, repetitive behaviors are usually exhibited to alleviate unpleasant sensations/premonitory urges, rather than obsessional thoughts. In general, OCRD-related rituals reduce anxiety, whereas tics reduce physical tension. Patients are often unaware of their tics, and they can have limited premeditation or thought processes involved in tic behaviors. OCRDs, on the other hand, typically involve a conscious link between the cognitive process of obsessions and compulsive behavior. This distinction becomes more difficult to determine, however, in the case of complex tics with multiple processes that may appear goal-directed as opposed to sudden, rapid, simple tic processes.

Hypochondriasis/Illness Anxiety Disorder.

Similar to compulsions in OCRDs, individuals with illness anxiety disorder (IAD; or "hypochondriasis") frequently engage in behaviors (such as reassurance seeking or body scanning) to reduce anxiety associated with the belief that they may have a disease or illness (Abramowitz, Schwartz, & Whiteside, 2002). Patients with IAD have thematically limited fears around disease and have less insight into the psychological cause of their distress than individuals with OCD, for instance, who are often eager to consider the irrationality of their obsessions. Patients with IAD have conviction about the feared disease and thus believe that any compulsive behaviors are justified. Additionally, patients with IAD are often worried about diffuse internal bodily sensations (e.g., headaches as potential signs of cancer), while patients with OCD are typically less preoccupied by physical sensations and have more varied obsessions and compulsions (e.g., sex, violence, harm, etc.).

Obsessive-Compulsive Personality Disorder (OCPD)

OCPD shares a preoccupation with perfection, order, and mental/interpersonal control with some of the OCRDs. Rigid behavior seen in OCPD, however, is usually as a result of a firmly held ego-syntonic belief (i.e., beliefs that are in line with the person's sense of self), rather than an intrusive unwanted (i.e., ego-dystonic) thought (Fineberg, Kaur, Kolli, Mpavaenda, & Reghunandanan, 2015). For instance, patients with OCPD may engage in ordering and arranging behaviors but describe such tasks as enjoyable and consistent with being an orderly person. Moreover, unlike OCD, repetitive behaviors in OCPD are not aimed at lowering obsession-related distress. For example, someone with OCPD might report that they need to maintain a certain routine because it is the "correct" and desirable thing to do rather than due to intrusive thoughts about something bad happening if they were to deviate from their routine.

Schizophrenia/Psychotic Disorders

Bizarre content of repetitive thoughts and overvalued ideas are present in both psychotic disorders and OCRDs (Kozak & Foa, 1994). Thus, obsessions (as seen in OCD) and delusions (as seen in psychotic disorders) may not be categorically distinct, but rather may exist on a continuum and vary by degree of insight (i.e., lower insight in psychotic disorders). However, distinctions can also be made, as the presence of compulsions or neutralizing behaviors indicates a diagnosis of OCD rather than a psychotic disorder, and other symptoms of psychosis (e.g., loose associations, negative symptoms) must additionally be present to diagnose schizophrenia.

Autism Spectrum Disorders (ASD)

ASD and OCRDs are similarly characterized by repetitive thoughts (i.e., fixated interests in ASD and obsessions in OCD) and strict adherence to routines and rituals. Furthermore, co-morbid OCD is common in ASD (Wu, Rudy, & Storch, 2014). However, when individuals with ASD become fixated on certain interests, they tend to enjoy the content of a particular topic (e.g., trains, dinosaurs). This is in contrast to obsessions and rituals and routines in OCD that are usually ego-dystonic (Wu et al., 2014). Similarly, an individual with ASD may engage in repetitive behaviors such as opening and closing a door repeatedly because he enjoys it, or it is calming, or in order to communicate something (e.g., that he wants to leave). In contrast, a patient with OCD may open and close the door a targeted number of times in order to neutralize an unwanted obsessional thought (e.g., about catastrophic consequences if the door is not closed in a way that is "just right").

Evaluation

Semi-Structured Diagnostic Interviews

The use of structured diagnostic interviews for the assessment OCRDs is common in research studies (but less common outside of a research setting). These interviews facilitate diagnostic decisions by utilizing specific questions to assess symptoms according to DSM criteria. The Structured Clinical Interview for DSM-V (SCID-5; First, Williams, Karg, & Spitzer, 2015) is a commonly used semi-structured clinical interview, which contains modules for OCD as well as the other OCRDs (BDD, HD, HPD, SPD as optional modules). The SCID is divided into sections by disorders and detailed questions regarding each disorder are administered as clinically indicated. These interviews usually take between 60 and 120 minutes to administer.

Clinician-Rated Symptom Severity Instruments

Individuals trained in the use of clinician-rated assessments utilize semi-structured interviews to gather severity ratings of OCRD-related distress and impairment. The gold standard clinician-rated instrument for assessing OCD symptom severity is the Yale-Brown Obsessive-Compulsive Scale (Y-BOCS; Goodman et al., 1989). The Y-BOCS examines the severity of obsessions and compulsions over the past week via the following five parameters: (a) the amount of time they occupy, (b) the degree to which they cause impairment in work, school, relationships, and activities, (c) the amount of distress they cause, (d) the frequency that patients attempt to disregard obsessions and refrain from compulsions, and (e) the level of control over these symptoms. Items are rated on a 5-point Likert scale from 0 (no symptomatology) to 4 (extreme symptomatology). Total scores on the Y-BOCS range from 0 to 40, and higher scores indicate greater symptom severity.

The Yale-Brown Obsessive-Compulsive Scale Modified for BDD (BDD-YBOCS) is an adapted version of this measure for BDD (Phillips et al., 1997). The BDD-YBOCS examines the severity of obsessional preoccupations about perceived appearance flaws (items 1–5), severity of BDD-related repetitive behaviors (e.g., comparing, mirror checking, camouflaging; items 6–10), insight into appearance beliefs (item 11), and avoidance due to BDD (item 12). Scores on the BDD-YBOCS range from 0 to 48, and higher scores indicate greater symptom severity.

Self-Report Instruments

In addition to clinician-rated measures, patient self-report measures are frequently used and provide several advantages in OCRD assessment: they can be completed quickly and independently of clinician time and thus are useful screening tools or markers of progress over treatment, and patients may feel more comfortable completing measures independently rather than in response to a clinician. Thus, used in conjunction with clinician-rated measures, self-report forms may add additional information to the clinical picture.

First, the Obsessive-Compulsive Inventory-Revised (OCI-R; Foa et al., 2002) is an eighteen-item measure of the degree to which patients are bothered or distressed by OCD symptoms in the past month (e.g., "I am upset by unpleasant thoughts that come into my mind against my will"). The OCI-R includes six dimensions: (1) Washing, (2) Checking/Doubting, (3) Obsessing, (4) Mental Neutralizing, (5) Ordering, and (6) Hoarding.[1] The BDD-Symptom Scale (BDD-SS; Wilhelm, Greenberg, Rosenfield, Kasarskis, & Blashill, 2016) rates the severity of specific BDD symptoms and associated thoughts, feelings, and behaviors including: checking rituals, grooming rituals, shape/weight-related rituals, hair pulling/skin picking rituals, surgery/dermatology seeking rituals, avoidance, and BDD-related cognitions. The Saving Inventory–Revised (SI-R; Frost, Steketee, & Grisham, 2004) is a twenty-

[1] Of note, given that hoarding is no longer considered a subtype of OCD (and is now its own diagnosis in DSM-5), previous studies examining the psychometric properties of the OCI-R subscales recommend removing the Hoarding subscale from the total score.

three-item self-report assessment of hoarding symptoms across three subscales: difficulty discarding, acquisition, and clutter. The Massachusetts General Hospital Hairpulling Scale (MGH-HPS; Keuthen et al., 1995) consists of seven items of HPD symptom severity in the past week, including frequency and intensity of urges to pull, perceived control over urges, frequency of hair pulling, attempts to resist and control over hair pulling, and associated distress. Finally, the Skin Picking Scale – Revised (SPS-R; Snorrason, Ólafsson, et al., 2012) is an eight-item self-report measure of skin-picking disorder severity in the past week, with items assessing the frequency and intensity of urges to pick one's skin; time spent and control over skin picking; associated distress, impairment, and avoidance; and resulting skin damage.

Treatment Approaches

In OCD, serotonin reuptake inhibitors (SRIs, often prescribed in relatively high dosages comparable to effective dosages for depression) and dopamine antagonists (i.e., antipsychotic/neuroleptics used mostly as an augmentation to SRIs) have been shown to be effective in decreasing symptom severity (Casale et al., 2018). Cognitive-behavioral therapy (CBT) with a prominent exposure and response prevention (ERP) component is also highly effective in treating OCD and is the gold-standard psychological intervention (Olatunji, Davis, Powers, & Smits, 2013). ERP entails repeated and prolonged confrontation with feared stimuli (that objectively pose no more than "everyday risk"; i.e., exposure), without attempting to reduce distress by withdrawing from the situation or performing compulsive rituals (i.e., response prevention). Comparisons indicate that ERP may be of equal or better efficacy compared to pharmacological treatment.

Cognitive therapy (CT) for OCD was also developed to directly address maladaptive belief domains in OCD (e.g., inflated sense of responsibility, perfectionism, over-importance of thoughts; Wilhelm & Steketee, 2006). CT for OCD serves to identify patients' cognitive interpretations and beliefs about intrusive thoughts and to instruct patients on how to modify distortions using techniques such as cognitive restructuring, behavioral experiments, and improved processing of emotional information. CT is a useful alternative to prolonged ERP for patients who are unwilling or unable to engage in exposure due to the provocation of high levels of discomfort (Wilhelm & Steketee, 2006). Initial research suggests CT for OCD is successful and well-tolerated and may provide an alternative or adjunctive treatment to ERP (Steketee, Siev, Yovel, Lit, & Wilhelm, 2018). Finally, deep brain stimulation (DBS) has been shown to be effective in treatment-refractory patients with severe illness who do not respond satisfactorily to other psychological/pharmacological interventions (B. D. Greenberg et al., 2010) and has earned humanitarian device exemption status with the FDA.

Similar to OCD, SRIs (also at high dosages) are also effective in treating BDD (Phillips & Hollander, 2008). Neuroleptic augmentation for SRIs was not found to be more effective than placebo; however, this is based on limited data and augmentation needs to be further studied in BDD. Again, CBT with a prominent component of both ERP and CT has been shown to be efficacious for BDD (Wilhelm et al., 2014). Notably, perceptual (i.e., mirror) retraining (i.e., helping patients learn to describe themselves more objectively and engage in healthier mirror-related behaviors) is a unique component of CBT for BDD, and additional time is often spent on cognitive interventions for patients with BDD with low insight.

Treatment efficacy for HD is less well-studied than the other OCRDs, given its new inclusion in DSM-V; however, some preliminary evidence from uncontrolled or waitlist comparison trials suggest that community-solicited individuals with HD may respond to SRIs (with as much efficacy as is seen in OCD), alone or in conjunction with CBT. CBT alone also is effective for individuals with HD (Williams & Viscusi, 2016).

In the treatment of HPD and SPD, the SRI clomipramine and the augmentation of SRIs with neuroleptics (dopamine blockers) have been shown to be effective for both disorders. Additionally, N-Acetylcysteine, a glutamate modulator, has been effective in clinical trials in HPD and case studies of SPD. Meta-analytic data show that SSRIs may not be an effective treatment for HPD or SPD. In terms of psychosocial interventions, empirical evidence has consistently shown that habit reversal training (e.g., teaching patients to perform a specific action – i.e., "competing response" – every time they have the urge to pick/pull; e.g., making a fist) and stimulus control techniques (i.e., eliminating triggers for picking/pulling; e.g., tweezers) are effective in reducing both hair pulling and skin picking. Some evidence indicates acceptance and commitment therapy (ACT) and dialectical behavior therapy (DBT) may also be effective for both HPD and SPD.

Future Directions

Significant research advances have been made over the last ten to twenty years in terms of elucidating the understanding and treatment of the OCRDs. That being said, there are still understudied research areas, such as neural substrates/neurobiology, genetic studies and biomarkers of the OCRDs, mechanisms of cognitive-behavioral interventions, as well as longitudinal data on HPD, SPD, and HD. This research is ongoing and will be important for adapting future treatments, as well as possible primary prevention programs.

First, the research improvements in the psychosocial and neurobiological underpinnings of OCRDs have inspired novel treatment approaches to date, including neurostimulation techniques such as transcranial magnetic stimulation (TMS) or repetitive transcranial magnetic stimulation (rTMS). TMS is a non-invasive meth-od that causes neurons in the neocortex under the site of stimulation to depolarize and discharge an action potential, and rTMS may produce longer-lasting effects. In OCD, TMS has been studied by targeting the stimulation of the dorsolateral prefrontal cortex (DLPFC) as well as inhibition of the orbitofrontal cortex (OFC) and supplementary motor areas (SMA; Blom, Figee, Vulink, & Denys, 2011). TMS may decrease symptoms of OCD by normalizing hypermetabolism in orbito-striatal circuits. This research is still preliminary because of the lack of comparison studies with sham stimulation but is a promising area for further study. TMS has been studied in OCD for the last fifteen years in treatment-refractory cases, and as of August 2018, deep TMS (which can stimulate areas deeper in the brain) was approved by the FDA for the treatment of OCD.

In the realm of psychosocial intervention research, Craske and colleagues (2008) have published novel theoretical models explaining the mechanisms for how ex-posure-based therapy works, building on laboratory research on fear learning and memory. According to this theory, original fear-based associations (e.g., bath-rooms are dangerous) are not corrected or replaced during exposure (as was orig-inally believed), and habituation of fear (i.e., subjective fear reduction) within and between sessions is not a reliable predictor of long-term outcome. Rather, this theory proposes that new inhibitory (i.e., safety) associations are formed via exposure (e.g., bathrooms are safe and tolerable). Therefore, the aim of CBT for OCRDs is to help maximize the recall of the new safety-based learning relative to the older, threat-based associations. This novel theoretical approach has important implications for the ways in which exposure is conducted (for instance, the theory purports that exposure may not need to be conducted in a gradual, hierarchi-cal approach, but can be done in a random/variable order), but more research is needed to extend these theoretical findings to the treatment of OCRDs (Jacoby & Abramowitz, 2016).

Other areas of novel research expansion include improving the accessibility of empirically supported treatments. Despite the effectiveness of cognitive-behavio-ral treatments for OCD, the majority of patients do not have access to this inter-vention due to a shortage of trained providers. Accordingly, technology-based and technology-enhanced interventions (e.g., internet-based CBT) aim to bridge this gap by providing CBT in a convenient and accessible format for patients. These treatments demonstrate promising feasibility, acceptability, and efficacy (Kyrios et al., 2018; Patel et al., 2018) and are being further investigated in ongoing studies. Additionally, in line with precision medicine initiatives at the National Institute of Mental Health, research on moderators and mediators of treatment outcome (e.g., depression symptom severity, obsessive beliefs) are currently being conduct-ed in order to help personalize existing treatment interventions to individual pa-tients. Specifically, given that not all patients benefit significantly from any one treatment approach, such work will help determine which treatments work best for whom (e.g., cognitive versus behavioral therapy; Steketee et al., 2018).

Finally, there has been a research focus on other OCRD diagnoses to consider for future iterations of the DSM. For example, olfactory reference syndrome (ORS) is an area of future research for inclusion in the OCRDs. ORS is a psychological disorder in which one erroneously believes that he/she is emitting a foul or offensive bodily odor (e.g., halitosis, genital odor, or flatulence; Feusner, Phillips, & Stein, 2010). ORS patients often report delusions of reference similar to those reported in BDD (e.g., believing that their offensive odor leads other people to take special notice of them). ORS may also lead to ritualistic and repetitive behaviors that alleviate anxiety or mask the perceived odor (e.g., checking/washing areas of concern). ORS shares phenomenology with other disorders, such as OCD, delusional disorder, social phobia, BDD, and IAD. The DSM Task Force considered ORS for inclusion with the OCRDs for DSM-V. However, given the general lack of research to date, especially in terms of the validators examined for inclusion in DSM-V, ORS will not be included until further research is done.

Additionally, new research, encouraged by case studies, is examining a potential psychiatric condition, body dysmorphic disorder by proxy (BDDBP). BDDBP is a condition by which an individual is overly concerned with someone else's (family member or friend's) appearance. BDDBP causes significant distress and impairment due to the intrusive and overwhelming thoughts about the other person's appearance, as well as interference due to obsessive behaviors, such as comparing their loved one's appearance to others. A preliminary internet study examined eleven individuals with self-reported BDDBP and found that most participants spent three to eight hours a day preoccupied by perceived defects in another person (mostly facial concerns) and all engaged in rituals similar to compulsions to alleviate distress (J. L. Greenberg et al., 2013).

Sample Interview Questions

Some important questions to ask when assessing an OCRD are:

1. What kinds of thoughts/impulses/images/doubts are bothering you?
2. What people, places, and things are triggers for these thoughts?
3. When these thoughts come up what do you do? Is there anything you have to do over and over again?
4. Is there anything you are avoiding because of these thoughts/behaviors?
5. How much time do these thoughts/behaviors take up?
6. How much distress do these thoughts/behaviors cause for you?
7. How well are you able to control the thoughts or resist the behaviors?

8. In what ways do these thoughts/behaviors interfere with your ability get to/be on time for your job/school/social events/other?

9. Do these thoughts/behaviors take away from your ability to concentrate or perform in your job/school/social, or other role obligations?

10. What do you think caused you to have these types of thoughts? Could there be a psychological cause?

11. What other medical conditions or psychological conditions have you been diagnosed with?

Case Examples

Obsessive-Compulsive Disorder (OCD)

Joe is a twenty-five-year-old man who presented for treatment due to his fears of contamination of contracting a disease. He reported fears of coming in contact with individuals he believed were contaminated. In particular, he believed homeless people had a high likelihood of having a disease and spreading it to him. He would avoid locations where he believed he was likely to encounter a homeless person, such as parks, crowded city corners, and public libraries. This meant taking indirect and much longer routes to places he needed to go. He also had difficulty in public restrooms and handling money (dollar bills or change). When feeling contaminated, Joe would repeatedly wash his hands with very hot water and scrub his hands and forearms until they were raw. Joe began to isolate himself socially in order to avoid the possibility of becoming contaminated by others.

Body Dysmorphic Disorder (BDD)

Sarah is an eighteen-year-old girl who describes her appearance as "monstrous" despite numerous people reassuring her that she is very physically attractive. She believes that her jaw is "too manly and square," and will spend three to five hours a day in front of the mirror checking her jawline and measuring her facial proportions. As part of these mirror-checking rituals, Sarah began to press firmly into her cheeks and jaw for long periods of time. Sarah's parents began to notice that her face was often red and swollen. Sarah also believes that anyone she comes in contact with will automatically notice her facial structure and judge her negatively. Sarah began wearing the same brightly colored scarf every day to distract from her jawline and hide her appearance. While Sarah had body image concerns to a lesser degree since approximately fifteen years old, these symptoms rapidly worsened, and she started to refuse to go to school all together.

Hoarding Disorder (HD)

Michael remembers first starting to collect trivial items following the end of his college romantic relationship. What began with saving items that reminded him of his ex-girlfriend (e.g., ticket stubs, receipts) evolved into collecting items more generally, such as half-eaten sandwiches and abandoned umbrellas or gloves found in the street. After living in his first apartment after college for six months, Michael's roommate confronted him about the smell of something rotting coming from Michael's room. His roommate found piles of garbage and demanded Michael throw them away. Michael refused and soon found a studio apartment he could afford to live in alone. Currently, the majority of the living space in Michael's apartment is occupied by staggering amounts of garbage. Neighbors have called the police due to the smell coming from his apartment. Michael is now worried he is in jeopardy of losing his apartment and all of his belongings he has worked so hard to amass.

Hair-Pulling Disorder (HPD)

Janet is a thirty-year-old woman who came to treatment by the urging of her mother because of her high levels of stress and noticeable hair loss from the right side of her scalp, above her ear, due to hair pulling. Janet had periods of hair pulling since age thirteen but was always able to conceal her bald patches through hair styling, hats, or wigs. Once her mother became aware of her pulling, Janet admitted she has been pulling for nearly ten years on and off, for periods of three to six months at a time. Janet most frequently pulls when sitting at her desk trying to write (she works as a freelance writer for several magazines) and while lying in bed. Janet reports feeling an intense urge to pull and a tingling in her scalp. She will spend time twirling her hair between her fingers and feeling through her hairs for more "course or kinky" hairs. After pulling a hair out, Janet feels great pleasure if the hair has an attached large "bulb." She then feels the bulb with her lips and bites it in half to study the interior pattern of the bulb. Janet reports that she often engages in this repeated pattern of hair pulling behavior for up to an hour and is horrified when she sees the pile of hairs next to her that she has pulled.

Skin-Picking Disorder (SPD)

Caroline is a forty-year-old mother of young twins who started treatment after being referred by her dermatologist. Caroline has been picking at minor bumps or scabs on her skin for as long as she can remember. She has never had periods longer than one month when she did not engage in picking behaviors. Caroline reports that she sees a direct correlation between the amount of stress she is under and her picking behavior. When feeling anxious, Caroline rubs her upper arms and legs, feeling for imperfections, and then uses her fingernails to pick at these areas.

This picking behavior has caused significant scaring on her arms and more than one infection that has required treatment from her dermatologist.

References and Selected Readings

- Abramowitz, J. S., and Jacoby, R. J. (2015). Obsessive-Compulsive and Related Disorders: A Critical Review of the New Diagnostic Class. *Annual Review of Clinical Psychology*, 11, 165–186.
- Abramowitz, J. S., Schwartz, S. A., and Whiteside, S. P. (2002). A Contemporary Conceptual Model of Hypochondriasis. *Mayo Clinic Proceedings*, 77(12), 1323–1330.
- American Psychiatric Association. (2013). *Diagnostic and Statistical Manual of Mental Disorders*, 5th ed. Arlington, VA: American Psychiatric Publishing.
- Bjornsson, A. S., Didie, E. R., and Phillips, K. A. (2010). Body Dysmorphic Disorder. *Dialogues in Clinical Neuroscience*, 12(2), 221–232.
- Blom, R. M., Figee, M., Vulink, N., and Denys, D. (2011). Update on Repetitive Transcranial Magnetic Stimulation in Obsessive-Compulsive Disorder: Different Targets. *Current Psychiatry Reports*, 13(4), 289–294.
- Buhlmann, U., Glaesmer, H., Mewes, R., Fama, J. M., Wilhelm, S., Brähler, E., and Rief, W. (2010). Updates on the Prevalence of Body Dysmorphic Disorder: A Population-Based Survey. *Psychiatry Research*, 178(1), 171–175.
- Casale, A. D., Sorice, S., Padovano, A., Simmaco, M., Ferracuti, S., Lamis, D. A., ... Pompili, M. (2018). Psychopharmacological Treatment of Obsessive-Compulsive Disorder (OCD). *Current Neuropharmacology*. https://doi.org/10.2174/1570159X16666180813155017.
- Craske, M. G., Kircanski, K., Zelikowsky, M., Mystkowski, J., Chowdhury, N., and Baker, A. (2008). Optimizing Inhibitory Learning during Exposure Therapy. *Behaviour Research and Therapy*, 46(1), 5–27.
- Dougherty, D. D., Brennan, B. P., Stewart, S. E., Wilhelm, S., Widge, A. S., and Rauch, S. L. (2018). Neuroscientifically Informed Formulation and Treatment Planning for Patients with Obsessive-Compulsive Disorder: A Review. *JAMA Psychiatry*. https://doi.org/10.1001/jamapsychiatry.2018.0930.
- Feusner, J. D., Phillips, K. A., and Stein, D. J. (2010). Olfactory Reference Syndrome: Issues for DSM-V. *Depression and Anxiety*, 27(6), 592–599.
- Fineberg, N. A., Kaur, S., Kolli, S., Mpavaenda, D., and Reghunandanan, S. (2015). Obsessive-Compulsive Personality Disorder. In K. A. Phillips and D. J. Stein (eds.), *Handbook on Obsessive-Compulsive and Related Disorders* (pp. 247–272). Arlington, VA: American Psychiatric Publishing.
- First, M., Williams, J., Karg, R., and Spitzer, R. (2015). *Structured Clinical Interview for DSM-V*. Arlington, VA: American Psychiatric Association.
- Foa, E. B., Huppert, J. D., Leiberg, S., Langner, R., Kichic, R., Hajcak, G., and Salkovskis, P. M. (2002). The Obsessive-Compulsive Inventory: Development and Validation of a Short Version. *Psychological Assessment*, 14(4), 485–496.
- Frost, R. O., Steketee, G., and Grisham, J. (2004). Measurement of Compulsive Hoarding: Saving Inventory-Revised. *Behaviour Research and Therapy*, 42(10), 1163–1182.

- Goodman, W. K., Price, L. H., Rasmussen, S. A., Mazure, C., Delgado, P., Heninger, G. R., and Charney, D. S. (1989). The Yale-Brown Obsessive-Compulsive Scale: II. Validity. *Archives of General Psychiatry*, 46(11), 1012–1016.
- Grant, J. E., and Chamberlain, S. R. (2016). Trichotillomania. *American Journal of Psychiatry*, 173(9), 868–874.
- Grant, J. E., Odlaug, B. L., Chamberlain, S. R., Keuthen, N. J., Lochner, C., and Stein, D. J. (2012). Skin-Picking Disorder. *American Journal of Psychiatry*, 169(11), 1143–1149.
- Greenberg, B. D., Gabriels, L. A., Malone, D. A., Rezai, A. R., Friehs, G. M., Okun, M. S., ... Nuttin, B. J. (2010). Deep Brain Stimulation of the Ventral Internal Capsule/Ventral Striatum for Obsessive-Compulsive Disorder: Worldwide Experience. *Molecular Psychiatry*, 15(1), 64–79.
- Greenberg, J. L., Falkenstein, M., Reuman, L., Fama, J., Marques, L., and Wilhelm, S. (2013). The Phenomenology of Self-Reported Body Dysmorphic Disorder by Proxy. *Body Image*, 10(2), 243–246.
- Jacoby, R. J., and Abramowitz, J. S. (2016). Inhibitory Learning Approaches to Exposure Therapy: A Critical Review and Translation to Obsessive-Compulsive Disorder. *Clinical Psychology Review*, 49, 28–40.
- Keuthen, N. J., O'Sullivan, R. L., Ricciardi, J. N., Shera, D., Savage, C. R., Borgmann, A. S., ... Baer, L. (1995). The Massachusetts General Hospital (MGH) Hairpulling Scale: 1. Development and Factor Analyses. *Psychotherapy and Psychosomatics*, 64(3–4), 141–145.
- Kozak, M. J., and Foa, E. B. (1994). Obsessions, Overvalued Ideas, and Delusions in Obsessive-Compulsive Disorder. *Behaviour Research and Therapy*, 32(3), 343–353.
- Kyrios, M., Ahern, C., Fassnacht, D. B., Nedeljkovic, M., Moulding, R., and Meyer, D. (2018). Therapist-Assisted Internet-Based Cognitive Behavioral Therapy versus Progressive Relaxation in Obsessive-Compulsive Disorder: Randomized Controlled Trial. *Journal of Medical Internet Research*, 20 (8), e242.
- Mataix-Cols, D., Frost, R. O., Pertusa, A., Clark, L. A., Saxena, S., Leckman, J. F., ... Wilhelm, S. (2010). Hoarding Disorder: A New Diagnosis for DSM-V? *Depression and Anxiety*, 27 (6), 556–572.
- Milad, M. R., Furtak, S. C., Greenberg, J. L., Keshaviah, A., Im, J. J., Falkenstein, M. J., ... Wilhelm, S. (2013). Deficits in Conditioned Fear Extinction in Obsessive-Compulsive Disorder and Neurobiological Changes in the Fear Circuit. *JAMA Psychiatry*, 70 (6), 608–618.
- Olatunji, B. O., Davis, M. L., Powers, M. B., and Smits, J. A. J. (2013). Cognitive-Behavioral Therapy for Obsessive-Compulsive Disorder: A Meta-Analysis of Treatment Outcome and Moderators. *Journal of Psychiatric Research*, 47(1), 33–41.
- Patel, S. R., Wheaton, M. G., Andersson, E., Rück, C., Schmidt, A. B., La Lima, C. N., ... Simpson, H. B. (2018). Acceptability, Feasibility, and Effectiveness of Internet-Based Cognitive-Behavioral Therapy for Obsessive-Compulsive Disorder in New York. *Behavior Therapy*, 49(4), 631–641.
- Phillips, K. A., and Hollander, E. (2008). Treating Body Dysmorphic Disorder with Medication: Evidence, Misconceptions, and a Suggested Approach. *Body Image*, 5 (1), 13–27.
- Phillips, K. A., Hollander, E., Rasmussen, S. A., Aronowitz, B. R., DeCaria, C., and Goodman, W. K. (1997). A Severity Rating Scale for Body Dysmorphic Disorder: Development,

Reliability, and Validity of a Modified Version of the Yale-Brown Obsessive-Compulsive Scale. *Psychopharmacology Bulletin*, 33(1), 17–22.

- Phillips, K. A., Pinto, A., Hart, A. S., Coles, M. E., Eisen, J. L., Menard, W., and Rasmussen, S. A. (2012). A Comparison of Insight in Body Dysmorphic Disorder and Obsessive-Compulsive Disorder. *Journal of Psychiatric Research*, 46(10), 1293–1299.

- Phillips, K. A., Stein, D. J., Rauch, S. L., Hollander, E., Fallon, B. A., Barsky, A., ... Leckman, J. (2010). Should an Obsessive-Compulsive Spectrum Grouping of Disorders Be Included in DSM-V? *Depression and Anxiety*, 27(6), 528–555.

- Snorrason, I., Belleau, E. L., and Woods, D. W. (2012). How Related Are Hair-Pulling Disorder (Trichotillomania) and Skin-Picking Disorder? A Review of Evidence for Comorbidity, Similarities and Shared Etiology. *Clinical Psychology Review*, 32(7), 618–629.

- Snorrason, I., Ólafsson, R. P., Flessner, C. A., Keuthen, N. J., Franklin, M. E., and Woods, D. W. (2012). The Skin Picking Scale-Revised: Factor Structure and Psychometric Properties. *Journal of Obsessive-Compulsive and Related Disorders*, 1(2), 133–137.

- Steketee, G., and Frost, R. O. (2014). Phenomenology of Hoarding. In R. O. Frost and G. Steketee (eds.), *The Oxford Handbook of Hoarding and Acquiring.* (pp. 19–32). New York: Oxford University Press.

- Steketee, G., Siev, J., Yovel, I., Lit, K., and Wilhelm, S. (2018). Predictors and Moderators of Cognitive and Behavioral Therapy Outcomes for OCD: A Patient-Level Mega-Analysis of Eight Sites. *Behavior Therapy.* https://doi.org/10.1016/j.beth.2018.04.004.

- Stewart, S. E., Yu, D., Scharf, J. M., Neale, B. M., Fagerness, J. A., Mathews, C. A., ... Pauls, D. L. (2013). Genome-Wide Association Study of Obsessive-Compulsive Disorder. *Molecular Psychiatry*, 18(7), 788–798.

- Wilhelm, S., Greenberg, J. L., Rosenfield, E., Kasarskis, I., and Blashill, A. J. (2016). The Body Dysmorphic Disorder Symptom Scale: Development and Preliminary Validation of a Self-Report Scale of Symptom Specific Dysfunction. *Body Image*, 17, 82–87.

- Wilhelm, S., Phillips, K. A., Didie, E., Buhlmann, U., Greenberg, J. L., Fama, J. M., ... Steketee, G. (2014). Modular Cognitive-Behavioral Therapy for Body Dysmorphic Disorder: A Randomized Controlled Trial. *Behavior Therapy*, 45(3), 314–327.

- Wilhelm, S., and Steketee, G. S. (2006). *Cognitive Therapy for Obsessive-Compulsive Disorder: A Guide for Professionals.* Oakland: New Harbinger.

- Williams, M., and Viscusi, J. A. (2016). Hoarding Disorder and a Systematic Review of Treatment with Cognitive Behavioral Therapy. *Cognitive Behaviour Therapy*, 45(2), 93–110.

- Wu, M. S., Rudy, B. M., and Storch, E. A. (2014). Obsessions, Compulsions, and Repetitive Behavior: Autism and/or OCD. In T. E. I. Davis, S. W. White, and T. H. Ollendick (eds.), *Handbook of Autism and Anxiety* (pp. 107–120). Cham, Switzerland: Springer.

Self-Assessment Questions

1. In DSM-V, OCD is included as part of an obsessive-compulsive spectrum of disorders. What are the other diagnoses in this spectrum?

A. Body dysmorphic disorder, hoarding disorder, hair-pulling disorder, and skin-picking disorder

B. Impulse control disorders, autism spectrum disorders, Tourette's disorder

C. Eating disorders, anxiety disorders, stress disorders

D. Schizophrenia, delusional disorder, psychotic disorders

2. OCD is characterized by:

A. Worries about one's physical symptoms of anxiety

B. Preoccupation with body appearance

C. Intrusive, unwanted thoughts, feelings, or behaviors

D. Delusional beliefs about thought insertion

3. In adults, OCD occurs:

A. More commonly in females

B. More commonly in males

C. Approximately equally in females and males

D. There is no data on the gender ratio of OCD

4. Body dysmorphic disorder (BDD) is typified by:

A. Preoccupation with one or more perceived flaws in physical appearance that are unobservable or slight

B. Preoccupation with accidentally causing harm to others

C. Preoccupation with one's body odor

D. Both A and C

5. In comparing delusional to nondelusional patients with BDD, research has shown that:

A. Delusional and nondelusional forms of BDD have many more similarities than differences and constitute the same disorder

B. Delusional and nondelusional forms of BDD are very different and likely represent different diagnoses

C. Delusional and nondelusional forms of BDD are both psychotic disorders

D. Both B and C

6. Hair-pulling disorder (HPD) and skin-picking disorder (SPD) tend to onset:

A. In infancy

B. In adolescence

C. In middle-age

D. In old age

7. What are trichobezoars?

A. Bald patches due to hair pulling

B. Large infected sores due to skin picking

C. Magnifying mirrors

D. Buildup of ingested hair in the gastrointestinal system

8. Olfactory reference syndrome (ORS) is a psychological disorder in which one
    ...
    A. Is fixated on negative interpretations of physiological sensations
    B. Erroneously believes that he/she is emitting a foul or offensive bodily
        odor
    C. Is preoccupied by the appearance of flaws in other people
    D. Believes that he/she has lost her sense of smell

Answers to Self-Assessment Questions

1. (A)
2. (C)
3. (C)
4. (A)
5. (A)
6. (B)
7. (D)
8. (B)

8 Disorders Related to Stress and Trauma

ERIC BUI, MEREDITH CHARNEY, MOHAMMED R. MILAD, DEVON HIN-
TON, FREDRICK STODDARD, TERENCE KEANE, ROGER PITMAN, AND
NAOMI M. SIMON

Introduction

Trauma derives from the Greek τραῦμα, meaning "wound." Although it has been used for centuries as a medical term to designate "*an injury to living tissue caused by an extrinsic agent,*" it was not until 1889 that this word endorsed a psychological meaning with the first clinical descriptions of "traumatic neuroses" in victims of railroad accidents by Oppenheim. Stress was first a mechanics term used to describe the pressure or tension exerted on a material object. It was then been applied to mental health to describe a feeling of psychological strain and pressure. Both psychological trauma and stress can result in psychiatric disorders.

The Spectrum of Disorders Related to Stress and Trauma

ASD, PTSD, Adjustment Disorders

Although the fourth edition of the *Diagnostic and Statistical Manual of Mental Disorders* (DSM-IV-TR), defined traumatic events as "events that involve actual or threatened death or serious injury, or a threat to the physical integrity of one-self or others" (criterion A1) that are accompanied by a feeling of "intense fear, helplessness, or horror" (criterion A2), its fifth edition (DSM-V) has dropped the required subjective reaction to the trauma (A2). Trauma can consist of direct exposure (i.e., being a victim), witnessing a traumatic event, or learning that it occurred to someone close. The new definition also includes extreme and repeated exposure to trauma details (e.g., first responders) but excludes exposure through the media.

Exposure to traumatic events can result in a variety of reactions, ranging from relatively mild, with no or minor disruptions, to more severe and debilitating. Most traumatized individuals will develop some level of a brief psychological stress response. However, for a minority of individuals, this stress response becomes clinically significant, persistent, and interfering. Reactions to trauma are defined according to their timeframe: immediate or peritraumatic reactions (lasting minutes to hours), acute stress disorder (ASD; between three days to one month), and posttraumatic stress disorder (PTSD; more than one month). Although exposure to trauma might induce other psychiatric disorders, including major depression and other anxiety conditions, those disorders are not specific to trauma and will not be reviewed in this chapter.

Similar to PTSD and ASD, adjustment disorder (AD) requires the presence of a stressful (yet not necessarily traumatic) event, which results in clinically significant distress or impairment.

Epidemiology and Impact

Traumatic Events

The lifetime prevalence of exposure to any traumatic event in North America has been estimated to range between 39 percent and 90 percent, depending on the study; however, different traumatic events confer different risks for PTSD. For example, learning about traumas to others is the most frequent traumatic event (approximately 60 percent) but is associated with a low risk for PTSD (about 2 percent), whereas being held captive, tortured, or kidnapped is much less frequent (approximately 2 percent), but is associated with a more than 50 percent risk for developing PTSD.

Acute Stress Disorder

Prevalence rates of ASD reported within a month of trauma exposure are somewhat inconsistent, with estimates ranging from 7 to 59 percent and a mean rate falling around 17 percent.

Posttraumatic Stress Disorder

In North America, 7 to 10 percent of individuals will suffer from PTSD in their lifetime, while the twelve-month prevalence rate is approximately 4 percent. Conditional rates of PTSD following a trauma vary based on a wide range of risk and protective factors, such as trauma type and severity, previous childhood or other trauma, the presence of prior mood or anxiety disorders, and social support. PTSD is associated with varying, and sometimes severe, impairment across domains of functioning. Specifically, PTSD has been associated with increased risk for academic failures, marital instability, and unemployment. In addition, PTSD is a risk factor for developing secondary psychiatric disorders including mood, anxiety, and substance use disorders, with an increased risk for suicide. In addition, PTSD is associated with a mean work loss of nine days per month. This level of associated impairment in occupational functioning is greater than that found in a number of somatic diseases including heart disease.

Adjustment Disorders

The prevalence of ADs in the general population has never been assessed in large epidemiologic studies of mental health conditions; however, some data suggest a prevalence rate of 1 percent. Despite the lack of robust epidemiological studies, it has been estimated that 9 to 36 percent of patients seen in psychiatry are diagnosed with an AD.

Some early evidence suggests that initial AD diagnosis in adolescents might precede the development of a major mental disorder, and it is possible that ADs may be a risk factor for other mood and anxiety disorders. ADs have also been shown to be associated with suicidality.

Clinical Features and Course

Acute Stress Disorder

The clinical features of ASD include exposure to a traumatic event, as defined previously. Whereas in DSM-IV, the diagnosis required at least three dissociative symptoms – one reexperiencing symptom, one avoidance symptom, and one increased arousal symptom – DSM-V no longer requires symptoms from each of these three clusters. To meet criteria, a person must now have nine of fourteen symptoms, including symptoms of *intrusion*, marked by recurrent distressing memories of the traumatic event(s), recurrent distressing dreams, dissociative reactions (e.g., flashbacks), intense or prolonged distress at exposure to reminders, physiological reactions to reminders; *dissociative symptoms*, marked by a persistent inability to experience positive emotions (e.g., emotional numbing), an altered sense of the reality of one's surroundings or oneself, inability to remember an aspect of the traumatic event(s) (typically dissociative amnesia); *avoidance symptoms*, marked by avoidance of internal, or external, reminders that arouse recollections of the traumatic event(s); and *arousal symptoms*, marked by sleep disturbance, irritable or aggressive behavior, hypervigilance, problems with concentration, and exaggerated startle. The duration of the symptoms runs from three days (formally two days in DSM-IV) to four weeks after trauma exposure, with clinically significant distress or impairment.

Posttraumatic Stress Disorder

The diagnosis of PTSD was modified in DSM-V to include the same exposure criteria as ASD (i.e., exposure to death or threatened death, actual or threatened serious injury, or actual or threatened sexual violation). In addition, the diagnosis requires (a) one symptom of intrusion as described above for ASD; (b) persistent avoidance of stimuli associated with the traumatic event(s) – reminders; (c) two symptoms of negative alterations in cognitions and mood associated with the traumatic event(s), such as persistent, distorted blame of self or others, persistent negative emotional state (e.g., fear, horror, anger, guilt, or shame), diminished interest or participation in significant activities, detachment or estrangement from others, or persistent inability to experience positive emotions (e.g., emotional numbing); (d) two symptoms of alterations in arousal and reactivity, such as irritable or aggressive behavior, reckless or self-destructive behavior, hypervigilance, exaggerated startle, problems with concentration, or sleep disturbance. The diagnosis also requires a duration of more than one month, and clinically significant distress or impairment, and that the symptoms not be associated with the effects of a substance or medical condition.

Course of ASD and PTSD
The course of both ASD and PTSD varies across the lifespan, with the effects generally longer lasting in younger individuals. Populations at risk also include the elderly, females, the injured or medically ill, refugees, survivors of genocide or disasters, combat veterans, and those with serious mental illness or economic disadvantage. In most studies, symptoms have been found to be most intense proximal to the time of the exposure, but for some individuals, the impact is chronic and resistant to existing treatments. Responses to trauma vary according to the degree of exposure, and to the stage of neurobiological, psychological, and overall development. Research has identified risk and protective factors, such as premorbid emotional functioning, prior trauma, level of social support, and psychiatric disorders.

Adjustment Disorders
In DSM-IV, adjustment disorders were conceptualized as a residual category for individuals who exhibit clinically significant distress without meeting diagnostic criteria for a discrete disorder. In DSM-V, they now comprise a heterogeneous group of stress-response syndromes that may occur after exposure to a distressing event, which may or may not be sufficiently severe to be termed traumatic. As opposed to most psychiatric disorders, no specific symptoms are required for the diagnosis of AD. Although this nonspecificity can make standardized assessments of AD difficult, it may provide a useful tool for clinicians to characterize individuals who are clinically distressed by a stressful event. The main requirements are that the symptoms must arise in response to a stressful event within three months of exposure to the stressor, be clinically significant, and resolve within six months of the offset of the stressor or its consequences. There are three subtypes, depending on the symptoms: (a) with depressed mood, (b) with anxious symptoms, and (c) with disturbances in conduct.

Differential Diagnosis

Contrary to PTSD diagnosis that requires four symptom clusters, including re-experiencing, avoidance, persistent negative alterations in cognitions and mood, and hyperarousal, ASD diagnosis requires nine out of fourteen symptoms. Further, the time frame differs between ASD and PTSD, with ASD diagnosed during the first month after trauma exposure, while PTSD is diagnosed beyond that.

The distinction between ADs and ASD/PTSD is that the diagnosis of AD does not require the stressor to be "traumatic," nor does it specify required symptoms. The ADs differ from normative stress responses in that they result in clinically significant symptoms (i.e., significant distress and/or functional impairment).

Although trauma exposure as well as other stressors can precipitate the onset of a range of mood or anxiety disorders, the causal nexus is not as tight as with PTSD, ASD, and ADs. Moreover, they can be differentiated from ASD and PTSD. For example, although patients with anxiety disorders, including panic disorder, general anxiety disorder, or social anxiety disorder, may exhibit hyperarousal and avoidance, the clinical presentation lacks both a focus around a traumatic event and re-experiencing symptoms. A major depressive episode triggered by a stressful experience may similarly include concentration difficulties, insomnia, social withdrawal or detachment, and anhedonia, but it will lack trauma re-experiencing or related avoidance.

Evaluation

An evaluation of a patient with possible PTSD should begin with a nondirective portion, in which the patient is encouraged to provide a history with only the minimum input from the interviewer necessary to keep the information flowing. This nondirective portion is useful in protecting against making a false PTSD diagnosis in persons who are motivated to appear to have this disorder in order to achieve some external incentive (e.g., recovery in a lawsuit or escaping criminal punishment). The reliability of the report of a patient who talks for fifteen or thirty minutes without mentioning a single symptom consistent with PTSD, but who then answers positively to all PTSD symptoms during subsequent direct questioning, should be regarded with caution.

An even greater potential problem, however, is missing PTSD in persons who really have it. Clinicians should be aware that talking about the traumatic event is almost always distressing to some degree in patients with PTSD. Because of their tendency to avoid painful traumatic memories, superficial questioning may fail to elicit symptoms or even to discover that a traumatic event occurred at all. It is not unheard of to encounter PTSD patients who have been in psychotherapy for years and never even told their therapist about the traumatic event. As a remedy to this pitfall, after the nondirective portion of the interview, a comprehensive psychiatric evaluation should include asking the patient whether they have ever experienced any of a range of various possible psychologically traumatizing experiences. Checklists for this purpose are available in the literature (e.g., the Trauma History Questionnaire). If a patient reports one or more such experiences, a thorough evaluation requires inquiring into at least a sufficient number of PTSD criteria to assure the interviewer that PTSD is not present. However, if PTSD is suspected, it is necessary to inquire into each and every DSM PTSD diagnostic criterion. In order to assist in this, "structured interview instruments" (originally designed for research use) are available to the clinician specifically for PTSD – for example, the Clinician-Administered PTSD Scale or the Posttraumatic Symptom Scale, Interview Version. Currently, these instruments are available for DSM-IV diagnostic criteria, but updated instruments for DSM-V should become available soon. In addition to providing a categorical (qualitative) determination of the presence or absence of the PTSD diagnosis, some structured interview instruments offer the advantage of providing a continuous measure of PTSD symptom severity in the form of a total score, as well as a subscore for each PTSD symptom cluster. This allows a dimensional (quantitative) approach to the disorder. Importantly, clinician-administered (as opposed to technician-administered) interview instruments do not require the interviewer to score an item positive just because the interviewee answers affirmatively. Rather, the clinician should probe to determine whether or not the detailed information the patient provides meet the symptom criterion in question.

While eliciting the history, close attention should be paid to the patient's behavior as part of the mental status examination, as certain PTSD symptoms, including irritability, difficulty concentrating, or exaggerated startle, may be directly observed, and to confirm that the patient's behavior and affect are consistent with the reported history.

Arguably more progress has been made in discovering the biology of PTSD than almost any other mental disorder. Unfortunately, however, as with almost all other mental disorders, there remains to date a dearth of diagnostically useful biomarkers for PTSD.

Treatment Approaches

ASD Treatment and PTSD Prevention

Most individuals will experience some psychological and/or somatic stress response symptoms in the acute aftermath of trauma. However, having these symptoms does not necessarily indicate a need for intervention, because they generally resolve on their own without professional intervention. For individuals presenting with acute symptoms that do not remit, recent literature indicates that brief (four to five sessions) cognitive-behavioral therapy appears to be effective in treating ASD and preventing the development of PTSD. These cognitive-behavioral interventions include education, breathing training/relaxation, exposure, and cognitive restructuring. The administration of these psychological interventions, however, requires trained therapists. Unfortunately, there remains insufficient availability of professionals trained to administer these types of treatments, and more dissemination of these evidence-based approaches is needed.

In contrast to cognitive-behavioral therapy, critical incident debriefing, which requires individuals to discuss trauma details, usually in a group setting, may not be effective and may even increase rates of PTSD and related distress. Thus, while those in distress or seeking assistance should be offered the opportunity to ventilate individually about the traumatic event if they wish to do so, forced debriefing is inadvisable. Instead, providing trauma survivors with "psychological first aid," including education about the usual course and reactions to trauma, assuring that basic medical and safety needs are met, and increasing access to social supports is recommended, with referral to clinicians as needed.

While another potential approach to the treatment of ASD and prevention of PTSD could be a pharmacological one, to date no data support the efficacy of any pharmacological agent for this indication. Of interest, some evidence suggests that benzodiazepines may worsen outcomes in trauma-exposed individuals, and they are thus not recommended for ASD and PTSD.

PTSD Treatment

The psychotherapeutic approaches that have yielded the most consistent findings in PTSD are cognitive-behavioral therapies (CBT). Individual CBT should be considered as a first-line treatment in PTSD when a suitable therapist is available. Prolonged exposure therapy (PE) and cognitive processing therapy (CPT) are the two types of CBT found efficacious in the treatment of PTSD. PE uses in vivo or (more often) imaginal exposure, the latter of which involves the repeated retelling and imagining of the traumatic event until distress subsides. When practical, in vivo exposure involves real-life exposure to situations that are avoided because they trigger traumatic reminders (e.g., being out after dark). Both forms of exposure promote extinction learning and, when effective, a reduction of PTSD symptoms. CPT employs predominantly cognitive interventions, including challenging and modifying dysfunctional beliefs related to the traumatic event (e.g., lack of safety, difficulty trusting others). CPT may include writing about the traumatic event as well. The goal is to help patients view the event in context and make sense of what happened.

Another technique that has been found to be effective in PTSD is eye-movement desensitization and reprocessing (EMDR), although the mechanism is unclear. According to its proponents, EMDR integrates elements of psychodynamic, cognitive-behavioral, cognitive, interpersonal, systems, and body-oriented therapies, as well as a bilateral brain stimulation component (e.g., eye movements). The current research suggests that EMDR is effective in the treatment of PTSD and may be considered a first-line psychological treatment. However, there is evidence that the eye movements may be an unnecessary part of the treatment, and the treatment effect may be a result of the exposure component. Although group CBT and stress management seem to be effective in PTSD, the effect has been reported to be weaker than individual CBT and EMDR.

In line with the treatment of other anxiety disorders, recommended pharmacological approaches to PTSD treatment include selective serotonin reuptake inhibitor antidepressants (SSRI), which, despite some associated side effects, are generally well tolerated and may also be useful to treat comorbid depressive disorders. Two SSRI agents are currently approved by the Food and Drug Administration for the treatment of PTSD – sertraline and paroxetine – although other serotonergic antidepressants are also commonly employed in clinical practice, and there is no evidence that they are less effective. Other newer antidepressants, such as the serotonin and norepinephrine reuptake inhibitor venlafaxine or mirtazapine, can also be effective. Because of a possible increase in anxiety symptoms at initiation, similar to practice in anxiety disorders, antidepressants should be titrated more slowly than in depression, and patients should be educated about initiation side effects as well as the delayed time course for efficacy and the need for daily dosing to enhance compliance. Sexual side effects remain a problem with these drugs, and there is a class warning for potential increased suicidal ideation in children and young adults. Finally, slow taper is recommended, as they can be associated with discontinuation side effects.

No robust data support the efficacy of benzodiazepines for PTSD. Further, individuals with PTSD are at heightened risk for substance abuse and dependence. The use of benzodiazepines may even interfere with extinction learning processes important to CBT efficacy, particularly when prescribed on an as-needed basis. In general, benzodiazepines are not recommended for PTSD, although selective patients with low abuse potential may sometimes benefit from them.

Randomized controlled study data suggest that prazosin, an alpha-1 adrenergic receptor blocker, may be helpful in the treatment not only of posttraumatic nightmares but also of other PTSD manifestations. Preliminary randomized controlled data suggest that eszopiclone might be efficacious in the treatment of PTSD with associated sleep disturbances. The potential efficacy of other pharmacological agents has been investigated with conflicting results, though research is ongoing.

Investigations of anticonvulsants in the treatment of PTSD have failed to provide strong support for their use in this indication. Taken together with the Food and Drug Administration class warning for elevated risk of suicidal ideation and behavior associated with them, anticonvulsants are generally not considered first-line treatments for PTSD.

Finally, an examination of the efficacy of antipsychotic agents, including olanzapine, quetiapine, and risperidone as monotherapy and/or augmentation for

PTSD, has yielded mixed results, including negative results from a large randomized controlled trial of risperidone in combat veterans. Newer antipsychotics may differ within class regarding efficacy and tolerability, and do not carry the risk of abuse of benzodiazepines. However, they are associated with short- and long-term side effects such as metabolic syndrome that warrant carefully longitudinal monitoring.

ADs Treatment

Although the research is limited, brief therapies are considered the most appropriate psychological interventions for AD. However, if the stressors are ongoing, prolonged supportive measures may be required. Some controlled data also suggest that cognitive therapy may be effective for AD. Pharmacological management of ADs traditionally includes the symptomatic treatment of insomnia and anxiety with benzodiazepines, although limited supportive data are available, and the cautions about these drugs expressed here are also relevant to AD.

Etiological Insights

Freud regarded traumatic neurosis as a fright-induced psychological phenomenon, in contrast to psychoneurosis, which he believed was caused by repressed sexual desires. Freud introduced the concept of *repetition compulsion*, as illustrated in recurrent traumatic nightmares. Kardiner coined the term *physioneurosis* following World War I, to emphasize the contribution of the autonomic nervous system, hyperarousal, and the startle response to what is now known as PTSD.

From a cognitive-behavioral standpoint, the development of PTSD is understood as a problem in natural recovery. As previously discussed, the experience of trauma does not necessarily lead to the development of PTSD. There are several impediments that tend to differentiate those who develop PTSD from those who do not. These include avoiding thoughts, feelings, and memories, as well as situations, activities, and people, that remind the patient of the traumatic event, and this avoidance retards adaptation. Unbalanced/unhealthy thinking (e.g., "I'm not safe," "The world is a dangerous place.") also contributes to a failure to recover. The goal of CBT is to kick-start the natural recovery process that has been stalled by the above impediments to help patients recover from PTSD and move forward in life.

Key brain regions involved in the neurobiology of PTSD appear to be the amygdala, hippocampus, ventral and dorsal regions of the anterior cingulate cortex, and the insular cortex. A currently predominant model posits that elevated fear and anxiety in PTSD is associated with increased activation of the dorsal anterior cingulate cortex (dACC) and insula. In contrast, the ventromedial prefrontal cortex (vmPFC), along with the hippocampus, appears to be hypoactive and fails to inhibit the amygdala.

Future Directions

In recent years, research has significantly furthered the understanding of the risk factors, phenomenology and biology, prevention, and treatment of ASD and PTSD. However, optimal identification of at-risk individuals, as well as optimal prevention and intervention strategies, are still needed.

Although significant advances in the treatment of PTSD have been made with the SSRIs and cognitive-behavioral therapy, the stigma and avoidance associated with PTSD still interfere with patients seeking treatment, and practitioners should screen for, and educate regarding, PTSD among trauma-exposed patients. Further, additional dissemination of evidence-based treatments to increase availability is needed.

PTSD is associated with high rates of psychiatric and medical comorbidities that should also be assessed and may require targeted treatment. More research is needed to increase the evidence base for commonly employed pharmacotherapies for PTSD, as well as to develop novel therapeutic approaches. Growing scientific knowledge from basic science and ongoing clinical research studies should lead to improved prevention, treatment options, and outcomes in the coming years.

Sample Interview Questions

- Have you ever been in a life-threatening situation? Or witnessed one? Or learned that someone close to you was a victim of one?
- Have you experienced any other trauma in your life?
- We don't need to go into detail right now, but can you tell me a little bit about what happened to you?
- How did you respond emotionally to this event?
- How does this event impact you today?
- Do you find yourself thinking about this event when you don't want to or when you are thinking of something else?
- Do you have bad dreams about this event or feel like you are reliving it when awake?
- Do you try not to think or talk about this event?
- Do you try to avoid situations or places that remind you of what happened?
- Do you find yourself very alert in new situations or places that make you anxious?
- Are you jumpy or easily startled?
- Have you had changes in your mood such as irritability or trouble feeling your emotions?

Case Examples

Ms. A is a forty-year-old woman who presented for therapy following a serious motor vehicle accident that occurred one year earlier. Ms. A has a history of childhood trauma, but had generally been functioning well until this car accident. After the accident, she was unable to drive, avoided crowded places such as restaurants and concerts, and was unable to think or talk about what happened without experiencing significant distress. She reported hypervigilance, poor sleep, and she isolated herself from friends and family. She received twelve sessions of prolonged exposure therapy with an individual therapist. This included imaginal exposure, which involved repeatedly retelling her memory of the motor vehicle accident during sessions and listening to recordings of the imaginal exposure between sessions. This also included graduated in vivo exposure, which for her consisted of starting to drive again, going to crowded places, and making plans with friends. By the end of treatment, she was driving regularly without distress, was reengaging with friends and family, and was making plans to engage in new activities such as traveling.

References and Selected Readings

- Alonso, J., Angermeyer, M. C., et al. (2004). Disability and Quality of Life Impact of Mental Disorders in Europe: Results from the European Study of the Epidemiology of Mental Disorders (ESEMeD) Project. *Acta Psychiatrica Scandinavica*, 420 (suppl.), 38–46.
- American Psychiatric Association (2000). *Diagnostic and Statistical Manual of Mental Disorders (Text Revision), DSM-IV-TR*, 4th edition. Washington, DC: American Psychiatric Publishing.
- American Psychiatric Association (2013). *Diagnostic and Statistical Manual of Mental Disorders*, 5th edition. Arlington, VA: American Psychiatric Publishing.
- Bryant, R. A. (2011). Acute Stress Disorder as a Predictor of Posttraumatic Stress Disorder: A Systematic Review. *Journal of Clinical Psychiatry*, 72(2), 233–239.
- Casey, P., and Bailey, S. (2011). Adjustment Disorders: The State of the Art. *World Psychiatry: Official Journal of the World Psychiatric Association*, 10(1), 11–18.
- Department of Veterans Affairs and Department of Defense (2010). *VA/DOD Clinical Practice Guideline for Management of Post-traumatic Stress*. Washington, DC: Department of Veterans Affairs & Department of Defense.
- Kessler, R. C. (2000). Posttraumatic Stress Disorder: The Burden to the Individual and to Society. *Journal of Clinical Psychiatry*, 61 (suppl. 5), 12–14.
- Kessler, R. C., Chiu, W. T., et al. (2005). Prevalence, Severity, and Comorbidity of 12-Month DSM-IV Disorders in the National Comorbidity Survey Replication. *Archive of General Psychiatry*, 62(6), 617–627.

- Kessler, R. C., Sonnega, A., et al. (1995). Posttraumatic Stress Disorder in the National Comorbidity Survey. *Archives of General Psychiatry*, 52(12), 1048–1060.
- Kilpatrick, D. G., Ruggiero, K. J., et al. (2003). Violence and Risk of PTSD, Major Depression, Substance Abuse/Dependence, and Comorbidity: Results from the National Survey of Adolescents. *Journal of Consulting and Clinical Psychology*, 71(4), 692–700.
- Pitman, R. K., Rasmusson, A. M., et al. (2012). Biological Studies of Post-traumatic Stress Disorder. *Nature Reviews Neuroscience*, 13(11), 769–787.

Self-Assessment Questions

1. Which of the following statements is true regarding the current DSM-V diagnosis of posttraumatic stress disorder (PTSD)?
   A. Symptoms of alteration in arousal and reactivity need not be present to meet criteria.
   B. Symptoms of negative alterations in cognition and mood associated with the traumatic event must be present.
   C. The diagnosis does not include a time duration requirement.
   D. Clinically significant impairment in function is not required to meet diagnostic criteria.
2. Which of the following brain regions have not been implicated in the neurobiology of PTSD?
   A. Hippocampus
   B. Amygdala
   C. Cerebellum
   D. Dorsal anterior cingulate cortex (dACC) and insula
3. Which of the following distinguishes between the diagnoses of acute stress disorder (ASD) and PTSD?
   A. Symptoms of hyperarousal and avoidance are present.
   B. The diagnosis requires a significant stressor.
   C. The duration is at least one month.
   D. The patient experiences significant distress or functional impairment.
4. Which of the following is an effective intervention in the treatment of PTSD?
   A. Critical incident debriefing in the group setting
   B. Benzodiazepines, such as clonazepam
   C. Cognitive-behavioral therapy
   D. Anticonvulsant
5. Which of the following pharmacological approaches are recommended in the treatment of PTSD?
   A. Benzodiazepines, such as clonazepam
   B. Selective serotonin reuptake inhibitors, such as sertraline and paroxetine

     C. Anticonvulsants, such as carbamazepine

     D. Atypical antipsychotics, such as risperidone

Answers to Self-Assessment Questions

1. (B)
2. (C)
3. (C)
4. (C)
5. (B)

9

Substance Use Disorders

HILARY S. CONNERY, MARK J. ALBANESE, JEFFREY J. DEVIDO,
KEVIN P. HILL, R. KATHRYN MCHUGH, DANA SARVEY, JOJI SUZUKI,
AND ROGER D. WEISS

*This chapter was created with the support of National Institute on Drug Abuse
UG1DA15831 and K24DA022288 (RW) and DA035297 (RKM).*

Overview of Substance Use Disorders

Classification of Commonly Misused Substances

Substance use disorders are highly prevalent, affecting millions of Americans directly (social, occupational, and health problems) and indirectly (billions of dollars in health care costs and lost revenues due to disability). This section briefly introduces the chemical classification and neurobehavioral properties of the most commonly misused substances.

Alcohol

Ethyl alcohol is the psychoactive ingredient in intoxicating beverages (beer, wine, and liquor) and fermented fruit. Alcohol has complex central neuromodulatory effects accounting for its psychoactive properties, including inhibition of NMDA-mediated glutamatergic excitatory neurotransmission and potentiation of inhibitory $GABA_A$-mediated neurotransmission, as well as potentiation of glycine, $5\text{-}HT_3$ serotonergic, and nicotinic cholinergic signaling. It also potentiates ion channel activity via effects on L-type calcium ion channels and G-protein inwardly rectifying potassium (GIRK) ion channels. In low doses, drinking alcohol results in euphoria, relaxation, and lowered inhibitions. Higher doses can result in sedation, slurred speech, nausea, emotional lability, loss of coordination, visual disturbances, impaired memory, sexual dysfunction, loss of consciousness, increased risk for injury or violence, fetal damage (in pregnant women), depression, neurologic disturbances, hypertension, liver and heart disease, and fatal overdose. Problematic drinking may take the form of either (1) drinking heavily most or all days of the week or (2) binge-pattern drinking, in which drinking episodes have high volume consumption but low frequency of occurrence. The abrupt cessation of problematic daily drinking can lead to life-threatening withdrawal seizures, thus necessitating medically supervised detoxification.

Patients typically seek medical care only after developing a relatively severe alcohol use disorder. Therefore, screening individual alcohol consumption patterns is routinely advised to detect opportunities for early intervention and prevention of alcohol use disorders, such as providing normative feedback and encouraging goal-setting or behavioral counseling to reduce drinking. Patients with severe alcohol use disorders may also benefit from adjunct medications that reduce heavy drinking days and improve abstinence outcomes.

Opioids

Opioids refer both to natural derivatives of the opium poppy plant as well as to synthetic and semi-synthetic ligands that activate central mu-opioid receptors (e.g., heroin and narcotic analgesics) and induce euphoria, sedation, and at high concentrations, respiratory depression. Opioid use disorders have increased tenfold in the past decade due to the prevalence of narcotic analgesic supplies (licit and illicit), the increased purity of heroin, and the rise of fentanyl, a highly potent synthetic opioid. According to the Centers for Disease Control and Prevention (CDC), 128 Americans die each day from opioid-related overdoses. Depending on the specific drug, opioids can be consumed by oral, sublingual, transdermal, and intranasal use; they may also be prepared to be smoked or injected subcutaneously or intravenously. Opioids may have additional health consequences including impaired coordination, dizziness, confusion, nausea, constipation, anorexia, and sexual dysfunction/hypogonadal syndrome. Injection drug use is associated with abscesses, cellulitis, endocarditis, hepatitis B and C, and HIV infection. Accidental overdose deaths have risen sharply with the increased prevalence of opioid use disorders but may be prevented by the timely administration of intravenous or intranasal naloxone. Although opioid withdrawal is very uncomfortable and marked by runny nose, muscle cramps, general aches, nausea/diarrhea, insomnia, opioid craving, and irritability, it is not typically life-threatening, allowing many patients presenting for treatment the option of outpatient detoxification. Medication maintenance therapies (opioid agonists or antagonists) that compete for central mu-opioid receptors are advised for severe opioid use disorders, as they roughly double a patient's chances of sustaining opioid abstinence following detoxification.

Tobacco

Although cigarette smoking has declined in the United States in recent years, smoking remains the number one preventable cause of morbidity and mortality in the United States and globally. The addictive component of tobacco, nicotine, is found in cigarettes, cigars, "hookah," electronic cigarettes, and smokeless tobacco products (chew, snuff). Short-term effects of tobacco use include increased blood pressure/heart rate and cognitive enhancement due to nicotine's activation of nicotinergic cholinergic receptors in the brain. Long-term effects of tobacco use include chronic lung disease; cardiovascular disease; cancers of the mouth, pharynx, larynx, esophagus, stomach, pancreas, cervix, kidney, and bladder; acute myeloid leukemia; and fetal growth restriction in pregnancy. A nicotine withdrawal syndrome will occur in abstinent chronic tobacco users, marked by irritability, anxiety, nicotine craving, poor concentration, and headaches. The unpleasant nature of nicotine withdrawal often leads to relapse, and this, along with greater social tolerance of nicotine use disorders compared with other substance use disorders, renders smoking cessation very challenging – the average smoker makes five or more quit attempts prior to successful cessation. Medications to assist cessation (nicotine replacement and other medications acting at central nicotinic cholinergic receptors) are routinely recommended to improve the probability of a successful quit attempt.

Cannabinoids

More people use marijuana than any other illicit drug, and trends of marijuana use among youth are concerning – use is on the rise, and perceptions of marijuana's harm are declining. Cannabinoids, which can be smoked or eaten, are derived from natural marijuana hemp plant parts, hydroponically engineered hemp plants, and synthetic compounds referred to variously as "K2," "Spice," and "Incense," among other names. Despite attempts by the US Food and Drug Administration (FDA) to limit exposure to synthetic cannabinoids, they remain illicitly available on the Internet and at some convenience stores (marketed as environmental incense or potpourri), and are a popular alternative to hemp cannabis in part because synthetic cannabinoids are not detectable by routine urine drug screens. Cannabinoid substances bind to central endocannabinoid receptors (primarily CB1 receptors, which are widely distributed, and also microglia CB2 receptors) to induce short-term effects of euphoria, slowed reaction time, relaxation, altered sensory perception, impaired coordination and balance, increased heart rate, increased appetite, impaired learning and memory, anxiety, panic attacks, and psychosis. Cannabis withdrawal in daily or near-daily users is marked by irritability, anxiety, insomnia, craving, and poor concentration, but it does not require medical attention. In contrast, synthetic cannabinoid intoxication can be life-threatening due to adrenergic dysregulation and psychosis, and may require supportive medical interventions during intoxication. To date, no medications have been approved by the FDA to assist in the treatment of cannabis use disorders.

Stimulants

Stimulants are popular drugs of abuse due to their powerful euphoric and cognitive-enhancing effects associated with central dopamine release. Commonly abused stimulants include cocaine, methamphetamine, prescription amphetamines, and synthetic cathinones referred to as "bath salts." Methamphetamine use has soared in rural communities in the United States in the last ten years, in part due to the wide availability of ingredients that can be readily used to synthesize the drug in makeshift "labs." "Bath salts" are sold illicitly disguised as potpourri, plant food, and bath additives in convenience stores, and consist of dried plant matter that has been sprayed with adherent stimulant chemicals. Stimulants may be smoked or taken by oral, intranasal, and intravenous routes. Short-term effects of stimulants may include increased heart rate, blood pressure, temperature, and metabolism; euphoria; increased energy and alertness; reduced appetite; increased libido; tremors; irritability; anxiety; panic attacks; paranoia; violent behavior; psychosis; cardiovascular spasm resulting in myocardial infarction and hemorrhagic stroke; and seizure. Long-term effects of stimulant use may include weight loss, insomnia, malnutrition and poor dentition, and nasal perforation. Stimulant users typically engage in binge-pattern use with episodes lasting days due to stimulant-induced insomnia, followed by a withdrawal syndrome consisting of severe dysphoria, dehydration, somnolence, and stimulant craving. Stimulant use is frequently paired with heightened sexual activity and is associated with risky sexual behaviors and HIV transmission. At this time, medications with established efficacy to assist the treatment of stimulant use disorders are unavailable.

Hallucinogens

Hallucinogens are popular among youth and include lysergic acid diethylamide (LSD), mescaline, psilocybin, methylenedioxymethamphetamine (MDMA), also known as "ecstasy," and dimethyltryptamine (DMT). They are predominantly serotonergic agonists, although some compounds such as MDMA also have stimulant properties via enhanced noradrenergic and dopaminergic neurotransmission. MDMA and DMT, especially, have been established as popular "club drugs." Hallucinogens can be ingested, smoked, inhaled, injected, or absorbed through the tissues of the mouth. Short-term effects of hallucinogens may include hallucination, altered states of perception, and nausea. Both LSD and mescaline can cause increased temperature, heart rate, and blood pressure; loss of appetite, sweating, insomnia, numbness, dizziness, weakness, tremors, impulsivity, and mood lability. Psilocybin use can result in nervousness, paranoia, and panic attacks. MDMA use can cause increased tactile sensitivity, empathic feelings, lowered inhibition, anxiety, chills, sweating, insomnia, muscle cramping, depression, impaired memory, and hyperthermia. Much of the risk that comes with hallucinogen use involves self-neglect or risky behavior during intoxication. Lasting effects of repeated hallucinogen exposure may include persistent perceptual disturbance disorder and problems with memory. There are no medical treatments specific to hallucinogen use disorders.

Dissociative Drugs

Dissociative drugs are notable for producing the feeling of being separate from one's body and surroundings; this is due to the activation of central sigma receptors (dextromethorphan [DXM] and salvia divinorum), NMDA receptor antagonism, and dopamine transporter antagonism (phencyclidine [PCP] and ketamine). These drugs can be chewed, ingested, smoked, inhaled, and injected. In addition to the sensation of dissociation, these drugs may cause impaired motor function, anxiety, nausea, tremors, numbness, and memory impairment. PCP and ketamine use may also produce analgesia, psychosis, aggression, violence, slurred speech, impaired coordination, hallucinations, respiratory depression, seizure, and death. Medical treatment is limited to supportive management of intoxication syndromes.

Anabolic-Androgenic Steroids

Anabolic-androgenic steroids are abused by professional and amateur athletes interested in boosting their athletic performance and/or appearance. Steroids may be ingested, injected, or applied to the skin. While the use of steroids does not produce euphoria, long-term effects of steroid use may include hypertension, left ventricular hypertrophy and cardiac dysfunction, changes in blood clotting and cholesterol, hostility and aggression, liver cysts, infertility, and acne. Steroid use in men may increase the risk of prostate cancer and may also lead to reduced sperm production, shrunken testicles, or breast enlargement. Steroid use in women (far less common) may lead to menstrual irregularities and increased masculine characteristics. Medical treatment is limited to the cessation of steroid use and supportive management of long-term sequelae.

Inhalants

Inhalants are popular among those looking for an easily accessible "high" and thus often used by adolescents and youth. Many household items, especially cleaning supplies, glues, gases, and paints may function as inhalants administered through the nose or mouth ("huffing"). While the effects of inhalants may vary by substance, they are all toxic chemical vapors with differing degrees of neurotoxicity. Short-term effects may include stimulation, loss of inhibition, headache, nausea, vomiting, slurred speech, or loss of coordination; long-term use may be associated with severe cognitive disorders, dementia, and death by suffocation. To date, there are no medical therapies to treat inhalant use disorders.

Sedative-Hypnotics

Sedative-hypnotics (benzodiazepines, barbiturates, and zolpidem-like drugs) potentiate central inhibitory γ-aminobutyric acid (GABA) neurotransmission by neuromodulatory binding to $GABA_A$ receptor subunits. They are typically ingested or injected and used for their anxiolytic and relaxation effects, or to augment other drug use (such as opioid use). Short-term use of sedative-hypnotics may cause sedation, muscle relaxation, confusion, memory impairment, dizziness, and impaired coordination. Chronic sedative-hypnotic misuse may be associated with impaired memory and impaired motor coordination. As with alcohol, abrupt cessation of daily sedative-hypnotic use can result in life-threatening withdrawal seizures. Thus medically supervised detoxification is recommended. Severe sedative-hypnotic use disorders are generally treated by gradual tapering of the misused drug under outpatient physician monitoring.

Epidemiology and Impact of Substance Use Disorders

In the early 1980s, the pioneering Epidemiologic Catchment Area (ECA) study provided the first systematic national assessment of the prevalence of substance use disorders in the United States. Subsequent to the ECA, several other studies have helped refine and track regional and national trends in substance use. These surveys consistently show that substance use disorders are (1) highly prevalent among all ages, beginning in late adolescence, and both genders; (2) frequently co-occur with significant medical and psychiatric illnesses; (3) are associated with high costs at both individual and societal levels; and (4) continue to be largely underdetected and undertreated, in part due to persistent cultural stigma and barriers to medical care, and in part due to the individual's minimization of symptoms deriving from substance abuse.

The World Health Organization (WHO) estimates that 5.4 percent of the total global disease burden results from alcohol and/or illicit drug use, and the mortality rate is highest for substance use disorder among all other mental health disorders. According to the 2016 National Survey on Drug Use and Health (NSDUH), 28.6 million Americans ages 12 and older reported past-month use of illicit drug(s), representing 10 percent of the population. Just over half of Americans in this age group (136.7 million) reported past-month alcohol use, with 48 percent of these reporting binge drinking (5 or more drinks within a few hours for men and 4 or more for women). An estimated 20.1 million Americans met DSM-IV criteria for a past-year substance use disorder (DSM-IV abuse + dependence, which should capture all in the substance use disorder category identified in DSM-5 updated criteria), with 2.3 million of these individuals having both alcohol and illicit drug(s) use disorders. Alcohol use disorder is twice as common as drug use disorder, with 15.1 million versus 7.4 million affected, respectively. Marijuana is the most commonly used drug among all age groups, with 24 million past-month users, of which 4 million met the criteria for past-year marijuana use disorder (1.5 percent of Americans). Prescription opioid use disorder was 2–3 times more commonly reported (1.8 million affected) than cocaine (900,000), methamphetamine (700,000), heroin (600,000), and prescription stimulant (500,000) use disorders. A total of 63.4 million Americans use a tobacco product, the majority (51.3 million) being cigarette smokers, making tobacco-related illnesses the most common preventable causes of morbidity, mortality, and societal health costs (estimated at $300 billion annually in the United States).

Substance use disorders frequently co-occur with other mental illnesses, and having any mental illness doubles an individual's lifetime risk for illicit drug use and/or having a substance use disorder. One in four suicides is associated with having an alcohol use disorder, and most accidental overdose deaths in the United States in 2016 were associated with opioids.

The World Health Organization reports that up to half of all tobacco users will die from tobacco-related causes, with 6 million deaths due to direct use of tobacco

and another 890,000 deaths due to second-hand smoke exposures. Second to tobacco use is alcohol use, with 5.9 percent of all deaths worldwide associated with
alcohol-induced injuries and accidents, cancers, cardiovascular diseases, and liver
cirrhosis. Among illicit drug users, injection drug use is most closely associated
with sexually transmitted disease and life-threatening blood-borne infections associated with needle sharing, such as HIV, HBV, and HCV. Illicit drug use is also
closely linked to tuberculosis infection and malnutrition. In addition to disease
burden, the socioeconomic impact of substance use disorders includes diminished
academic achievement, lower vocational level, and greater on-the-job injuries,
as well as increased violence, domestic abuse and neglect, and incarceration for
drug-related crimes.

Public prevention efforts include raising the perception of risk associated with
substance use, diminishing easy access to substances as defined by legal age limits, policies limiting the geographic density of sales, higher sales taxes imposed
on drugs of abuse, and recent mandates to support smoke-free public environments. Other prevention efforts specifically target vulnerable populations, such as
campus security enforcement directed toward underage drinking and illicit drug
use, mandated substance screening on parole and drug court-mandated treatment
for individuals whose crimes are largely substance-related, safer opioid treatment
interventions for those with co-occurring pain disorders, and culturally sensitive
interventions for at-risk populations (e.g., American Indians, native Alaskans, LG-
BTQ, and chronically homeless individuals).

Etiology of Substance Use Disorders

Substance use disorders, like many other illnesses, have a variety of determinants,
including genetic and psychological vulnerability, the nature of the drug and its
effect on a specific individual, cultural mores, the availability and legality (or lack
thereof) of a particular substance, and the context in which an individual takes a
drug (e.g., morphine administered after major surgery versus oxycodone taken at
a party). Given the complexity of the etiology of substance abuse and substance
use disorders, one way to increase our understanding of this phenomenon is to
invoke the classic public health perspective typically used in the context of infectious disease: that the development of a substance use disorder, like an infectious
disease, involves an interaction between (1) host, (2) agent (in this case, a specific
substance), and (3) environment. The following sections review how each of these
three factors may influence the probability that an individual will engage in substance abuse or develop a substance use disorder.

The Host

Both biological and psychological characteristics of an individual will influence
the probability of substance abuse or expressing a substance use disorder. For

example, having a family history of alcohol use disorder substantially increases the lifetime probability of expressing an alcohol use disorder, and this is due to multiple factors. Studies show that having a parent with severe alcohol use disorder roughly quadruples the risk for alcohol use disorder, and having a sibling with alcohol use disorder is also predictive of increased risk. Yet the fact that alcohol use disorder runs in families does not tell us whether this occurs as the result of genetic or environmental influences, or both; we know that both hemophilia and speaking English runs in families, for example, but the former is genetically transmitted and the latter is an environmentally acquired behavior.

To determine mediators, twin studies have been informative in that monozygotic (identical) twins show a higher concordance rate for severe alcohol use disorders than dizygotic (non-identical) twin pairs, suggesting an etiologic role of genetic heritability. It could be argued, however, that monozygotic and dizygotic twins have differing environmental experiences (i.e., they may be treated differently); therefore these data alone cannot fully inform etiology. Adoption studies help discern genetic from environmental influences, as these studies examine individuals who are adopted soon after birth and thus carry a potential genetic risk for alcohol use disorder from biological parents who do not raise them and an environmental risk from adoptive parents with no biological relationship. Interestingly, studies of this type generally demonstrate that biological children of parents with severe alcohol use disorder retain a greater lifetime risk of expressing alcohol use disorder, regardless of environmental upbringing, confirming the heritability of alcohol use disorder.

What is it about this complex neurobehavioral disorder that could be inherited? Differential neurobiological sensitivity to alcohol exposure appears to be one heritable factor that confers either risk or protection. A series of seminal studies conducted by Schuckit and colleagues compared alcohol responses in young, healthy men with a family history of severe alcohol use disorder to an age-matched group of men without this family history. The two groups had significant differences in both subjective and objective response to alcohol: those with a positive family history had *attenuated* responses to alcohol at equivalent blood alcohol levels, compared with those with a negative family history. Those at-risk appear to have a higher tolerance to the effects of alcohol, which would be predicted to lead to increased alcohol consumption in order to achieve feedback that one is intoxicated. Considering this, intoxication perception serves as a satiety feedback signal (i.e., "I have now had enough to drink."). Malfunction of this feedback loop would cause an individual to perceive intoxication only after blood alcohol levels are well beyond low-risk levels; health consequences along with social/occupational consequences will more likely occur, and impaired executive functioning during intoxication will facilitate perseverative consumption, leading over time to increased tolerance and physiologic dependence.

Subsequent studies have examined potential genetic factors contributing to the differential response to alcohol. One area of intense interest has been the metabolic pathway for alcohol, specifically the enzymes alcohol dehydrogenase and aldehyde dehydrogenase. Since aldehyde dehydrogenase is responsible for the oxidation of acetaldehyde, deficiencies in this enzyme cause an accumulation of acetaldehyde with alcohol ingestion, which can lead to aversive symptoms such as flushing, headache, and tachycardia (not unlike the mechanism of action of the medication disulfiram, as discussed later in the section "Disulfiram in the Treatment of Alcohol Use Disorders"). A substantial minority of the Asian population has reduced aldehyde dehydrogenase activity, resulting in aversive conditioned response to alcohol consumption and thus avoidance of drinking. This genetic variant would be protective against developing alcohol use disorder.

Other biological factors that appear to influence the treatment of alcohol use disorder involve the mu-opioid receptor system. Genetic variance in the mu-opioid receptor OPRM1 gene affects the response to the opioid antagonist, naltrexone, an evidence-based medication used to treat severe alcohol use disorders. Patients in whom aspartic acid (Asp) replaces asparagine (Asn) at position 40 of the mu-opioid receptor are more likely to respond beneficially to naltrexone than those who are homozygous for the Asn40 allele.

The Agent

The principle of reinforcement plays an important role in the development of substance use disorders. Common drugs of abuse are all highly reinforcing, meaning that subjectively perceived reward facilitates and trains repeated drug-taking behaviors. Solid evidence supporting the reinforcing properties of substances of abuse is derived from both animal and human self-administration research. In the classic laboratory paradigm, an animal is trained to "work" for a substance by performing a particular behavior (e.g., pressing a lever) that results in the administration of a drug. The animal may then be required to increase the frequency of that behavior to obtain the drug again; the strength of the reinforcing property of that drug can be measured as a function of the number of times an animal is willing to press the lever to obtain the drug (how hard the animal will "work" for reward). Reinforcement can also be examined in studies in which the animal presses one lever to receive a drug and a different lever to receive food, a natural reinforcer; comparative strength of the two reinforcing stimuli can thus be measured. An extreme example of drug reinforcement is that rhesus monkeys given free access to intravenous cocaine will self-administer the drug until it results in death. In this case, the supernatural strength of the stimulant reward essentially "hijacks" all natural survival behaviors, including rest and seeking nourishment.

Although the common drugs of abuse vary in their effects, the method by which they exert their reinforcing effects share some similarities. Specifically, many substances of abuse exert their reinforcing properties by amplifying dopamine neurotransmission or direct release within areas of the mesolimbic dopaminergic pathways, particularly the nucleus accumbens and amygdala. Other neurotransmitters implicated in reward/reinforcement include glutamate, endorphins and enkephalins (endogenous opioids), norepinephrine, and serotonin.

The Environment

Substance use and misuse occur within a context of familial, regional, and national culture, social attitudes and mores, laws, religious beliefs and practices, and varying accessibility. All of these factors influence the regional prevalence of substance use and misuse, and some of these factors, particularly accessibility, will influence the probability of a higher frequency of substance use, a risk factor for developing a substance use disorder. For instance, the two substances with the highest rates of physiologic dependence and substance use disorder in the United States are alcohol and nicotine, largely due to high accessibility by virtue of being legally available to adults. Additionally, the competitive market within legal sales drives down cost, another factor increasing accessibility to the average individual. It has been repeatedly demonstrated in studies throughout the world that increasing cost of substances effects use: restricting the accessibility of alcohol and cigarettes through increased taxes leads to reduced consumption, while increasing accessibility by extending the hours during which one may purchase alcohol and cigarettes leads to increased sales and higher consumption.

Perceptions of substance use risk also substantially influence substance use prevalence and initiation of substance use. For example, in the mid-1980s, public perceptions of cocaine shifted from that of a relatively harmless "party drug" to a potentially dangerous drug that could lead to overdose and death; the number of people who used cocaine during that time declined accordingly. In 2012, cannabis use among adolescents and young adults increased with reduced perceptions of cannabis risk among these cohorts. The decreased perception of risk is occurring within the cultural context of the medical marijuana and recreational legalization movement; here, a cultural influence (medical marijuana and legalization promotion) both increases access directly to the consumer (especially in states with approved recreational legalization and/or broad indications for being recommended medical marijuana) and indirectly via lowered perceptions of harm with use (in this case, also with increased perceptions of safety and benefit with use).

The context in which a drug is taken also influences the natural history of its use. At no time was this more clearly demonstrated than when large numbers of members of the United States military used heroin while fighting in the Vietnam War. There was substantial concern that when these troops returned to the United States, there would be a dramatic increase in the rate of heroin addiction in this country; however, that did not occur. Interestingly, only a small percentage of those who used heroin while in Vietnam continued to do so after returning to the United States. The role of context was critical here. In Vietnam, heroin was easily available, highly pure, and inexpensive. Moreover, for US troops the setting was uniquely stressful. Upon their return to the United States, many military personnel would have encountered access barriers, including challenges of obtaining an illicit drug, lower purity (i.e., lower quality of reinforcement) and higher cost, cultural disapproval, as well as competing factors against drug-taking, such as access to college or work-study programs through veterans benefits. Additionally, the home environment was completely different, such that cue-conditioned and stress-conditioned drug-taking associated with the Vietnam combat theater would be substantially diminished.

The role of context is important in the transition from substance use to substance use disorders in another way, namely through classical (Pavlovian) conditioning. When people use reinforcing substances within a particular environment (e.g., a neighborhood), they are likely to experience a strong desire or craving to use that substance again upon re-entry to that environment. Indeed, this type of conditioned response that triggers substance craving remains for a substantial time after cessation of substance use (i.e., it extinguishes slowly). Other conditioned cues associated with substance use (e.g., hearing someone open a can or bottle of beer, smelling cigarette smoke, seeing a hypodermic needle) may provoke thoughts and cravings to use that substance, or even another substance of abuse. Over time, these conditioned associations will weaken, but they endure in learned memory, and thereby constitute an enduring risk factor for relapse to substance use.

In sum, the development of substance use disorders represents a complex interplay between individual biological vulnerability, the reinforcing properties of a substance taken, the frequency and quantity of a substance taken repeatedly, the ease of access to the substance, and sociocultural and environmental context. The complexity of these interactions helps to explain the heterogeneity of substance use disorders observed in community populations.

Clinical Features and Course

Core Clinical Features

Problematic substance use can range from discrete episodes of hazardous or harmful use to a pattern of substance use meeting diagnostic criteria for substance use disorder according to the *Diagnostic and Statistical Manual of Mental Disorders*, 5th edition (DSM-5). A universal clinical feature of all problematic substance use is either the occurrence or a credible threat of an unintended negative consequence directly caused by or related to substance use. Examples of this would include any of the following occurring in the context of substance use: operating machinery or a motor vehicle while intoxicated, risky sexual behavior, uncharacteristic interpersonal altercation or fight, absenteeism from work or school, physical injury (such as a fall or hypothermia), and acute medical or psychiatric illness exacerbation caused by substance use. Substance use also significantly increases the risk for both suicide and violent behavior, including homicide, as well as increasing the risk of becoming the victim of a violent act.

Core features of a substance use disorder are defined by maladaptive patterns of substance use (episodic or daily) associated with predictable biological, cognitive, and behavioral changes. These changes manifest as (1) the development of tolerance (increased self-dosing in order to achieve a desired effect) or a characteristic withdrawal syndrome in the absence of the substance, (2) anticipation and craving for the substance and preoccupation with obtaining the substance, (3) loss of self-regulation over substance use (using greater amount or more frequently than intended), and (4) increased time spent in obtaining, using, or recovering from substance use, at the cost of time spent engaged in healthy behaviors and interests. It is worth emphasizing that individuals can meet criteria for having a substance use disorder without developing physiologic tolerance or withdrawal. Typically, individuals having a substance use disorder can recognize negative consequences related to their patterns of substance use, yet substance use persists because of more powerful neurobiological incentives to use substances, either for pleasure/reward or to experience relief from stress or withdrawal syndromes. These natural incentives frequently override judgment or otherwise interferes with efforts to stop using substances, particularly when access to substances is readily available.

It is important to note that substance use disorders occur along a continuum of severity; it is thus possible to have a mild, moderate, or severe substance use disorder. Moreover, some but not all substance use disorders progress; some individuals have mild problems for many years without developing more serious consequences.

Acute Intoxication

Individuals acutely under the influence of a substance display recognizable clinical signs and symptoms of substance intoxication evident on mental status exam and physical exam. Acute intoxication states are specific to the substance being used (as noted previously) and are described in terms of neurological depressant, stimulant, or hallucinogenic effects. Polysubstance use produces mixed effects; severe medical sequelae (e.g., cardiac arrhythmia, seizure, autonomic instability, respiratory depression) are seen with polysubstance use, high-dose or intravenous substance use, and substance use in medically compromised individuals.

Abstinence Syndromes

Abstinence syndromes are characteristic of individuals with physiological dependence as part of a substance use disorder. With repeated substance use, the brain will compensate for abnormal neurochemical signaling induced by substance exposure via adjustments in inhibitory and excitatory neurotransmission (primarily gamma-aminobutyric acid (GABA) and glutamate, respectively), a process referred to as *allostasis*. Abrupt cessation of substance use results in physiological and psychological signs and symptoms reflecting allostatic changes in neural signaling, with recognizable "rebound" syndromes that typically oppose the acute effects of the substance (e.g., hyperexcitability with CNS depressant use and fatigue with CNS stimulant use).

Physical Examination and Biomarkers

Physical examination is helpful not only in detecting acute intoxication and abstinence syndromes associated with substance use but also in detecting chronic health effects and/or social harm related to substance use. The following sections describe substance-specific signs and symptoms and laboratory tests that can assist diagnosis and direct treatment interventions.

Alcohol Use

Heavy drinking is defined as having at least four (women) or five (men) drinks per drinking episode and is correlated with increased medical consequences and risk for several cancers. Alcohol is neurotoxic, and overuse may lead to peripheral neuropathies, cerebellar degeneration with gait instability and abnormal reflexes, loss of cerebral gray matter and cognitive decline, and in pregnant women, fetal alcohol spectrum disorders. Chronic heavy alcohol use may be associated with high blood pressure, thiamine deficiency and poor nutrition, gastrointestinal bleeding and gastroesophageal reflux, pancreatitis, fatty liver and hepatic cirrhosis, cardiomyopathy, and stigmata of the skin including flushing and spider angiomas. Abnormalities in complete blood count (enlarged mean corpuscular volume and decreased hematocrit), hepatic panel (elevated AST, ALT, GGT, and CDT), elevated serum amylase, and decreased serum magnesium may be seen in individuals with more advanced alcohol use disorders. A smell of alcohol on the breath may be confirmed with a calibrated breathalyzer to determine blood alcohol levels, conferring risk for impaired driving, alcohol poisoning, or alcohol withdrawal syndrome.

Tobacco Use

Cigarette smoking and the use of smokeless tobacco products are significantly associated with increased cancer risk of multiple types, especially of the lung and oropharynx, due to "tar" contaminants that are carcinogenic, particularly upon combustion with cigarette smoking. Smoking is associated with respiratory compromise (asthma, emphysema, chronic obstructive pulmonary disease) and significantly increases an individual's risk for coronary artery disease, high blood pressure, cerebrovascular accidents, blood clotting, peripheral vascular compromise, and poor wound healing. Second-hand smoke exposure is associated with increased risk for lung cancer, respiratory compromise, and cardiovascular disease in adults; in children, passive exposure to second-hand smoke is associated with respiratory compromise (especially asthma), increased incidence of respiratory viral illness and ear infections, and sudden infant death syndrome. Tarry yellowing of fingers, smoke on breath, abnormalities on pulmonary auscultation and pulmonary function testing, and subjective symptoms of shortness of breath are common indicators of nicotine dependence and tobacco use. Pregnant women who smoke are at greater risk for miscarriage, intrauterine growth restriction, and premature labor.

Cannabis Use

Like cigarette smoking, chronic heavy use of smoked marijuana is associated with increased risk for respiratory illnesses, cancer, and heart attack. Daily or near-daily cannabis use has been associated with negative effects on learning, memory, mood, and capacity to engage in normal pleasurable activities. Heavy use of cannabis in adolescence has been associated with an increased risk for having a lifetime psychotic episode. The neuropsychiatric risks of cannabis use are greatest for heavy daily smokers, those who begin smoking in early adolescence, and babies exposed to intrauterine cannabis due to mother's use during pregnancy. A pungent cannabis odor and glassy, injected sclerae on physical exam are signs of acute cannabis intoxication, which more than doubles the risk of having a motor vehicle accident. Urine toxicology in daily users may remain positive for cannabinoids for up to thirty days.

Opioid Use

Accidental overdose fatalities due to respiratory depression with illicit and prescribed opioid use quadrupled in the last decade, in parallel with national increases in prescription opioid prescribing. Prescription opioid use is associated with the majority (62 percent) of reported overdoses compared with heroin use alone; more recently, illicitly manufactured fentanyl analogs contribute to rising rates of opioid overdose deaths. On physical exam, drowsiness and pupillary constriction with depressed vital signs (decreased pulse, respiratory rate, and blood pressure) are suggestive of acute use, while the appearance of "track marks" (erythema at injection sites) and/or a history of opioid withdrawal symptoms and doctor-shopping or "lost" prescriptions suggest a more chronic opioid use disorder. Babies with intrauterine opioid exposure are at risk for low birth weight and neurodevelopmental abnormalities, and may require medical treatment for opioid abstinence syndrome upon birth. Urine toxicology will detect codeine and morphine metabolites of heroin within one to three days of use, but routine panels will not identify many prescription opioids; clinical suspicion warrants a specially ordered narcotic panel.

Cocaine/Stimulant Use

Cocaine, methamphetamine, and prescription stimulant (e.g., amphetamine, dexedrine, methylphenidate) use may be oral, intranasal, smoked (crack cocaine), or intravenous and is associated with significant increases in risk for elevated heart rate, temperature and blood pressure, cardiac arrhythmias, abdominal pain and vomiting, stroke, seizure, aggressive behavior, hallucinations/paranoid ideation, and sudden death. Increasing access to higher-purity methamphetamine has significantly contributed to increasing drug overdose death rates. Stimulant use during pregnancy significantly increases the fetal risk of abruptio placentae, low birth weight, and neurodevelopmental abnormalities. Chronic use is associated with gingivitis and tooth decay, sinus infection and perforated nasal septum, and depressed mood with increased risk for suicide. Intravenous use increases the risk of blood-borne infections. Concurrent cocaine and alcohol use produces the hepatic metabolite, cocaethylene, which increases the risk of sudden cardiac death, seizure, and hemorrhagic stroke.

Urine toxicology detects use within one to three days. Since many stimulant users have an episodic binge pattern of use, hair sampling toxicology may be more useful for detecting less frequent episodes during the previous ninety days.

Hallucinogens and Synthetic Drug Use

A variety of dangerous synthetic drugs, primarily used by teenagers and young adults, are commonly referred to as "club drugs" due to the proclivity to use these drugs within social gatherings. This category includes many drugs – for example, stimulants such as methamphetamine, MDMA ("ecstasy"), and synthetic cathinones ("bath salts"); hallucinogens and dissociative drugs such as LSD, GHB, ketamine, salvia, and synthetic cannabinoids such as "K-2" and "spice" – with potent hallucinogen effects and varying physiological effects including vomiting, insomnia, temperature dysregulation and dehydration, autonomic instability, psychosis, delirium, and sudden death. In the past decade, a sharp rise in the accessibility of new synthetic compounds has posed problems to clinical detection, as many compounds are not detectable with routinely available toxicology panels, and clinical presentation is variable and often confounded by polysubstance use. Seeking data from collateral sources (friends and family) is imperative if clinical suspicion is high and toxicology is unrevealing.

Heterogeneous Course of Illness

Substance use disorders range in both severity and chronicity and the majority of individuals with problematic substance use or substance use disorder never receive medical treatment. For example, a large national epidemiologic database revealed five distinct subtypes of DSM-IV alcohol dependence, with a majority of individuals experiencing natural remission and a small fraction progressing to persistent disease. Diagnosis of the individual phenotype is critical to developing appropriate-level treatment interventions.

Epigenetic Factors

Substance use disorders are heritable, multifactorial disorders, defined as the result of multiple genes interacting with environmental and lifestyle factors. As such, the phenotype spectrum is broad, and within any individual, the frequency of substance exposures determines neuroadaptive molecular and cellular changes that may result in stable alterations of gene expression, termed *epigenetic mechanisms of functional plasticity*. The good news here is that no matter how vulnerable a person's genetic predisposition to substance use disorders, disease is not expressed if substance exposure is prevented.

Individual Protective Factors

Many factors have been identified in youth and adults that protect against the initiation of substance use and/or support efforts to stop using substances. These include older age at first use, lack of immediate access to substances in social networks and environment, higher educational achievement, close family supports, after-school monitoring and structure, being employed, and having cultural and spiritual values and beliefs that promote abstinence from substance use or use in moderation, whereby drinking is viewed as acceptable but getting drunk is not.

Individual Risk Factors

Risk factors for problematic substance use are both biological and environmental. Biological risk factors include a family history of substance use disorders and psychiatric disorders, having a chronic pain disorder or psychiatric disorder, and temperamental factors such as impulsivity and aggressiveness. Other risk factors include young age of first use, easy access to substances in social networks and environment, any history of childhood trauma, lack of social supports and structured activity, poverty, and acute negative life events or loss such as the death of a spouse or sudden loss of employment.

Clinical Evaluation and Differential Diagnosis of Substance Use Disorders

According to the 2016 National Survey on Drug Use and Health, the vast majority (89 percent) of Americans with a substance use disorder report no treatment in the past year. Having an untreated substance use disorder increases the likelihood of developing other illnesses or failing to respond adequately to treatment aimed at other illnesses. Thus it is recommended that every clinician screen for problematic substance use at every clinical encounter. It is also helpful for clinicians to be trained in interviewing styles, such as motivational interviewing, that are designed to elicit self-report data on sensitive topics for which collaborative behavioral change goals may be advisable, and to support patient-clinician collaboration.

Acute Syndromes: Intoxication, Impairment, and Injury

Substance intoxication is often suspected in a patient who presents to a clinical setting with an altered mental status. The patient may appear confused, "high," drowsy, irritable, euphoric, anxious, paranoid, disoriented, and so forth. In such situations, clinicians screen for substance use as a contributing factor by:

- Asking about recent use of substances, both licit and illicit, in a non-judgmental and empathic manner
- Looking for signs and symptoms expected with substance use during the physical examination
- Performing toxicological analysis for suspected substances of abuse
- Performing other laboratory or imaging studies to confirm or rule out a substance-related condition
- When necessary or appropriate, asking significant others about the possibility of substance use

Patients may be reluctant to fully disclose substance use to clinicians due to stigma about substance use, fear of being negatively evaluated or treated, having previous negative experiences with health care, or concerns about confidentiality and/or liability. With this in mind, a patient's denial of substance use is insufficient to rule out substance use contributing to altered mental status. Similarly, a patient's self-report endorsing substance use may be incomplete in the type of substance or quantity/frequency of substance consumed. Patients may knowingly omit a history of illicit drug use while endorsing alcohol use, or they may intend to disclose fully but be unaware of having consumed adulterant drugs (e.g., cannabis adulterated with stimulants). Finally, patients frequently use multiple substances concurrently (e.g., heroin and cocaine, known as "speedballing") or sequentially (e.g., drinking heavily and then using stimulants to remain awake), making the differential diagnosis challenging at times.

The consumption of alcoholic beverages, non-ethanol alcohols (e.g., antifreeze, rubbing alcohol, methanol fuel), as well as non-beverage ethanol (e.g., hand sanitizers, mouthwash) all produce similar signs and symptoms of intoxication. These signs and symptoms are overlapping with those seen with the use of sedatives and hypnotics (benzodiazepines, barbiturates, "z-drugs" such as zolpidem, and gamma-hydroxy-butyrate). Typically, a patient exhibits dose-dependent changes in mood and affect (initially social disinhibition, followed by dysphoric presentations upon larger volume consumption and increased blood alcohol levels), slurred speech, motor incoordination, flushed faces, disinhibited and/or perseverative behavior, red conjunctivae, and odors of alcohol that may be detectable on breath and perspiration. Ingesting toxic amounts ("alcohol poisoning") leads to acute confusion, stupor, unconsciousness, and respiratory depression, especially if alcohol is combined with sedatives. A serum alcohol level or a breathalyzer should be obtained to determine the blood alcohol content (BAC). A patient who appears acutely intoxicated from alcohol but with a negative BAC should prompt serum analysis for isopropyl alcohol (rubbing alcohol), methanol, and ethylene glycol (antifreeze). Methanol ingestion is important to identify in a patient presenting with intoxication and acute visual changes, as permanent loss of vision may occur without emergency management of acute metabolic acidosis.

Although positive toxicology does not establish causality about altered mental status, a positive drug screen for benzodiazepines or other sedatives in an acutely intoxicated individual is important data informing risk for respiratory depression (especially with longer-acting sedatives) as well as the risk of future withdrawal seizure (especially with shorter-acting sedatives). It is important to note that routine urine toxicology may not reliably identify commonly misused sedatives (e.g., clonazepam is frequently not detected).

Acute opioid intoxication is important to recognize since respiratory depression with overdose may be rapidly reversed with the opioid antagonist, naloxone. In addition to experiencing analgesia, patients will present with dose-dependent changes in mood (relaxation to euphoria), level of consciousness (mild sedation to "nodding off" to unresponsive), constricted pupils, hypoventilation, and reduced gut motility. Additionally, patients may experience bradycardia, nausea, vomiting, hypothermia, and itching. "Nodding off" is a characteristic finding in opioid intoxication – the patient appears asleep but may be subjectively aware of the surroundings, is able to respond when spoken to, but is self-absorbed with the feelings of euphoria and relaxation. Obtaining a toxicology test for opioids is important, although caution is needed in the interpretation. Standard immunoassays are calibrated for detecting morphine and codeine (two metabolites of heroin), and other brief opioid panels may be calibrated to detect methadone, but routine assays may not detect opioid analgesics commonly associated with opioid use disorders (hydrocodone, oxycodone, fentanyl, and tramadol). Special order narcotic panels are recommended for suspected opioid misuse and overdose.

In contrast, acute stimulant (e.g., cocaine, methamphetamine, bath salts) intoxication induces dose-dependent cognitive enhancement, euphoria, psychomotor agitation, restlessness, hypersexuality, teeth grinding, and other sympathomimetic signs, such as tachycardia, hypertension, dilated pupils, and sweating. At very high doses, paranoia, hallucinations, delusions, seizure, and hyperthermia may be observed. Smokers of crack cocaine may present with acute injury to their lungs, complaining of fever, hemoptysis, shortness of breath, and cough ("crack lung"). Routine urine toxicology is generally sensitive for detecting the cocaine metabolite, benzoylecgonine. In contrast, urine testing for amphetamines is less reliable due to a large number of compounds that cross-react, resulting in high rates of false-positive results.

Intoxication from dissociative drugs (e.g., phencyclidine, ketamine, dextromethorphan) can produce signs and symptoms similar to alcohol and sedative intoxication – alterations in mood (i.e. euphoria, irritability, anxiety), ataxia, nystagmus, slurred speech, red conjunctivae, and motor incoordination. They can also produce sympathomimetic signs similar to those produced by cocaine and other stimulants – tachycardia, hypertension, flushing, and sweating. However, at higher doses, hypotension and bradycardia may be noted, as well as motor disturbances such as dystonia, tremors, seizures, and coma. Other notable changes include a sense of derealization or detachment from the world, numbness in extremities, agitation, hallucinations, paranoia, disorganized thought process, and violence toward the self or others. Persistent psychosis warrants testing for these substances.

Hallucinogens (e.g., LSD, psilocybin, mescaline) may produce an intoxication characterized by profound alterations in mood, perceptions, thought process, and behavior. Moods may vary tremendously from calm to agitated. Hallucinogen intoxication is heavily influenced by the psychological ("set") and physical ("setting") environment of the user. Therefore, a depressed patient taking LSD in an unsafe environment may experience a worsening of depression and anxiety. When dysphoria, paranoia, or anxiety is significant, the intoxication may lead to a "bad trip," characterized by panic attacks. Autonomic changes are often noted, especially dilated pupils, tachycardia, and hyperthermia, sweating, and tremors. Routine toxicology will not detect these substances.

Polysubstance use is a lead cause of accidental fatalities presenting to emergency care and trauma units. Differential diagnosis of emergency presentations of accident or violent injury includes screening for substance abuse, which may be associated with such presentations in all age cohorts.

Stabilization of Withdrawal Syndromes

Withdrawal syndromes occur when a substance used chronically is abruptly stopped or reduced. Stabilization is achieved by administering controlled doses of agonist substitutes.

Alcohol withdrawal symptoms typically begin six to twelve hours after the last drink ingested. Symptoms vary individually but will most consistently include elevations in heart rate, blood pressure, and temperature. A minority of patients will develop more severe forms of alcohol withdrawal, such as tonic-clonic seizures and delirium tremens (DTs), which generally occur during the first forty-eight to seventy-two hours after the last drink. Patients developing DTs may exhibit hallucinations (auditory, visual, and tactile), but disorientation is more of a hallmark of DTs, typically accompanied by severe autonomic disturbances. DTs is a life-threatening medical emergency treated with aggressive benzodiazepine therapy that may require intensive care support.

If delirium or seizure develops greater than one week after the last drink, other etiologies or contributing factors should be sought. A challenge for clinicians is to distinguish between patients delirious from an underlying medical issue (e.g., sepsis or metabolic disturbances) and those delirious due to DTs. A known history of alcohol use disorder, prior episodes of DTs, history of detoxification, and absence of any underlying medical disturbances, should all prompt the clinician to consider DTs as the etiology for the change in mental status. Conversely, a patient younger than age thirty, or those without a prolonged drinking history (>10 years), are less likely to experience DTs. In some instances, scoring the revised Clinical Institute Withdrawal Assessment for Alcohol (CIWA-Ar) can assist in assessing the risk for DTs.

Withdrawal from sedative and hypnotics (benzodiazepines, barbiturates) may produce a similar syndrome to alcohol withdrawal or may first manifest with only neuropsychiatric disturbances (severe anxiety, confusion, hallucinations, or paranoia) and without prominent psychomotor or autonomic signs. While alcohol withdrawal is rare among youth, sedative-hypnotic withdrawal may be experienced in much younger patients. The pharmacokinetic profile of the substance determines the time course of the withdrawal syndrome. For example, withdrawal from long-acting benzodiazepines and barbiturates may begin much later than withdrawal from a short-acting benzodiazepine. Patients maintained on therapeutic levels of benzodiazepines can experience withdrawal, and overuse increases this risk.

Opioid withdrawal presents a predictable constellation of signs and symptoms. For short-acting opioids (heroin, morphine, oxycodone), withdrawal begins about eight to twelve hours after last use, and may be characterized by irritability, anxiety, cravings for opioids, insomnia, nausea, diarrhea, muscle and joint pains, rhinorrhea, lacrimation, yawning, goose flesh, tremors, dilated pupils, fever, tachycardia, hypertension, fatigue, and hot and cold flashes. These signs and symptoms tend to increase in intensity over the course of several days, and may take seven to ten days to resolve. Long-acting opioids (buprenorphine, methadone, fentanyl) may lead to the emergence of withdrawal two to five days after the last use, and may take up to several weeks to resolve completely, with mild residual subjective symptoms (fatigue, malaise) remaining for months. Confusion, disorientation, and seizures are not experienced with opioid withdrawal, and their presence should prompt the evaluation for other etiologies. The Clinical Opiate Withdrawal Scale (COWS) may be helpful in the assessment.

Screening Assessments for Office-Based Detection of Substance Use

Not all problematic substance use will meet the criteria for a DSM-5 substance use disorder, and early detection of hazardous substance use (defined by the World Health Organization as a pattern of substance use that increases the risk for harmful health consequences to the user) is an important goal for preventing harmful use and the development of substance use disorders. It is recommended that all health care settings incorporate screening assessments for hazardous and harmful substance use. It is also recommended that all clinicians be trained to be able to deliver simple brief interventions (such as providing normative feedback and advice to reduce substance use) and to have a referral option for more complex needs. A comprehensive assessment of substance use and referral algorithm is referred to as SBIRT (screening, brief intervention, and referral) and is coded as a reimbursable health care service.

Many validated screening assessments exist for tobacco, alcohol, and drug use (see the National Institute on Drug Abuse [NIDA] online tools at www.drugabuse. gov/nidamed-medical-health-professionals/screening-tools-resources/chart-screening-tools). The most commonly used assessments are those that are publicly accessible, have properties that fit well into routine clinical care settings, and are appropriate to the population being served. Generally, single-item screening questions or very brief (three items or fewer) assessments begin the process and further screening follows if the initial screen is positive. For instance, the Heaviness of Smoking Index is an abbreviated aspect of the Fagerstrom Test for Nicotine Dependence:

1. How soon after you wake up do you smoke your first cigarette?
   3– Within 5 minutes
   2– 6–30 minutes
   1– 31–60 minutes
   0– After 60 minutes
2. How many cigarettes/day do you smoke? (1 pack equals 20 cigarettes)
   0– 10 or less
   1– 11–20
   2– 21–30
   3– 31 or more

The sum of points for both questions interprets the results of the assessment as "low addiction" (0–2), "moderate addiction" (3–4), and "high addiction" (5–6). Since tobacco use is carcinogenic and has other health consequences, any use would warrant brief education and advice to stop smoking, and heavy use would warrant smoking cessation treatment/referral and support.

For alcohol use, two brief screens are commonly used. There is a single-question screen, "How many times in the past year have you had five or more (men)/four or more (women) drinks in a day?" Any score other than zero is a positive screen, indicating the need for further assessment and discussion. The gold standard alcohol use assessment is the ten-item Alcohol Use Disorders Identification Test (AUDIT), which can be used as a follow-up to the single-question screen noted previously. Items score volume and frequency of drinking, alcohol dependence, and lifetime problems associated with alcohol use. The AUDIT and its scoring is available at www.who.org. An abbreviated three-item version, the AUDIT-Consumption

(AUDIT-C), is a screen frequently used in primary care, shown here with scoring points where 3 or more is positive for women and 4 or more is positive for men, unless all points are scored only in item 1.

1. How often do you have a drink containing alcohol?
   0– Never
   1– Monthly or less
   2– 2–4 times a month
   3– 2–3 times a week
   4– 4 or more times a week
2. How many standard drinks containing alcohol do you have on a typical day?
   0– 1 or 2
   1– 3 or 4
   2– 5 or 6
   3– 7 to 9
   4– 10 or more
3. How often do you have 6 or more drinks on one occasion?
   0– Never
   1– Less than monthly
   2– Monthly
   3– Weekly
   4– Daily

In each of these examples, the clinician must be trained in proper interpretation of assessment scoring and be prepared to translate medical advice to the patient regarding "low-risk" drinking patterns and "high-risk" drinking patterns, or patterns consistent with alcohol use disorder. Since low to moderate alcohol consumption may also provide health benefits in healthy adults without risk factors, individualized assessment is necessary. Providing patient feedback and advice is best delivered in an engaging, non-judgmental manner that allows the patient to feel comfortable asking follow-up questions. The National Institute on Alcohol Abuse and Alcoholism provides patient-friendly online tools for "Rethinking Drinking" at www.rethinkingdrinking.niaaa.nih.gov/how-much-is-too-much/.

Illicit drug screening also may use a single-question screen: "How many times in the past year have you used an illegal drug or used a prescription medication for nonmedical reasons?" Any score other than zero is a positive score requiring further assessment, especially screening for injection drug use, which can pose serious health consequences with even a single use. A common screen is the ten-item Drug Assessment Screening Tool (DAST-10), in which a score of 2 or more is a positive screen. Several abbreviated versions may be used, including the following three questions:

- Do you abuse more than one drug at a time?
- Have you ever neglected family or missed work because of your use of drugs?
- Have you ever experienced withdrawal problems as a result of heavy drug intake?

Brief interventions for illicit drug use are always recommended, as there is no known "safe" or "low-risk" pattern of drug use and there are significant legal risks associated with illicit drug use (including felony offense with a diversion of controlled prescription medications, such as opioid analgesics).

Special Populations: Screening for Substance Use in Adolescents and Pregnant Women

Two clinical populations at risk for harmful substance use are adolescents, whose use patterns tend to be impulsive/experimental and often ignorant of health and neurodevelopmental risks, and pregnant women, for whom there is no known safe amount of any substance use (tobacco, alcohol, and most drugs of abuse have demonstrated teratogenicity). Therefore, unique screening assessments have been designed for these at-risk populations, outlined as follows.

Adolescent Substance Use: The CRAFFT

The CRAFFT screen is named for the six-item question content that was developed to be sensitive to detecting hazardous alcohol or drug use in adolescents, who frequently engage in episodic substance use that may be high risk, but often does not meet medical criteria for a DSM-5 substance use disorder. The screening questions are as follows, and any answer "Yes" indicates problematic substance use requiring brief intervention; a score of 2 or more "Yes" responses warrants referral to substance abuse treatment.

- Have you ever ridden in a CAR driven by someone (including yourself) who was high or had been using alcohol or drugs?
- Do you ever use alcohol or drugs to RELAX, feel better about yourself, or fit in?
- Do you ever use alcohol or drugs while you are by yourself, ALONE?
- Do you ever FORGET things you did while using alcohol or drugs?
- Do your family or FRIENDS ever tell you that you should cut down on your drinking or drug use?
- Have you ever gotten into TROUBLE while you were using alcohol or drugs?

Pregnant Women and Those Planning A Pregnancy: The T-ACE and TWEAK

Pregnant women often under-report substance use for reasons associated with stigma, shame, and fears about mandated reporting of substance use during pregnancy (required in most states) that may affect child custody postpartum and that in some states has been considered a criminal act of child abuse. It is imperative that screening be delivered with respect and concern for supporting positive maternal-fetal outcomes. The risks associated with screening in a judgmental manner or omitting screening altogether include dropout from prenatal care and/ or continued substance use and fetal exposure that may result in fetal malformations or growth restriction. Additionally, it is critical to safe birthing and infant care to know in advance whether or not the newborn is likely to require treatment for a neonatal abstinence syndrome.

The T-ACE (tolerance, annoyed, cut down, eye-opener) is a four-item assessment very similar in content to the standard CAGE screen for heavy alcohol use (cut down, annoyed, guilty about drinking, eye-opener); exchanging the "guilt" item for the "tolerance" item improves the assessment utility among pregnant women. A score of 2 or more is positive (all items "yes" are 1 point except the first item on tolerance, which is 2 points).

- How many drinks does it take you to get high? (>2 is positive for tolerance)
- Have close friends/relatives ever been annoyed with you because of your drinking?
- Have you ever felt the need to cut down your drinking?
- Do you sometimes take a drink in the morning?

The TWEAK (tolerance, worried about drinking, eye-opener, amnesia, "kut" back) is a similar five-item screen where a score of 2 or more is positive (items one and two are 2 points and three through five are 1 point).

- How many drinks does it take you to get high? (>2 is positive for tolerance)
- Have close friends/relatives worried or complained about your drinking in the last year?
- Do you sometimes take a drink in the morning?
- Has a friend or family ever told you something you said or did that you didn't remember?
- Have you ever felt the need to cut down your drinking?

The 4Ps Plus is a validated proprietary screen that comprehensively asks pregnant women about risk factors for all substance use (tobacco, alcohol, and drugs), including asking for information about family history of substance use problems, past use and recent use (prior to pregnancy awareness) of substances, partner use of substances, and social factors affecting stress (e.g., single parenting, interpartner violence).

Pregnant or pre-conception women who score significantly on these screens are best referred to specialized treatment, with the goal of achieving total abstinence from all substances. National self-report data indicate that most pregnant substance users are motivated to reduce use significantly once a pregnancy is known and prenatal counseling has advised abstinence. Engaging expecting fathers in abstinence support enhances a pregnant woman's probability of abstaining from substance use.

Biomarkers and Immunoassay in Substance Use Screening

Laboratory analyses of biomarkers are most useful in monitoring health concerns related to chronic substance use, but may sometimes be useful as part of a comprehensive assessment to assist in diagnosis. For instance, several biomarkers of alcohol use can be assessed at baseline and periodically during follow-up to monitor progress with abstinence. Chronic alcohol use may result in elevated gamma-glutamyl transferase (GGT >40 u/L) and increased mean corpuscular volume (MCV >90). Aspartate aminotransferase (AST) and alanine aminotransferase (ALT) elevations are reflective of more recent heavy alcohol use, with an AST:ALT >2 suggestive of alcohol-induced liver damage. Note that elevated transaminase is frequently unobserved in younger, healthy populations, even with heavy drinking patterns; a normal result should not be interpreted as reassurance that drinking patterns are not medically harmful.

Less frequently tested biomarkers for alcohol use include elevated carbohydrate-deficient transferrin (CDT), ethyl glucuronide (EtG), and ethyl sulfate (EtS). The latter two markers are highly sensitive, becoming positive with even very low-level recent exposure to alcohol. They are controversial markers because products of routine daily use (e.g., antiseptic hand sanitizers) can yield a false-positive result. Even less frequently utilized is phosphatidyl ethanol (PEth), which can persist for three weeks after a few days of moderate alcohol intake. Since treatment-seeking patients frequently self-report accurately about their progress or challenges with achieving drinking reduction goals, these sensitive biomarkers have not been considered cost-effective options for routine care of patients with alcohol use disorders who are actively participating in treatment to reduce drinking.

In addition to the above biomarkers, a number of bodily fluids and tissues (e.g., hair follicles) can be tested for alcohol and drugs and their metabolites. The most common fluids tested are urine and saliva samples. The initial testing procedure is a screening immunoassay. Cross-reactivity is a major limitation of immunoassay, so positive tests may need to be confirmed by a second procedure. Gas chromatography is often combined with mass spectroscopy (GC/MS) as the confirmatory procedure. It is important to know the cutoff of whatever test is being used to measure a substance. The cutoff is the concentration of the substance above which the result is considered to be positive, and below which it is interpreted as negative. If, for example, a hospital has calibrated an assay to assess for overdose (i.e., a supratherapeutic dose), subtherapeutic or therapeutic levels may not result in a positive result, even though the patient is taking the medication as prescribed.

Also, it is important to understand which substances within a class are detected by an assay. For example, many benzodiazepine immunoassays detect only the oxazepam molecule, which is not a component of some commonly used and misused benzodiazepines, such as clonazepam. Similarly, an opiate assay typically will detect the morphine molecule, which means that synthetic opioids, such as methadone, oxycodone, and buprenorphine, are not detected. There are specific assays for these drugs that must be requested by name or panel (i.e., a "full narcotic panel").

A positive drug screen does not alone define a diagnosis of drug misuse, nor does a negative screen indicate drug abstinence; this result must be carefully interpreted within the comprehensive clinical context.

Providing Medical Advice When Screening Reveals Problematic Substance Use

The FRAMES Model of Brief Interventions

Brief interventions refer to educational counseling sessions of two- to fifteen-minute duration that have demonstrated efficacy in office-based settings, especially for promoting alcohol reduction. FRAMES is an acronym standing for *feedback, responsibility, advice, menu of options, empathy,* and *self-efficacy/support follow-up.* These are the components that comprise an effective brief counseling intervention. Feedback to the patient should be individualized and ideally include normative comparisons (e.g., "Your binge drinking pattern places you in the top 10 percent of heavy drinkers, and also puts you at greatest risk for alcohol-related health problems."). Responsibility recognizes patient autonomy in decision-making ("Have you ever worried about your drinking or had ideas about cutting down?"). Advice is medically directed toward safety and risk prevention, and is succinct and unambiguous ("Continuing to binge drink will increase your current cardiovascular risks, whereas reducing your drinking may improve your blood pressure significantly."). The menu of options should be as broad as possible, since the more choices a patient is presented with, the more likely that patient will view at least one of the options as an acceptable next step toward reducing health risk ("There are many ways we can help you to stop or reduce your drinking. There are safe medications that can help, experienced counselors who can work with you to set achievable goals, and there are a lot of things you can do on your own, such as keeping a calendar of your drinking days and writing down reasons you'd like to stop drinking. There are also mutual support groups like Alcoholics Anonymous and SMART Recovery that many people find particularly helpful. Would you be interested in learning more about any of these supports?"). Maintaining an empathic stance is critical; clinical studies demonstrate that interventionist empathy is correlated with positive patient change ("Stopping drinking is really challenging, and the key thing is that you don't get so discouraged that you give up. We can always add more support to help you reach your goals, and it's clear you've already been making healthier choices recently."). Supporting self-efficacy – the individual's confidence about being able to refrain from taking a drink or a drug – and ensuring an appropriate follow-up to assess progress are also critical components of an effective brief intervention ("You were able to do more than you initially thought you could; I can see how important this is to you. Let's make sure we meet again in two weeks to help you keep moving forward successfully!").

Patient Readiness to Change

The Transtheoretical Stages-of-Change Model can help classify where a patient is on the continuum of (1) recognizing a problem with substance use and (2) readiness to take action toward behavioral change to resolve the problem. The application of this model is helpful because it predicts which interventions a clinician may introduce that will have the best probability of patient follow up. For instance, a patient who sees no problem with his drinking patterns is unlikely to change his drinking just based on clinical advice to stop drinking. In this instance, introducing a motivational intervention that helps the patient consider how his drinking patterns may conflict with his life goals and personal values, and asking permission to review this with him at a follow-up visit, is more likely to initiate recognition of a problem and to evoke concern about the need for behavioral modification. According to this model, the readiness continuum moves fluidly between five cognitive/motivational stages:

- *Precontemplation.* Patients are unaware of a problem and therefore see no need to make any changes (sometimes referred to as "denial" of a problem).
- *Contemplation.* Patients are evolving awareness of a problem and therefore contemplating the need for change.
- *Preparation.* Patients acknowledge a problem and are planning behavioral change.
- *Action.* Patients have chosen a path to change and are taking behavioral steps toward change.
- *Maintenance.* Patients have achieved change geared toward the resolution of a problem and conform behavioral patterns to sustain successful change.

Identifying the stage of change during the assessment interview directs the appropriate intervention selection, and a self-report assessment such as the SOCRATES (Stages of Change Readiness and Treatment Eagerness Scale) may be used to assist in determining the patient's stage of change. If a patient is in the precontemplation stage, the clinician's goal is to help the patient discern problem behavior and its negative impact on individual life goals and values. Note, this requires the clinician to accurately elicit what life goals and values are of greatest importance to the presenting patient. In contemplation, the clinician works to help the patient consider and resolve ambivalence about making change, strengthen thoughts and ideas about making a positive change, and feel confident that change is possible to achieve. In preparation, the clinician helps to evoke commitment to taking action; in action, the clinician is supportive and may assist the patient with problem-solving challenges; maintenance is supportive and affirmative to the patient's success in change, reflecting especially ways in which change has achieved important health goals.

Clinicians must empathically anticipate fluctuations in patient readiness, since behavior change is challenging, and levels of commitment or confidence can shift with life events or mood changes. It is not uncommon for a patient to initiate change and then fall back to the precontemplation stage under stressful circumstances. (This is very common with smoking cessation quit attempts, for example.) Clinicians must be prepared to adjust interventions to shifts in natural cycling rather than to feel discouraged or to conclude that treatment has been ineffective. Behavioral change is often an incremental or iterative process.

Treatment Approaches

Pharmacotherapy

Medications are helpful for both the acute treatment of substance use syndromes as well as for maintenance therapies of substance use disorders. The two major applications are:

- *Medical withdrawal management.* Physiological stabilization of acute withdrawal syndromes
- *Relapse prevention therapies* for alcohol, opioid, and nicotine use disorders.

Throughout this section, keep in mind that no medication therapies have demonstrated efficacy without being paired with educational interventions targeting cognitive and/or behavioral changes necessary to achieve and sustain abstinence, and all efficacy studies have been conducted in actively treatment-seeking patients, which limits our knowledge of how effective they may or may not be in individuals who are not actively seeking treatment.

Detoxification from Alcohol and Sedative-Hypnotics

The prompt recognition of early symptoms of withdrawal from chronic alcohol or sedative-hypnotic use and treatment with a benzodiazepine prevents life-threatening conditions, including withdrawal seizure, hypertensive crisis, and delirium tremens. During detoxification, vital signs and other symptoms of autonomic hyperactivity are monitored at least every two to four hours, more often if the patient is unstable, and patients are dosed using standardized protocols to remission of symptoms. Medication selection and dosing route will vary depending on the medical setting (e.g., oral use is common in outpatient settings and intravenous use is common in hospital settings) and the severity or complexity of the withdrawal presentation. After the patient is stabilized (typically within twenty-four to forty-eight hours), a tapering schedule is set with daily decreasing doses until the benzodiazepine is tapered to zero. In the setting of alcohol withdrawal, this is usually achieved within two to five days. Sedative-hypnotic use disorders may require longer tapering, lasting weeks to months, typically completed in an outpatient setting.

Benzodiazepine selection depends on patient characteristics. For instance, a patient with a respiratory disorder will require a benzodiazepine with a short half-life, such as lorazepam, to reduce the risk of benzodiazepine accumulation that could precipitate respiratory failure. Lorazepam metabolism does not require hepatic oxidation and is also a good medication choice if hepatic functioning is impaired. Patients with a high tolerance for alcohol or a history of withdrawal-related complications, such as delirium tremens or seizures, may benefit from a longer-acting agent (e.g., chlordiazepoxide). Its effective half-life extends beyond the short length of an acute inpatient admission, thanks to its multiple active metabolites. When treating sedative-hypnotic dependence, it is important to take into consideration that benzodiazepine cross-reactivity is imperfect; thus selection is preferred to most closely match the substance(s) being taken chronically, in order to achieve optimal coverage for withdrawal syndrome prevention.

When working in a medical or surgical inpatient service, keep in mind that some patients at risk for withdrawal may not be aware of their substance dependence ("I'm not an alcoholic. I just relax after work with a few drinks."). Beta-adrenergic antagonists (e.g., propranolol) and similar medications prevent elevations of heart rate and blood pressure, and thus may mask symptoms of alcohol or sedative-hypnotic withdrawal, but they do not prevent the medical dangers of untreated withdrawal. If a history of daily drinking of two to four drinks or more is established, prophylactic treatment with benzodiazepines during hospitalization may be indicated to prevent withdrawal, even prior to the onset of symptoms of withdrawal. It is easier and less dangerous to prevent alcohol withdrawal than to treat it.

Although the use of benzodiazepines is the primary treatment for alcohol withdrawal in most settings, alternative options may include the use of long-acting barbiturates or carbamazepine. The benzodiazepine class is generally preferred because of its safety, optimal efficacy for preventing both withdrawal seizures and delirium tremens, and its cost-effectiveness.

Detoxification from Opioids
Opioid withdrawal is unpleasant, painful, and anxiety-provoking but mostly not medically dangerous on its own (exceptions include cases vulnerable to dehydration or cardiovascular/autonomic instability, as well as fetal vulnerability in

pregnant women). Some patients do not bother with any treatment and simply stop using "cold turkey," but this approach carries the highest rate of relapse and recidivism. Symptomatic treatment that does not prevent opioid withdrawal may be used, although it is not recommended because patient discomfort is greater and treatment dropout rates are high. In turn, rates of opioid relapse are high. The typical symptomatic regimen includes an alpha-2 adrenergic agonist (clonidine or lofexidine), plus medication that treats joint and body pain (e.g., ibuprofen). Attempts to relieve other symptoms, such as stomach cramps (dicyclomine), nausea and vomiting (anti-emetics), diarrhea (loperamide), and insomnia/anxiety (hypnotic aids and other non-benzodiazepine sedatives, such as low-dose quetiapine), are frequently included in the standard symptomatic detoxification regimen.

Most patients seeking treatment prefer detoxification with mu-opioid receptor agonists. Traditionally, inpatient detoxification was achieved with decreasing doses of methadone. Since the FDA approved the opioid partial agonist, buprenorphine, in 2002 for the treatment of opioid withdrawal and the maintenance treatment of opioid use disorder (discussed in more detail later), its use in opioid detoxification has steadily expanded. Buprenorphine is highly efficacious but safer and more tolerable, with fewer drug-drug interactions, compared with methadone. Advances in research on the safety and efficacy of buprenorphine maintenance during pregnancy have provided a second option for treatment of opioid use disorder for pregnant women, in addition to methadone maintenance.

Detoxification from Other Drugs

There are no effective agents for the detoxification from other substances of abuse except nicotine, where nicotine agonist replacement therapies (as discussed later) are frequently utilized in acute care settings for substitution, detoxification, and treatment of nicotine use disorder. No FDA-indicated treatment for cannabis withdrawal is yet available, despite multiple research efforts to design an endocannabinoid receptor agonist that could address cannabis use disorder. Stimulant and hallucinogen use disorders require supportive interventions during withdrawal and abstinence for behavioral safety and control of autonomic dysregulation, but likewise, no safe, effective substitution therapies have yet been demonstrated.

Naltrexone in the Treatment of Alcohol Use Disorders

Alcohol does not directly activate opioid receptors but does disinhibit endogenous opioid neurotransmission, and this activation contributes to the experience of pleasure associated with alcohol consumption. Opioid signaling also mediates anticipatory aspects of pleasure when a person is planning to drink alcohol. Therefore, opioid antagonism may effectively reduce cravings for alcohol and decrease the reinforcing effects of alcohol in those attempting to abstain from drinking (with high inter-individual variability in efficacy).

The opioid antagonist, naltrexone, is a first-line FDA-approved medication for the treatment of alcohol use disorder, and may be taken in oral formulation daily (50–150 mg) or by monthly intramuscular injection (380 mg) for improved adherence. The COMBINE study, the largest federally funded trial of the pharmacotherapy of alcohol dependence, compared combinations of naltrexone, acamprosate (discussed later), and placebo with or without adjunctive specialized addiction counseling on drinking reduction outcomes. Results showed that oral naltrexone administered in the context of "medical management" (i.e., no specialized addiction counseling) was most effective in helping patients successfully reduce or stop drinking. Medical management is a brief manualized treatment, which structures a twenty-minute health practitioner follow-up visit to include assessment of sobriety, encouragement of abstinence, assessment of medication adherence and side effects, and brief education about alcohol use disorders and the health benefits of achieving abstinence. In COMBINE, all interventions, including placebo plus medical management and specialized addiction counseling alone, decreased drinking over the twelve-month follow-up period, but naltrexone paired with medical management was significantly more effective than the other treatments.

Prospective patients must not take opioid agonists (prescribed or illicit) seven to fourteen days prior to initiation of treatment with naltrexone, as naltrexone administered in this context will precipitate opioid withdrawal. Naltrexone is typically discontinued three to fourteen days prior to elective surgery requiring prescription opioid analgesia. Common side effects include transient headache and nausea, and reversible increases of hepatic transaminases have been reported, but it is safely used in patients with substance use and active HCV infection. Adverse injection site reactions are a risk with depot naltrexone.

Acamprosate in the Treatment of Alcohol Use Disorders

Acamprosate is an NMDA-glutamate receptor modulator that may reduce cravings for alcohol and help normalize allostatic changes related to chronic alcohol use. Multiple placebo-controlled trials have shown modest efficacy in prolonging time to first drink, especially among heavy drinkers who are committed to abstinence and have already achieved a full week of sobriety at the initiation of acamprosate. All trials with positive results were conducted in Europe. In large US studies, acamprosate was not more effective than placebo, and in COMBINE, acamprosate was ineffective alone and, when added to naltrexone, did not confer any additional benefit compared with naltrexone monotherapy. Acamprosate is not metabolized in the liver but excreted through the kidneys, making it a good option for patients with hepatic failure.

Acamprosate has poor bio-availability and must be taken three times daily at a maintenance dose of 2 grams daily. Best practice instructs the patient to improve adherence by scheduling before meals and taking a few minutes to reflect on sobriety goals at dosing. It is well-tolerated, and initial dosing titration is recommended over a one-week period in order to avoid the most common side effect, diarrhea.

Disulfiram in the Treatment of Alcohol Use Disorders

Disulfiram, FDA approved in 1951, inhibits the conversion of acetaldehyde, the toxic metabolite of alcohol, to acetate. Alcohol consumption after inhibition of acetaldehyde-dehydrogenase results in an aversive syndrome of headaches, flushing, nausea, and vomiting, and a more severe reaction may include hypertensive crisis and death. Although this mechanism is an aversive conditioning paradigm, likely the most effective aspect of disulfiram therapy is the cognitive shift to alcohol as an inaccessible substance, since a patient taking disulfiram anticipates a disulfiram response should s/he plan to drink. The perceived reduction in alcohol's availability also reduces anticipatory cravings for a drink (also called *reduced expectancy*). It takes up to two weeks to regenerate sufficient acetaldehyde-dehydrogenase, and patients are warned that stopping the medication will not offer them immediate freedom to drink without health consequences. Taken together, medication adherence is a critical factor in disulfiram efficacy, and monitored dosing in reluctant or ambivalent patients is recommended (e.g., those mandated to treatment and those in family treatments because of problematic drinking).

Daily dosing is recommended at 125–500 mg. Unfortunately, disulfiram is associated with rare instances of serious and idiopathic side effects, including potentially irreversible fulminant hepatitis (1 in 25,000 patients per year) and optic neuritis, even in the absence of alcohol relapse. This risk renders disulfiram a second-line treatment option in many cases, especially for patients actively engaged in seeking help and reasonable candidates for naltrexone or acamprosate.

Off-Label Use of FDA-Approved Medications for Alcohol Use Disorders

The antiseizure medication topiramate demonstrates replicated benefit in controlled clinical trials that target reduced drinking among those with severe alcohol use disorders. While the evidence base is strong for topiramate use in alcohol dependence, FDA indication to treat alcohol use disorder was not requested since the medication was already available in generic formulation. It is notable that topiramate is the only medication shown to be effective even among patients still actively drinking at the time of initiation. Studies pair the administration of topiramate in increasing doses (target dose 200–300 mg daily) with medical management, facilitation of patient goal-setting for drinking reduction targets, and referral to Alcoholics Anonymous. Topiramate is contraindicated in those with glaucoma or a history of renal calculi, and it is commonly associated with both benign (tinny taste in mouth, mild paresthesia) and more serious adverse effects (metabolic acidosis, cognitive impairment), especially if titration is rapid and the target dose is higher than 300 mg.

Newer research suggests the antiseizure medication gabapentin to be effective in preventing relapse in the treatment of patients with severe alcohol use disorders. One placebo-controlled study in patients with alcoholic cirrhosis found the GABA$_B$ agonist baclofen to be well-tolerated and associated with maintenance of abstinence.

Agonist Therapy of Opioid Use Disorders: Methadone

More than 90 percent of patients who undergo medically supervised detoxification from opioid use will relapse within the first three months without medication maintenance, and the institution of agonist treatments at least doubles the probability of maintaining opioid abstinence. Methadone maintenance treatment was introduced in New York City in 1966, against considerable public resistance and legal challenges. Methadone maintenance clinics are federally regulated clinics ("opioid treatment programs") and are the only places in the United States where methadone may be legally prescribed and dispensed for the purpose of addiction treatment. Methadone maintenance treatment, although maintaining physiological opioid dependence, breaks the addiction cycle by maintaining steady-state opioid levels and thus reducing cravings to use opioids, risk behaviors associated with injection use, risky sexual behavior, crime associated with drug dependence, and medical morbidity and mortality associated with illicit opioid use and needle-sharing. According to federal regulations, methadone dosing must occur under daily monitoring during the stabilization phase of treatment. With continued treatment adherence and reduction of illicit substance use, patients may earn privileges to have up to thirty daily doses of methadone dispensed to self-administer at home. Participation in psychosocial counseling and toxicological screens are required as part of opioid treatment programs.

Methadone has good oral bioavailability and is most frequently administered in liquid form to prevent drug diversion. Typical maintenance doses are between 60 and 150 mg, though some patients require higher doses. Serum levels peak within 4 hours (variability 1–6 hours) after ingestion. The metabolism of methadone is complex and involves several cytochrome P450 liver enzymes, most prominently CYP2B6 and CYP2D6. The average half-life is 22 hours, with a range of 5 to 130 hours, and is subject to changes due to drug-drug interactions. While the long half-life facilitates daily dosing and minimizes withdrawal symptoms with regular dosing, it is also associated with the risk of accumulation and accidental overdose if doses are increased rapidly without adequate medical monitoring. This risk is compounded by the interference of methadone with cardiac conduction in vulnerable individuals, which can be detected by QT interval prolongation in the ECG. Opioid relapse rates upon discontinuation are greater than 80 percent within one year (in the absence of initiating buprenorphine or naltrexone following discontinuation).

Agonist Therapy of Opioid Use Disorders: Buprenorphine

The promise of the partial opioid receptor agonist, buprenorphine, as a treatment for opioid use disorder was first demonstrated in humans by Mello and Mendelson at McLean Hospital in 1980. These seminal experiments demonstrated that IV heroin users, when premedicated with buprenorphine, chose dose-dependent decreases in self-administered heroin. Two decades of subsequent clinical trials and one act of congress later (DATA 2000), buprenorphine was FDA approved as an office-based maintenance therapy alternative to methadone for the treatment of opioid dependence.

Federal law currently restricts buprenorphine prescribing for addiction to medical prescribers who complete an approved eight-hour training course that qualifies them for a Drug Enforcement Agency waiver to prescribe buprenorphine ("x-license"). As with methadone maintenance, educational adjuncts to medical management are required ("medical counseling") and toxicological screening for adherence and assessment of substance use is strongly recommended.

Buprenorphine has partial agonist pharmacology, giving it distinct advantages in safety and tolerability compared with methadone maintenance. In particular, its agonist effects alleviate opioid cravings and symptoms of withdrawal but are not sufficiently potent to induce respiratory depression owing to a "ceiling effect" of partial agonism at the mu-opioid receptor. Furthermore, buprenorphine has the highest affinity for the mu-opioid receptor, as well as a slow receptor dissociation rate. Thus it binds tightly and at therapeutic doses (8–32 mg daily) effectively acts as a competitive antagonist which protects against the reinforcing effects of relapse to illicit opioid use. Conversely, if buprenorphine is used while opioid receptors are still occupied by a full agonist, most agonists are rapidly displaced by buprenorphine, resulting in a precipitous decline in opioid receptor activation and abrupt onset of opioid withdrawal syndrome. Unlike full agonists, doses above 32 mg daily are not associated with increased agonist effects. In the absence of other sedating agents, healthy adults will not die of an overdose of buprenorphine. Due to its high first-pass metabolism in the small intestine and the liver, the oral bioavailability of buprenorphine is low and thus it is administered sublingually. As a precautionary measure against potential misuse, in the United States, transmucosal buprenorphine preparations are typically combined 4:1 with the opioid antagonist naloxone. Naloxone is not absorbed sublingually or orally. It is active when used intravenously and thus competitively antagonizes opioid effects if the combined medication is dissolved and injected in an attempt to get high. Newer depot buprenorphine formulations lasting weeks are available to improve adherence and reduce misuse.

Buprenorphine treatment is composed of an induction phase, during which a patient in moderate opioid withdrawal (COWS > 8) takes 2–4 mg of buprenorphine with subsequent dose increases to a typical daily maintenance dose between 8 mg and 24 mg, after which it is adjusted accordingly during maintenance treatment. If necessary or desired, buprenorphine may be tapered off, though rates of relapse to opioid use following discontinuation of buprenorphine stabilization and maintenance are high.

As with all opioid agonist medications, common side effects of maintenance therapy include nausea, constipation, headache, sedation, sexual dysfunction, and possible hypogonadal syndrome. Sedative-hypnotics and alcohol are relatively contraindicated during maintenance due to the risk of synergistic effects on sedation, cognition, and respiratory depression.

Antagonist Therapy of Opioid Use Disorders: Naltrexone
The opioid antagonist, naltrexone, was developed as a treatment for opioid dependence in the 1980s. Naltrexone effectively blocks the reinforcing effects of opioid agonists during relapse to opioid use, and thereby also indirectly reduces cravings by reducing expectancies about relapse to opioid use. Unfortunately, adherence rates are notoriously poor with daily oral naltrexone dosing (50 mg daily), and unless daily dosing is monitored (as in certain mandated treatments or family behavioral contracts, similar to the use of disulfiram for alcohol use disorder), individuals with opioid use disorder are very likely to stop taking naltrexone when they wish to relapse. Therefore, the extended-release depot formulation of naltrexone (380 mg per month) is recommended for the treatment of opioid use disorder, and was FDA-approved for this indication in 2010. Results of clinical trials demonstrate that if a person completes the process of naltrexone induction and remains adherent to monthly dosing, its efficacy is comparable to that of daily buprenorphine maintenance; however, preventing drop-out remains a challenge. Note that naltrexone is not used in pregnant women.

In all cases of medical treatment for opioid use disorders, it is essential to warn patients that extended periods of abstinence result in loss of opioid tolerance, and relapse to opioid use is more likely to have a lethal effect in this context. Patients are also warned that attempts to "override" medical therapies with greater amounts of illicit opioids may result in respiratory depression and death. Patients on agonist therapies that are self-administered are instructed to store medication in a lockbox to prevent accidental exposures to children, youth, pets, and vulnerable adults. Finally, intranasal naloxone spray rescue kits for accidental overdose are recommended to patients and families to reduce opioid overdose lethality.

Pharmacotherapy for Nicotine Dependence
Smoking cessation is very challenging; it often takes five or more quit attempts before a person achieves sustained abstinence. Medications can double the

probability of successfully quitting and remaining abstinent. Varenicline is the most effective FDA-indicated medication for smoking cessation in individuals with or without co-occurring psychiatric illness, followed by equivalent efficacy of FDA-approved nicotine replacement or bupropion. Nicotine replacement is most effective when combining long-acting and short-acting formulations (for example, transdermal nicotine patch plus as needed nicotine gum or lozenges).

Nicotine replacement therapies (NRT) are available both over-the-counter and by prescription. NRT comes in multiple formulations (OTC gum, lozenge, transdermal patch, and inhaler; prescribed inhaler and nasal spray) and doses. The strategy is the prevention of cravings and symptoms of nicotine withdrawal, coupled with cessation of the behaviorally cued habits associated with smoking. Following stabilization, nicotine therapies are then gradually weaned off. This is often a preferred first intervention since no new substance is being introduced to the brain, and the main side effects are either local irritation of mouth and throat with gum/lozenges or, with patches, nightmares when worn overnight. Electronic cigarettes, though increasingly popular and widely accessible, are not yet FDA-regulated and are as such not yet recommended for nicotine replacement due to lack of data indicating safety and efficacy, and lack of quality control.

The antidepressant bupropion is an effective adjunct to smoking cessation therapy, alone or in combination with NRT. The sustained-release formulation is preferred and it is dosed to 150 mg twice daily two weeks prior to the quit date. A common adverse effect is unpleasant jitteriness if titration is too rapid. Bupropion lowers the seizure threshold and is contraindicated in those with epilepsy or other risk factors for seizures. As with all antidepressants, bupropion may be associated with an increased risk of suicidal ideation and a trial should be monitored closely for neuropsychiatric side effects.

Varenicline is a partial agonist at central $\alpha_2\alpha_4$ nicotinic acetylcholine receptors and is a full agonist at α_7 neuronal nicotinic receptors. At daily oral doses of 1–2 mg, it prevents cravings and symptoms of nicotine withdrawal but does not produce the euphoric reinforcing effects of nicotine. Its partial agonist properties also render it a competitive antagonist to the reinforcing effects of smoking relapse, similar to buprenorphine with opioid relapse. Initiation is frequently complicated by gastrointestinal side effects, especially nausea and diarrhea.

No Pharmacotherapy for Cocaine, Cannabis, and Other Drug Use Disorders

Despite significant research investments, to date no medication has shown replicable efficacy in the treatment of cocaine, cannabis, or other drug use disorders besides opioids and nicotine.

Behavioral Therapy

Behavioral therapies are commonly used for the treatment of substance use disorders, either alone or in combination with pharmacotherapy. These approaches draw from theoretical perspectives on behavioral processes (e.g., learning via rein-forcement, interpersonal, or emotion regulation skills deficits) that contribute to disorder development and maintenance. Behavioral therapies are typically brief in nature (1–20 sessions) and can be administered in individual, couples/family, or group formats. The goals of therapy vary, from reducing substance use or harmful behaviors associated with use (e.g., sharing needles) to achieving and maintaining complete abstinence from all harmful substances.

Although there are several different categories of behavioral therapies, all share a focus on modifying thoughts, behaviors, and lifestyle choices contributing to maladaptive substance use patterns. Commonly used techniques include (1) psych-oeducation and individualized feedback on substance use and its consequences, (2) introduction of self-monitoring substance use patterns, (3) identification of "high risk" situations and other environmental and emotional triggers for use, (4) skill development and rehearsal for avoiding use and high-risk situations, (5) altering environmental cues (e.g., removing alcohol from one's home), (6) introducing posi-tively reinforcing, safe (i.e., substance-free) activities and leisure, and (7) providing incentives (e.g., vouchers, family-mediated contingencies) for achieving periods of abstinence or progression in treatment. This section provides an introductory overview of evidence-based behavioral therapies for substance use disorders.

Motivational Enhancement Therapies

Even in the context of significant negative consequences due to substance use (e.g., impaired social relationships, employment difficulty, health problems), the decision to reduce substance use can be particularly difficult due to the perceived benefits of continued use (e.g., enhancement of social interactions, avoidance of negative emotions or withdrawal symptoms). Accordingly, uncertainty or ambiva-lence about the desire to change patterns of substance use is common among those with substance use disorders. Motivational enhancement therapies, based on moti-vational interviewing, are used to facilitate decision-making about change, with the goal of enhancing motivation and readiness for change. Motivational therapies place significant emphasis on a clinician style that is nonjudgmental, empathic, and respectful of autonomy and patient resourcefulness. This patient-centered approach is believed to be a critical component of enhancing motivation and has been demonstrated to be more effective than a confrontational or authoritative approach to encouraging patients to change. Other elements include identifying discrepancies between behavior and elicited goals and values ("While you enjoy drinking, you are also concerned about how it is affecting your health and rela-tionships right now"), providing feedback about the individual's pattern of use ("Sometimes you have difficulty remembering what you talked about at dinner when you've had more than one drink"), and placing focus on a patient's state-ments that are consistent with change ("Getting along better with your husband is important to you").

Motivational therapies are typically used as a platform to engage patients in either a brief educational intervention or a referral to a specific treatment, such as medication, self-help, or psychotherapy. For instance, Screening, Brief Intervention, and Referral to Treatment (SBIRT) interventions are widely used in opportunistic settings to address substance-related health problems. SBIRT entails (1) an assessment of the presence and severity SUD symptoms (screening), (2) a brief (often single-session) intervention delivered in a motivational interviewing style, and (3) a referral to a treatment facility for further evaluation and intervention, when indicated. SBIRT is demonstrated to be effective for reducing alcohol-related risks when used in primary care and emergency settings, but it has less evidence for effectiveness at reducing illicit drug use. The efficacy of motivational interventions improves with clinician training and skill, and in most contexts, multiple sessions are more effective and enduring than single-session interventions.

Psychoeducational and Counseling Therapies

Individual and group counseling interventions are among the most commonly used behavioral therapies for substance use disorders. In the United States, these approaches emphasize abstinence as the long-term treatment goal. These treatments are often paired with pharmacotherapy, either to directly treat the substance use disorder or to treat a co-occurring psychiatric disorder, as lifetime rates of co-occurrence are two to eight times greater than in the general population. Treatments focus on providing education about substance use and abuse, identifying high-risk situations and triggers for use, and avoidance of environmental cues that increase the probability of use. Daily self-monitoring of use patterns is encouraged and reviewed in each session to set target reduction goals. Early treatment sessions focus on the identification of risky people, environments (e.g., neighborhoods, bars), and things (e.g., drug paraphernalia), and the development of strategies to avoid or replace these cues is a major focus of treatment. Many counseling approaches also strongly encourage attendance at mutual-help meetings, such as Alcoholics Anonymous and Narcotics Anonymous (twelve-step programs) or SMART Recovery (a program based on cognitive-behavioral principles for reducing substance use). Research suggests that these treatments are helpful for reducing tobacco, alcohol, and drug use; however, response rates are modest with these approaches, particularly if used in isolation (i.e., without medication or other therapeutic adjuncts).

Behavioral Learning Theory Interventions

Contingency management and cue exposure are behavioral treatments that draw directly from basic behavioral theories of addiction. These treatments attempt to modify alcohol and drug use based on the learning processes (operant and classical conditioning) that are thought to contribute to the development and maintenance of maladaptive substance use.

Contingency management (CM) capitalizes on models of reinforcement of behavior and has been particularly successful in the treatment of substance use disorders, particularly for drug dependence. CM involves providing patients with a non-drug reinforcer (e.g., money, vouchers) for abstinent behavior (typically confirmed with some form of biological test, such as a urine drug screen). The principle underlying this approach is that the psychoactive effects of alcohol and drug use are powerful reinforcers of drug use behaviors, which makes discontinuing use extremely difficult. CM involves providing a reinforcer for alternative (i.e., non-drug) behaviors to increase the likelihood of these behaviors and to break habitual patterns of use. The implementation of CM can include monetary (cash or vouchers) or non-monetary incentives (prizes or treatment privileges) intended to be desirable to the patient. Incentives can be administered either for each episode of behavior or can be administered in a "lottery" format, where opportunities to earn incentives (e.g., tickets for a monthly drawing) are provided for desired behaviors.

CM has demonstrated success for reducing tobacco, alcohol, and drug use. Its application has been expanded to other adaptive behaviors, such as medication adherence and attendance at medical appointments. CM is also often combined with other behavioral or pharmacological strategies and seems to have additive benefits for those approaches, with combination CM strategies demonstrating some of the largest treatment effect sizes across behavioral treatment approaches. CM is intended to initiate reduction in substance use, and eventually incentives are tapered or discontinued. Although relapse to use has been observed with the discontinuation of CM, many patients maintain gains past the end of treatment. Despite the success of this approach in clinical trials, its adoption into clinical practice settings has been limited. However, a common application of this principle is often seen in methadone maintenance treatment facilities, where patients can "earn" the opportunity to receive take-home doses of methadone in return for providing negative urine drug screens.

Cognitive-Behavioral Therapies
Cognitive-behavioral therapies vary in their specific components but share the use of a combination of behavioral and cognitive interventions to reduce substance use. A core element of these approaches is functional analysis, a detailed assessment of the process surrounding substance use patterns. Functional analysis provides information about the contexts (internal and external), thoughts, behaviors, and consequences associated with substance use. For example, an argument with a family member may lead to feelings of stress, then the thought, "I can't handle this stress," then drinking alcohol to relieve stress, and then guilt or continued interpersonal difficulty related to alcohol use. Patterns such as these provide a basis for building alternative skills that are non-substance related, such as improving interpersonal skills or generating alternate strategies to reduce and relieve stress.

Cognitive-behavioral therapies, much like other behavioral therapies, typically encourage a balance of avoidance (e.g., staying away from substance-using peers, avoiding places associated with substance using) and the development of adaptive skills for managing risks that are either unavoidable or that the patient does not wish to avoid. Unavoidable triggers may include important social relationships (e.g., family members), environments that are common (e.g., restaurants), and internal states, such as stress, pain, and negative emotions. These therapies will often target building interpersonal skills, such as substance refusal skills, the ability to decline a drink or drug when offered. Skill development typically includes a rehearsal component, such as role-play with a therapist or with group therapy peers, to enhance mastery and confidence in one's capacity to implement the new skill outside of a therapy session. Practice in executing the skill in real-life situations is encouraged as "homework" and results reviewed with the therapist in follow up sessions.

Cognitive strategies involve the identification and modification of maladaptive, distorted thought patterns that may contribute to use. A common example of this is "may-as-well thinking" – that is, "I've just blown my sobriety, so I may as well keep drinking," or "Even though I've stopped using I still fight all the time with my wife, so I may as well go back to using, since it hasn't made a difference." The therapist assists the patient in identifying such thought patterns and then encourages him to challenge the veracity and effectiveness of these thought patterns, with an ultimate goal of normalizing thought patterns into more reasonable, adaptive ones ("cognitive restructuring"). In the example provided, cognitive restructuring might be, "Although I feel badly about blowing my sobriety, if I stop drinking now I can get back on track with recovery."

Cognitive-behavioral therapies are effective for reducing alcohol and drug use and for improving other areas of life functioning; they are also very effective treatments for commonly co-occurring psychiatric disorders, such as depression and anxiety disorders. The combination of cognitive-behavioral therapy with contingency management has been shown to be a particularly effective behavior therapy option for drug dependence.

Family and Couples Therapy

Treatments that involve family, partners, or other significant others within social support networks focus on the substance-using individual's interactions within social networks, and leverage these networks to support the individual's achieving and maintaining abstinence. Behavioral couples therapy (BCT) is an evidence-based approach to treating alcohol dependence when one partner is using and the other does not have an alcohol use disorder; it also shows some promise with drug use disorders. BCT and other couples-based and family-based treatments focus on the interaction of interpersonal functioning and substance use, with maladaptive patterns in each domain negatively affecting the other. Accordingly, treatment aims to address both interpersonal functioning within the relationship as well as the substance use through providing education and introducing adaptive skills with both the patient and partner/family member(s). A number of behavioral strategies are used and may include the identification and implementation of alternative non-substance behaviors and activities, reinforcement (e.g., praise) for abstinence by the partner, communication exercises, and education about substance use and relational functioning. Evidence for the use of BCT and other couples- and family-based therapies suggest that these are efficacious treatments for substance use as well as interpersonal functioning (relationship effectiveness and satisfaction). In addition, the incorporation of a partner or family member may enhance treatment retention by providing an additional source of accountability, support, and investment in the treatment.

Maximizing the Effectiveness of Behavioral Therapies

Attempts to compare types of behavioral therapies for substance use disorders and to identify predictors of treatment response (to allow for "matching" of patients to treatments) have been largely inconclusive. Large-scale multi-site clinical trials of treatments for cocaine dependence and alcohol dependence have found superiority of some treatments relative to others on some, but not all outcomes. Consideration of smaller studies comparing therapy types has similarly yielded mixed results. Overall, it appears that when studies use clearly defined manualized behavioral therapies, outcomes tend to be similarly improved across therapy types. An exception is drug dependence, in which contingency management appears to be associated with the best outcomes, particularly when combined with another behavioral therapy or pharmacotherapy.

Behavioral Therapy Plus Pharmacotherapy

Behavioral therapies are often administered concurrently with pharmacotherapy for substance use disorders. Presuming that behavioral therapies and pharmacotherapies act on different neurocognitive mechanisms underlying substance use disorders, the hope has been that the combination of these therapies would result in enhanced outcomes (i.e., at least an additive effect, if not synergistic). Yet research on this issue has demonstrated mixed results. Several large-scale trials have failed to find any benefits for the addition of behavioral therapy to medication, and other studies demonstrate the benefit of combining pharmacotherapy and behavioral therapy. For example, the addition of behavioral therapy to nicotine replacement therapy for smoking cessation yields improved rates of treatment response. Combination therapy may be particularly indicated for those with co-occurring psychiatric disorders, for enhancing non-substance outcomes, such as interpersonal or employment functioning, and for enhancing medication adherence.

Although the utilization of some form of psychosocial intervention is common across substance use treatment settings, access to evidence-based behavioral therapies, such as those described herein, is limited. Moreover, even though many of the behavioral treatments described here have demonstrated efficacy in improving substance use outcomes, many patients will not adequately respond to these treatments. Much work remains to be done to improve patient access to treatment and individual treatment response.

Future Directions

There are two primary areas of growth in the treatment of substance use disorders, providing integrated behavioral health care, and the research and development of pharmacogenomics for individualizing medical management.

Integrated Behavioral Health Care

Historically, the treatment of mental illnesses has been considered a specialty practice beyond the scope of primary care systems. Yet, according to national community sample studies, the 12-month prevalence of mental illnesses in the United States is high, including depressive disorders (9 percent), anxiety disorders (depending on subtype, 3–9 percent), and substance use disorders (drug use 1.4 percent; alcohol use 3.1 percent). Furthermore, most of these have greater than 90 percent lifetime co-occurrence with another major health disorder. This means that a majority of patients with mental illnesses are being seen by other medical specialties, and there are insufficient mental health specialists available to serve this volume of community patients. Finally, having an inadequately treated mental health or substance use disorder greatly impairs treatment adherence for other illnesses, increases recurrence of symptoms, reduces self-care capacity, and ultimately is very costly to society. To address this, the medical field is re-designing its delivery practices to training basic competency in all health care clinicians for the detection of common mental health and substance use disorders, and providing a capacity within the system to treat common mental health and substance use disorders. We are currently in an era of health care re-organization to meet these needs. Training programs are incorporating more training and experience in this, board examinations have increased behavioral health content among all specialties, and health care systems are determining which models will best provide for cost-effective integration of behavioral health and physical health care. The Substance Abuse and Mental Health Services Agency (SAMHSA) provides online toolkits for clinicians learning and adjusting to the new standards of integrated health care (Center of Excellence for Integrated Health Solutions, www.thenationalcouncil.org/integrated-health-coe/).

Among behavioral health specialists, the development of new treatments that integrate care of mental illness and substance use continues to demonstrate improved outcomes. Commonly referred to as "dual diagnosis" treatment, patients are able to access integrated care in one setting and therapies focus on education and skill development for managing the interactive aspects of co-occurring disorders.

Pharmacogenomics

Pharmacogenomics is the study of how an individual's genes may affect that individual's response to medications and other chemical substances, such as alcohol, nicotine, and drugs. The study of neuropharmacology combined with the study of behavioral genetics creates a scientific pathway for the development of (1) diagnostic tests that may help to predict a person's sensitivity and response to a chemical substance or medication, and (2) new medications to better target identified genetic vulnerabilities. For instance, pharmacogenomics may be used to predict in childhood who is at increased risk for developing a substance use disorder; high-risk individuals could receive more intensive preventive counseling and behavioral interventions. It may also be used to help guide medication selection in someone with a known substance use disorder, as has been suggested for alcohol dependence and naltrexone response (i.e., the single polymorphism A118G, or "G" allele, of the mu-opioid receptor predicts beneficial response to naltrexone). Further, it may be used to predict which individuals are at risk for having a serious adverse response to medication, which could prove helpful in avoiding idiopathic responses such as fulminant hepatitis with disulfiram. It may also be used to assess metabolic pathways which would help predict dose and drug-drug interactions prior to medication initiation. An advance of this type would have a high impact on patient care with medications such as methadone, notorious for drug-drug interactions. As the pharmacogenomics evidence base expands, it is imaginable that patients entering treatment may experience a faster pathway to health due to optimal medication selection, dosing, and minimization of side effects or extended morbidity due to "trial and error" prescribing.

Sample Interview Questions

In addition to implementing evidence-based screening assessments reviewed previously, it is helpful to consider sample interview questions that will assist in the domains of assessing volume and frequency of use, identifying consequences of use, and assessing interest and motivational incentives to change, as well as the perceived capacity to change behavior. Given the increased prevalence of prescription drug misuse and use disorders, routine assessment of misuse of prescribed drugs is recommended.

Assessment of Substance Use Patterns

- Do you drink alcoholic beverages, such as wine, beer, or liquor? Have you ever in the past?
- Have you ever used any illicit or non-prescribed drugs? When was the last time?
- Have you ever smoked cigarettes or use any tobacco products? When was the last time?
- Have you ever used more of a prescribed medication than your doctor told you to, or used a medication more often than you were supposed to?
- How many days in the past month have you used (alcohol, drugs, tobacco)?
- How much do you drink/use when you typically drink/use? Is this more than you used when you first started using?

Substance Use History

- How long have you been using alcohol/drugs/tobacco?
- How old were you when you first tried alcohol/drugs/tobacco?
- Have you ever been in treatment for substance use? If yes, did you find it helpful?
- Has anyone ever recommended that you attend treatment?

Consequences of Substance Use

- Have any friends, family members, or significant others in your life expressed any concerns about your drinking or drug use?
- Have you ever had any problems with others, like getting in arguments, about your use or when you were using?
- Have you ever had any legal problems related to alcohol or drug use?
- Does your alcohol or drug use interfere with daily responsibilities at work or home, or interfere with things you like to do like social activities and hobbies?
- What do you like about using alcohol or drugs? Are there any downsides?
- How does your substance use impact your mood or your physical health?

Controllability of Substance Use and Motivation

- Have you ever wanted to cut back on your alcohol/drug/tobacco use?
- Have you ever had trouble cutting back or stopping your alcohol/drug/tobacco use?
- Do you use alcohol/drug/tobacco even when you know that it might have negative effects on your health, work, or relationships?
- How often do you experience cravings or urges for alcohol/drugs/tobacco that are difficult to control?
- How often do you think about using alcohol/drugs/tobacco? Do you ever notice thinking about it when you are trying to do other things, such as work or social activities?

- Do you ever notice feeling sick after you stop using alcohol/drugs/tobacco, like feeling nauseous, anxious, shaky, or irritable?
- What time do you usually have your first drink/drug/cigarette of the day?
- Have you ever thought about cutting back your alcohol/drug/tobacco use?
- How important is it to you to reduce your alcohol/drug/tobacco use?
- How confident are you that you could reduce or stop using alcohol/drugs/tobacco if you decided today that this is something important for you to do?

Prevention and Early Intervention in Children and Adolescents

Epidemiology and Risk Factors

More than 70 percent of adults with an identified substance use disorder retrospectively report that their first initiation of substance use occurred during the period of adolescence. Both late childhood and early adolescence are therefore critical time periods in the life cycle for intervention. Specifically, the current literature points to a significantly elevated risk for those who initiate substance use in early adolescence, leading not only to a greater likelihood of the development of a substance use disorder, but also to a greater risk of a range of physical and mental health difficulties, such as aggressive behavior, involvement with the criminal justice system, driving while under the influence, as well as an increased likelihood of academic failure.

Adolescents use a variety of substances. The most commonly used substances for adolescents ages twelve to seventeen (in order of prevalence) are cannabis, alcohol, and the nonmedical use of prescription stimulants. By the time an adolescent is preparing to graduate from high school within the United States, almost 70 percent have experimented with alcohol, almost 20 percent will have tried a prescription drug for a nonmedical purpose, and more than 40 percent will have tried a nicotine-based product. Although the current prevalence data indicate that illicit substance use among adolescents is staying the same or trending downward, there is increasing concern about the low perception of harm for some substances, especially with cannabis use and nicotine use through vaporizing devices. This shift may be a prognostic signal of a future increase in the prevalence of use of these substances. Among adolescents who do use cannabis, there has been an increase in heavy (>3 times per week) use over the past decade. Use of almost all substances (tobacco, alcohol, stimulants, cocaine, cannabis, and inhalants) during adolescence has been shown to lead to an increased risk of developing a subsequent substance use disorder. Cannabis is the most common first substance used for those with substance use disorders who initiated use at age fourteen or younger. After age fifteen, alcohol is the most common first substance used.

It is challenging to determine what drives some adolescents to begin using earlier and more heavily than others. One theory is that youth who are genetically and environmentally more vulnerable are more likely to move toward substance use as a means of coping. This would assume that substance use is, in fact, a proxy for underlying psychiatric difficulties that are already present, with the use then continuing to negatively shape an adolescent's trajectory by leading to secondary difficulties. This may explain why adolescents with externalizing behavior disorders (oppositional defiant disorder and attention deficit disorder) have been shown to possess a greater likelihood of developing a substance use disorder, as compared to adolescents who do not suffer from these illnesses. The second theory is that the early onset and heavy substance use itself leads to negative outcomes and an altered trajectory. This implies that a gateway hypothesis exists, in which an adolescent begins using one substance, then progresses over time to more substances, with increasing frequency, and that significant challenges result. An example of this is the correlation between early tobacco use and the increased likelihood of later progression to illicit substance use (as compared to adolescents who do not use tobacco products). As is true for the etiology of many other medical illnesses, it is likely a combination of these factors, rendering substance use a multifactorial process, with both genetic and environmental influences playing a role.

Risk factors that have been correlated with the later development of a substance use disorder are listed in Figure 9.1.

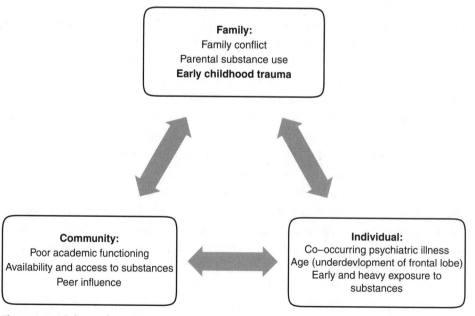

Figure 9.1 Risk factors for substance misuse

Given the time frame within which many of these risk factors develop, initiation of substance use may be best viewed through a developmental lens. In fact, studies demonstrate that substance use is more likely to begin during periods of life transition. Adolescence is naturally a time of experimentation and risk taking, based on the predictable process through which brain development occurs (neuronal maturation and pruning proceeds in a caudal to rostral direction, with the maturation of the frontal lobes and prefrontal cortex – the brain parts involved in executive functioning and self-control – being last in the sequence). It is also a time in which peer groups become a very significant and influential part of adolescents' lives, which can then strongly influence their experience with substance use.

Most of the risk factors listed here should be considered modifiable rather than fixed, and they also frequently overlap or become additive, in that one risk factor being present then increases the likelihood of another being present. Youth with parents who suffer from substance use disorders are not only more likely to have a heritable risk but also are at risk for family conflict, which itself is another known risk factor. In terms of co-occurring disorders, the most significant risk is associated with externalizing disorders, namely oppositional defiant disorder and attention deficit disorder. However, major depressive disorder and anxiety disorders (to a lesser degree) have also each been correlated with a greater risk of developing a substance use disorder. While co-occurring disorders could be thought of as an individual, nonmodifiable risk factor, it is very important to recognize and treat these disorders when present, as outcomes improve when a co-occurring illness is recognized and treated. It should also be noted that early childhood trauma has been established as a particularly strong and independent risk factor for the development of a substance use disorder during adolescence. Even after controlling for other environmental and genetic factors (age, gender, ethnicity, income, parental substance use), traumatic events, particularly interpersonal violence prior to age eleven, remains significant in the increased risk it poses for later development of a substance use disorder.

Screening Tools

Based on the heterogeneity of risk factors, and it being a critical time of intervention, it is recommended that health providers screen adolescents regularly for substance use disorders. The National Institute on Drug Abuse has launched two online screening tools, the BSTAD and S2BI, which can be used to quickly assess an adolescent's risk for a substance use disorder (www.drugabuse.gov/nidamed-medical-health-professionals/screening-tools-resources/screening-tools-for-adolescent-substance-use). Both can be easily accessed and administered within two to five minutes, categorizing an adolescent's risk into one of three categories: no reported use, low risk, and high risk. After scoring, clinicians then receive information and recommendations about the next course of action, based on the risk category.

Evidenced-Based Prevention Programs

School-based prevention programs are an obvious choice for targeting a large audience of at-risk adolescents. Programming can be initiated as early as preschool and typically involves the identification of modifiable risk factors (such as aggressive episodes, family conflict, and poor social skills). By elementary school, the focus is largely on the development of social skills, emotional awareness, and self-regulation. In middle and high school, the prevention shifts toward education on different types of substances and how they affect the body, as well as navigating peer interactions, teaching assertiveness, and drug-refusal skills. Traditional models of lecturing students on the dangers of substance use have largely fallen out of favor, as they have been proven ineffective at reaching an adolescent audience. Instead, programs have focused on social skills training, appropriate psychoeducation, and problem-solving/decision-making skills. Specifically, focusing on ways in which adolescents naturally interact with one another, helping them become more aware of how and when they might make healthy decisions, as well as equipping them with the tools to understand how the use of substances can quickly lead to adverse outcomes can increase awareness and prevention of substance use.

Family-based interventions aim to affect modifiable risk factors within the family unit, which can be highly influential. Increased parental monitoring and supervision at home is critical, in addition to educating parents and caregivers about how their approach to substances can strongly influence their children's attitudes. Interventions can be brief and often focus on rule-setting and consistency at home.

Community-based programs offer targeted secondary prevention at critical times of transition, such as intervening when middle school students transition to high school or high school students are preparing to graduate. Because adolescents who delay initiation of substance use are at markedly less risk than those who initiate earlier, many preventative efforts are focused on delaying the onset of use and incorporate this developmental aspect. For example, an adolescent who smokes cannabis for the first time at fourteen years old is six times more likely to develop a later substance use disorder, as compared to an adolescent who smokes cannabis for the first time at eighteen years old.

Evidence shows that programs that combine elements of both family involvement and education-based interventions are more effective than a single program targeting just students. Programs that incorporate an interactive element, such as a group discussion, have also been found to be much more effective than those that do not.

There are also specific challenges associated with identifying and treating adolescents who are at heightened risk of developing psychosis, within the setting of ongoing cannabis use. Heavy cannabis use is associated with an increased risk of developing a psychotic disorder, and that risk is exacerbated in the setting of early initiation, as well as a family history of psychotic disorders. However, most adolescents with a cannabis use disorder do not seek treatment, despite being at elevated risk. Identifying and treating such adolescents is critical, given the long-term academic, financial, and social consequences that can evolve in the absence of such interventions. A targeted screening and brief intervention tool called Teen Marijuana Check-Up has been developed for this purpose, and its administration to select at-risk high school students has been demonstrated to reduce cannabis use among adolescents with past heavy use. It utilizes a motivational interviewing framework, in which adolescents are asked about their cannabis use in a nonjudgmental fashion to elicit thought about how their use might be problematic, and takes an inventory of any adverse consequences of use that the teen would like to change.

Case Examples

Alcohol use disorders and opioid use disorders are the most common substance use disorders seen in most treatment settings. This section presents an example of each of these disorders.

Case 1: Treatment of Alcohol Use Disorders

Mr. A., a fifty-five-year-old married father of three children and an executive at a financial company, visits you, his primary care physician, for follow-up for hypertension. Six months ago, his atenolol dose was increased to 25 mg twice daily, and he reports that his home blood pressure readings have been 140/90 for the last few weeks. Mr. A. also has a history of anxiety disorder, for which he sees a psychiatrist monthly, who prescribes clonazepam 1 mg twice daily. You ask him about how things are going at work and at home, and you learn that he has been told that he will likely lose his job soon due to company restructuring. You also learn that he is drinking almost a quart of vodka daily in an unsuccessful attempt to manage his anxiety and stress, and his wife has threatened to force him to leave the family home if he does not stop drinking.

You have a conversation with Mr. A. about his drinking, and he reluctantly agrees that his drinking has worsened and it may be contributing to his problems at work. He counters that he often entertains clients in the evenings as a part of his job, and drinking is involved in those social events. He says that he is not sure how he would be able to do his job without drinking. You reply that you are concerned about his heavy drinking, and you understand that his job poses some real challenges to reducing drinking. You ask permission to speak with his psychiatrist, and you also worry that clonazepam may be a more risky medication for him given the volume of alcohol he is consuming daily.

Mr. A. allows you to speak with his psychiatrist, who was aware of his drinking but unaware of the change in volume and frequency. He, too, is very concerned, especially since he recently increased the prescribed dose of clonazepam to 3 mg daily in response to Mr. A.'s increased anxiety symptoms. You both agree that a consultation with an addiction specialist is advisable, and he is instructed to reduce his clonazepam dose back to 2 mg daily.

Mr. A. sees an addiction psychiatrist for an initial consultation and a subsequent family meeting, where Mr. A. declines a referral for inpatient detoxification and anxiety stabilization, citing concern about his career. He agrees he needs to stop drinking and says that he has tried to cut back, unsuccessfully. Following an alcohol-related event at work, Mr. A. is hospitalized for detoxification and is given a chlordiazepoxide taper alongside a gradual reduction in his clonazepam dosing. Both are weaned off and he is discharged to outpatient follow-up with his regular psychiatrist, who prescribes naltrexone for relapse prevention and initiates daily therapy with a selective serotonin reuptake inhibitor for anxiety, with a temporary adjunct of hydroxyzine 25 mg every 4 hours as needed until SSRI titration is complete. He also initiates gabapentin 600 mg at night to assist with sleep, as he is concerned about prescribing any sedative-hypnotics having pharmacological cross-reactivity with alcohol. Mr. A. complains of persistent insomnia, and low-dose clonazepam (0.5 mg at bedtime) is transiently re-introduced to assist with first-month recovery stabilization. He begins attending AA meetings five mornings per week and there meets another professional, who has been sober for six years, who agrees to sponsor him in recovery. Mr. A. and his psychiatrist meet more frequently and focus on strategies to avoid drinking and to manage stress more effectively; his wife participates in some treatment sessions and learns more about alcohol use disorders.

Eight weeks after his detoxification, he returns to see you, and his blood pressure is much improved. He is down to 0.25 mg clonazepam at night and has remained sober on most days, but last night he drank a pint of vodka and is afraid to tell his wife or psychiatrist. You acknowledge that the choice is up to him, but encourage him to disclose, as they have both been supportive of his recovery. He agrees and says he prefers to call his psychiatrist himself.

He does call, but only after drinking for two more days until his wife noticed. Together, they call his psychiatrist, who refers him back to the addiction psychiatrist consultant. Mr. A. is then referred to an intensive outpatient therapy and daily contacts with his AA sponsor, and he and his wife are counseled on monitoring naltrexone adherence, as Mr. A. stopped taking it ten days prior. Mr. A. achieves abstinence again, and at a follow-up visit, he shows you his AA six-month abstinence chip, thanking you for helping him. He has weaned off clonazepam completely.

Case 2: Treatment of Opioid Use Disorders

Ms. O., a thirty-five-year-old married mother of two young children, has no previous psychiatric history and presents to you for her annual physical examination. After asking her about her recent health, a careful physical examination reveals signs of intravenous drug use on her arms ("track marks"). She bursts into tears and tells you that she has been injecting heroin daily for the past month. She was initially prescribed oxycodone following a whiplash injury when she was rear-ended while driving her children home from school. She had been experiencing increased family stressors and insomnia. Oxycodone not only helped her pain, but she slept better at night and felt it gave her energy during the day. She sought a second prescription at an urgent care center, stating that she reinjured her neck picking up one of her children. After her prescription ran out, she complained about her neck pain at her exercise class, and a woman there offered to sell her some of hers; soon this was a regular exchange and she developed tolerance.

After she began to need three or four 30 mg oxycodone tablets per day to get the same effect that she did when she first started using, she found that she could no longer afford to buy oxycodone to use daily. She withdrew money from the family vacation account to pay for more oxycodone, and when this was noticed by her husband, he became suspicious of the problem, asked his sister to take care of the children, and demanded she stop using or he would leave her and take the children. She threw out half a bottle of pills in front of him and promised she wouldn't use anymore, but she had another full bottle in her car that she continued to use. Her source for oxycodone offered her a less expensive but even more powerful alternative, heroin, telling her that she never needed to use a needle; she could just "snort" it. She began snorting, and one month later, she had her first injection use, seeking greater effects at a lower cost.

You discuss treatment options for Ms. O., who reports using 0.5–1 grams of intravenous heroin daily. Ms. O. opts for a brief inpatient admission for opioid detoxification. After a four-day buprenorphine taper, she is discharged from the inpatient unit and starts an intensive outpatient program (IOP) that she attends three days a week for three hours at a time over the next two weeks. The treatment team on the inpatient unit discusses the three FDA-approved medications for the treatment of opioid use disorders – buprenorphine, methadone, and naltrexone– and, after a more in-depth discussion of the pros and cons of buprenorphine maintenance, Ms. O. decides to attempt to remain abstinent from opioids without the help of medication.

After finishing the IOP, she begins seeing a social worker with experience treating addictions on a weekly basis. In addition, she attends Narcotics Anonymous (NA) meetings two to three times weekly as a supplement to her individual psychotherapy. In her second week of IOP, she tells her counselor that she is having very intense cravings to use heroin and she fears she will do so. With her permission, her counselor calls you, and you schedule an urgent visit during which you and Ms. O. agree that it would be safest for her to begin a trial of depot naltrexone. She sees you for monthly injections, and six months after her annual physical exam visit, she remains active in treatment and abstinent from opioids, although she reports that her life remains stressful. She continues to work on alternative coping strategies in her psychotherapy while getting support from her husband at home and others in recovery at NA meetings.

References and Selected Readings

Recommended Textbooks
- Galanter, M., and Kleber, H. D. (eds.) (2015). The American Psychiatric Publishing Textbook of Substance Abuse Treatment, 5th ed. Arlington, VA: American Psychiatric Publishing.
- Miller, W. R., and Rollnick, S. (2013). *Motivational Interviewing:* Helping People Change (Applications of Motivational Interviewing), 3rd ed. New York: Guilford Press.

Selected Articles
- Anton, R. F., O'Malley, S. S., Ciraulo, D. A., Cisler, R. A., Couper, D., and the COMBINE Work Group (2006). Combined Pharmacotherapies and Behavioral Interventions for Alcohol Dependence: The COMBINE Study: A Randomized Controlled Trial. JAMA, 295 (17), 2003–2017.
- Anton, R. F., Oroszi, G., O'Malley, S., Couper, D., Swift, R., Pettinati, H., and Goldman, D. (2008). An Evaluation of Mu-Opioid Receptor (OPRM1) as a Predictor of Naltrexone Response in the Treatment of Alcohol Dependence: Results from the Combined Pharmacotherapies and Behavioral Interventions for Alcohol Dependence (COMBINE) Study. Arch Gen Psychiatry, 65 (2), 135–144.
- Carliner, H., Keyes, K., and McLaughlin, K. (2016). Childhood Trauma and Illicit Drug Use in Adolescence: A Population-Based National Comorbidity Survey Replication-Adolescent Supplement Study. J Am Acad Child Adolesc Psychiatry 55 (8), 701–708.
- Fudala, P. J., Bridge, T. P., Herbert, S., Williford, W. O., Chiang, C. N., and the Buprenorphine/Naloxone Collaborative Group (2003). Office-Based Treatment of Opiate Addiction with a Sublingual-Tablet Formulation of Buprenorphine and Naloxone. N Engl J Med, 349 (10), 949–958.
- Project MATCH Research Group (1998). Matching Alcoholism Treatments to Client Heterogeneity: Project MATCH Three-Year Drinking Outcomes. *Alcoholism:* Clinical and Experimental Research, 22, 1300–1311.
- Substance Abuse and Mental Health Services Administration, Center for Behavioral Health Statistics and Quality (July 17, 2014). The TEDS Report: Age of Substance Use Initiation among Treatment Admissions Aged 18 to 30. Rockville, MD.
- Weiss, R. D., Potter, J. S., Fiellin, D. A., Byrne, M., Connery, H. S., et al. (2011). Adjunctive Counseling during Brief and Extended Buprenorphine-Naloxone Treatment

for Prescription Opioid Dependence: A 2-Phase Randomized Controlled Trial. Arch Gen Psychiatry 68 (12), 1238–1246.

Guidelines

- Kleber, H. D., Weiss, R. D., Anton, R. F., George, T. P., Greenfield, S. F., et al. (2007). Work Group on Substance Use Disorders; American Psychiatric Association; Steering Committee on Practice Guidelines. *Treatment of Patients with Substance Use Disorders*, 2nd Edition. American Psychiatric Association. *Am J Psychiatry*, 164 (4 suppl.), 5–123.

Online Resources

- Alcoholics Anonymous, www.aa.org
- Narcotics Anonymous, www.na.org
- National Institute on Alcohol Abuse and Alcoholism (NIAAA), www.niaaa.nih.gov/
- National Institute on Drug Abuse (NIDA), www.drugabuse.gov
- SAMHSA-HRSA Center for Integrated Health Solutions (CIHS), http://wwwwww.integration.samhsa.gov
- SMART Recovery, www.smartrecovery.org
- Smokefree.gov, www.smokefree.gov

Self-Assessment Questions

1. Which of the following statements is false regarding the heritability of alcohol use disorders?
   A. Men with a family history of severe alcohol use disorder have attenuated responses to alcohol at equivalent blood alcohol levels compared with those individuals without such a history.
   B. Having a parent with severe alcohol use disorder quadruples the risk for alcohol use disorder.
   C. Adoption studies show that biological children of parents with severe alcohol use disorder retain a greater lifetime risk of developing alcohol use disorder regardless of environmental upbringing.
   D. Individuals at risk for alcohol use disorder have a lower tolerance for the effects of alcohol.
   E. Individuals with genetically reduced alcohol dehydrogenase activity have an accumulation of acetaldehyde with alcohol ingestion, leading to aversive symptoms such as flushing, headache, and tachycardia, and thus should avoid alcohol consumption.

2. Which of the following statements is false regarding substance use disorders (SUDs)?
   A. Marijuana is the most abused illicit drug in the United States.
   B. Cigarette smoking has increased in recent years.

C. Routine drug screens do not detect synthetic cannabinoids such as "K2".

D. There is a cannabis withdrawal syndrome characterized by irritability, anxiety, insomnia, and poor concentration.

E. Synthetic cannabinoid intoxication can be life-threatening due to adrenergic dysregulation and psychosis.

3.   Which of the following statements is true of opioid use disorders?

A. Opioid use disorders have increased in the United States in the past decade.

B. Heroin use is associated with the majority of reported opioid overdoses in recent years.

C. The physical examination in a patient with opioid overdose includes findings of pupillary dilation and elevated respiratory rate.

D. Opioid withdrawal is a potentially lethal syndrome.

E. There is no medical treatment for opioid withdrawal with an established safety profile for pregnant women.

4.   Which of the following would be used in the case of a heroin overdose?

A. Naltrexone

B. Naloxone

C. Clonazepam

D. Buprenorphine

E. Bupropion

5.   Which of the following hallucinogens have both serotonergic and noradrenergic properties?

A. Lysergic acid diethylamide (LSD)

B. Methylenedioxymethamphetamine (MDMA)

C. Psilocybin

D. Mescaline

E. Dimethyltryptamine

Answers to Self-Assessment Questions

1. (D)
2. (B)
3. (A)
4. (B)
5. (B)

10 | Personality Disorders

LOIS W. CHOI-KAIN, ANA M. RODRIGUEZ-VILLA, GABRIELLE S.
ILAGAN, AND EVAN A. ILIAKIS

The Concept of Personality Disorders

At the turn of the twenty-first century, our understanding of personality disorders radically evolved as research on their biological characteristics and effective evidence-based treatments (EBTs) emerged to challenge preexisting notions of these syndromes as defensive, psychologically determined, and untreatable. Reflecting the turmoil of a paradigm shift, intense controversy raged in attempts to revise the diagnostic system for personality disorders in the transition from the DSM-IV to the DSM-5. Proposed changes included both the elimination of five of the ten existing DSM personality disorders (narcissistic, histrionic, schizoid, paranoid, and dependent) and the implementation of a complex diagnostic system involving the evaluation of both categorical prototypes and dimensional traits of personality. The extremity of these proposed changes in the diagnostic system provoked major opposition among prominent experts, ultimately leading to the retention of the existing set of personality disorder criteria and relegation of the proposed alternative model to a section calling for further research. One prominent change in the transition to the fifth edition of DSM was the elimination of the multi-axial system, ending the segregation of Axis II disorders from Axis I disorders. Consistent with research implications and treatment advances, the collapse of the multiaxial system overturned the perceived dividing lines between so-called conditions that may be the focus of clinical attention and the peculiar grouping of personality disorders with intellectual disability. What we know now is more about the importance of recognizing and treating personality disorders, which should eventually overturn the tradition of deferring their diagnosis.

A second significant change in the DSM-5 is that personality disorders are identified as primarily disorders of the self and interpersonal relationships. This is a valuable and overdue change that distinguishes personality disorders from all other major forms of mental illness. Personality disorders are prevalent, cause major morbidity and mortality, and contribute to a substantial economic burden on society (Soeteman et al., 2008; van Asselt et al., 2007). Personality disorders exist in approximately one-tenth of the general population, constitute up to half of the psychiatric population in hospital units and clinics, and are highly co-morbid with Axis I disorders (Lezenweger et al., 2007; Torgersen, 2009; Gunderson, 2011;

Table 10.1 Estimated prevalence in general population and heritability of personality disorders

Diagnosis	Prevalence of disorder (percent)	Heritability
Paranoid	0.4–5.1	.34
Schizoid	0.4–4.9	.43
Schizotypal	0.1–4.6	.61
Antisocial	0.2–4.5	.69
Borderline	0.7–5.9	.67
Histrionic	0.0–3.0	.63
Narcissistic	0.0–6.2	.71
Avoidant	0.7–5.2	.42
Dependent	0.1–1.8	.56
Obsessive-Compulsive	0.7–9.3	.60

Source. DSM-5; Lenzenweger et al., 2007; Torgersen, 2009; Torgersen, 2012

Skodol & Gunderson, 2011; see Table 10.1). All clinicians are guaranteed to encounter patients with personality disorders and the failure to make a diagnosis may leave patients' symptoms untreated in the best of cases and exacerbated or reinforced in the worst.

The complex interaction of personality disorders with other psychiatric and medical conditions presents clinical challenges, since the symptoms of these disorders impact the therapeutic alliance and efficacy of treatment. Research confirms that the presence of co-morbid personality disorders lengthens time to remission, increases risk of relapse, and decreases response to otherwise effective treatments for other psychiatric illnesses. Individuals with personality disorders suffer from instabilities of behavior and interpersonal functioning, that is, tendencies of avoidance, dependence, mistrust, and impulsivity complicate treatment interactions, increasing the likelihood of poor compliance with prescribed treatments and recurrent conflicts with clinicians.

Considering the prevalence, co-morbidity, dysfunction, and therapeutic challenges associated with personality disorders, it is not surprising that they pose a significant economic burden to society. The costs associated with health care and lost productivity of individuals with personality disorders, particularly borderline personality disorder (BPD) and obsessive-compulsive personality disorder (OCPD), exceed such costs associated with major depressive (MDD) or generalized anxiety disorders (GAD; Soeteman et al., 2008). This finding suggests that the failure of both clinicians to diagnose and treat personality disorders as well as insurance companies to reimburse care for these disorders is costly to society.

The evaluation and treatment of these disorders sometimes require more time than a generalist practitioner can independently provide. However, once a clinician suspects a personality diagnosis, evaluations of interpersonal, behavioral, affective, and cognitive tendencies require only a simple review of diagnostic criteria. Personality disorders involve pervasive patterns in affect, behavior, cognition, and interpersonal functioning that cause significant distress or dysfunction. Generally, clinicians can quickly construct a concise differential diagnosis when they evaluate the degree to which a person's thoughts and emotions become dysregulated – that is, either constricted or exaggerated – in addition to their tendencies toward interpersonal preoccupation or avoidance (see Figure 10.1). Making a treatment plan for any major psychiatric disorder without considering the differential diagnosis and common co-morbidities that involves personality disorders can lead to misdiagnosis, the prescription of ineffective treatments, and sometimes even iatrogenic outcomes.

In general, the treatment of personality disorders is both simple and complex. While some evidence for the efficacy of pharmacologic treatments for personality

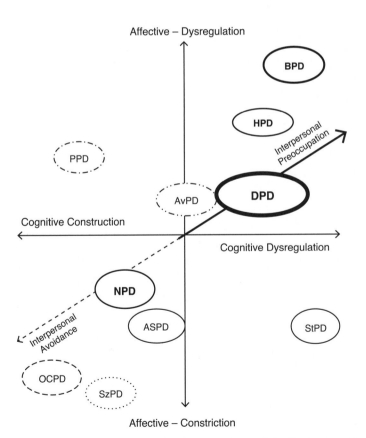

Figure 10.1 DSM-5 personality disorders according to their affective, cognitive, and interpersonal features

Table 10.2 Common differential diagnoses and co-morbidities of personality disorders

Diagnosis	Differential diagnosis	Common co-morbidities
Paranoid (PPD)	Delusional Disorder, Persecutory Type	PTSD
	Schizophrenia, Paranoid Type	Social Phobia
	Mood Disorder with Psychotic Symptoms	Schizophrenia
	Schizotypal PD	Alcohol Use Disorders
	Schizoid PD	
	Narcissistic PD	
	Antisocial PD	
	Borderline PD	
	Avoidant PD	
	Core Distinguishing Features →mistrust and suspicion	
Schizoid (SzPD)	Schizophrenia	MDD
	Depression	
	Autism and Asperger's Disorder	
	Schizotypal PD	
	Avoidant PD	
	Core Distinguishing Features →disinterest in others	
Schizotypal (StPD)	Schizophrenia	MDD
	Schizoid PD	Substance Use Disorders
	Paranoid PD	
	Core Distinguishing Features →eccentric ideas and behavior	
Antisocial (AsPD)	Substance Use Disorders	Impulse Control Disorders
	Bipolar Disorder	Borderline PD
	ADHD	ADHD
	Intermittent Explosive Disorder	Substance Use Disorders
	Autistic Spectrum Disorder	
	Narcissistic PD	
	Core Distinguishing Features →social irresponsibility, disregard, and secondary gain	

Table 10.2 (cont.)

Diagnosis	Differential diagnosis	Common co-morbidities
Borderline (BPD)	Bipolar Disorder	MDD/Dysthymia
	Antisocial PD	Substance Related Disorders
	Core Distinguishing Features →intolerance of aloneness, emotional dysregulation	Eating Disorders
		PTSD
		ADHD
		Narcissistic PD
		Antisocial PD
Histrionic (HPD)	Dependent PD	MDD/Dysthymia
	Borderline PD	Somatization Disorder
	Narcissistic PD	Conversion Disorder
	Core Distinguishing Features →attention seeking	Borderline PD
		Antisocial PD
Narcissistic (NPD)	Bipolar Disorder	MDD/Dysthymia
	Histrionic PD	Anorexia Nervosa
	Antisocial PD	Substance Related Disorders (esp. cocaine)
	Core Distinguishing Features → dysregulated, fragile self-esteem	Histrionic PD
		Borderline PD
		Paranoid PD
Avoidant (APD)	Social Phobia	MDD/Dysthymia
	Schizoid PD	Social Phobia
	Core Distinguishing Features → avoidance, rejection sensitivity	Panic Disorder
		OCD
Dependent (DPD)	Mood Disorders	MDD/Dysthymia
	Panic Disorder	Anxiety Disorders
	Agoraphobia	Alcohol Use Disorders
	Borderline PD	Borderline PD
	Histrionic PD	Histrionic PD
	Avoidant PD	
	Core Distinguishing Features → submissiveness, dependency	

Table 10.2 (cont.)		
Diagnosis	Differential diagnosis	Common co-morbidities
Obsessive-Compulsive (OCPD)	OCD	MDD/Dysthymia
	Schizoid PD	Alcohol Use Disorders
	Avoidant PD	OCD
	Narcissistic PD	
	Core Distinguishing Features ➜ need for control, perfectionism, rigidity, obstinacy	

ADHD = attention deficit hyperactivity disorder, MDD = major depressive disorder, OCD = obsessive-compulsive disorder, PD = personality disorder, PTSD = post-traumatic stress disorder

disorders exist, medications tend to target only manifest symptoms, not underlying mechanisms or personality traits. For example, mood stabilizers may mitigate mood swings or improve depressive symptoms, but do not change intolerance of aloneness or deep mistrust of others. Furthermore, few medication trials have been conducted and results are inconsistent (see Choi-Kain et al., 2017 for review).

The gold standard of treatment for personality disorders is psychotherapy. Psychotherapy increases the rate of remission of symptoms significantly in this group of disorders (Perry, Banon, & Ianni, 1999). When the patient is seeking treatment and is motivated to change, both individual and group psychotherapy are effective for many of these disorders. In relationships with therapists and with other patients in group therapy, individuals with personality disorders are able to see and hear feedback about how they interact with others. More recently, generalist approaches to treating BPD have been developed and proven as effective as more intensive specialized psychotherapies (see Choi-Kain et al., 2017 for review). These approaches prioritize diagnosis, psychoeducation, and clinical management, rather than psychotherapy, which might render them more accessible for psychiatrists and other clinical professionals who either do are not psychotherapists, or cannot implement lengthy and more time-intensive interventions. Table 10.3 summarizes treatment approaches.

The following chapter will review the current literature on the classification, epidemiology, etiology, longitudinal course, differential diagnosis, evaluation, and treatment of personality disorders. While there is burgeoning empirical literature on some disorders (e.g., borderline, schizotypal, antisocial) there is a paucity of research on others (e.g., paranoid, schizoid, histrionic). This chapter will integrate clinical theories and approaches with relevant empirical bases where available.

Table 10.3 Treatment of personality disorders: Pharmacologic and psychotherapeutic interventions

Diagnosis	Pharmacology	Psychotherapy
Paranoid (PPD)	Antidepressants	Supportive
		CBT
Schizoid (SzPD)		Supportive
		Social Skills Training
Schizotypal (StPD)	Antipsychotics	Supportive
		Social Skills Training
		CBT for anxiety management
Antisocial (AsPD)	Antidepressants (SSRIs)	Early Intervention
	Mood stabilizers (lithium, valproate)	CBT for impulsivity and behavioral shaping *controversy over treatability*
Borderline (BPD)	*Mood symptoms, impulsivity, anxiety*	*Generalist approaches*
	Mood stabilizers (lamotrigine, topiramate)	GPM, SCM, and other structured clinical management approaches
	Transient psychotic symptoms, anger problems	Supportive
	Atypical antipsychotics	*Specialist approaches*
	Not harmful but limited efficacy	DBT
	Antidepressants	MBT
	Minimize due to risk of dependency	TFP
		SFT
	Benzodiazepines	STEPPS
	Stimulants	
Histrionic PD (HPD)		Psychodynamic psychotherapy
Narcissistic (NPD)		Psychodynamic psychotherapy
		DBT
		MBT
		TFP
Avoidant (APD)	Antidepressants (MAO-Is, SSRIs)	Psychodynamic psychotherapy
	Anxiolytics	Supportive psychotherapy
		CBT

Table 10.3 (cont.)

Diagnosis	Pharmacology	Psychotherapy
Dependent (DPD)	Antidepressants (MAO-Is, SSRIs) *may have increased risk for benzodiazepine dependency*	Psychodynamic psychotherapy CBT
Obsessive-Compulsive (OCPD)	Antidepressants (SSRIs)	Psychodynamic psychotherapy CBT

CBT = cognitive-behavioral therapy; GPM = general psychiatric management; SCM = structured clinical management; DBT = dialectical behavioral therapy; MBT = mentalization based treatment; SFT = schema-focused therapy; SSRI = Selective Serotonin Reuptake Inhibitor; STEPPS = Systems Training for Emotional Predictability and Problem Solving; MAO-I = Monoamine oxidase inhibitors; TFP = transference based psychotherapy

Cluster A: Paranoid, Schizoid, and Schizotypal Personality Disorders

Cluster A disorders, referred to as the "odd, eccentric" cluster of personalities, are characterized primarily by the social withdrawal and cognitive-perceptual distortions or eccentricities seen in more psychotic proportions in schizophrenia and its related disorders. Historically, in the earliest efforts toward the classification of major mental illnesses, the subtypes coined as descriptors of what was thought to be variations of schizophrenia, such as "pseudoquerulant type," "shut-in personality," and "borderline schizophrenia," recognizably represent these Cluster A disorders. The overlap of the Cluster A disorders with major thought disorders has led to conceptions of a schizophrenia spectrum where the personality diagnoses represent shared underlying biological vulnerabilities phenotypically expressed in more muted forms or as pre-morbid precursors to more severe symptoms. Akin to schizophrenia, symptoms in this cluster range from "positive" or psychotic-like symptoms (e.g., paranoia and disorganized thinking in paranoid and schizotypal personality disorder) to "negative" or deficit symptoms (e.g., constricted affect and social apathy in schizoid personality disorder). Shared tendencies of interpersonal mistrust and detachment lend toward the low prevalence of patients with these disorders seeking treatment, as well as subjects willing to engage in research.

There is an overall dearth of academic literature, but of the three, research on schizotypal personality disorder is most robust, showing both strong evidence of familial aggregation and shared genetic vulnerabilities with schizophrenia as well as distinctive structural brain abnormalities and impaired areas of performance on cognitive tasks in common with schizophrenia. Nonetheless, very little is known about response to treatment and longitudinal course of these disorders. Further investigation is needed to assess the validity of both the paranoid and schizoid diagnoses, as they uncommonly exist by themselves and the schizotypal diagnosis so strongly overlaps with features of both.

For individuals with Cluster A disorders, their tendencies may be ego-syntonic and not cause distress. Oftentimes, these patients will present with chief complaints of depression or anxiety or because concerned family members insist on treatment. Clinicians should determine the chronicity, severity, and bizarreness of symptoms and interpersonal functioning to contrast these disorders to their "Axis I" (DMS-IV) cousins. One can then evaluate the function or core mechanisms underlying the symptoms to differentiate these disorders from other personality diagnoses (Table 10.2). Treatment of these individuals is impeded by their paranoia, social cognitive deficits, and phobic or disinterested attitudes toward others. Individual therapy with Cluster A patients works best when not overly probing or confrontational, but rather supportive and structured. These individuals are often unable to tolerate or navigate more open-ended group therapy approaches as their understanding of themselves and others is grossly impaired. However, individuals with these disorders can sometimes benefit from cognitive-behavioral or psychoeducational skills-based groups.

Paranoid Personality Disorder (PPD)

Clinical Features
The hallmark of paranoid personality is pervasive and unwarranted suspicion and mistrust of others as bearing malevolent motives. Individuals with PPD assume that others intend to harm or deceive them. They are hypervigilant and hypersensitive to any signs that confirm their suspicions and remain socially aloof out of fear of being exploited or betrayed by those with whom they get close. They are quarrelsome and litigious, bearing grudges persistently. Persons with paranoid personality are therefore prone to self-fulfilling prophecies, where their prediction of others acting unfavorably toward them is often realized when others are provoked by their suspicious hostility.

The prevalence of PPD is estimated between 0.4 to 5.1 percent of the general population (Lenzenweger et al., 2007) and 9.7 percent of the clinical population (Triebwasser et al., 2013). Of all personality disorders, PPD ranks among the top diagnoses associated with a reduction in functioning and quality of life (Triebwasser et al., 2013). Clinical theories implicate feelings of anger and inadequacy developed from early experiences of excessive parental rage and recurrent humiliation. The primary defense mechanism at hand is projection, where intolerable emotions or thoughts within one's self are split off and attributed to others. The limited empirical literature confirms a significant association between PPD and childhood emotional and physical abuse and victimization (Triebwasser et al., 2013). While literature on the biological features of this illness is sparse, there are patterns of familial aggregation that are unlikely to be caused by shared environmental effects and more likely to arise from gene-environment interactions. PPD's estimated heritability ranges from .28 to .66 (Triebwasser et al., 2013). Limited evidence indicates that first-degree relatives of individuals with delusional disorder are at greater risk for developing PPD, suggesting these two disorders may be genetically related.

Treatment

Given their pervasive mistrust, individuals with PPD tend not to seek clinical help. The evaluation of PPD is complicated given the ego-syntonic nature of its features. Patients with PPD are unlikely to see their problems as internal and instead rigidly blame others. Since their symptoms limit the scope of their interpersonal world, the accessibility of family members or spouses to provide collateral information is often lacking. When clinicians detect global suspiciousness without frank psychosis, they might inquire about close relationships and how the patient interacts with others. The differential diagnosis includes paranoid schizophrenia; delusional disorder, paranoid type; and schizotypal, schizoid, borderline, narcissistic, antisocial, and avoidant personality disorders. Both schizophrenia and delusional disorder differ from PPD in the persistence, prominence, and proportion of their paranoid beliefs, which are exclusively interpersonal, less bizarre, and harder to disprove in PPD. Individuals with PPD often meet criteria for other personality diagnoses, but these persons can be distinguished by the pervasiveness of their paranoia regarding others (as opposed to the more transient paranoia characteristic of borderline personality) and by its organizing core of mistrust of others as opposed to disinterest (schizoid), dependency (borderline), grandiosity (narcissistic), exploitation (antisocial), or fear of rejection (avoidant). Discerning the differences between these diagnoses is complicated by the high rate of co-morbidity with other psychiatric disorders ranging from thought disorders to anxiety disorders (PTSD, social phobia) to other personality disorders (BPD). Rarely is PPD the sole diagnosis.

No controlled studies have been completed for the treatment of PPD. In approaching treatment, whether medical or psychiatric, a non-confrontational, respectful, straightforward manner should be used to minimize the aggravation of symptoms so that enough trust can be generated for the patient to cooperate in treatment. Efforts to appreciate any validity in the patient's suspicions may facilitate an alliance between patient and treater. This alliance may then enable the patient to make use of cognitive-behavioral treatments or atypical antipsychotics, which may work to decrease anxiety for individuals with PPD. However, mistrust often interferes with adherence to such measures, and their sensitivity to criticism and perceiving slights interferes with what is, in the best-case scenario, a long course of treatment. Little is known about PPD's longitudinal course, but considering the low likelihood that individuals with PPD will seek treatment, and endure relationships long enough to change core beliefs about others, their paranoia seems likely to sustain itself for life.

Schizoid Personality Disorder (SzPD)

Clinical Features

Schizoid personality disorder (SzPD) is marked by pervasive detachment from and general disinterest in social relationships. Individuals with SzPD show limited expression of affect regarding others and limited skill in relating to others meaningfully. It is the least studied of all personality disorders and also one of the least common, with its prevalence estimated at less than 1–4.9 percent of the general population (Triebwasser et al., 2012). Clinical theories posit that persons with SzPD have histories of experiencing caregivers as emotionally cold, neglecting, and detached, fueling the schizoidal individual's attitude that relationships are ungratifying. There is some evidence that this disorder runs in families as the disorders on the schizophrenia spectrum as a group demonstrate familial aggregation. The heritability of SzPD is estimated at .28 (Triebwasser et al., 2012).

Treatment

Like individuals with PPD, those with SzPD seldom seek psychiatric treatment due to their general disinterest in interacting with others. The evaluation of the disorder relies on a review of the diagnostic features in the DSM, which may take time to collect in the form of both clinical observation and self-report by the patient. The absence of any cognitive or perceptual disturbances such as paranoia or hallucinations, distinguish this disorder from schizotypal disorder and other schizophrenia spectrum disorders. Schizoidal individuals can be distinguished from those with high functioning variants of autism, like Asperger's syndrome, by the degree of social impairment and stereotyped behaviors or interests, which are more severe in autistic disorders. The social awkwardness in Asperger's syndrome is considered "active but odd," whereas in SzPD the social awkwardness is inactive and disinterested. Careful evaluation of depression is needed to discern whether the social apathy and anhedonia as well as the constricted affect are stable or episodic in conjunction with other neurovegetative features. While both schizoid and avoidant personality disorders present with social isolation, the schizoidal patient's withdrawal is driven by disinterest whereas the avoidant patient's is rooted in rejection sensitivity. Phobic avoidance related to feeling overwhelmed in relationships with others may underlie the schizoidal patient's disinterest in other people.

No controlled research has been published on either manualized psychotherapies or psychopharmacology for SzPD. Schizoid patients will have no interest or skills to form a therapeutic relationship, but may in crisis or in seeking treatment for other psychiatric problems be able to use a treatment relationship as an exposure to increase the tolerability of emotions and intimacy. In general, efforts to share interest in non-human topics like objects or hobbies that appeal to those preferring solitary pursuits can help in the navigation of a therapeutic interaction. Cognitive-behavioral approaches that focus on the acquisition of social skills may also facilitate change. While little is known about SzPD's course, limited research suggests that traits of SzPD are among the most stable over time of all the personality disorders (Triebwasser et al., 2012).

Schizotypal Personality Disorder (StPD)

Clinical Features

Individuals with StPD are distinguished from their Cluster A cousins by both the variety of cognitive-perceptual distortions other than paranoia and anxious affect. Their cognitive experiences reflect a more florid departure from reality (e.g., ideas of reference, paranoid ideas, bodily illusions, magical thinking) and a greater level of disorganization when compared to other personality disorders. The likelihood that other individuals or communities might share some of their odd or eccentric beliefs as well as the less enduring quality of these symptoms distinguish it from schizophrenia proper.

StPD occurs in less than 1 percent of the general population and has an estimated heritability of .61 (Torgersen et al., 2000). Family history studies demonstrate an increased risk for disorders related to schizophrenia in probands with StPD and vice versa. The etiology of the disorder is thought to be primarily biological, as it shares many of the brain-based abnormalities characteristic of schizophrenia. Its attenuated manifestations of clinical and biological features associated with schizophrenia have led to questions of whether or not StPD should be grouped with personality disorders or with schizophrenia and its related illnesses. In fact, in the ICD-10, a diagnostic system used widely internationally, StPD is classified with schizophrenia, and not with other personality diagnoses. In the DSM-5, it is listed in the schizophrenia spectrum section but discussed in full detail in the personality disorders section. Of all the personality disorders, it is least associated with defense mechanisms. It is associated with persistent substance use disorders (Hasin et al., 2011), but otherwise is not associated strongly with Axis I disorders.

Treatment

Individuals with StPD will rarely seek treatment independently, particularly if they are paranoid. However, concerned family members are likely to bring them to seek professional evaluation given the resemblance of their symptoms to schizophrenia. The primary diagnostic task is to differentiate schizotypal individuals from those with major thought disorders in terms of the severity, bizarreness, and duration of symptoms. The presence of odd and disorganized thought and behavior will differentiate StPD from PPD and SzPD, where the social withdrawal is not accompanied by the range of unusual cognitions and behaviors characteristic of StPD.

Psychological formulations of the disorder and evidence of the efficacy of psychotherapeutic interventions are limited. Given its biological similarities with schizophrenia, StPD is primarily treated with medications. Antipsychotic medications are shown to decrease anxious and psychotic-like symptoms and antidepressants may be helpful to ameliorate the anxiety experienced by those with StPD. A supportive and psychoeducational approach may assist individuals with this disorder in orienting them to social skills and increased awareness of how their own behavior may be perceived. Compared to those with other Cluster A disorders, individuals with StPD may be more able to engage in and benefit from a group therapy structured either around cognitive-behavioral techniques or psychoeducation.

Cluster B: Histrionic, Borderline, Narcissistic, and Antisocial Personality Disorders

Of all the personality disorders diagnoses, those within Cluster B may be the most clinically relevant as they are prevalent in treatment settings, have symptoms that are high risk for self-harm or harm toward others, and have effective treatment approaches devoted to them. They are referred to as the "dramatic" cluster, as they tend to be either attention-seeking (i.e., histrionic, narcissistic, borderline) or impulsive (i.e., antisocial and borderline). Individuals with Cluster B disorders are among the most interpersonally interactive of the personality disordered population, as their core characteristics involve specific preoccupations with others, whether it be via attention-seeking or exploitation and manipulation (Figure 10.1). Because of their interpersonal orientations, they are likely to seek care in most cases or come for care at the behest of others via the interpersonal problems they create.

In contrast to the Cluster A disorders, there is a wealth of literature, both clinical and empirical, dedicated to these disorders and their treatments. These disorders often co-occur with other major psychiatric disorders in virtually all major categories (e.g., mood, anxiety, substance use, eating, etc.) and complicate their treatment. In addition, diagnoses within this cluster often co-occur with other personality disorders. Their evaluation is therefore complicated, as many of the diagnoses implicated in the differential (e.g., depression or substance abuse) may in fact be co-morbid with these Cluster B diagnoses. Despite this complication, a simple but systematic review of symptoms listed in the DSM criteria may be all that is required to make a diagnosis. Oftentimes simply handing a patient a list of diagnostic criteria will lead to self-diagnosis, developed out of recognition of features in themselves.

There is significant psychoanalytic literature devoted to the formulations and conceptualizations of the personality diagnoses in this cluster, and relevant treatment techniques and approaches have stemmed from these formulations. In addition, the overt behavioral symptoms and cognitive distortions have been the focus of a growing cognitive-behavioral literature. Several empirically validated techniques now exist for managing borderline personality disorder (BPD), and these same techniques are thought to be effective in treating most of the diagnoses in this cluster. While there are some medications that help alleviate elements of these disorders, they are adjunctive at best. Psychotherapeutic approaches are considered the gold standard. Still, treatment with patients in this population will challenge the most astute clinicians, as the interpersonal features distinctive of these disorders play themselves out robustly in therapeutic relationships.

Antisocial Personality Disorder (ASPD)

Clinical Features

Central to the antisocial personality disorder (ASPD) diagnosis is a pervasive disregard for consequences and the rights of others in favor of personal profit or pleasure. Antisocial persons will commit unlawful, deceitful, reckless actions without remorse. They justify their behavior and remain indifferent to the harmful effects of their actions on others. While they may be cold and dispassionate in their attitude toward the suffering of others, individuals with antisocial personality can become irritable and aggressive, prone to fighting and assaultive action. The presentations of these individuals vary. Some are more impulsive and disorganized; the crimes and harmful acts committed by these individuals stem from a failure to inhibit drives or consider consequences. Other individuals with ASPD are more psychopathic and their behaviors are calculated such that self-serving consequences are intended or consequences that are harmful to others are disregarded. Some antisocial persons are more callous than others, and in severe cases of psychopathy, pleasure is sadistically derived from inflicting pain on others.

ASPD exists in 1 to 4.5 percent of the general population and is more common in men than in women. While some of these individuals seek treatment, frequently aimed at secondary gain, many are not bothered by their antisocial tendencies and have little internal motivation to change. These individuals are commonly seen in the penal system, and therefore bear a significant burden on public services. The heritability of ASPD is estimated at .69 (Torgersen et al., 2012). Externalizing, action-oriented disorders, such as substance abuse and ASPD, run in the families of individuals with ASPD. The scientific literature suggests that genetic factors combined with environmental factors (i.e., childhood maltreatment) converge in the etiology of ASPD. Impulsive aggression, connected to abnormal serotonin transporter functioning, is hypothesized as one core biological mechanism underlying the disorder. In addition, neglectful or aggressive parenting behavior is also found more commonly in individuals with ASPD. Prospective research suggests disregard for the pain of others in early childhood predicts antisocial behavior in late adolescence.

Treatment

The evaluation of this group is complicated by its characteristics of deceitfulness, motivation for secondary gain, and the high rates of co-morbid substance use disorders. Individuals with ASPD are often charming and convincing. They enlist others, including medical professionals, in efforts to promote their own agendas.

These individuals can be disruptive to clinical settings, in terms of their influence on other patients and the operations of the clinical team. A majority of individuals with ASPD have substance use problems and approximately half of those with substance use problems meet the criteria for ASPD. Discerning the differences between the impulsivity and irresponsibility resulting from substance use versus ASPD can be difficult, but inquiry into the timeline of periods of sobriety, including early history, may clarify the primary diagnosis. Sometimes making the diagnosis of ASPD after the substance use disorder is treated may be more accurate, but ASPD is diagnosable even when a co-occurring substance use disorder is active. Conduct disorder is defined by a pervasive pattern of violating social norms and laws, so it overlaps a great deal with ASPD criteria, but it must be present before the age of fifteen.

Both clinical experience and empirical evidence suggest that most people with ASPD are not treatable. In theory, individuals who are exploitative and maintain a primary focus on personal gain in their core orientation to others are likely to use a treatment relationship in the same vein. In other words, treatment may be pursued for secondary gain, meaning the treatment is instrumental in achieving some other personal goal, such as disability or avoidance of legal consequences, rather than internal change. In the empirical literature of treatment interventions for adult patients, there is no evidence that any treatment leads to long-term gains.

There is some controversy about the traditional therapeutic nihilism associated with this group. There is evidence that some antisocial individuals have a capacity to form a therapeutic alliance, experience guilt and depressive symptoms in confined settings, and change when confronted in group situations. Although there are some predatory and sadistic individuals with ASPD who show an inability to learn and low motivation for change, there also exists a subset of more impulsive, affectively dyscontrolled, and disorganized individuals who may be motivated to learn skills for self-control in order to avoid aversive consequences. In theory, those individuals may benefit from cognitive-behavioral or pharmacologic (i.e., lithium, valproate, and serotonin reuptake inhibitors) interventions for impulsive aggression. However, no evidence exists supporting the efficacy of these interventions for adults with ASPD. The longitudinal course showing that the prevalence declines with age suggests the possibility that individuals can learn over time to change. Individuals meeting criteria for ASPD who seek treatment should be treated for co-morbid disorders with evaluation of risk for suicidality, aggression, and secondary gain.

Borderline Personality Disorder (BPD)

Clinical Features
Patients with borderline personality disorder (BPD) abound in all clinical settings. They are distinguished by their extreme mood fluctuations, self-destructive

tendencies, and interpersonal hypersensitivity. Their dysregulation spans all four sectors of personality functioning and can swing between states of underregulation and overregulation. A patient with BPD can at times appear shutdown, avoidant, and helpless, and at others seem enraged, reckless, and demanding. At their core, individuals with BPD suffer from an intolerance of aloneness. They frantically avoid abandonment and will generate crises – that is, with aggression, recklessness, and suicidality – in a way that invites rescue or hostile engagement by others. Some experts have criticized the borderline concept because of its wide-ranging symptoms and presentations, calling it a "wastebasket diagnosis." However, BPD's symptoms have a distinctive organization where the constellation of symptoms is reactive to interpersonal situations. For instance, when a patient with BPD feels connected and cared for, they will present as anxious, depressed, and collaborative. But when the same patient perceives criticism, rejection, or abandonment, she may become enraged, reckless, and threatening. In more extreme circumstances, when the borderline patient is truly alone and disconnected from others, she may become dissociated, paranoid, and suicidal. Thus, there is an oscillation in symptoms according to the patient's state of attachment. Those who interact with patients with BPD become either idealized as benevolent caretakers or devalued as cruel punishers. This oscillation reflects the phenomenon called *splitting*. The extreme swings in opinions of others can match the evaluations that the borderline patient has of herself as either worthy of being saved or essentially bad and broken beyond repair.

Every clinician will encounter patients with BPD. Patients with BPD are both highly prevalent in and high utilizers of health care. Its prevalence in the general population is 1 to 5.9 percent (Table 10.1) but can be up to an estimated 20 percent in mental health treatment settings. Individuals with BPD are frequently seen in primary care providers' offices as well as in emergency rooms. In clinical settings, 75 percent of patients with BPD are female.

Previously, BPD was thought to be the product of early childhood trauma. While individuals with BPD in particular and personality disorders in general have been shown to have high rates of early childhood abuse, trauma is neither necessary nor sufficient in the development of this disorder. More recently, research has accumulated to confirm BPD's significant biological basis. The heritability of BPD is estimated at .67 and family studies demonstrate the likelihood that the heterogeneous features of the disorder (e.g., behavioral, cognitive, emotional, interpersonal instability) are transmitted via a single common pathway. In the neuroimaging literature, early studies reported hyperreactivity in limbic areas of the brain (i.e., amygdala), while later studies began to describe distinct dysfunction in prefrontal and frontolimbic activity as the larger mechanism behind emotional dysregulation in BPD. These data support the notion that emotional intensity and dysregulation in BPD is the manifestation of failures of top-down frontal control processes that should modulate the effects of the bottom-up hyperreactive limbic structures. Differences in the functioning of neurohormone systems, like opioids and oxytocin, have also been associated with problems of pain perception as well as trust and collaboration in individuals with BPD. While early childhood adversity, dysfunctional caretaking, and general early life stress may function as major etiological forces in the development of BPD, genetics, in addition to disturbed regulatory functions of brain and neuropeptide systems, may prime individuals to be more prone to pathological responses to environmental life stress.

Treatment

Historically, individuals with BPD were identified by their poor responses to treatments that were generally effective for patients with other disorders. In the clinical community, they became stigmatized as treatment resistant. Psychiatry's view on the course and treatability of the disorder has been radically revised by research that has shown both the efficacy of a number of manualized psychotherapeutic treatments for BPD (Table 10.3), as well as rates of remission of up to 85 percent by ten years of follow-up, even without specialized treatments.

The treatment of borderline patients is commonly complicated by both under- and misdiagnosis. However, the evaluation of BPD can be simple. Handing a patient a list of the diagnostic criteria can lead to self-diagnosis and relief, as these patients have commonly experienced multiple failed treatments for either co-morbid illnesses, like depression, or for diagnoses they do not have, like bipolar disorder. Making the BPD diagnosis and providing psychoeducation about its symptoms can in itself improve symptoms, as it raises the patient's awareness to the nature of their difficulties. BPD has a complex pattern of comorbidity, commonly co-occurring with a number of other disorders, particularly depression and anxiety disorders like post-traumatic stress disorder or panic disorder as well as eating and substance use disorders (Table 10.3). The identification of BPD and its co-morbidities are important. The course of MDD can be prolonged significantly when BPD is co-morbid, and will respond more readily to treatment if BPD is treated. Conversely, it may be difficult to treat BPD when there is co-occurring substance abuse or anorexia, which must be stabilized before a patient can effectively engage in treatment for their BPD.

BPD is most commonly misdiagnosed as bipolar disorder, due to the wide fluctuations in mood, behavior, and sleep that are in BPD related to problems of self-regulation. What distinguishes the borderline from the bipolar individual is the reactivity of the borderline's symptoms; their mood and behavioral swings are reactive to stressors, especially interpersonal. The mood fluctuations of BPD happen over minutes to hours and are generally among states of depression, anxiety, and anger rather than depression and elation. The interpersonal symptoms of BPD are most distinguishing from other disorders, as the negative self-image, insecure attachment, and rejection sensitivity are generally absent in patients with other mood or anxiety disorders.

In differentiating BPD from other personality disorders, one can determine the primary functions of interpersonal patterns. Narcissistic, histrionic, dependent, and borderline individuals are all attention seeking, but persons with BPD often engage with others in a hostile dependency, where negative attention is preferable to no attention at all. Additionally, those with BPD will see themselves as bad and experience emptiness, while those with histrionic or narcissistic personality disorders do not characteristically (Table 10.2).

There are now many treatments proven to improve the suicidality, depression, and functioning of individuals with BPD (Table 10.3). Some of these evidence-based treatments (EBTs) are cognitive-behavioral in orientation – such as dialectical behavioral therapy (DBT) and systems training for emotional predictability and problem solving (STEPPS) – and construct BPD as a problem primarily of emotional dysregulation and deficit in emotional and social skills. Both DBT and STEPPS provide skills training to mitigate symptoms in all four sectors of instability in BPD, and DBT additionally provides individual therapy formatted as skills coaching and driven by principles of behavioral shaping. Mentalization-based treatment (MBT), transference-focused psychotherapy (TFP), and schema-focused therapy (SFT) all formulate interpersonal disturbances as the basis of BPD, and focus on stabilizing the ways patients emotionally experience themselves and others. These three treatments utilize the patterns observed both in the patient's life and in the therapy relationship to raise awareness to and change interpersonal patterns and sensitivities.

There are common features of all these EBTs that contribute to their effectiveness. All these EBTs except STEPPS involve an individual therapy component and all but TFP involve a group therapy component. Therapists in all modalities are active and focused on the here and now, rather than on past experiences that contribute to the patient's problems.

All of the EBTs mentioned so far primarily target the problems of BPD, they are specialized approaches and are proven to work better than general psychiatric approaches that are not informed by an understanding of BPD. An unanticipated byproduct of the randomized controlled trials for DBT, TFP, and MBT is the finding that structured clinical management and supportive therapy approaches provided by clinicians either experienced with BPD or educated about the basic features of BPD are also highly effective in decreasing symptoms. While the more specialized EBTs require specialized training and treatment resources, there are now EBTs such as general psychiatric management (GPM), designed for the generalist practitioner that can be employed without teams or group therapy by a general psychiatrist in outpatient practice.

There is limited scientific literature on the efficacy of pharmacologic approaches to managing BPD. In clinical practice, as these patients frequent acute settings such as emergency rooms and inpatient hospitals, mental health professionals may attempt to temporize crises by adding medications in an unsystematic fashion. This tendency increases the risk for significant morbidity and mortality from medical problems (e.g., obesity) as well as decreased functioning related to significant side effects of medications. Optimally, medications work best when used sparingly and systematically for specific symptoms. Antipsychotics are most effective in ameliorating anxious, angry, and cognitive symptoms of BPD. While serotonin reuptake inhibitors and mood stabilizers like lamotrigine are usually well-tolerated and of minimal lethality in overdose, research shows they are only marginally effective. Still, when such medications are associated with sustained monitoring of BPD signs and symptoms, they can be associated with strong benefits (Gunderson & Choi-Kain, 2018).

The longitudinal course of BPD has been elucidated by studies that have more than 10 years of follow-up data, showing that individuals with BPD usually remit with very low relapse rates. However, their functional status does not generally improve as dramatically. While many self-destructive events for individuals with BPD are not aimed to end life, the risk of suicide in BPD is forty-fold that of the general population and older studies on suicide indicate a 10 percent prevalence among those with the disorder. Thus, while individuals with BPD largely get better over time, better-informed treatments are necessary to prevent suicide, increase functioning, and decrease the recurrent use of high-cost health care resources.

Histrionic Personality Disorder (HPD)

Clinical Features
Individuals with histrionic personality disorder (HPD) are distinguished by excessive emotionality and attention-seeking. They use their physical appearance to gain the attention of others, interacting in inappropriately seductive or provocative ways. While dramatic and theatrical, histrionic individuals lack depth in emotional experiencing, as the flamboyance of their expressions function to evoke reactions in others. Persons with HPD lack a sense of self-direction and are highly suggestible, often acting submissively to retain the attention of others. They conceive of situations and express themselves impressionistically, lacking attention to details and a comprehensive reality.

Histrionic personality disorder has an estimated prevalence between 1 and 3 percent in the general population, occurring more commonly in women than men. The heritability of HPD is .63 and co-aggregates with other Cluster B personality disorders in families, particularly ASPD. There is very little empirical literature dedicated primarily to HPD, but there is a rich psychoanalytic literature conceptualizing the disorder. The conceptualization of HPD derived from the earlier concept of hysteria, which described patients who displayed physical symptoms (e.g., paralysis) that were inconsistent with any medically sound explanation. The hysterical presentation was, in the early psychoanalytic literature, related to unconscious conflict and early psychological trauma. Hysteria is no longer used in the medical lexicon as a diagnostic term. The presentations of unexplained somatic complaints thought to be a manifestation of split off and repressed distress from psychic conflict or early trauma were diagnostically reclassified under categories of somatoform disorders and dissociative disorders. The personality thought to be associated with hysteria was captured in the criteria for HPD.

Treatment

The evaluation of histrionic personality is complicated by the lack of self-awareness individuals with this disorder have. While those with ASPD may recognize the way they meet diagnostic criteria but remain indifferent to the implications, those with HPD in general have poor insight into their own tendencies as they are externally oriented (i.e., focused on appearance, dramatic action, and others' attention) and may have limited capacities for deep reflection and critical self-analysis. Just as their somatic complaints may have no deeper roots to a discernable anatomically or physiologically driven source, their emotional displays may have no obvious root to deeper emotional sources (at least not to the patient herself). The diagnostic evaluation might be triggered by the presentation of somatization disorder, which is known to co-occur with the disorder (Table 10.2).

HPD is also often co-morbid with other Cluster B personality disorders, causing researchers to wonder whether a shared biological vulnerability exists or alternatively whether HPD even exists as an independent entity. Nonetheless, clinicians can differentiate HPD from other personality disorders by identifying the core mechanisms behind their symptoms (Table 10.2). While both histrionic and narcissistic individuals seek attention, the narcissist needs adulation or to feel elevated by it. The histrionic individual is not so selective about the kind of attention he or she gets and does not mind being regarded as cute or silly. Borderline individuals regard themselves as bad and experience emotions intensely and deeply, whereas individuals with HPD do not see themselves as bad, even though their dependence on the reaction of others may be rooted in poor self-esteem. Lastly, individuals with dependent personality seek proximity with others like the individual with HPD, but the dependent person is more anxious and inhibited.

Whether the disconnection between how the histrionic individual acts and feels is (1) driven by conflict and repression or (2) reflecting a deficit in recognizing emotions, clinicians must determine what the histrionic patient is capable of using in terms of treatment. A therapist might start by encouraging the patient with HPD to emote verbally rather than behave physically. Once the patient can engage in less dramatic ways of both understanding themselves and communicating with others, the therapist can help the patient to realize how their "histrionics" functions maladaptively to attract the attention of others to manage their self-esteem. Ultimately, the patient can be oriented to how this tendency results in shallow relationships and emotional experience, and therefore works against developing emotional skills and meaningful deeper commitment in relationships. No systematic treatment research exists, so little is known about the efficacy of pharmacologic interventions or cognitive-behavioral approaches.

Narcissistic Personality Disorder (NPD)

Clinical Features
Individuals with narcissistic personality disorder (NPD) are known for their tendencies toward grandiosity, need for adulation, and lack of empathy. Behind their arrogant and haughty behaviors is often a fragile sense of self and self-esteem. The basic difficulties narcissistic persons have with sustaining a sense of superiority drive both the need for praise and their affiliations with special people or institutions as well as the tendency to devalue others. While people with NPD need the admiration of others and can exploit people to promote themselves, they lack empathy and otherwise remain interpersonally distant. When individuals with NPD experience rejections, criticisms, or defeat, they react angrily, feeling deeply wounded. In these states, narcissistic individuals may become severely depressed and sometimes dangerously suicidal.

The prevalence of NPD is estimated at approximately 0.5 percent and occurs more commonly in men than women. Its heritability is high at .71, but there is a dearth of scientific research elucidating biological factors that contribute to the symptoms of NPD. Clinical theories have pointed to early experiences of failures to be accurately attuned by caregivers. Some individuals with NPD in fact have special gifts or talents, and become accustomed to having their self-image and sense of self tied to the admiration and esteem of others. When their sources of admiration recede, narcissistic crises result, including self-destructive tendencies.

Treatment
Like with HPD, there is a significant and rich psychoanalytic literature on the formulation and treatment of NPD. However, there is very little treatment research on this disorder. In clinical settings, patients with NPD often present with depression and in some cases are misdiagnosed as bipolar because of their grandiosity. They may suffer from co-morbid depression but are distinguished from those with bipolar disorder by the persistence of their need for elevating themselves above others.

The mood reactivity of the individual with NPD is triggered by insults to their self-esteem. They exploit others to promote themselves like those with ASPD, but the aims of the narcissist center around sustaining one's sense of superiority. The narcissistic person may seek the attention of others, but unlike histrionic individuals, those with NPD would have disdain for being considered cute or silly.

Because individuals with NPD experience deep shame behind their pompous symptoms, they are often reluctant to seek treatment. When they do, they are often sensitive and reactive to perceived criticism when clinicians point to problems in an attempt to promote change. Individuals with NPD may hold therapists at arm's length, appearing to have intellectually sophisticated understandings of themselves which may bear no relationship to their real experiences or deeper feelings. For this reason, treatment may be challenging. The bulk of the treatment literature on NPD comes from psychoanalytic experts who describe effective approaches using psychodynamic psychotherapy. Some approaches developed for BPD may be adapted for use with NPD. With CBT approaches, NPD patients may find the opportunity to increase mastery as appealing and their need for praise may enable a therapist to shape their behavior. Other interpersonally focused approaches, such as transference-focused psychotherapy (TFP) and mentalization-based treatment (MBT) may also be effective for patients with NPD.

Cluster C: Avoidant, Dependent, and Obsessive-Compulsive Personality Disorders

Cluster C disorders have an anxious affective component with concurrent cognitions, behaviors, and interpersonal tendencies shaped by doubt and worry. They are therefore referred to as the "anxious" or "worried" group of personality disorders. Both avoidant and dependent personality disorders are organized around severe rejection sensitivity and excessive need for reassurance from others. Those with avoidant personality cope by avoiding situations that might involve criticism or rejection, while those with dependent personality indiscriminately seek relationships and act submissively in the service of maintaining access to support. In contrast, those with obsessive-compulsive personality disorder are worried about making mistakes and defensively adapt through the use of controlling tendencies like perfectionism. All of these disorders tend to be co-morbid with anxiety disorders. Empirical inquiry has focused on elucidating the convergences and divergences between the Cluster C disorders and anxiety disorders, testing the hypothesis that both sets of disorders exist on a single spectrum that are more related biologically than Cluster C disorders are to other personality disorders.

The treatment of these disorders optimally involves some combination of medications and psychotherapy. In themselves, antidepressants and anxiolytic medications can diminish the anxious state of cluster C disorders, but therapy is needed to manage characterologic traits and adaptive defenses central to these diagnoses. In general, individuals with Cluster C disorders are less impaired than those with Cluster A or B personality disorders. These individuals also are more likely to respond to and be retained in more general psychotherapeutic treatments. There are no evidence-based treatments (EBTs) specially designed for these disorders. Because anxiety and coping strategies are central to these diagnoses, standard approaches suited to anxiety management or defensive adaptations to anxiety can work well for this population. Longer-term therapies are indicated for these patients, rather than just brief treatments that might suffice for their axis I co-morbidities.

Avoidant Personality Disorder (AVPD)

Clinical Features

The hallmark of AVPD is the avoidance of social situations or interactions where there is a risk for rejection, criticism, or humiliation. Individuals with AVPD suffer from intense feelings of inadequacy and cope maladaptively through avoiding any situations in which they may be evaluated negatively. The world of avoidant individuals become highly constricted, due to their pervasive hypersensitivity to being shamed or ridiculed, and consequently, their opportunities to challenge or test their assumptions about themselves are limited. Not surprisingly, when these individuals do engage in social situations, they are often inhibited, self-conscious, and shy; thus their experience of social activity can remain unsatisfying and fuel further avoidance.

The prevalence of AVPD ranges from 1 to 5.2 percent, and the heritability is estimated at .28 (Table 10.1). It is more common in women than men and is found to be associated with increased risk for suicide. Research on the etiology of the disorder implicates the role of experiences of rejection and marginalization in early life as well as of innate traits of social anxiousness and avoidance. These traits are detectable as early as around age two, when physiological arousal and avoidant tendencies have been observed in social situations. AVPD symptoms appear more stable over the course of a year after diagnosis than do the symptoms of BPD, StPD, and OCPD. Little else is known about the course of the disorder.

Treatment

The main differential diagnosis with AVPD includes SzPD and social phobia. Those with SzPD are more disinterested in than hypersensitive to others. The differences between AVPD and social phobia are subtler. AVPD involves more pervasive anxiety and avoidance than social phobia, which is commonly specific to situations that involve the possibility of public embarrassment. There is a "generalized" form of social phobia that appears similar to AVPD. Social phobia is also highly co-morbid with AVPD, and studies show those with both disorders have more severe symptoms and disability than those with either disorder alone.

Those with AVPD will often avoid treatment. Individuals with both social phobia and AVPD can respond to social skills training groups and other group therapies that are homogenous – in other words, composed of others with the same difficulties. Those with AVPD respond to individual therapies that are supportive and understanding of the avoidant person's hypersensitivities toward others. Eventually, once an alliance can be developed, reflection about the nature and effectiveness of their defensive avoidance can be broached. Clinicians sometimes respond to these patients with either excessive protectiveness or expectations for change, and are cautioned to attempt a balance between accommodation of patient's limitations and gradual exposure to social situations.

Pharmacologically, these patients respond to monoamine oxidase inhibitors (MAO-Is) or selective serotonin reuptake inhibitors (SSRIs) as well as anxiolytics, which help reduce anxiety enough to allow them to expose themselves to new social situations. However, therapies are needed to help patients manage their interpersonal fears and behavioral tendencies, so that beliefs about one's self as inept in social situations can be challenged and change.

Dependent Personality Disorder (DPD)

Clinical Features
The core feature of those with dependent personality disorder (DPD) is the pervasive and excessive need to be taken care of, which fuels clinging behaviors at the expense of one's own autonomy and independent interests. The dependent personality needs others to provide enough reassurance and guidance in order to make decisions or initiate projects. Individuals with DPD rely on others to assume responsibility in all areas of life, and so go to excessive lengths to maintain the support of others. These individuals manage their intense anxieties about taking care of themselves through excessive dependency and submissiveness.

The prevalence of DPD is 0.7 percent (Table 10.1) of the general population and is more common in women than men. The heritability is estimated at .57, and familial traits such as submissiveness, insecurity, and self-effacing behavior may contribute to the liability toward developing DPD. There is limited clinical and empirical literature on the etiology of this literature. Cultural factors, negative early experiences, biological vulnerabilities associated with anxiousness contribute to the development of DPD. Little is known about the course of the disorder.

Treatment
The evaluation of excessively rejection-sensitive and dependent individuals invokes the differential diagnosis of BPD, HPD, and AVPD. While individuals with DPD, AVPD, and BPD are all interpersonally and rejection sensitive, those with BPD and AVPD would be too frightened to submit to the degree of control the

dependent personality invites from others. The individual with BPD would vacillate between submissiveness and rageful hostility, the latter of which distinguishes these two disorders. Lastly, the individual with HPD will seek attention rather than reassurance and is more disinhibited.

Those with DPD can be easily engaged in treatment, and often present with increased anxiety or depression in the context of relationship difficulties, real or perceived. Both psychodynamic and cognitive-behavioral psychotherapeutic approaches aimed at examining fears of independence and difficulties with assertiveness help those with DPD. Clinicians should be cautious about promoting dependency in the therapy relationship, as in those cases the treatment itself can regenerate the kind of interpersonal interaction central to the disorder.

The evidence basis for psychopharmacologic interventions for DPD is sparse. MAO-Is have been found effective in AVPD and disorders like atypical depression, which also involve rejection sensitivity. One study demonstrated an association between DPD and benzodiazepine dependence, suggesting medications of this class may become addictive for these patients.

Obsessive-Compulsive Personality Disorder (OCPD)

Clinical Features

Individuals with obsessive-compulsive personality disorder (OCPD) exhibit a pervasive tendency toward orderliness, perfectionism, and control in a way that overshadows the point of any activity at hand and ultimately slows or interferes with getting anything done. The need for control in OCPD leads to tendencies to be solitary in their endeavors and to mistrust the aid of others. They are miserly and hoard out of worry for future needs. Ultimately, persons with OCPD have very constricted interpersonal orbits as they become preoccupied with work and alienate others with their stubbornness and rigidity. Their outward affect is also highly constricted, but their experience of anxiety related to their compulsive perfectionism is intense.

OCPD is common, occurring in up to 9.3 percent of the general population (Table 10.1). It is more common in men than in women. The heritability is high at .78, and familial traits of compulsivity, restricted range of emotion, and perfectionism may be related to this disorder. The symptoms of OCPD have been found to decline over the period of a year, but longer-term studies are lacking.

Treatment

Patients with OCPD may present in treatment settings with anxiety, depression, and difficulties with sleep. They may appear similar to patients with obsessive-compulsive disorder (OCD), but lack the repetitive thoughts and ritualistic behaviors characteristic of OCD. The need for control is driven by a preoccupation with order in itself and is ego syntonic in those with OCPD, in contrast with those with OCD who are often distressed by their lack of control over compulsive drives. The social isolation of the individual with OCPD differs from that seen in SzPD and AVPD, as the obsessive-compulsive personality will prioritize work and productivity to relationships, and only mistrusts others in terms of their potential to intrude on their perfectionism.

The treatment of OCPD is complicated by the need for control and rigidity central to the disorder. Their controlling tendencies may confuse clinicians who may misdiagnose them with NPD. Patients with OCPD are highly intellectualized and on guard for any suggestion that they are wrong. They do not show much emotion and tend to not be naturally self-disclosing, especially not of vulnerabilities. Their rigidity often elicits boredom or frustrations in therapists. In some cases, their interesting, detailed intellectualized conversation may seem psychologically minded but are void of affect, and do not promote change. Little empirical literature exists on the treatment of these disorders.

Future Directions

The status of personality disorders in the DSM will remain uncertain until further research on the validity, course, and treatment of all the DSM-IV disorders can be completed. While the growth of empirical literature on BPD has clarified and enriched the existing clinical knowledge on the disorder, the scientific literature on disorders such as PPD, SzPD, HPD, AVPD, DPD, and OCPD is scarce. More research is needed about the relationship Cluster A disorders have to psychotic disorders and also the relationship between Cluster C personality and anxiety disorders to assess what latent neurobiological features may confer liability toward these illnesses previously divided by the multiaxial diagnostic framework. Currently, we have the personality disorders conceptualized as a discrete group, but biological mechanisms underlying these diagnoses yet to be discovered may reveal that personality disorders group more coherently with other categories of illness as we have seen with StPD and schizophrenia. However, retaining the sense that disorders distinctively reflect character pathology, which responds more to psychotherapeutic measures than somatic therapies, may sustain an argument for the need for long-term psychotherapies as central to their medical management.

Sample Interview Questions

In the evaluation of patients with personality disorders, clinicians need to consider both what the patient reports and also how he behaves, especially how he behaves in the interpersonal interaction with the clinician. Open-ended questions are generally where psychiatric interviews begin, and both the review of symptoms and the level of organization and coherence in thought will reveal cognitive and emotional coping resources. For instance, if a patient is constricted in his report and perspective of his problems, probing for cluster A disorders, NPD, AVPD, or OCPD may lead to a diagnosis. If the patient is disorganized and effusive, making little meaning of sense, probing for StPD, BPD, or HPD may clarify the diagnosis. The most revealing inquiry will be in asking the patient about what their relationships are typically like particularly why or how important relationships have ended. Patients with personality disorders will have varying levels of insight, with those with NPD, ASPD, PPD, and SzPD being least distressed or bothered by their personality symptoms. Directness or confrontation may reveal some of these patients' more dysfunctional interpersonal traits but should be employed thoughtfully as these moves might disrupt treatment alliance in those with cluster A personality disorders in particular. The following questions are fairly simple and are derived from Kernberg's structural interview of personality.

Sample Questions:

1. What brought you to treatment? What is the nature of your difficulties? *Assess insight, organization of thought, ability to reflect about oneself, ability to admit flaws, black-and-white thinking, internalizing versus externalizing problems. Other ways to inquire the same thing include:* What are you motivated to change in yourself? What are your goals in treatment? What gets in the way of your happiness or achieving your goals in life?
2. What is your personality like? How do you describe yourself? How would others describe you? *This provides a sense of the patient's self-image (how insecure or grandiose as well as how realistic) and also their capacity to mentalize, that is, understand themselves and others in terms of mental states.*
3. Who are the most important people in your life? How would you describe your relationships with those people? How well do you get along with others? *Assess stability of relationships, insecurities, entitlements, fears, anxieties as well as how realistically they portray others.*

Case Examples

Sarah

Sarah is a nineteen-year-old single, otherwise healthy woman with a history of bulimia and non-suicidal self-injury. She is brought in for evaluation by her mother who shares that Sarah has relapsed and is "purging again." "I don't know what else to do," she adds.

Sarah had recently returned home to live with her parents and younger brother, leaving college mid-way through her second semester of freshman year. Though academically successful in high school, Sarah struggled to organize her assignments and stay up to date with her college course work. Overwhelmed by the pace of the academic work and stress related to making new friends, Sarah would retreat to her dorm room, skipping classes and avoiding calls from family. When she did call her parents, she was often tearful describing worries that she would not be accepted in the sorority of her choosing and concerns that her parents did not miss her. To Sarah, taking time off from school seemed "the only solution."

At home, Sarah began to suspect that her parents were planning to divorce and her bulimic and self-harming behaviors returned. If she heard her parents fighting, she felt an immediate need to purge and would do so in an adjacent bathroom, easily overheard by her parents. Her family had always been very responsive to her bulimia. In the past, her parents always mobilized following stretches of bulimia or superficial cutting and Sarah received attention and uniform support that she found comforting and reassuring.

While at a family reunion over the winter holiday, Sarah was discovered cutting her wrists in her bedroom and was hospitalized. She attended an intensive outpatient program for two weeks, where she excelled in group therapy sessions, participating consistently, completing all assignments thoroughly, and receiving positive feedback from her providers that seemed to buoy Sarah's self-confidence. She expressed a goal of establishing a more honest relationship with her parents and a hope that they could learn to discuss feelings and emotions openly.

Despite this goal and the efforts made in her program, Sarah continued to passively express distress at home, engaging in purging behaviors openly and evading questions about her urges to self-harm. If her parents did not immediately respond to her phone calls, her anger would escalate quickly and she would claim they "don't care" or make threats to leave home. Whenever she felt that her parents did not give her what she "needed," she would feel intense anger and sadness. Her impulsivity when angry and her intentional withholding of information caused her parents to feel like they were "walking on eggshells" and could not directly discuss any issue which may upset her. You hope that a treatment informed by knowledge of personality disorders can help her manage her symptoms.

References and Suggested Reading

- American Psychiatric Association (2000). *Diagnostic and Statistical Manual of Mental Disorders: DSM-IV-TR.* Washington, DC: American Psychiatric Association.
- Choi-Kain, L. W., Finch, E. F., Masland, S. R., Jenkins, J. A., and Unruh, B. T. (2017). What Works in the Treatment of Borderline Personality Disorder. *Current Behavioral Neuroscience Reports*, 4, 21–30.

- Gunderson, J. G. (2011). Borderline Personality Disorder. *New England Journal of Medicine*, 364, 2037–2042.
- Gunderson, J. G., and Choi-Kain, L. W. (2018). Medication Management for Patients with Borderline Personality Disorder. *American Journal of Psychiatry*, 175(8), 709–711.
- Hasin, D., Fenton, M. C., Skodol, A., et al. (2011). Personality Disorders and the 3-Year Course of Alcohol, Drug, and Nicotine Use Disorders. *Archives of General Psychiatry*, 68, 1158–1167.
- Kernberg, O. F. (1981). Structural Interviewing. *Psychiatric Clinics of North America*, 4, 169–195.
- Lenzenweger, M. F., Lane, M. C., Loranger, A. W., and Kessler, R. C. (2007). DSM-IV Personality Disorders in the National Comorbidity Survey Replication. *Biological Psychiatry*, 62, 553–564.
- Lilienfeld, S. O., Van Valkenberg, C., Larntz, K., and Akiskal, H. S. (1996). The Relationship of Histrionic Personality Disorder to Antisocial Personality and Somatization Disorders. *American Journal of Psychiatry*, 143, 718–722.
- Perry, J. C., Banon, E., and Ianni, F. (1999). Effectiveness of Psychotherapy for Personality Disorders. *American Journal of Psychiatry*, 156, 1312–1321.
- Ronningstam, E. (2005). *Identifying and Understanding the Narcissistic Personality*. Oxford: Oxford University Press.
- Shea, M. T., Stout, R. L., Gunderson, J. G., et al. (2002). Short-Term Diagnostic Stability of Schizotypal, Borderline, Avoidant, and Obsessive-Compulsive Personality Disorder. *American Journal Psychiatry*, 159, 2036–2041.
- Shea, M. T., Stout, R. L., Yen, S., et al. (2004). Associations in the Course of Personality Disorders and Axis I Disorders Over Time. *Journal of Abnormal Psychology*, 4, 499–508.
- Skodol, A. E., and Gunderson, J. G. (2011). Personality Disorders. In Hales, R. E., Yudofsky, S. C., and Gabbard, G. O. (eds.), *Essentials of Psychiatry*, 3rd ed. Arlington, VA: American Psychiatric Publishing.
- Soeteman, D. I., Hakkart-van Roijen, L., Verheul, R., and Busschbach, J. J. (2008). The Economic Burden of Personality Disorders in Mental Health Care. *Journal of Clinical Psychiatry*, 69, 259–265.
- Torgersen, S. (2009). The Nature (and Nurture) of Personality Disorders. *Scandinavian Journal of Psychology*, 6, 624–632.
- Torgersen, S., Lygren, S., Oien, P., Skre, I., Onstad, S., Edvardsen, J., and Kringlen, E. (2000). A Twin Study of Personality Disorders. *Comprehensive Psychiatry*, 6, 416–425.
- Torgersen, S., Myers, J., Reichborn-Kjennerud, T., et al. (2012). The Heritability of Cluster B Personality Disorders Assessed by Both Personal Interview and Questionnaire. *Journal of Personality Disorders*, 26, 848–866.
- Triebwasser, J., Chemerinski, E., Roussos, P., and Siever, L. J. (2012a). Schizoid Personality Disorder. *Journal of Personality Disorders*, 6, 919–926.
- Triebwasser, J., Chemerinski, E., Roussos, P., and Siever, L. J., (2013). Paranoid Personality Disorder. *Journal of Personality Disorders*, 27(6), 795–805.
- van Asselt, A. D., Dirksen, C. D., Arntz, A., and Severens, J. L. (2007). The Cost of Borderline Personality Disorder: Societal Cost of Illness in BPD-Patients. *European Psychiatry*, 22, 354–361.

Self-Assessment Questions

1. In the preceding vignette, Sarah presents with symptoms most consistent with which of the following personality diagnoses:
    A. Antisocial personality disorder
    B. Obsessive-compulsive personality disorder
    C. Borderline personality disorder
    D. Schizoid personality disorder

2. Which of the following interventions are found to be the most effective for personality disorders?
    A. Medications
    B. Electroconvulsive therapy
    C. Hospitalization
    D. Psychotherapy

3. Which of the following statements about medication management applies to the treatment of personality disorders?
    A. Medications are used adjunctively to treat symptoms and co-occurring disorders, but have not been found to be consistently effective for personality disorders.
    B. Adequate research exists to support the use of medications as a definitive treatment for personality disorders.
    C. Medications should never be used in the treatment of personality disorders.
    D. Medications should be used as a last resort in the treatment of personality disorders.

Answers to Self-Assessment Questions

1. (C)
2. (D)
3. (A)

11 Neurocognitive Disorders

BRENT P. FORESTER, FEYZA MAROUF, BEN LEGESSE, OLIVIA I.
OKEREKE, AND DEBORAH BLACKER

Delirium, Major or Mild Neurocognitive Disorders

Classification

Cognitive disorders in the DSM-IV-TR included delirium, dementia, amnestic disorder, and cognitive disorders not otherwise specified. DSM-V retains the diagnosis of delirium and introduces the term *neurocognitive disorder* (NCD), dividing NCDs into major NCD or mild NCD and unspecified NCD. The diagnostic category of major NCD encompasses syndromes that were previously categorized as dementia and amnestic disorder. Memory loss is no longer an essential criterion for major NCD in DSM-V as it was for dementia in DSM-IV-TR. Major NCD also includes progressive neurodegenerative dementias, as well as static cognitive disorders that are not expected to worsen over time. The term *dementia* is retained in DSM-V because of familiarity of the term to the public and medical practitioners.

According to DSM-V, the two core features of delirium are impairment in awareness (reduced orientation to the environment) and disturbance in attention (impaired ability to direct, focus, sustain, or shift attention). Diagnosis of major NCD, in contrast, requires a significant decline in at least one cognitive domain sufficient to interfere with independence in everyday activities (see Table 11.1). Mild NCD requires the presence of a modest decline in cognitive function not severe enough to interfere with independence in everyday living and to meet criteria for major NCD. Mild cognitive impairment (MCI) will be diagnosed as mild NCD under DSM-V.

DSM-V links neuropathological etiology with clinical diagnosis of NCD. Major or mild NCD can be due to Alzheimer's disease, frontotemporal lobar degeneration, Lewy bodies, vascular disease, traumatic brain injury, substances/medications, HIV infection, prion disease, Parkinson's disease, Huntington's disease, or another medical condition. Unspecified NCD is applied in situations where symptoms of NCD are present but full criteria for major or mild NCD have not been met.

Delirium

Epidemiology and Impact

Delirium is a very common psychiatric disorder in hospital settings, occurring in up to 24 percent of patients on general medicine floors and almost half of

Table 11.1 DSM-V criteria for major neurocognitive disorder

A. Evidence of significant cognitive decline from a previous level of performance in one or more cognitive domains (complex attention, executive function, learning and memory, language, perceptual-motor, or social cognition).
    1. Concern of the individual, a knowledgeable informant or clinician that there has been a SIGNIFICANT decline in cognitive function; and
    2. A SUBSTANTIAL decline in cognitive performance, documented by standardized neuropsychological testing or, in its absence, another quantified clinical assessment
B. The cognitive deficits interfere with independence in everyday activities.
C. The cognitive deficits do not occur exclusively in the context of delirium.
D. The cognitive deficits are not better explained by another mental disorder (e.g., major depressive disorder).

post-operative surgical patients. Delirium is often unrecognized during hospitalization and can persist for weeks to months after the initial episode. Indeed, for almost half of delirious patients, symptoms do not fully resolve until six months after the episode. Older adults, especially those with preexisting cognitive impairment, are more vulnerable to developing delirium.

The long-term complications of delirium include acceleration in cognitive decline and poor functional outcomes, with double the risk of discharge to a nursing home compared to similar hospital patients without delirium. Mortality rates associated with delirium are high, comparable to patients suffering a myocardial infarction or sepsis. The one-year mortality rate attributed to delirium is 35 to 40 percent. Given the difficult hospital course, longer length of stay, frequent need for nursing home and rehabilitation placement as well as home health care services, the health care costs associated with delirium are more than double the costs for comparable patients without delirium.

Clinical Features and Course

As discussed previously, the core features of delirium include (1) inability to direct, focus, sustain, and shift attention and (2) disturbance in awareness (reduced orientation to the environment). Attentional impairments often manifest as distractibility by irrelevant environmental stimuli, difficulty staying on the topic of conversation or the task at hand. Sensorium changes range from lethargy, stupor, obtundation, and may even progress to coma. However, delirium should not be diagnosed in comatose patients. Patients with delirium may appear excessively somnolent or have difficulty staying awake. Sleep-wake cycle is usually disrupted, with patients staying awake at night and sleeping during the day.

The onset of delirium symptoms occurs over the course of hours to days. Symptoms of delirium fluctuate within a twenty-four-hour period and do so more dramatically than seen in other neuropsychiatric disorders. Patients may appear to be at their baseline on cross-sectional examination but can be markedly symptomatic a few hours later. Thus it is important to obtain collateral information from nurses and family members who tend to spend more time with the patient. While patients with more dramatic presentations get diagnosed early, hypoactive symptoms of delirium may be misattributed to depression, leading to a delay in diagnosis.

Patients with delirium usually have significant impairment in multiple cognitive domains, including memory, language, orientation, and executive functions. Abnormalities in thought process may range from mild circumstantiality to disorganized and disjointed speech in more severe cases. Alterations in affective regulation are also common in delirium. Rapid dramatic shifts in affective states (i.e., mood lability) can be quite striking. Patients may appear anxious, apprehensive, and hypervigilant, or withdrawn and apathetic. Hyperactive delirium presents with increased psychomotor activity with agitation and restlessness while hypoactive delirium is characterized by slowed motor activity often with apathy and withdrawal, though it is common to alternate between varying levels of psychomotor activation (mixed delirium).

More than two-thirds of patients with delirium demonstrate psychotic symptoms. Hallucinations may be visual, auditory, or tactile. Unlike in schizophrenia, visual hallucinations are more common than auditory hallucinations in delirium. Delusions due to delirium usually have persecutory themes, tend to be fragmented (non-systematized), and are rarely bizarre. Together with agitation and aggression, psychotic symptoms can pose a risk for patient safety and may result in the disruption of the patient's medical care (pulling out IV lines or Foley catheter).

Major or Mild Neurocognitive Disorders

Epidemiology and Impact

Age is the most significant risk factor for developing dementia (or major NCD), a disease that increases in prevalence from 3 percent for those aged 65–74 to almost 50 percent in those aged 85 or older. Studies estimate that an additional 14 percent of people over 70 meet criteria for mild cognitive impairment (mild NCD). Of this population, 7–10 percent are estimated to progress to dementia each year. Alzheimer's disease is the most common cause of dementia (or major NCD), accounting for more than 60 percent of cases and currently affecting 5.8 million Americans. In addition to AD, other important causes of major NCD include vascular dementia (20 percent), dementia with Lewy bodies (15 percent), and frontotemporal dementia (2 percent).

According to the Alzheimer's Association, the overall cost of health care for patients with dementia, including Medicare and Medicaid spending as well as out-of-pocket costs, will increase from $305 billion in 2020 to $1.1 trillion in 2050. This number does not include the billions of hours of unpaid care provided by family, friends, and neighbors (an average of 21.9 hours per caregiver per week) to patients with Alzheimer's disease. Many caregivers experience very high levels of emotional stress and are vulnerable to declines in their own physical health. In fact, more than half of caregivers demonstrate significant symptoms of depression, with at least a quarter meeting criteria for major depressive disorder. Providing individual and family counseling and encouraging participation in support groups not only alleviates depressive symptoms in caregivers but can help delay residential care placement for patients themselves.

Mild Neurocognitive Disorder

There is increasing evidence that the neuropathological changes of AD begin well in advance of the onset of clinical symptoms, perhaps decades before a diagnosis of dementia is made. Recent advances in neuroimaging, cerebrospinal fluid analysis, and other biomarkers point to evidence that AD may be best described as a progression along a clinical continuum, from preclinical or pre-symptomatic stages of disease through mild NCD, and then to major NCD. As defined by the guidelines developed by the National Institute of Aging and the Alzheimer's Association in 2011, the preclinical stage begins with asymptomatic functional and structural brain alterations, including cerebral amyloidosis, synaptic dysfunction, and neurodegeneration that lead to subtle cognitive decline, which can occur years before patients meet criteria for mild NCD. The identification of this preclinical stage is especially important, as it provides a critical opportunity for potentially more effective intervention (Figure 11.1; Table 11.2).

In progressive dementias, mild NCD can be the intermediate stage between normal cognitive function and major NCD. Mild NCD is defined by modest cogni-

Table 11.2 Three stages of Alzheimer's disease, as proposed by the NIA and Alzheimer's Association

Preclinical Alzheimer's disease	Mild cognitive impairment (MCI) due to Alzheimer's disease	Dementia due to Alzheimer's disease
Measurable biomarker changes (e.g., amyloid accumulation on PET, atrophy on volumetric MRI) occur years before subtle cognitive impairment	Mild changes in memory and thinking are noticeable and can be measured on mental status tests, but are not severe enough to disrupt daily life	Impairments in memory, thinking, and behavior decrease the ability to function independently in everyday life

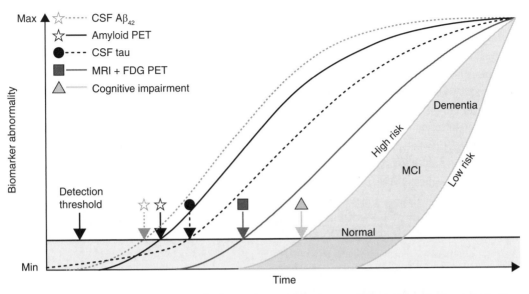

Figure 11.1 Model integrating Alzheimer's disease immunohistology and biomarkers. The threshold for biomarker detection of pathophysiological changes is denoted by the black horizontal line. The gray area denotes the zone in which abnormal pathophysiological changes lie below the biomarker detection threshold. In this figure, tau pathology precedes Aβ deposition in time, but only early on at a subthreshold biomarker detection level. Aβ deposition then occurs independently and rises above the biomarker detection threshold (arrows with a star). This induces the acceleration of tauopathy and CSF tau and then rises above the detection threshold (arrow with circle). Later still, FDG PET and MRI (arrow with square) rise above the detection threshold. Finally, cognitive impairment becomes evident (arrow with triangle), with a range of cognitive responses that depend on the individual's risk profile (light-gray-filled area). Aβ = amyloid β. FDG = fluorodeoxyglucose. MCI = mild cognitive impairment. From Jack, C. R., Jagust, W. J., Petersen, R. C., Weiner, M. W., Aisen, P. S., et al. (2013), Tracking Pathophysiological Processes in Alzheimer's Disease: An Updated Hypothetical Model of Dynamic Biomarkers, *Lancet Neurology*, 12, 207–216.

tive impairment in at least one cognitive domain, not severe enough to affect independence in everyday functions of the individual. Although the day-to-day function is largely intact, a decline in cognitive function can be demonstrated by neuropsychological testing. These cognitive dysfunctions may involve a single domain of cognition (e.g., memory) or multiple cognitive domains (see Table 11.3). It is estimated that as many as 15 percent of those who bring themselves to a physician's office with symptoms of mild NCD go on to meet criteria for major NCD per year, while others may remain stable or even resolve.

Mild NCD must also be distinguished from normal age-associated cognitive decline. As speed of processing, attention span, working memory, and speed of learning decline with normal aging, some individuals worry that these changes may be heralding symptoms of a neurodegenerative disease. The diagnosis of mild NCD is warranted only if the severity of cognitive impairment exceeds what would be expected from normal aging.

Table 11.3 DSM-V criteria for mild neurocognitive disorder

A. Evidence of modest cognitive decline from the previous level of performance in one or more cognitive domains (complex attention, executive function, learning and memory, language, perceptual-motor, or social cognition).

 1. Concern of the individual, a knowledgeable informant, or clinician that there has been a MILD decline in cognitive function; and

 2. A MODEST decline in cognitive performance documented by standardized neuropsychological testing or, in its absence, another quantified clinical assessment

B. The cognitive deficits DO NOT interfere with independence in everyday activities.

C. The cognitive deficits do not occur exclusively in the context of delirium.

D. The cognitive deficits are not better explained by another mental disorder (e.g., major depressive disorder).

Major Neurocognitive Disorders

The diagnosis of major NCD requires a significant decline in one or more cognitive domains (complex attention, executive function, learning and memory, language, perceptual-motor, or social cognition). These changes can be discerned from the history and clinical observations, or demonstrated in quantified clinical assessment or neuropsychological testing. Cognitive deficits in major NCD interfere with independence in everyday activities. Now let us briefly discuss the different etiologic subtypes of NCDs.

Neurocognitive Disorder Due to Alzheimer's Disease (AD)

Symptoms of AD usually begin after fifty years of age and increase in prevalence with advancing age. The initial manifestation of AD is rapid forgetting of newly acquired information. Memory for recent events is impacted early in the course of illness, with increasing difficulty remembering past events as the dementia advances. In AD, the cognitive and functional impairment is insidious in onset and progresses gradually, often over several years.

In the mild stages of AD, the person may recognize his/her memory difficulties. As the illness progresses, others close to the patient will begin to notice memory impairment. Symptoms can include name and word-finding difficulties. Executive deficits may also appear early and worsen with the progression of the illness. Misplacing items, planning, and organizational difficulties for more complex tasks are detected. Forgetfulness for more recent autobiographic events and conversations becomes increasingly apparent.

At the mild stages of the illness, patients can function nearly independently for less complex and routine day-to-day activities. As AD progresses to the moderate stages of the illness, disorientation to time and place and more pronounced autobiographic memory loss (e.g., birth date) become more evident. Day-to-day activities become noticeably impaired at this stage of the illness. In the late stage of the illness, patients become increasingly dependent on others for even basic care (feeding, toileting, etc.). Patients may fail to recognize close family members. In the advanced stage of AD, basic bodily functions such as swallowing and ambulation deteriorate, leading to aspiration pneumonia, decubitus ulcers, and malnutrition. Patients may also develop seizures. These medical co-morbidities ultimately lead to the patient's demise.

In addition to cognitive decline, patients with AD often develop behavioral and psychological disturbances. These symptoms may first manifest in the mild NCD stage and become more common as the disease progresses. Neuropsychiatric manifestations of AD can include anxiety, depression, mood lability, hallucinations, delusions, agitation, or aggression. Apathy and social withdrawal manifest early in the disease course but become increasingly common as dementia progresses. Patients may appear uninterested in the environment and others around them. In the moderately severe stages of the illness, irritability, agitation, combativeness, wandering, and psychotic symptoms are common.

Psychotic symptoms occur in up to 40 percent of patients with AD and develop often in the moderate stage of illness, while depression occurs in up to 50 percent of patients with AD, often beginning in the early stages of AD. Together with the cognitive impairment and inability to perform activities of daily living, these behavioral and psychological symptoms of AD cause significant distress for the patient, earlier institutionalization, and increased caregiver burden. The average length of survival after diagnosis of Alzheimer's dementia is four to eight years (although some people live with AD for as long as twenty years).

Vascular Neurocognitive Disorders (VNCD)

VNCD is caused by cerebrovascular insult. VNCD can present with a range of cognitive and clinical symptoms, with complex attention, executive function, and processing speed being typically impaired. Unlike AD, in patients with VNCD, cued recognition memory is better than un-cued recall. Depressive syndromes commonly accompany VNCD. Other features such as personality changes, irritability, and lack of motivation are often seen in VNCD. The course of vascular NCD is also variable. Some patients may exhibit the classic "step-wise" progression, with periods of acute worsening followed by plateaus of relatively stable cognition, while others show a progressive decline.

Neurocognitive Disorder Due to Lewy Bodies (NCDLB)

Although clinically underdiagnosed, NCDLB is the second most common cause of late-onset (onset after sixty-five years of age) neurodegenerative dementia, occurring in up to 15–20 percent of patients. NCDLB has an insidious onset with gradual progression. Typically, there is wide symptom fluctuation that can mimic delirium. A careful medical and neurological assessment of these episodes does not find a specific, acute etiology. In addition, patients with NCDLB exhibit recurrent formed visual hallucinations and spontaneous parkinsonian symptoms. REM sleep disorders, common in NCDLB, may precede the development of cognitive symptoms. In contrast to AD, memory impairment is less severe early in NCDLB and the cognitive fluctuations are more pronounced. Hallucinations appear earlier in the disease process in NCDLB than AD. Anxiety, depressive, and other neuropsychiatric symptoms are more common in NCDLB compared to AD. Other features of NCDLB include repeated falls, syncopal symptoms, unexplained loss of consciousness, and increased sensitivity to antipsychotic medications. Due to increased sensitivity to extrapyramidal side effects and falls, antipsychotics should be avoided if possible in patients with NCDLB.

Frontotemporal Neurocognitive Disorder (FTNCD)

FTNCD is a group of neurodegenerative dementias characterized by localized atrophy of frontal and/or temporal lobes. Symptoms usually begin in the forty-five to sixty-five years of age range and gradually progress from mild to severe. There are two different subtypes of FTNCD: (1) the frontal (behavioral) variant and (2) the language variant (primary progressive aphasia). In the frontal variant, behavioral symptoms predominate. These behaviors can range from apathy and social withdrawal to increased impulsivity, irritability, and disinhibited behaviors. Patients with the behavioral variant of FTNCD often demonstrate socially inappropriate, disinhibited behavior that commonly results in a psychiatric evaluation. Compared to AD, executive dysfunction is disproportionately affected early in the behavioral variant of FTNCD, while memory functions are relatively preserved until later stages of the illness. Decline in language ability is the early presenting symptom in the language variants of FTNCD. The language variant is subdivided into semantic, agrammatic/nonfluent, and logopenic variants, based on relative impairments in comprehension, fluency, and syntax. Behavioral symptoms are seen in the later stages of the language variant of FTNCD.

Neurocognitive Disorder Due to Traumatic Brain Injury

Traumatic brain injury (TBI) can lead to a NCD. TBI may cause posttraumatic amnesia, confusion, or loss of consciousness, as well as focal neurologic deficits. Inattentiveness, executive dysfunction, and personality changes may also be present. The severity of cognitive impairment due to TBI can range from mild to severe and cause disabling symptoms. NCD due to TBI may be transient or persistent, and varies depending on the severity of trauma, age, and other factors related to the individual or the nature of the trauma.

Neurocognitive Disorder Due to Prion Diseases

Protein-like infectious agents cause prion diseases. The transmission of prion diseases via body fluids is well documented. However, sporadic and familial cases are known to occur. Multiple prion diseases have been described, with Creutzfeldt-Jakob disease (CJD) being the most common. CJD typically presents with rapidly progressing cognitive decline often accompanied by gait abnormalities, myoclonus, and seizures. As a group, these diseases tend to be rapidly progressive and fatal within several months.

Neurocognitive Disorder Due to HIV Infection

The prevalence and severity of cognitive symptoms increase in the later stages of HIV disease. A syndrome of mild NCD due to HIV disease (also called minor motor/cognitive disorder) includes mental slowing, impaired attention and memory, slowed movements, incoordination, and mood and personality changes. Late-stage HIV disease and AIDS can also cause major NCD. In HIV dementia (major NCD), MRI of the brain shows increased hyperintensities on T2 weighted images in subcortical gray and white matter. It is important to rule out opportunistic infections (e.g., herpes simplex encephalitis, progressive multifocal leukoencephalopathy, and toxoplasmosis) and primary or secondary malignancies or stroke, which may cause cognitive symptoms in patients with AIDS, before making a diagnosis of NCD due to HIV.

Neurocognitive Disorder Due to Parkinson's Disease

Mild NCD is common in Parkinson's disease, and in 20–40 percent of patients, the cognitive symptoms progress to major NCD. Spontaneous parkinsonian symptoms may be seen in NCDLB, FTNCD, and some cases of AD. The onset of parkinsonian symptoms relative to cognitive symptoms helps inform the etiology of the dementia diagnosis. Major NCD due to Parkinson's disease is characterized by the presence of parkinsonian motor symptoms preceding the onset of the cognitive symptoms by at least one year. However, the development of cognitive impairment prior to the onset of parkinsonian symptoms raises the possibility of other NCD diagnostic considerations, particularly NCDLB.

Neurocognitive Disorder Due to Huntington's Disease

Huntington's disease (HD) is caused by CAG trinucleotide expansion. Although motor symptoms are often the hallmark of HD, mood, psychotic, and cognitive symptoms are also common. Cognitive symptoms are mild at first but are often progressive. Advancing disease is characterized by progressive motor and cognitive symptoms leading to profound disabilities, ultimately resulting in death.

Neurocognitive Disorder Due to Another Medical Condition

Cognitive symptoms may accompany many systemic and brain diseases. The severity and functional consequences of these cognitive disturbances can range from mild to severe. The progression and outcomes of these NCDs are also variable depending on the etiology. Untreated neurosyphilis may lead to severe and progressive cognitive decline. Hypoxic brain injury, malignancies, epilepsy, and multiple sclerosis may result in varying severity of static or progressive cognitive impairment. Systemic inflammatory conditions (such as lupus), electrolyte abnormalities (e.g., hypercalcemia), and system-organ failures can also cause cognitive dysfunction. Normal pressure hydrocephalus (NPH) is a syndrome characterized by cognitive impairment, gait disturbance, and urinary incontinence. CT or MRI of the brain demonstrates an enlarged ventricular system out of proportion to cortical atrophy.

Medication/Drug-Induced Neurocognitive Disorders

Prescription medications, alcohol, and other drugs of abuse can cause profound cognitive dysfunction. The NCD due to alcohol can be mild and reversible with abstinence, but persisting deficits are well known to occur. Wernicke-Korsakoff syndrome, encountered in malnourished alcoholic patients, is one example. Wernicke's encephalopathy (delirium, gait abnormalities, and ophthalmoplegia) may be followed by Korsakoff's syndrome, characterized by persisting amnesia and confabulation.

Differential Diagnosis

The differential diagnosis of cognitive impairment is extensive and requires a systematic approach to elicit signs and symptoms. Physical examination and additional laboratory and neuroimaging studies help identify the etiology of cognitive impairment. Given that major NCD and delirium can have overlapping symptoms and that patients with preexisting cognitive impairment are at higher risk of developing delirium, it is important to rule out delirium before making the diagnosis of a dementia.

Cognitive symptoms occur in many psychiatric and neurologic disorders. Psychotic, mood, and anxiety disorders often include cognitive dimensions, but unlike NCD, they do not require the presence of cognitive symptoms for diagnosis. Intellectual development disorder should be differentiated from NCD. NCD represents a decline from a previously attained cognitive and functional level, while patients with intellectual development disorder do not reach the age-appropriate cognitive and functional milestones. Some conditions such as Down's syndrome cause intellectual development disorder (mental retardation) and later result in deterioration in cognition from the patient's established baseline, in which case an additional diagnosis of major or mild NCD can be made. Schizophrenia can also be associated with cognitive impairment and a decline in functioning. Unlike NCD, schizophrenia has an earlier age of onset, different clinical features and course, and less severe cognitive impairment.

Differentiating cognitive impairment secondary to depression from primary NCD is clinically challenging. Individuals with mild or major NCD can develop depressive disorders. Therefore, to clarify this differential diagnostic conundrum, depression should be excluded as a cause of cognitive impairment, and individuals with established major or mild NCD should be monitored for the development of depression. Furthermore, studies have demonstrated that older individuals with cognitive impairment due to depression are at higher risk of subsequently developing a dementia syndrome, even after the depression remits. Cognitive impairment associated with depression also predicts poorer response to antidepressant treatment in late-life depression.

Evaluation

A comprehensive evaluation of cognitive impairment includes a careful history, physical examination, and laboratory assessment. Due to difficulties eliciting accurate and reliable history in patients with significant cognitive impairment, information from collateral sources such as a family member or health care providers is invaluable. See Table 11.4 for elements of the history and mental status examination of particular importance when evaluating patients with potential NCD. Further testing should be guided by the history and examination.

Table 11.4 History and mental status items in evaluating neurocognitive disorders

History
- The onset, progression, and timeline of cognitive symptoms
- Impact on daily functioning systematically evaluated
- Pre-morbid (baseline) level of functioning (educational, occupational, hobbies)
- Safety assessment (Can the patient drive; call for help; manage finances, medications, appointments, mobility, past or present suicidal and aggressive thoughts and acts?)
- Psychiatric symptoms (mood, anxiety, psychotic symptoms)
- Prenatal, birth, and developmental history
- Past medical, surgical history with a comprehensive review of systems
- Medication history (prescription, over-the-counter, and herbals)
- Seizure symptoms
- History of head trauma, drug and alcohol use
- Family medical history
- Personal and social history

Mental status examination
- Physical malformations, asymmetric body features, and dysmorphic features
- Speed and quantity of motor movements
- Affective facial expressions and gestures
- Rate, rhythm, tone, inflictions of voice should be carefully documented
- Abnormal movements (tremors, tics, myoclonus, and choreiform movements)
- Thought form, process, and content
- Insight and judgment
- Cognitive function: brief evaluation of orientation memory, spatial function, executive function, ideally using a scored test such as the Montreal Cognitive Assessment (MoCA)

Evaluation of Delirium

It is important to keep in mind that delirium is a medical and psychiatric emergency, requiring urgent evaluation and intervention. The diagnosis of delirium is based on history, mental status, and cognitive examination. However, physical examination can reveal clues as to the cause of delirium. Here are some examples:

- Hypotension can imply cardiovascular, medication/toxic, or infectious etiologies.
- Fever can point to infectious causes.
- Lung, cardiac, or abdominal examinations may reveal evidence of pneumonia, congestive heart failure, or acute abdomen, respectively.
- Neck stiffness and meningeal signs point to meningeal irritation either due to infection or subarachnoid bleeding.
- Focal neurologic signs suggest stroke or injury to the relevant nervous system structures.
- Asterixis and myoclonus may indicate toxic/metabolic causes such as renal or hepatic failure.

Bedside observation of mental status and cognitive function is important in patients with suspected delirium. Since delirium causes impairment in arousal and attention, reliable assessment of more complex elements of the cognitive exam, such as memory and executive function, will be challenging. Due to symptom fluctuation in delirium, it is important to obtain additional information from family members or health care providers and serial bedside examinations rather than entirely excluding the diagnosis of delirium on a single evaluation.

Due to the multi-factorial etiology of delirium, diagnostic evaluation should be guided by history and physical examination. Initial laboratory testing for delirium should include (1) complete blood count, (2) comprehensive metabolic panel, (3) urinalysis and culture, (4) serum and urine drug screen, and (5) EKG and chest x-ray, when clinically indicated. Serum levels of certain medications with a defined therapeutic index should be assessed (e.g., lithium, digoxin, carbamazepine).

Head imaging (CT or MRI) is not necessary in all patients with delirium, unless warranted by clinical findings. However, it is reasonable to obtain at least a CT-scan of the head to rule out an intracranial bleed or mass, if the etiology of delirium is still unclear after the initial workup. MRI of the brain may also be considered in selected patients, such as those with abnormal neurologic examinations or to better characterize CT scan findings. Typical EEG findings associated with delirium include non-specific diffuse slowing of background rhythm. An EEG is indicated if seizures are suspected as the cause of the mental status changes. More invasive testing, such as lumbar puncture, may be pursued to rule out an infectious or inflammatory condition of the central nervous system. Additional laboratory and imaging tests may be undertaken based on clinical suspicions.

Evaluation of Patients with Major or Mild NCD

The objective of the diagnostic workup in major or mild NCD is to determine the etiology of the NCD. Initial laboratory testing for major or mild NCD should include complete blood count, comprehensive metabolic panel, urinalysis and culture, urine and serum drug screen, TSH, vitamin B12 level, and CRP or ESR. HIV and syphilis serology should also be done if indicated. The American Academy of Neurology recommends at least one neuroimaging study as part of the dementia evaluation. MRI has better spatial resolution and is more sensitive to detect white matter disease compared to CT scan. Brain CT or MRI may give clues to the cause of dementia, and help rule out treatable causes of cognitive impairment, including NPH (normal pressure hydrocephalus). Mesial temporal lobe atrophy can be seen in AD, while focal frontal and/or temporal atrophy suggests FTNCD on head CT/MRI.

Lumbar puncture is not a routine procedure in the evaluation of NCD, but it can help in ruling out infectious, inflammatory, and malignant causes of NCD. In patients with Alzheimer's disease, CSF levels of β-amyloid (1–42) are lower compared to cognitively healthy individuals while phosphorylated tau and total tau levels are higher. Brain fluorodeoxyglucose positron emission tomography (FDG PET) scan can aid in the differential diagnosis of atypical cases of NCD. In early AD, FDG PET scan of the brain will show hypometabolism of temporal and parietal lobes, while hypometabolism of temporal and/or frontal regions of the brain suggest FTNCD. Brain PET scans utilizing amyloid tracers are used in research settings to quantify brain amyloid deposition in clinical trials and may ultimately have more widespread clinical utility.

Treatment

Treatment of Delirium

The key steps in the management of delirium are to address all precipitating causes, provide supportive care, and consider both non-pharmacologic and pharmacologic strategies to treat behavioral and psychotic symptoms.

A thorough evaluation of potential precipitants of delirium begins with a careful review of medications, looking particularly for those with psychoactive properties (opiates, corticosteroids, benzodiazepines) or anticholinergic side effects. Careful examination for common medical precipitants, including infection, pain, constipation, and urinary retention, should also be part of this initial review. Supportive care, which minimizes the risk of complications from delirium, includes protecting the patient's airway, maintaining hydration and nutrition, and positioning and mobilizing the patient to prevent pressure sores and deep venous thrombosis.

Non-pharmacologic approaches to managing the behavioral symptoms of delirium include efforts to optimize the environment by providing cues to orientation, minimizing disruptions, and facilitating a regular sleep schedule. In a hospital setting, patients are subjected to many unfamiliar sounds, staff shift changes, room changes, and interruptions for vital sign checks and medication administration that can cause significant confusion for elderly patients. The use of calendars, clocks, and familiar objects from home helps to orient patients to their surroundings. Familiar staff and family members who provide reassurance will further re-orient patients. Fostering an uninterrupted period for sleep at night by decreasing ambient noise and lighting is also important to avoid behavioral complications of delirium. Normal sleep-wake cycles can be encouraged by opening blinds and encouraging wakefulness and mobility during the day. For many patients, the impact of environmental modifications and staff training can be as effective as psychoactive medications in reducing behavioral symptoms of delirium.

When hallucinations, delusions, and agitation are severe, pharmacological management of delirium may become necessary. Antipsychotic agents have long been used in the treatment of delirium. For most patients, low dose haloperidol is a reasonable choice, starting at 0.5 mg to 1 mg up to twice daily as a standing dose. Its onset of action is 10 to 30 minutes, and it can be administered again within an hour. The effectiveness and safety of low-dose haloperidol (less than 3.0 mg per day) are comparable to atypical antipsychotics, such as risperidone (at 0.5 mg–2.0 mg per day) and olanzapine (at 2.5 mg–10 mg per day). Because antipsychotic medications can interfere with cardiovascular function by causing orthostasis and prolonging the QTc interval, predisposing patients to dizziness, syncope, and even sudden death, obtaining a baseline EKG and continuing periodic monitoring during treatment is recommended.

For patients with relative contraindications to antipsychotics, such as those with Parkinson's disease, Lewy body dementia, or neuroleptic malignant syndrome, behavioral agitation due to delirium may be better managed with benzodiazepines. Benzodiazepines are also indicated in treating delirium due to alcohol or chronic sedative withdrawal. However, benzodiazepines may precipitate behavioral disinhibition and paradoxical agitation, exacerbating or prolonging the course of delirium. In older patients, benzodiazepines can cause excess sedation and respiratory depression.

Treatment of Major or Mild NCD

The goals of treatment for dementia include slowing cognitive decline, improving daily functioning (getting dressed, shopping, cooking, handling money), reducing behavioral complications, and enhancing or maintaining quality of life. Because there are no curative treatments in most cases, one of the key aspects of treating dementia is to set realistic expectations for therapeutic outcomes. The main benefit of pharmacotherapy is an attenuation of cognitive decline over time. This is important to discuss with patients and their families, who may expect improvement rather than relative stability.

Cognitive Symptoms

Acetylcholinesterase inhibitors (ACHEIs) represent the first-line treatment for the mild to moderate cognitive decline of Alzheimer's dementia. This class of medications currently includes donepezil (Aricept), galantamine (Razadyne), and rivastigmine (Exelon). There is no evidence to suggest any difference in efficacy among these medications. ACHEIs are titrated slowly in order to minimize gastrointestinal side effects, including nausea, vomiting, and diarrhea. These medications also increase the risk of bradycardia or heart block. Therefore, heart rate should be carefully monitored, especially for individuals with preexisting cardiac disease or concurrently treatment with medications that slow heart rate (e.g., beta-blockers).

Memantine (Namenda) is an NMDA-receptor antagonist that decreases glutamate-induced excitotoxicity in the brain. Among patients with moderate to severe AD, combination treatment with ACHEI and memantine more effectively slows cognitive decline than ACHEI monotherapy. There is also some evidence that combination therapy may prevent the emergence of behavioral symptoms, including agitation and aggression.

Current pharmacotherapies target the symptoms of dementia rather than the underlying neuropathological changes. The effects of these interventions are modest and vary among individuals. During the initial 6 to 12 months of treatment, patients' performance on measures of cognition, activities of daily living, behavioral symptoms, and overall clinical impression may significantly improve in a minority (10–20 percent), plateau in nearly half, or continue to deteriorate in a third.

Prevention strategies may minimize the risk of cognitive decline or dementia. Growing evidence suggests that cognitive functioning is closely linked to cerebrovascular health. Adequate management of vascular risk factors such as hypertension, hyperlipidemia, diabetes, obesity, and smoking may help minimize the risk of cerebrovascular lesions and postpone the clinical manifestation of dementia. Regular physical activity and exercise can reduce the risk of cognitive decline. Both aerobic exercise and strength training have been shown to have benefits in this regard. The Mediterranean diet has also been associated with a lower risk of Alzheimer's dementia. Although individuals with advanced education or higher "cognitive reserve" have been found to experience slower cognitive decline as they age, it is not clear that adding intellectual stimulation in the form of puzzles and games leads to generalized gains in cognitive functioning.

Behavioral and Psychological Symptoms

Behavioral agitation, mood, and psychotic symptoms are common in all types of dementia. Common triggers of agitation and aggression in patients with dementia include confusion or noisy environments, pain, constipation or fecal impaction, medical illness, boredom, loneliness, depression, arguments with caregivers, or exacerbation of co-morbid illness. Identifying the underlying precipitant allows for the treatment of any contributing medical problem and modification of the environment, and can minimize the need for psychiatric medications. Non-pharmacologic interventions can be as simple as redirecting and refocusing the patient, increasing social interaction, initiating enjoyable activities, and eliminating sources of conflict. Establishing routines and providing comforting stimulation, such as the patient's favorite music or films, are often beneficial in decreasing behavioral agitation. Caregivers can be taught strategies to modify their style of interaction, minimizing the caregiver's own level of frustration and distress.

When neuropsychiatric symptoms persist in a severe and disruptive manner, disrupting functioning and interfering with the provision of care, or raising the possibility of self-injury or harm to others, the use of psychiatric medications may be considered. Such medications are most effective for specific psychiatric syndromes, including psychosis or depression, although no medications have ever been FDA approved to treat the behavioral and psychiatric symptoms of dementia.

Atypical Antipsychotics
Atypical antipsychotics are the most commonly prescribed medications for the treatment of dementia-associated neuropsychiatric syndromes, and confer modest improvements in aggression and psychosis. Atypical antipsychotics (risperidone, olanzapine, quetiapine, and aripiprazole) are preferred over typical agents like haloperidol, which have a less-favorable side-effect profile, including a higher risk of extrapyramidal syndromes and tardive dyskinesia. Common atypical antipsychotic medication dose ranges in dementia are 0.25–2 mg daily of risperidone, 2.5–10 mg daily of olanzapine, 12.5–200 mg daily of quetiapine, and 2–10 mg daily of aripiprazole. In clinical practice, patients are often maintained on antipsychotics for long periods of time, so it is important to re-evaluate these medications regularly to reduce or even discontinue an antipsychotic. In addition to their side effect profile in adults, both typical and atypical antipsychotics have been shown to be associated with increased risk of cerebrovascular accidents and mortality, the latter leading the FDA to impose a black box warning on all antipsychotics for the treatment of dementia-related psychosis.

Pharmacotherapy for Behavioral Symptoms of Dementia, Beyond Antipsychotics
Despite the significant safety concerns of antipsychotics, limited evidence exists to recommend alternative psychotropic medications. Several small trials suggest that anti-epileptics like carbamazepine are effective for neuropsychiatric symptoms in dementia, whereas valproate, which is still widely used, has no clear benefit in randomized studies. Future investigation of gabapentin and lamotrigine, which have more favorable side effect profiles, is needed. Cholinesterase inhibitors may contribute to improvements in apathy, dysphoria, and anxiety, but there is no evidence to suggest a benefit for agitation or aggression. Retrospective analyses of memantine, on the other hand, suggest some benefit in mild to moderate irritability,

lability, agitation, and aggression in patients with Alzheimer's disease, but randomized controlled trials data are lacking. Most evidence for antidepressants relates to SSRIs such as citalopram and sertraline, but studies are quite small. Tricyclic antidepressants are generally poorly tolerated due to anticholinergic side effects, and trazodone has shown limited evidence in randomized trials. Benzodiazepines are best avoided among demented patients, given the risk of disinhibition, gait instability, falls, and delirium, although they may be useful at times for severe anxiety or infrequent agitation (see Table 11.5 for a detailed summary of non-psychotic medications that are used in the treatment of AD).

Table 11.5 Medications to treat Alzheimer's disease

Medication	Indication	Dosing	Comments
Donepezil (Aricept)	Mild, moderate, and severe dementia	Start 5 mg daily, increase to 10 mg daily after 1 month, consider 23 mg after 3 months	Selective, reversible non-competitive inhibitor of Acetylcholinesterase
			Once-daily dosing simplifies regimen, increases adherence
			Gradual dose titration minimizes risk of GI side effects (nausea, vomiting, diarrhea)
Rivastigmine (Exelon)	Mild to moderate dementia	Start 1.5 mg twice a day with meals, increase by 3 mg/day every 2–4 weeks up to 6 mg twice a day	Pseudo-irreversible inhibitor of Acetylcholinesterase and Butyrylcholinesterase
			FDA approved for dementia of Parkinson's disease
		Patch: increase monthly to 9.5 mg/d, then 13.3 mg/d	Available as a daily transdermal patch (4.6–13.3 mg)
			Side effects: nausea, vomiting, diarrhea, loss of appetite, weight loss, muscle weakness
Galantamine (Razadyne)	Mild to moderate dementia	Start 4 mg twice a day with meals, increase by 8 mg every month up to 12 mg twice a day	Reversible inhibitor of Acetylcholinesterase, presynaptic modulator of Nicotinic acetylcholinesterase
			Side effects: nausea, vomiting, diarrhea, loss of appetite, weight loss
Memantine (Namenda)	Moderate to severe dementia	Start 5 mg daily, increase by 5 mg per week as twice a day dosing, up to 10 mg twice a day	Noncompetitive NMDA antagonist, blocks toxic effects of excess glutamate and regulates glutamate activation
			New extended-release tablet starts at 7 mg daily, increase weekly by 7 mg up to 28 mg
			Side effects: dizziness, headache, constipation, confusion

Depression is common in AD, and often is undiagnosed and untreated. If behavioral problems appear to be more mood-oriented (e.g., the patient shows significant irritability or tearfulness), a trial of an antidepressant such as a selective serotonin reuptake inhibitor may be clinically effective. Although generally well-tolerated and used in clinical practice, recent treatment studies of sertraline and mirtazapine for depression in dementia have not demonstrated significant antidepressant efficacy. For patients with severe depression in the setting of dementia, electroconvulsive therapy may be effective and well tolerated.

Etiological Considerations

Delirium

The etiology of delirium is likely complex and multifactorial. Known risk factors for delirium include very young or advanced age, preexisting dementia, and medical co-morbidities, in particular acute precipitants, such as infections or medications (Table 11.6). The more risk factors that are present, the more likely delirium is to occur. Moreover, an individual with multiple predisposing factors may develop delirium in the context of few precipitants. For example, a frail, medically ill older

---

Table 11.6 Delirium: Risk factors

Predisposing factors
Age >65
Dementia
Sensory impairment
Chronic physical illness
Dehydration, malnutrition
Multiple medications
Substance use
Depression
Neurological impairment

Precipitating factors (pneumonic: AEIOU TRIPS)
A→ Alcohol or other drug (benzodiazepines, opiates) intoxication or withdrawal
E→ Electrolyte imbalance (hyponatremia, hypoglycemia) and environmental changes
I→ Iatrogenic (anticholinergics, steroids, antibiotics)
O→ Oxygen (hypoxia)
U→ Uremia/hepatic encephalopathy
T→ Trauma (head injury, subdural hematoma, surgery)
R→ Restraints
I→ Infection (urinary tract, pneumonia, meningitis, sepsis)
P→ Pain
S→ Seizures and stroke

adult may develop delirium in the setting of an uncomplicated urinary tract infection, a stressor far less severe than what would precipitate delirium in a younger, healthier person.

Dementia is one of the strongest predisposing factors for delirium; more than two-thirds of delirium cases occur in patients with cognitive impairment. Delirium and dementia are both associated with cholinergic deficiency, decreased cerebral metabolism, and inflammation, reflecting overlapping clinical, metabolic, and cellular mechanisms. Notably, patients without dementia who develop delirium are at increased risk of incident dementia over the next several years. For many patients, it remains unclear whether delirium exposes previously unrecognized cognitive impairment or whether the delirium itself initiates a neurobiological cascade of events that leads to dementia. Regardless, even cognitively intact patients who develop delirium need to be monitored closely for dementia, even if the acute symptoms of delirium resolve entirely.

Medications commonly precipitate delirium, especially those with anticholinergic effects. Medications with strong anticholinergic effects include antihistamines, antipsychotics, tricyclic antidepressants, digoxin, furosemide, isosorbide dinitrate, warfarin, dipyridamole, codeine, and captopril. Opiates frequently cause delirium. However, finding a balance in terms of adequate pain management is essential, because high levels of postoperative pain have also been associated with delirium.

Although the precise pathophysiology of delirium is still poorly understood, cholinergic neurons are known to play a central role. In addition, other neurotransmitter systems, including dopamine, norepinephrine, and serotonin pathways, are also implicated. These monoamines are involved in regulating arousal and the sleep-wake cycle, modulating physiological responses to stimuli, and balancing cholinergic activity. Increases in dopamine may underlie agitation and delusions. The increased cerebral secretion of cytokines and the resulting inflammation in cases of trauma, infection, or surgery are also proposed as an explanatory model for delirium. Finally, clinical factors associated with greater oxidative stress (e.g., sepsis or pneumonia) occur more frequently among those diagnosed with delirium.

Major or Mild NCD

Pathology
The senile plaques and neurofibrillary tangles first identified by Alois Alzheimer in 1907 are considered the hallmark neuropathologic features of AD. Discovery of the beta-amyloid protein as the key component of the senile plaques led to the development of the "amyloid hypothesis," which emphasizes the deposition of beta-amyloid as the initial pathological trigger leading to intracellular tangles, neuronal cell death and ultimately dementia.

Small vessel disease, multiple infarcts, and cortical stroke are seen in many cases of VNCD, while NCDLBD is characterized by Lewy body formation and abnormal alpha-synuclein metabolism. It is important to note that mixed pathology (e.g., Alzheimer-type pathology with vascular pathology or Lewy body pathology) is not uncommon.

Genetics

The majority of AD cases are sporadic. In very rare cases, early-onset disease is seen in an autosomal dominant inheritance pattern in families with mutations in one of three genes: amyloid precursor protein and the presenilin 1 and presenilin 2 proteins. Individuals with a first-degree relative with Alzheimer's are two to four times more likely to develop the disease, and those who have more than one first-degree relative with AD are at even higher risk of developing the disease. The APOE4 allele is the only major genetic risk factor for both early- and late-onset AD. It is a susceptibility gene, being neither necessary nor sufficient for Alzheimer's development. With an increasing number of APOE4 alleles, the risk of dementia increases and the age of onset decreases. Patients with Down's syndrome begin to show neuropathological features of AD relatively early in life and are vulnerable to developing early dementia.

On the other hand, up to 40 percent of patients with FTNCD have a positive family history of illness, and approximately 10 percent show an autosomal dominant inheritance pattern. Familial FTNCD was first linked to chromosome 17. Familial cases of NCDLBD have been related to the alpha-synuclein gene on chromosome 4. Cerebral Autosomal Dominant Arteriopathy with Subcortical Infarcts and Leukoencephalopathy (CADASIL) syndrome, a cause of VNCD, is attributed to the Notch3 gene mutation.

Vascular disease

Growing evidence suggests that cognitive functioning is closely linked to cerebrovascular health. Vascular risk factors (smoking, obesity, high cholesterol, high blood pressure, diabetes, infarcts, and white matter lesions) are associated with an increased risk of dementia. Unlike genetic risk factors, many of these vascular disease risk factors are modifiable.

Other factors

The "cognitive reserve" model attempts to explain how advanced education may provide compensatory mechanisms to reduce the impact of degenerative pathological changes in the brain, and therefore delay the onset of dementia. Head injury has also been proposed as contributing to the development of dementia.

Future Directions

Increasing dementia prevalence rates and associated financial and psychosocial impact on families threaten to become the signature health care crisis of the baby boomer generation. Absent a cure or therapeutic interventions that delay the onset of Alzheimer's disease progression, the stability of our health care system is in jeopardy. The United States adopted its first National Alzheimer's Plan in 2011. The goal of this policy is to develop methods of prevention and/or a cure for AD by the year 2025. Federal funding for dementia research must increase substantially to meet this challenge and prevent potentially devastating economic, social, and personal consequences of maintaining the status quo.

Current efforts to redefine the approach to early recognition of dementia pathophysiology prior to the onset of clinically relevant or apparent symptoms represent the first step in a path to dementia prevention. Advancing technologies in neuroimaging and genetics have the potential to identify at-risk individuals most likely to benefit from disease-modifying interventions. Scientists collaborating with clinicians in the fields of neurology, geriatric medicine, and geriatric psychiatry will help further refine the association between biomarkers of AD, such as CSF amyloid-beta and tau protein, genetic markers, and neuroimaging evidence of amyloid plaque pathology identified with PET scans, and the development of clinical symptoms of cognitive impairment. Although the initial amyloid-targeted therapies have largely failed to slow disease progression, enrolled subjects were in the moderate stages of illness when treated. Study designs have now shifted to include pre-clinical AD or the MCI of AD subjects in clinical trials to improve the chances of demonstrating disease modification and prevention. The first proof of this concept will be the results of a clinical trial of a monoclonal antibody targeting amyloid plaque aggregation in a sample of young Columbians who have an autosomal dominant inherited mutation that predicts a 100 percent risk of AD development at an early age. Two other landmark prevention trials also began subject recruitment in 2014: the Dominantly Inherited Alzheimer's Network (DIAN) and the Anti-Amyloid Treatment in Asymptomatic Alzheimer's Disease (A4) studies.

Our success in utilizing prevention and disease-modifying treatments, however, depends on the early identification of individuals with underlying AD pathology. Currently, more than half of individuals with dementia are not diagnosed until reaching moderate stages of illness, at which time an individual frequently is unable to drive a car, manage finances, or safely self-administer and monitor medications. Specialists will need to work with primary care physicians to develop methods for accurate and reliable early detection using structured history gathering techniques, cognitive assessments, and neurobiological testing. In the meantime, dementia complications, such as behavioral disturbances and increased risk for delirium, will persist and drive premature institutionalization and mortality. We must develop a better understanding of the pathophysiology of psychiatric syndromes of dementia so that our treatments can be neurobiologically-targeted and effective while limiting the substantial toxicity of current treatments. Furthermore, non-pharmacological strategies to reduce agitated behaviors must be examined in well-controlled studies to improve the array of evidence-based interventions that may reduce the development of, or adverse impact from, the neuropsychiatric syndromes of dementia.

Sample Interview Questions

Assessment of cognitive impairment requires detective work involving patient and family member/informant interview, medical records review, and detailed cognitive assessment. The Montreal Cognitive Assessment (MOCA) is a sensitive tool to objectively assess cognitive impairment and differentiate normal aging, MCI, and dementia. Furthermore, this instrument includes measures of executive functioning absent in the more widely used Mini-Mental Status Examination. Examples of interview questions for patients and caregivers are as follows.

Interviews with the patient can occur alone or with a family member present. It is important for the clinician to ask the identified patient questions first while acknowledging to both that you will also seek input from the family member/informant and recognize that their perspectives may differ. Similar questions are also relevant for the informant.

- What is your understanding of why you are here today?
- Have you noticed any changes in your ability to remember new information including appointments, familiar names, or recent events?
- Are you concerned about changes in your memory or have others expressed their concern?
- How do you spend your typical day?
- Are there any recreational or work activities or hobbies that you have cut back on? If so, try to determine why.
- Do you feel that changes in your memory have impacted your ability to function day to day? If so, how? Are you noticing any changes in your driving skills, such as accidents, getting lost, or starting the engine and not remembering where you were supposed to be going?
- Are you able to manage your own finances, or has a family member or friend begun to help you pay bills or balance the checkbook?
- Have you noticed any recent changes in your mood, level of anxiety, or disturbances in your sleep, appetite, or energy?

Sample Cases

Mrs. Smith is a fifty-two-year-old divorced, Caucasian female with a history of hyperlipidemia. She presents with a two-year history of increasing forgetfulness, including misplacing personal objects around her home, forgetting appointments, and difficulty with recalling familiar names. She has gotten lost driving back home from her sister's home on one occasion. Her sister has noticed that she has been adding instead of subtracting in her checkbook after paying a bill. Since her divorce, she has been despondent, tearful, and has disrupted sleep, with a ten-pound weight loss in the past year. She has a twelfth-grade education, has been unable to hold down a job for the past two years, and has a paternal uncle who had AD in his late seventies. On the MOCA, she scores a 22/30, with deficits in visuospatial skills, executive functioning, and delayed recall, though she is fully oriented.

What further historical information, lab testing, or cognitive assessment will help elucidate the differential diagnosis? How would you differentiate depression, MCI, and dementia? If further neuropsychological testing indicates findings consistent with the MOCA but mentions that attentional impairment may be depression-related, would you first treat depression or begin cholinesterase inhibitor therapy or both? What further follow-up would be required?

References and Suggested Readings

- Alexopoulos, G. S., Meyers, B., Young, R. C. et al. (2000). Executive Dysfunction and Long-Term Outcomes of Geriatric Depression. *Arch Gen Psychiatry*, 57, 285–290.
- Alzheimer's Association (2020). *Alzheimer's Disease Facts and Figures*. New York: Alzheimer's Association.
- American Psychiatric Association (2013). *Diagnostic and Statistical Manual of Mental Disorders*, 5th edition. Arlington, VA: American Psychiatric Association.
- Banerjee, S., Hellier, J., Dewey, M., et al. (2011). Sertraline or Mirtazapine for Depression in Dementia (HTA-SADD): A Randomised, Multicentre, Double-Blind, Placebo-Controlled Trial. *Lancet*, 378, 403–411.
- Ballard, C., Creese, B., Corbett, A., and Aarsland, D. (2011). Atypical Antipsychotics for the Treatment of Behavioral and Psychological Symptoms in Dementia, with a Particular Focus on Longer Term Outcomes and Mortality. *Expert Opin Drug Saf*, 10, 35–43.
- Cummings, J., and Mega, M. (2003). *Neuropsychiatry and Behavioral Neuroscience*. New York: Oxford University Press.
- Gitlin, L. N., Kales, H. C., and Lyketsos, C. G. (2012). Non-Pharmacologic Management of Behavioral Symptoms in Dementia. *JAMA*, 308 (19), 2020–2029.
- Inouye, S. K. (2006). Delirium in Older Persons. *NEJM*, 354 (11), 1157–1165.
- Jack, C. R., Jagust, W. J., Petersen, R. C., et al. (2013). Tracking Pathophysiological Processes in Alzheimer's Disease: An Updated Hypothetical Model of Dynamic Biomarkers. *Lancet Neurol*, 12, 207–216.

- Kales, H. C., Kim, H. M., Zivin, K., et al. (2012). Risk of Mortality among Individual Antipsychotics in Patients with Dementia. *Am J Psychiatry*, 169, 71–79.
- Kavirajan, H., and Schneider, L. S. (2007). Efficacy and Adverse Effects of Cholinesterase Inhibitors and Memantine in Vascular Dementia: A Meta-Analysis of Randomised Controlled Trials. *Lancet Neurol*, 6 (9), 782–792.
- Lacasse, H., Perreault, M. M., and Williamson, D. R. (2006). Systematic Review of Antipsychotics for the Treatment of Hospital-Associated Delirium in Medically or Surgically Ill Patients. *Ann Pharmacother*, 40 (11), 1966–1973.
- Petersen, R. C. (2011). Mild Cognitive Impairment. *NEJM*, 364, 2227–2234.
- Rolinski, M., Fox, C., Maidment, I., and McShane, R. (2012). Cholinesterase Inhibitors for Dementia with Lewy Bodies, Parkinson's Disease Dementia and Cognitive Impairment in Parkinson's Disease. *Cochrane Database Syst Rev*, 3, CD006504.
- Schulz, R., and Beach, S. (1999). Caregiving as a Risk Factor for Mortality: The Caregiver Health Effects Study. *JAMA*, 282, 2215–2219.
- Seitz, D. P., Adunuri, N., Gill, S. S., et al. (2011). Antidepressants for Agitation and Psychosis in Dementia. *Cochrane Database Syst Rev*, CD008191.
- Tariot, P. N., Farlow, M. R., Grossberg, G. T., et al. (2004). Memantine Treatment in Patients with Moderate to Severe Alzheimer Disease Already Receiving Donepezil: A Randomized Controlled Trial. *JAMA* 291 (3), 317–324.
- Vigen, C. L., Mack, W. J., Keefe, R. S., et al. (2011). Cognitive Effects of Atypical Antipsychotic Medications in Patients with Alzheimer's Disease: Outcomes from CATIE-AD. *Am J Psychiatry*, 168, 831–839.
- Witlox, J., Eurelings, L. S., de Jonghe, J. F., et al. (2010). Delirium in Elderly Patients and the Risk of Postdischarge Mortality, Institutionalization, and Dementia: A Meta-analysis. *JAMA* 304, 443–451.
- Yaffe, K., Blackwell, T., Gore, R., et al. (1999). Depressive Symptoms and Cognitive Decline in Nondemented Elderly Women: A Prospective Study. *Arch Gen Psychiatry*, 56 (5), 425–430.
- Yudovsky, S., and Hales, R. (eds.) (2007). *The American Psychiatric Publishing Textbook of Neuropsychiatry and Behavioral Neurosciences*, 5th edition. Arlington, VA: American Psychiatric Publishing.

Self-Assessment Questions

1. Which of the following findings are not a criterion for the diagnosis of mild cognitive disorder?
    A. The deficits do not interfere with independence in everyday activities.
    B. The severity of cognitive impairment exceeds what would be expected from normal aging.
    C. Quantified neuropsychological testing does not reveal a decline in cognitive function.
    D. Cognitive deficits do not occur exclusively in the context of delirium.

    E. Decline from previous level of performance on complex attention, executive function, learning and memory, and language are present.

2.   M. G. is a forty-five-year-old male who comes to his internist at the urging of his wife because of problems with memory and concentration. The patient works as an electrician. He has noted that he has begun to misplace tools and confuse his daily schedule of appointments. He describes occasional "tics and shaking," which have at times made it difficult to complete his work projects. His sleep and appetite are normal and his mood is good, though he worries about the symptoms he is experiencing. He has no history of psychiatric disorders or medical problems. His family history includes a neurological disorder that his father, who died when the patient was a young teenager, developed when he was fifty years old. What is the most likely cause of the patient's neurocognitive presentation?

    A. Alzheimer's disease

    B. Major depressive disorder

    C. Huntington's disorder

    D. Mild cognitive impairment

    E. Lewy body dementia

3.   Which of the following is false regarding the symptoms of Alzheimer's disease (AD)?

    A. Symptoms usually begin after age 50.

    B. Memory for recent events is an early manifestation of the illness.

    C. The patient typically does not recognize cognitive impairments.

    D. In the later stages of AD, seizures may develop.

    E. Behavioral and psychological disturbances are a prominent problem and include mood and anxiety symptoms, as well as psychosis.

4.   Which of the medications listed below have shown efficacy in the treatment of symptoms of dementia?

    A. NMDA-receptor agonists such as memantine

    B. Atypical antipsychotics such as risperidone and olanzapine

    C. Acetylcholinesterase inhibitors, including donepezil and galantamine

    D. Benzodiazepines

    E. Antiepileptics such as carbamazepine

5.   Which of the following medications are contraindicated in the management of delirium in the elderly patient?

    A. Haloperidol

    B. Benzodiazepines such as clonazepam

    C. Olanzapine

    D. Risperidone

Answers to Self-Assessment Questions

1. (C)
2. (C)
3. (C)
4. (D)
5. (B)

12 | Feeding and Eating Disorders

ANNE E. BECKER, KAMRYN T. EDDY, DAVID C. JIMERSON,
AND JENNIFER J. THOMAS

The Spectrum of Eating Disorders

Classification

DSM-5 describes three eating disorders (anorexia nervosa, bulimia nervosa, and binge-eating disorder), three feeding disorders (avoidant/restrictive food intake disorder, pica, and rumination disorder), and two residual feeding and eating disorder categories (APA, 2013). Although these disorders contain some overlapping features, an individual can receive just one feeding or eating disorder diagnosis at a time. The only exception is pica, which can be diagnosed concurrently with another feeding or eating disorder if the pica behavior is severe enough to warrant additional clinical attention.

Eating Disorders

The hallmark feature of anorexia nervosa (AN) is a significantly low body weight, accompanied by an intense fear of weight gain, and body image disturbance (for example, feeling "fat" while very thin, or an inability to recognize the self-relevance of health consequences associated with low weight). Although clinical judgment is necessary to determine whether low body weight reaches clinical significance, it would conventionally fall below the 18.5 kg/m^2 lower limit of normal weight range for adults and below the fifth percentile for sex, height, and age for children. Individuals with AN may maintain their low weight by eating very little (AN restricting type) or by attempting to compensate for any episodes of actual or perceived overeating by engaging in purging behaviors such as self-induced vomiting or misuse of laxatives, diuretics, or other medications (AN binge-eating/purging type; APA, 2013).

In contrast, individuals with bulimia nervosa (BN) are typically normal-weight or overweight. BN is characterized by recurrent binge eating (i.e., consuming large amounts of food while feeling out of control) and inappropriate behaviors intended to compensate for the potential impact of these binge episodes on one's body weight. Such compensatory behaviors can take the form of self-induced vomiting; misuse of laxatives, diuretics, or other medications; fasting; or excessive exercise. Binge eating and compensatory behaviors must occur, on average, at least once per week for at least three months before a diagnosis of BN can be conferred. Individuals with BN also base their self-worth primarily or even exclusively on their current body shape or weight, resulting in fluctuating or poor self-esteem (APA, 2013).

Binge-eating disorder (BED) is also characterized by recurrent binge eating, but in the absence of the compensatory behaviors that are the *sine qua non* of BN. The majority of individuals with BED are overweight or obese. Although many individuals with BED also overvalue their shape and weight, this is not a diagnostic criterion. Instead, the ascertainment of BED focuses on distinguishing binge eating from episodes of ordinary overeating. Specifically, to meet diagnostic criteria for BED, binge episodes must be characterized by three or more of the following key features: rapid eating, eating beyond satiety to the point of discomfort, eating alone due to guilt or shame, eating in the absence of hunger, and/or feeling dysphoria or self-reproach because of the overeating. Binge eating must be associated with significant distress, and occur, on average, at least once per week for at least three months, before a BED diagnosis can be made (APA, 2013).

Feeding Disorders

DSM-5 avoidant/restrictive food intake disorder (ARFID) is a revision of the *DSM-IV* category of feeding or eating disorder of infancy or early childhood, which has been expanded to account for similar presentations in adolescents and adults. Individuals with ARFID are unable to meet their nutritional needs as evidenced by low weight, nutritional deficiency, reliance on enteral feeding/ nutritional supplements, and/or psychosocial impairment. In contrast to the body weight concerns observed in AN and BN, body shape or weight concerns are not present in ARFID. Instead, persons with ARFID typically exhibit a lack of interest in feeding, avoidance of food due to sensory features (e.g., texture, temperature), or a fear of a traumatic eating-related experience (e.g., choking, involuntary vomiting). To meet diagnostic criteria, food avoidance cannot be associated with a normative cultural practice (APA, 2013).

Individuals with pica engage in the persistent consumption of nonnutritive, non-food substances, such as paper, cloth, or dirt. A minimum duration of one month is required before the diagnosis can be made. Commonly ingested non-nutritive substances (e.g., low- or no-calorie foods) do not meet the non-food requirement. To qualify for a diagnosis of pica, the behavior cannot be part of normative development or a locally accepted cultural practice. DSM-5 therefore suggests a minimum age of two, as non-aberrant mouthing behaviors are common during infancy and toddlerhood (APA, 2013).

Rumination disorder is characterized by the persistent and effortless regurgitation of food over a period of at least one month. After regurgitating, individuals with rumination disorder typically re-chew, re-swallow, or spit out the previously ingested food. Although the regurgitation may be at least partially voluntary, it is distinct from the self-induced vomiting characteristic of BN, because the latter is intended to compensate for calories ingested during a binge-eating episode. It can also be distinguished (by physical examination or testing) from esophageal reflux and other gastrointestinal conditions (APA, 2013).

Other Feeding and Eating Problems

Some feeding or eating disturbances are associated with clinically significant distress and/or impairment but do not meet criteria for one of the specific diagnoses described above. This residual category was previously termed eating disorder, not otherwise specified (EDNOS) until the nomenclature changed in DSM-5. A new term, other specified feeding or eating disorder (OSFED), now captures these residual cases, and includes five example presentations. Atypical anorexia nervosa describes anorexic features at normal or above-normal weight. Bulimia nervosa (of low frequency and/or limited duration) and binge-eating disorder (of low frequency and/or limited duration) are appropriate diagnoses when individuals have engaged in relevant behaviors less frequently than once per week or for fewer than three months. Purging disorder describes a symptom profile that includes self-induced vomiting and/or misuse of laxatives, diuretics, or medications at least once per week for three months, in the absence of frank binge episodes. Night eating syndrome comprises either recurrent evening or nocturnal eating (e.g., a large amount of food consumed after dinner or eating after awaking from sleep) that results in distress or impairment. Lastly, if insufficient information is available to confer a definitive feeding or eating disorder diagnosis (e.g., in an emergency room setting) and/or the reasons that a clinical presentation does not meet diagnostic criteria for a feeding or eating disorder remain unspecified, a diagnosis of unspecified feeding or eating disorder (UFED) may be applied.

Epidemiology and Impact

Although eating disorders do affect boys and men, available data indicate that these disorders are significantly more common in girls and women. In a recent epidemiological study of women in the United Kingdom, 15.3 percent had experienced a DSM-5 eating disorder by the fourth or fifth decade of life, with the most common presentation being other specified feeding or eating disorder (Micali et al., 2017). Aggregated data from the United States and Western Europe indicate that, among young females, AN has a 12-month prevalence of 0.4 percent, while BN is two to three times more common, with a 12-month prevalence of 1.0–1.5 percent (APA, 2013). The sex ratio of BED is more balanced; with BED affecting 1.6 percent of females and 0.8 percent of males in a 12-month timeframe (APA, 2013). ARFID may be equally common in both females and males, but less is known about its prevalence in the general population. The prevalence of pica and rumination disorder is similarly unknown, but both disorders are thought to be more common among individuals with intellectual disabilities. Eating disorders also have global distribution, and although prevalence is highest across North America, Europe, Australia, and New Zealand, evidence supports that prevalence has been increasing more rapidly in regions in the Global South over the past decade (IHME, 2018).

Course, Mortality, Recovery

Course and Outcome

The long-term course and outcome of eating disorders is variable. Many individuals with an eating disorder will achieve full remission or substantial improvement, while others will have an illness course marked by chronicity, fluctuation in symptoms with periods of improvement punctuated by relapse, or even fatality. Although the course and outcome of eating disorders have been the focus of many longitudinal and treatment studies, interpretation of the literature is challenged by methodological variability across investigations and inconsistent operationalization of outcome. Taken together, extant work suggests the longitudinal course may be influenced by factors including age at onset, diagnosis, symptom presentation, treatment participation, and comorbidity, among others.

Recovery and Relapse

Anorexia nervosa. Anorexia nervosa (AN) typically onsets during adolescence or early adulthood. Considerable longitudinal research has described the long-term course and outcome of anorexia nervosa. Comprehensive reviews of outcome studies have suggested that half of surviving patients achieve full recovery, one third improve but continue to experience symptoms, and approximately 20 percent persist in chronic illness (Steinhausen, 2009). However, a more recent study showed more promising outcomes, with 62.8 percent of women with anorexia nervosa classified as recovered after an average of 22 years of study follow-up (Eddy et al., 2017). Younger age at illness onset was associated with improved outcomes, and indeed, research suggests that rates of recovery are generally higher among adolescents than adults. Taken together, data suggest that the majority of adolescents will achieve full recovery, depending on the definition of outcome used, with weight remission preceding the resolution of cognitive symptoms.

In addition to younger age, a shorter duration of illness and a milder illness (e.g., higher body weight, less entrenched cognitive symptoms) have been associated with improved outcomes. Lower body weight and the presence of bulimic symptoms may mark a more severe course. Whereas the subject of relapse has received less research attention, studies of clinical samples suggest that approximately one-third of patients treated for anorexia nervosa who recover will relapse.

Notably, understanding the course and outcome of AN comes primarily from studies of treatment-seeking individuals, which may reflect a selection bias. The findings from the National Comorbidity Survey Replication (NCS-R) suggested that spontaneous recovery from AN in non-treatment seeking individuals may occur often, although an understanding of factors contributing to this outcome is incomplete (Hudson et al., 2007).

Bulimia nervosa. Bulimia nervosa onsets in late adolescence or early adulthood. The longitudinal course of bulimia nervosa is also variable, most often marked by recovery or substantial improvement, but for some patients, it is characterized by chronicity or relapse. Reviews indicate 50–75 percent will achieve full recovery and that 20–25 percent will have a chronic protracted illness course (Steinhausen, 2009). For example, in a recent study, 68.2 percent of individuals with bulimia nervosa were classified as recovered after an average of 22 years of study follow-up (Eddy et al., 2017). As in the studies of anorexia nervosa, reconciliation of the findings in bulimia nervosa was challenged by variable definitions of recovery. Longer duration of illness, history of treatment refractoriness, comorbid impulsive-spectrum problems (e.g., substance abuse, borderline personality disorder) may be associated with poorer outcome. Approximately one-third of those who recover will relapse. Persistent cognitive eating disorder symptoms, including body image disturbance or overvaluation of weight and shape, may increase the likelihood of behavioral relapse.

Binge-eating disorder. Less research exists describing the longitudinal course and outcome of binge-eating disorder (BED). Community-based research suggests that the diagnosis is unstable over time, with some data indicating that over six months nearly half of those with BED no longer met full criteria for the disorder. Prognosis is generally positive, with other findings suggesting that fewer than one-fifth of those with BED still having clinically significant eating disorder symptoms by five years of follow-up. However, rates of concomitant obesity increase in these samples over time, which may be an important health outcome to assess in addition to the eating disorder. Relapse appears to be less likely for those with BED compared to those with anorexia nervosa or bulimia nervosa.

Mortality

Eating disorders are associated with an increased risk of premature death. In spite of diagnostic and treatment advances, the prognosis for adult anorexia nervosa does not seem to have improved during the twentieth century. Recent meta-analytic findings indicate standardized mortality ratios (SMRs) of 5.9 overall among patients with anorexia nervosa (Arcelus et al., 2011), and of 31.0 for death by suicide specifically (Preti et al., 2011). Factors noted to predict death in anorexia nervosa include lower body weight, longer duration of illness, comorbid substance use disorders, poorer social functioning, and history of suicidality. Death is often ascribed to medical complications of the illness, including cardiac failure, as well as suicide. SMRs among those with bulimia nervosa are estimated to be lower than those in anorexia nervosa at 1.9 overall (Arcelus et al., 2011) and 7.5 for suicide (Preti et al., 2011). Whereas mortality among other types of eating disorders has received less research attention, some data suggest SMR for those with low weight EDNOS may be comparable to that observed in anorexia nervosa. However, those with low weight EDNOS may constitute a heterogeneous group as other research (e.g., focused on non-fat phobic AN) has suggested prognosis may be more favorable (Becker, Thomas, & Pike, 2009). Across diagnoses, the prognosis is better for child and adolescent patients (Rome et al., 2003).

Diagnostic Crossover

The course of eating disorders is characterized by symptom fluctuation and, frequently, diagnostic crossover. Crossover between the anorexia nervosa subtypes, and from anorexia nervosa to bulimia nervosa, appears to be the most common. Approximately 50 percent of those with anorexia nervosa will develop regular binge eating and/or purging behaviors, crossing between the subtypes (e.g., from restricting type to binge/purge type) or to bulimia nervosa if the development of these symptoms is concomitant with weight gain. Research suggests that crossover from primary restriction to binge/purge symptoms most commonly occurs within the first three to five years of illness, although longitudinal data do suggest that crossover is frequent, bi-directional, and can occur even many years into illness (Eddy et al., 2008).

Crossover from bulimia nervosa to anorexia nervosa is less common and generally limited to individuals who had a previous history of anorexia nervosa. Further, diagnostic migration from binge-eating disorder to bulimia nervosa or anorexia nervosa appears to be rare, but prospective research in this area is limited.

Given that symptom fluctuation is common, achievement of symptomatic improvement – even in the absence of full remission – is common across eating disorder diagnoses. This can give the impression of crossover from anorexia nervosa, bulimia nervosa, and binge-eating disorder, to the range of OSFED presentations (e.g., those that narrowly miss full criteria for AN or BN). However, these transitions most often resemble the initial eating disorder diagnosis and are associated with improvements in psychosocial functioning, suggesting that they may be better conceptualized as a transition to a partially recovered state, rather than to a new eating disorder diagnosis (Eddy et al., 2010).

Feeding Disorders

Less is known about the course and outcome of the feeding disorders including pica, rumination disorder, and ARFID. Pica can onset in early childhood and also can be observed in school-age children as well as adults. Rumination disorder often begins during the first year of life and can occur in the context of developmental delays; however, it can be diagnosed across the lifespan and does also occur in typically developing individuals. Spontaneous remission occurs for many, but for those with co-occurring intellectual disabilities, a more protracted course may be expected (APA, 2013). ARFID is a newly revised, heterogeneous diagnosis and thus the long-term course and outcome have not yet been reported on. While some of those youth with selective eating or failure to thrive may receive early intervention and achieve healthy growth and development over time, others will persist in feeding or eating problems. There is some suggestion that those with early feeding problems may be at increased risk for the development of eating disorders over time, but further research about the longitudinal relationship between early feeding and prospective eating disorders is needed.

Differential Diagnosis

Differential diagnosis of a clinical presentation falling within the broad category of feeding and eating disorders is rendered especially challenging for several reasons. First, there is potentially moderate phenomenologic overlap in presentation across the diagnostic categories, ARFID, anorexia nervosa, bulimia nervosa, and binge-eating disorders, as well as other specified feeding and eating disorders (OSFED) and unspecified feeding and eating disorders (UFED). As noted previously, some patients migrate from one diagnostic category to another during their longitudinal course, and definitions of remission, partial remission, and recovery are not well-established empirically. Second, medical illness needs to be considered as potentially driving some or all of the signs and symptoms such as appetite, weight, and gastrointestinal discomfort or dysfunction, and then also rigorously evaluated, excluded, and/or managed when appropriate. Next, observed, collateral, and longitudinal data are often indispensable to establishing an eating disorder diagnosis, depending on the patient's capacity for insight and willingness to share important diagnostic information during an initial clinical encounter. Limited insight especially characterizes child and adolescent patients who may not formulate their behaviors as motivated (e.g., by weight or shape concerns) or even as voluntary at all. Patients with an eating disorder are commonly reluctant to disclose symptoms to a clinician because of associated shame or stigma, or perceived secondary gains associated with the disorder. Finally, eating disorders are highly comorbid with other mental disorders – and particularly with mood and anxiety disorders – and symptoms and signs such as appetite and weight changes might be partially attributable to the comorbid disorder in some cases.

Although AN is characterized by low weight, intense fear of weight gain (and/or behaviors undermining appropriate weight gain), and body image disturbance, it overlaps phenomenologically with BN with respect to clinically significant concerns about weight and behaviors that prevent weight gain – or at least are intended to prevent it by compensating for calories consumed during a binge eating episode. Both patients with AN and BN can meet criteria for these respective disorders through dietary restriction, purging (vomiting), laxative use, and excessive physical activity, among other behaviors or a combination of these. For example, an estimated one half of individuals with AN engage in regular binge-eating and/or purging, and conversely, some individuals with BN engage in fasting and/or exercise to neutralize calories taken in during a binge, but do not induce vomiting or misuse laxatives. In this respect, a useful clinical sign distinguishing AN from BN is a significantly low weight. Likewise, because both AN and ARFID are characterized by low weight, the two can be difficult to distinguish clinically. Whereas the onset of ARFID, which can begin in infancy, tends to be younger than AN, which has its peak onset in adolescence, underweight adolescent patients who disavow an intense concern with fatness or weight gain may eventually meet diagnostic criteria for either disorder. A key distinguishing characteristic would be that a patient with AN may present as unable to recognize or accept the medical risks of the behavior, whereas a patient with ARFID will often be distressed by the behavior and may have more overt fears that underlie food avoidance. As noted previously, patients may not receive a concurrent diagnosis of more than one feeding or eating disorder, with the exception of pica. As a result, if criteria are met for both AN and BN, a diagnosis of AN is made. BN and binge-eating disorder are mutually exclusive; the latter is distinguished by the absence of routine compensatory behaviors to prevent weight gain after a binge.

Atypical depression with weight loss is generally distinguishable from AN by the actual loss of appetite; by contrast, individuals with AN typically override hunger in order to restrict their diet. In addition, whereas individuals with atypical depression commonly lose interest in food and eating, individuals with AN may show interest in preparing food for others and may experience eating or mealtimes as unpleasant or affectively charged. Body image disturbance and distress associated with AN and BN can be similar to the intense scrutiny and distress associated with an imagined defect in physical appearance as seen in body dysmorphic disorder. When the attention is focused on weight or shape and other associated criteria are met, a diagnosis of either AN or BN should be made. Although the body image disturbance associated with AN can result in distortions that can present in similar ways as do somatic delusions, they do not typically warrant a separate diagnosis of delusional disorder.

Food-related anxiety and/or aversions to particular tastes/textures/temperatures common to ARFID may also be present in certain specific phobias or in those with autism spectrum disorders. If the food avoidance behaviors are sufficiently significant to warrant independent treatment, an ARFID diagnosis is appropriate.

Differentiating an Eating Disorder from a Medical Disorder
Patients presenting with failure to gain weight or new-onset weight loss should be evaluated for medical causes or contributions to weight or appetite loss, hypermetabolic states, or failure to thrive, as well as for an eating disorder. Occult

malignancies, thyroid and other autoimmune disease, diabetes, infectious and parasitic diseases, and gastrointestinal disease should be considered in the differential diagnosis of weight loss. Anorexia nervosa not infrequently follows a medically precipitated weight loss, so the course and its relation to known medical illness may yield important clinical data that would lead a clinician to consider anorexia nervosa in the differential diagnosis. Weight and shape concerns are prevalent among adolescent and adult women, so clinicians should take care not to prematurely attribute profound weight changes solely to dietary restriction or exercise. Likewise, clinicians should not prematurely exclude eating pathology based on patient self-report alone, but rather should seek corroborating diagnostic data through judicious deployment of appropriate medical diagnostic testing, clinical records detailing past medical and psychiatric history as well as treatment, and should systematically aim to reconcile any incongruities among clinical history, patient report, physical exam, laboratory tests, and observed behavior. If nutritional rehabilitation is indicated, clinicians should assess whether the patient is able to progress with weight gain as expected (for example, outpatient treatments typically aim for a weight gain of 1–2 lbs/week), and if not, whether and how these longitudinal data are informative to the diagnosis. If a patient chooses either to conceal or not disclose weight concerns, dietary restriction, binge eating, purging, and other behaviors preventing weight gain, an eating disorder may be a diagnosis of exclusion after medical causes are evaluated and ruled out and the longitudinal course supports that the patient is undermining weight gain. Sometimes laboratory tests can be informative when they are suggestive of chronic vomiting or laxative abuse (e.g., if there is an unexplained hypokalemia or hyperamylasemia) but they are neither sensitive nor specific for an eating disorder. Bulimia nervosa commonly presents without any physical abnormalities on examination, so is an even more difficult diagnosis to establish if a patient does not disclose symptoms. That said, a dental exam revealing a wear pattern consistent with chronic exposure to vomitus and Russell's sign (excoriation on the back of the hand from trauma after chronic scraping against the incisors) are suggestive of BN, but do not offer a highly sensitive test for BN. Their prevalence is unknown; the former is not readily visible in the context of a mental health examination and the latter is relatively uncommon. Finally, patients with BED are frequently overweight or obese, but rarely have non-weight related medical complications related to binge eating per se.

Differentiating an Eating Disorder from Normative Behaviors

For some underweight and overweight patients, the diagnostic criteria related to cognitive or affective symptoms (e.g., intense fear of weight gain, marked distress following a binge eating episode) must be assessed against the local social context and associated norms governing diet, exercise, and weight management behavior. Some patients will present their behaviors as motivated by a desire to achieve a "healthy lifestyle" or become more competitive athletically (e.g., through implementing rigid dietary rules or a rigorous exercise regimen). Under such scenarios, clinicians need to discern whether the behaviors have resulted in clinically significant distress or impairment or carry medical risks or result in complications that the patient is unable to recognize or accept.

Evaluation

Evaluation of a known eating disorder will almost always comprise psychological/psychiatric, medical, and nutritional dimensions. Indeed, since signs can potentially first manifest as psychological, medical, or nutritional or, in some cases, can be absent or subtle, primary care clinicians, medical sub-specialists (including gastroenterologists and cardiologists), or general psychiatrists may be the first to detect an eating disorder. This chapter focuses on the psychiatric or psychological component of the evaluation and we emphasize that the psychiatrist or psychologist is often the clinician who coordinates team communications, referrals, and the management plan and thus should have an excellent grasp of the spectrum of clinical evaluation and care required.

The evaluation of a patient with an eating disorder will be very different for a patient who has – versus one who has not – acknowledged symptoms and accepts the importance of providing a candid history in order to evaluate their clinical significance. If an eating disorder is unconfirmed, but suspected because of the history, the initial evaluation will focus on ascertaining and piecing together relevant clinical and collateral data. These sources include history of present illness and presenting symptoms, past medical and psychiatric history, physical and mental status examination, and laboratory and/or findings from other diagnostic testing, as well as collateral sources of information from family members, teachers, and chart review with particular attention to unexplained changes in weight, diet, and possible physiologic sequelae of chronic purging (e.g., perimolysis, hypokalemia, hyperamylasemia or poor nutrition). For children and adolescents in particular, who may have limited insight into their motivations or behaviors due to cognitive maturity and therefore find it challenging to self-report on symptoms, collateral assessment of parents or other caretakers is critical.

An eating disorder will often first come to light in a primary or specialty medical care setting. That being said, the diagnosis is easily missed as well. Studies show that up to half of eating disorder cases are not recognized in primary care settings. Moreover, an estimated one half of individuals with an eating disorder have not received specialty care for this problem. In primary care settings, patients may not manifest any clinical signs of an eating disorder, except low weight, in the case of anorexia nervosa. Further, unless a patient is motivated to seek treatment for symptoms – or an accompanying family member requests an evaluation on his or her behalf – the eating disorder may not be easily apparent. For these reasons, primary care clinicians and mental health generalists should maintain vigilance for undisclosed eating disorder symptoms and understand that patients are frequently reluctant to seek care for this problem. There is typically a several-year delay between onset and treatment seeking; postponement of treatment allows the physiologic and psychological impacts of the disorder to accrue. Although patients may be reluctant to volunteer information about these symptoms, evidence also supports that doctors frequently fail to inquire. When doctors do ask, patients often will admit to symptoms and a more thorough and prompt evaluation can ensue. It is understandable that busy primary care clinicians must be selective in screening questions they pose to their patients and therefore may choose to focus screening for eating pathology in the demographic that they believe will yield the greatest number of cases. Whereas it is undeniably important to exercise watchfulness for eating pathology in the evaluation of adolescent and young adult women, the demographic in which eating disorders are most likely to onset, clinicians should recognize that eating disorders can present in childhood through late adulthood, in both men and women and across all major US ethnic groups.

The eating disorder screening questionnaire, the SCOFF, has clinical utility as a self-report first stage screener (Hill et al., 2009), though importantly it may not identify feeding disorders such as ARFID, pica, or rumination disorder. Alternatively, posing a general screening question, such as "Do you have any concerns (or has anyone else expressed concerns) that you might have an eating disorder or problems with your eating?," may be useful but has uncertain yield. In the absence of a patient report, clinicians may look for clinical signs heralding an incipient or occult eating disorder, such as low weight, poor weight gain, weight losses and gains, signs of poor nutrition or evidence of potassium wasting (possibly indicative of chronic vomiting, laxative, or diuretic use), or physical signs consistent with chronic vomiting, as noted previously.

Evaluating a Suspected Eating Disorder

If a new-onset eating disorder is suspected, a directed history should ascertain the timeline and severity of weight loss, weight gain, or weight cycling. Clinicians should take special note of rapid and substantial weight loss while ascertaining any of its precipitants. A previous history of the weight nadir at the patient's present height is an informative benchmark that will guide urgency of intervention, as will history of weight loss or decline in BMI centile with respect to the patient's growth trajectory. A targeted review of systems should identify signs and sequelae of poor intake, undernutrition, and/or purging and other compensatory behaviors, such as lightheadedness, palpitations, syncopal episodes, seizure, and skipped or irregular menstrual periods. Patients often feel reluctant or ashamed to describe purging symptoms, so it is advisable for clinicians to inventory the type, duration, and frequency of inappropriate compensatory behaviors in an empathic, non-judgmental way that optimally elicits pertinent history. In some cases, patients may not recognize the extreme medical risk posed by purging behavior (e.g., inducing vomiting through syrup of ipecac use or by underdosing or withholding insulin) and prompt education about serious health impact and appropriate intervention is imperative. On the other hand, clinicians should be mindful that their history taking could potentially suggest modes of purging to some patients (e.g., withholding of insulin dose by a patient with insulin-dependent diabetes) and should exercise appropriate caution in evaluating these possibilities.

Medical history and physical and laboratory examination should consider and exclude medical conditions that might have precipitated or exacerbated weight loss. These include gastrointestinal, infectious, rheumatologic, and endocrine disorders. Physical and laboratory exam should also evaluate the potential manifestations and medical consequences of low weight and chronic undernutrition, as well as chronic purging and other compensatory behaviors, including any history of ipecac use. Physical findings rarely confirm a diagnosis of an eating disorder, but they can augment the clinical data informing the differential diagnosis of weight loss. They are also essential in determining the urgency of and optimal setting for therapeutic intervention. Anorexia nervosa and bulimia nervosa are associated with potentially serious medical comorbidity as well as elevated mortality, as noted previously. Because some patients first present with severe illness, the initial evaluation should ascertain whether the patient requires immediate inpatient medical or psychiatric admission for safety and optimal management. For example, rapid and substantial weight loss or a body weight below 75 percent expected for height and age; marked hypotension, bradycardia, or hypothermia; cardiac dysrhythmia or markedly abnormal serious electrolyte derangement such as marked hypokalemia or hypomagnesemia; or other serious complications such as a seizure or syncope are each an indication for inpatient medical care to stabilize and manage medical complications that are either manifest, or that could imminently emerge. Clinicians should be aware that nutritional rehabilitation can precipitate the refeeding syndrome. The refeeding syndrome is a potentially life-threatening condition involving cardiac, respiratory, hematologic, and neuromuscular complications arising during the course of nutritional rehabilitation in severely emaciated individuals. The syndrome is commonly associated with hypophosphatemia, hypomagnesemia, and hypokalemia, and at-risk patients may therefore require intensive monitoring with clinical evaluation, serial laboratory examination, and telemetry for their medical safety.

Because eating disorders commonly have physiological impacts, a comprehensive clinical evaluation of an eating disorder comprises psychological, nutritional, and medical dimensions. Nutritional assessment and management are beyond the scope of this text, but all health professionals treating patients with an eating disorder should be familiar with weight parameters that signal medical risk.

Patients with AN require laboratory examination to evaluate additional medical complications. A comprehensive examination includes screening for (1) electrolyte abnormalities, hypoglycemia, elevated transaminases, elevated amylase and lipase, anemia, leukopenia, thrombocytopenia; (2) electrocardiographic abnormalities, including low voltage, bradycardia, QT interval prolongation, and irregular rhythm; and (3) osteopenia with bone densitometry. Targeted evaluation of endocrine function to evaluate weight changes and menstrual abnormalities may be indicated as well. Patients with BN as well as patients with OSFED/UFED who purge by induced vomiting, laxative, and/or diuretic misuse require evaluation of electrolytes, including potassium and magnesium.

Patients with BED can present with or develop overweight and obesity, which are associated with substantial medical comorbidity and require medical evaluation and management. In addition, because BED can develop subsequent to overweight or weight gain, clinicians should consider medical causes of increased appetite, weight gain, and obesity in their differential diagnosis of patients presenting with BED when clinically appropriate.

Treatment Approaches

Psychotherapy is the best-studied treatment for eating disorders, with cognitive and behavioral treatments having the greatest evidence base. Although new psychosocial therapies are beginning to be evaluated for efficacy for avoidant/restrictive food intake disorder (Thomas & Eddy, 2019) and rumination disorder (Murray & Thomas, 2017), the most is known about the treatment of anorexia nervosa, bulimia nervosa, and binge-eating disorder.

Cognitive-Behavioral Approaches

Cognitive-behavioral therapy (CBT) has the greatest evidence base for the treatment of adults with eating disorders. In its most recent "enhanced" format (i.e., CBT-E), this 20-session treatment (40 sessions for those who are underweight) is transdiagnostic in its application to individuals across the spectrum of eating disorders, including those with AN, BN, BED, and OSFED (Fairburn, 2008). In the first of four phases, the therapist and patient co-create a personalized formulation of the illness, highlighting the maintaining mechanisms of the disorder, and identifying potential areas to intervene. The patient is also encouraged to keep detailed self-monitoring records of meals, snacks, and associated thoughts and feelings to identify triggers (e.g., negative mood, breaking a dietary rule) for engaging in restricting, binge eating, and purging. Although self-monitoring has traditionally been done by paper and pencil, more recently, specialized mobile applications have become widely available for this purpose. In the second phase, the patient works to replace the disordered pattern of eating – typically characterized by fasting for long periods or bingeing outside of mealtimes – with a pattern of regular eating comprising three meals and two snacks per day. The third phase focuses on the overvaluation of shape and weight that is conceptualized to be the core psychopathology of the eating disorder. Rather than directly challenging the patient's distorted thoughts about "feeling fat," the therapist encourages the patient to reduce body checking behaviors, stop avoiding valued activities (e.g., going to the beach) due to body shame, and re-engage in marginalized areas of life (e.g., relationships, hobbies). The fourth and final phase focuses on preventing relapse by forecasting and problem-solving potential triggers for symptom recurrence.

In a study of 154 patients with BN, BED, and subthreshold presentations (which DSM-5 would now characterize as OSFED) who received CBT-E, more than half had eating disorder features within one standard deviation of community norms at post-treatment. Of the subset with BN, 39 percent had achieved abstinence from bingeing and purging at post-treatment. Therapeutic gains were maintained at 60-week follow-up (Fairburn et al., 2009). In some cases, lower doses of CBT may be just as effective as the full version. For example, patients with BN, BED, and subthreshold presentations who received ten sessions of CBT achieved similar levels of remission at post-treatment (Waller et al., 2018) as those who, in prior studies, received CBT for twice as long. Similarly, eight sessions of guided self-help, in which the therapist uses brief sessions to support the patient in working independently through the CBT self-help manual *Overcoming Binge Eating*, has resulted in abstinence rates of up to 64 percent among individuals with BED and recurrent binge eating (Wilson & Zandberg, 2012).

Although these data are promising, the obvious corollary is that one-half to one-third of patients are not likely to benefit from CBT adequately. In particular, there is less evidence for the efficacy of CBT for AN; in a recent uncontrolled trial, average BMI remained in the underweight range (increasing from 16.1 to 17.9 in the intent-to-treat sample) after 40 sessions of CBT-E (Fairburn et al., 2013). Moreover, its efficacy for children and adolescents is largely unknown. In addition, the efficacy of CBT in patients with co-occurring problems such as acute non-eating-disorder psychopathology (e.g., substance use disorder depression with suicidality) or medical instability is unknown because such patients are typically excluded from randomized controlled trials (Fairburn, 2009). In such cases, other approaches, including hospitalization, interpersonal psychopathology, dialectical behavioral therapy, psychodynamic therapy, and supportive therapy, may be viable alternatives.

Family-Based Treatment

Family-based treatment (FBT) is an intensive outpatient approach for adolescent eating disorders in which parents are recognized as integral participants in the recovery process. First developed by clinicians and researchers at the Maudsley Hospital in London for the treatment of adolescent anorexia nervosa, FBT has been adapted for the treatment of the broad spectrum of child and adolescent eating disorders, as well as for young adults with anorexia nervosa. The treatment draws on a number of different family therapy models, and the keys to its success are likely the active involvement of all family members and the direct targeting of eating disorder symptoms from the outset of treatment. FBT takes an "agnostic" view as to the cause of the eating disorder and is explicitly non-blaming, but rather empowering, of the parents. In FBT, the clinician brings an expertise about eating disorders, and the parents are regarded as experts on their own children; the therapist becomes an expert coach in helping the parents restore their ill child's health. The treatment proceeds through three phases that are typically carried out over six to twelve months. The first phase empowers the parents adequately to take charge of the ill patient's eating by viewing food as medicine, with a focus on goals of weight restoration and re-establishment of healthy eating behaviors. As healthy weight and eating patterns develop, control of eating is returned to the patient. The final treatment phase focuses on establishing a healthy adolescent identity and preparing for future challenges.

Review of the literature indicates that FBT is the best-studied treatment for eating disorders in adolescence and has demonstrated efficacy in clinical trials (Couturier et al., 2013); it is regarded as the first-line treatment approach for adolescents with anorexia nervosa. Among those with anorexia nervosa, approximately 50 percent will achieve full recovery and two-thirds will attain substantial improvement post-treatment; rates of recovery and improvement increase over time. A recent case series demonstrated similarly positive outcomes for adolescent anorexia nervosa with FBT delivered remotely via telemedicine (Anderson et al., 2017). For those with bulimia nervosa, fewer studies have been conducted but preliminary findings suggest that FBT is also useful. Adaptations of FBT to the treatment of subthreshold eating disorders are also underway.

Residential and Inpatient Treatment

For patients who are very unwell or have not responded to outpatient treatments, a higher level of care may be indicated. Potential options include intensive outpatient treatment (e.g., three hours/day including supervision of one meal), partial hospitalization (e.g., six to twelve hours/day including multiple supervised meals), residential care (twenty-four-hour supervision), and inpatient care (twenty-four-hour supervision with intensive medical oversight). In light of limited data to support the efficacy or selection of specific levels of care, the American Psychiatric Association has provided guidelines based on expert consensus (2006). These guidelines recommend intensive outpatient treatment for patients with fair motivation who are medically stable and able to maintain their weight above 80 percent expected body weight (EBW), but who need additional structure to refrain from symptomatic behavior such as restricting intake, binge eating, or purging. In contrast, partial hospitalization should be considered for patients who have only partial motivation, struggle with intrusive thoughts for more than three hours per day, and/or require additional mealtime structure to gain weight. Residential care is appropriate for patients who are medically stable but who may be <85 percent EBW, have poor motivation, and/or need close supervision at all meals to prevent restricting, bingeing, or purging. Lastly, inpatient hospitalization is necessary for patients who are medically compromised or unstable (e.g., individuals with clinically significant bradycardia, hypotension, cardiac dysrhythmias, or hypokalemia), very underweight, at risk for re-feeding syndrome, and/or have suicidal ideation with plan or intent. Although this clinical guidance uses particular percent expected body weights as a means of choosing a safe and effective level of care for patients with an eating disorder, it is important to evaluate the clinical salience of low weight and weight loss in the full clinical context of a patient's medical and psychological history, presentation, and needs.

Pharmacologic Management of Eating Disorders

In aggregate, clinical trial data evaluating the efficacy of pharmacologic agents for the treatment of eating disorders are somewhat limited in comparison with clinical data relevant to many other categories of mental disorders. Whereas medication management can be recommended for the management of bulimia nervosa and binge-eating disorder in adult patients, it is generally considered adjunctive to psychotherapeutic management and many caveats apply. Notably, although there are a number of pharmacologic therapies for eating disorders shown to have efficacy in randomized controlled trials (RCTs; Hay & Claudino, 2012), only two pharmacologic agents have US Food and Drug Administration (FDA) approval for an eating disorder indication (i.e., fluoxetine for bulimia nervosa and lisdexamfetamine dimesylate for BED). That being said, other agents may have clinical utility and are in routine clinical use, even if off-label.

With the exception of fluoxetine, the efficacy of pharmacologic agents has been studied for only short-term treatment of eating disorders. Clinical trial data on pharmacologic agents are generally disorder specific within the eating disorders, with important differences in efficacy across AN, BN, and BED. There are no published RCTs evaluating pharmacologic agents for the treatment of a heterogeneous EDNOS or OSFED study sample. Finally, there are few trials in children and adolescents to guide clinical management. No RCT data support the management of ARFID, rumination disorder, or pica with pharmacologic agents.

Anorexia Nervosa

Despite a number of clinical trials evaluating antidepressants, antipsychotic, and other pharmacologic agents, there is insufficient support to recommend any one agent for the treatment of the primary symptoms of AN. Of these, the atypical antipsychotic agent olanzapine (with a dosage range of 2.5–10 mg/day), had shown some promise, but the aggregate evidence does not offer consistent enough findings upon which to base general recommendations for the treatment of AN. A meta-analysis, moreover, did not find that atypical antipsychotics were superior to placebo in either increasing BMI or in reducing symptoms relating to body dissatisfaction or drive for thinness for patients with AN, although there was a significant reduction in the level of depression among those on an active drug (Lebow et al., 2013). Given the potential for serious medical side effects associated with atypical antipsychotic medications, caution is warranted in prescribing these medications for anorexia nervosa. RCT data evaluating fluoxetine for the treatment of weight recovered patients with AN have also yielded mixed findings. It should be noted from RCTs that while SSRI antidepressants such as fluoxetine do not significantly accelerate the rate of weight gain in hospitalized patients with anorexia nervosa, they may be useful for the treatment of comorbid psychiatric disorders such as major depression.

Bulimia Nervosa

Antidepressants from several classes have demonstrated efficacy for the treatment of BN via the reduction of bingeing and purging behaviors. These include the aforementioned fluoxetine, which is the best-studied agent for the treatment of BN and the only agent studied in the treatment of an eating disorder for longer-term use (over the course of one year); the effective dose is 60 mg/day. If this agent is not effective or well-tolerated, other agents with demonstrated efficacy may be useful in reducing symptoms. In the absence of comparative effectiveness data, the choice of an agent may be guided by side effect profiles, patient preference, comorbid illness, and history of response to previous therapies. Sertraline, another serotonin specific reuptake inhibitor, has established efficacy at a dosage of 100 mg/day for the short-term treatment of BN, based on one RCT. Other classes of agents with efficacy in the treatment of BN include topiramate (in dosages of up to 250 mg/day and up to 400 mg/day, respectively, in two RCTs) and ondansetron (24 mg/day in six divided doses for severe BN in one RCT), although the latter agent is not commonly used in clinical practice and the former associated with adverse side effects that limit its clinical utility (Hay & Claudino, 2012).

Other medications have shown efficacy in treating bulimia nervosa (fluvoxamine, desipramine, imipramine, and trazodone) but are not recommended as first-line agents, given their side-effect profiles and reports of adverse events during clinical trials among patients with bulimia nervosa. In addition and notably, bupropion was associated with a higher than expected – and unacceptable – risk for seizure in one clinical trial, and there are case reports of hypertensive crises in patients with BN taking MAOIs. Given alternative therapeutic agents and modalities for managing BN, these agents should not be selected to treat BN and should be avoided for the treatment of other disorders in patients with an eating disorder when possible. If there is a compelling rationale to consider their use for another indication, a careful review of benefits, risks, and precautions should be discussed with the patient.

Binge-Eating Disorder

Treatment of the patient with BED often involves a combination of interventions targeting symptoms of binge eating and medical comorbidities associated with obesity, when present. As noted previously, CBT represents an effective intervention for binge eating, but has limited benefit in facilitating weight loss. It should also be noted that behavioral weight-loss interventions targeting obesity have limited efficacy for symptoms of binge eating. Lisdexamfetamine dimesylate (LDX) at a dosage of 50 mg to 70 mg daily has been shown to be effective in achieving remission and reducing symptoms associated with moderate BED (McElroy et al., 2016) and is the only medication with an FDA indication for BED. Additional pharmacological approaches (e.g., topiramate and second-generation antidepressants [SGAs] as a group) appear to decrease binge eating in BED when compared to placebo, but remain off-label for this indication; unlike CBT and SGAs, LDX and topiramate have been associated with weight loss in individuals with BED (Brownley et al., 2016). Whereas studies to date, however, provide little evidence that antidepressant medication plus CBT is superior to CBT alone for the treatment of BED, some evidence supports that topiramate combined with CBT is superior to CBT alone in binge eating remission and weight loss (Hay & Claudino, 2012).

Treatment of Other Mental Disorders Comorbid with an Eating Disorder

Mental disorders commonly comorbid with eating disorders include mood disorders, anxiety disorders, obsessive-compulsive disorder, substance use disorders, and personality disorders. Suicide risk is high among patients with eating disorders as well, as noted previously. Since patients with eating disorders frequently have comorbid mental disorders, clinicians will want to consider side effect profiles of pharmacologic agents that could impose medical risk or discomfort to patients with an eating disorder. For example, patients will want to be informed of the known possible weight impacts of medications. Medications that can prolong the QT interval should be avoided or used with caution in patients with a risk of hypokalemia secondary to purging. Medications associated with orthostasis should be avoided in patients with poor fluid intake. Of note, patients with major depression comorbid with AN appear to respond less well to antidepressant therapy than normal-weight patients.

In summary, the overall clinical utility of pharmacologic agents for the management of eating disorders is limited. Only one agent is FDA approved for bulimia nervosa and only one agent is FDA approved for BED; none has been FDA approved for AN or OSFED. Other pharmacologic agents in routine clinical use achieve a reduction in symptoms, but remission rates are suboptimal. That being said, adjunctive therapy with medication can provide relief from some symptoms. Patient preference and comorbidities may steer clinicians either toward avoiding medications or augmenting other treatment modalities for a more aggressive approach to symptom reduction.

Coordination of the Management Team

Eating disorders impose risks and consequences across psychological, nutritional, and medical domains. For this reason, the core team that anchors treatment ideally comprises a mental health specialist, primary care clinician, and, if needed, a dietitian. In addition, medical and nutritional complications may fluctuate over the course of the disorder as behavioral symptoms wax and wane or take new forms. Tight integration of care management across medical, nutritional, and psychological domains of treatment is therefore optimal for safe and effective treatment. Care teams may coordinate care across different clinical services or even across different institutions for outpatient management. Composition of this care team may also vary and expand to include appropriate subspecialists (e.g., a psychopharmacologist, family therapist, gastroenterologist, cardiologist, etc.).

At the onset of treatment, the clinical team should establish treatment goals and processes, roles of each clinician (e.g., who will monitor the patient's weight, who will monitor dietary intake, who will monitor the frequency and/or severity of behavioral symptoms, etc.) and how they will communicate with one another so that all members are promptly apprised of clinical problems requiring attention or adjustment in the care plan. If the patient has a history of or risk for severe symptoms that may require future inpatient or residential care, the team should agree upon which parameters will be followed as indicators of a need for adjusting to a more intensive level of care. Splitting among care providers is not uncommon during the course of managing a patient with an eating disorder – sometimes because clinical information becomes fragmented and sometimes because there are differences of opinion – so a candid discussion of an agreed plan can preempt disagreement during a crisis and can be referred to in communicating a consistent and clear message of the team's expectations and plans to the patient. Patients should know about the plans and means of sharing information. Consent should be obtained that allows the exchange of clinically relevant information. If electronic communication will be used, consent should be obtained for that as well. For some patients, it is helpful to summarize the care plan, roles, and indicators for the need to add treatment, increase the level of monitoring, or increase the level of treatment intensity. When there is disagreement among the care team, team consultation is recommended.

Etiological Insights

As is the case for most other major psychiatric disorders, specific etiological factors have not been identified for eating disorders. For the purpose of this brief review, we will focus on risk factors for anorexia nervosa, bulimia nervosa, and binge-eating disorder, considering psychosocial and cultural, genetic, and neurobiological perspectives.

Indirect evidence suggests that cultural and social ideals associating feminine beauty with slenderness can contribute to the preoccupation with body shape and weight that is a frequent precursor to the onset of bulimia nervosa and anorexia nervosa among young women. Performing arts fields and sports involving a focus on body weight and shape (e.g., ballet dancing and wrestling) are associated with an increased prevalence of eating disorders. In recognition of the risks associated with severe dietary restriction, a number of jurisdictions have moved toward formal guidelines for minimal BMI for fashion models. Evidence also supports an association between mass media exposure and eating disorder risk. The increase in eating disorder symptoms following the introduction of broadcast television to Fiji, a region in which eating disorders had been reportedly rare, illustrates the potential impact of Western media content on risk (Becker et al., 2002).

Conversely, there has been increasing awareness and public-health-related concern regarding social and cultural factors that may contribute to the rising prevalence of overweight status and obesity in children and adults. Along with genetic and metabolic factors, consumption of high calorie fast-foods or sedentary lifestyle may sometimes play a role. In children, for example, this might include more time devoted to electronic social media and less time devoted to sports or other physical activities. In addition to raising the risk for medical comorbidities, obesity is thought to represent a major risk factor for the development of a binge-eating disorder. Moreover, the current trend toward increased population body weight may also contribute to an increasing number of individuals at risk for the development of an eating disorder by virtue of their participation in prolonged and/or recurrent periods of dieting.

Clinicians and researchers have long recognized that heritable factors can contribute to the risk for developing an eating disorder, reflecting a substantial role for genetic risk factors. In anorexia nervosa, for example, there is significantly increased concordance for monozygotic as opposed to dizygotic twins. Estimates place genetic heritability in the range of 0.5 to 0.6 for anorexia nervosa; in a similar range for bulimia nervosa; and in a somewhat lower range for binge-eating disorder. There is ongoing interest in candidate gene studies spanning a broad spectrum of neurotransmitters and neuromodulators in eating disorders.

Research on neurobiological risk factors for eating disorders has been informed by a number of clinical and behavioral models. Proposed models have encompassed abnormalities in central nervous system (CNS) pathways involving hunger and satiety; reward circuits (similar to alterations postulated in substance abuse); mood and anxiety; cognition; and energy metabolism / body weight regulation. Methodologies employed in clinical investigations have included measurement of cerebrospinal fluid metabolites, functional assessment of neuroendocrine regulation, pharmacological / behavioral challenge studi / and functional brain imaging with magnetic resonance imaging (fMRI), magnetic resonance spectroscopy (MRS) and positron emission tomography (PET). There has also been interest in preclinical research / an animal model for anorexia nervosa ("activity based anorexia") as well as multiple animal models for obesity and binge eating.

Major targets in clinical and preclinical neurobiological studies have included the neurotransmitters serotonin and dopamine; the hypothalamic neuropeptides NPY and alpha-MSH; the fat-derived hormone leptin; and the gut-related peptides cholecystokinin, ghrelin, and PYY. Clinical studies have frequently tested hypotheses based on the neurobiology of hunger and satiety. Thus, hypothalamic serotonin and gut-derived cholecystokinin (CCK) contribute importantly to post-ingestive satiety. Clinical investigations indicate that CNS serotonin function and CCK release from the gut are in fact diminished in patients with bulimia nervosa, suggesting that associated impairment in satiety may play a role in binge eating episodes. Medications that augment serotonin function, indirectly reinforcing meal-related satiety, have for many years been candidates for the treatment of bulimia nervosa (e.g., fluoxetine) and obesity (e.g., dexfenfluramine and lorcaserin in the past).

Because changes in nutritional status can have wide-ranging effects on CNS neurocircuitry and on peripheral hormone levels, clinical investigators strive to differentiate neurobiological alterations representing risk factors that predate the onset of an eating disorder from alterations which may emerge over the course of the disorder and serve to perpetuate eating disorder-related symptoms. Blood levels of the fat-derived, pro-satiety hormone leptin, for example, are markedly reduced in anorexia nervosa and markedly elevated in obesity. Normal-weight women with bulimia nervosa (as well as women with the OSFED subtype purging disorder) have circulating leptin levels that are significantly lower than control values, suggesting a possible role in abnormal eating patterns (Jimerson et al., 2010). Even modest restriction in caloric intake can lower circulating leptin levels, however, creating demanding methodological requirements for matching nutritional status in studies comparing patients and controls.

Future Directions

The global burden of disease imposed by eating disorders is increasingly recognized. Notwithstanding considerable advances in understanding their complex biosocial etiology and in the development of new therapeutic and preventive

Table 12.1 Priorities and promising directions for research

Classification and etiology	• Characterization of the distinctive clinical course and health impacts of purging disorder, night eating syndrome, and other specified feeding and eating disorders • Identification of underlying neurobiological abnormalities that are either unique to eating disorders or common to other forms of mental illness • Longitudinal studies to help clarify risk factors, as well as risk mediators and moderators and maintaining factors
Epidemiology and impact	• Documentation of the prevalence and associated burden of disease for the eating disorders in low- and middle-income regions • Characterization of the prevalence, course, and health impacts of pica and rumination disorder in the general population
Clinical features and course	• Identification of predictors of diagnostic crossover in order to prevent the onset of binge-eating/purging among individuals with restrictive disorders • Clarification of the temporal relationship between childhood feeding disorders and adolescent or adult eating disorders
Differential diagnosis and evaluation	• Diagnostic assessment and other tools that can be deployed by community mental health workers and non-specialist health professionals to detect, respond to, and refer individuals with an eating disorder in community and collaborative care settings • Assessment tools and strategies to differentiate ARFID from non-fat phobic AN in clinical settings • Incorporation of feeding disorder probes into widely used eating disorder screening measures
Novel preventive and treatment approaches	• Preventive approaches that can be integrated with other health priorities (such as obesity) in school-based and other community settings and that are scalable • Creation of "personalized medicine" assessments to allow individualized treatment approaches • The development of novel and more effective psychotherapies for adult anorexia nervosa and their rigorous evaluation in large, representative study samples • Development of novel pharmacologic approaches for AN (e.g., targeting the endocannabinoids) that are associated with fewer adverse effects • Identification of mediators and moderators of CBT/FBT treatment response, to enhance symptom reduction among non-responders • Evaluation of novel brain-directed treatments (e.g., repetitive transcranial magnetic stimulation [rTMS]) for eating disorders, particularly severe and enduring variants of illness • Rigorous evaluation of low-cost and low-intensity treatments in low- and middle-income regions within community and collaborative care settings, as well as guided self-help delivered in print and electronic media platforms
Expanding access to quality care	• More effective uptake of evidence-based approaches such as cognitive-behavioral therapy (CBT) and family-based treatment (FBT) beyond academic medical or eating-disorder specialty settings • Services utilization and implementation research aimed at understanding and reducing ethnic disparities in care access for eating disorders

approaches, critical gaps in scientific knowledge remain and must be addressed to achieve more acceptable levels of effectiveness and scale that these prevalent and potentially lethal disorders require. Table 12.1 lists high priority areas for research to address these.

Sample Interview Questions

Assessing a Patient without a Known Eating Disorder

- Do you have any concerns – or has anyone else expressed a concern – that you might have an eating disorder?
- Have you had any recent changes in your weight? How much weight did you lose [gain]? Over what period of time? What caused the change? What is your weight now? What is the lowest weight you have been at this height? (When was that?) What is the most you have weighed? (When was that?) What do you think is the best weight for you?
- Are you getting your menstrual periods every month? Have you ever skipped a period? How many? When was that?
- Are there any foods that you have cut out of your diet? Which foods and why? Does it bother you if you eat too much or if you eat foods that you consider to be too high in fat, sugar, or calories?
- What is your usual routine for meals? Do you eat three meals a day? How frequently do you skip meals? Do you snack in the evenings? Do you ever feel that you lose control of your eating?
- Have you ever made yourself vomit after overeating to prevent weight gain? Have you ever used laxatives, over-the-counter "nutraceuticrals," supplements, diet pills, teas, or water pills to manage your weight? When did this start? How frequently do you do this? Have you tried to stop?
- [If too thin] Your weight is actually low. How would you feel about working together to establish a healthy diet and gain to a healthy weight?
- [To parents/caretakers of children/adolescents] Have you noticed any changes in your child's eating patterns/moods? Has he or she made comments about his or her appearance that are concerning to you?

Supplemental Questions for Patients with a Known Eating Disorder

- Have you ever had low potassium or other laboratory abnormalities? [Probe further]
- Have you ever fainted or had a seizure? [Probe further]
- Have you ever had refeeding syndrome? [Probe further]

- Have you ever had palpitations, skipped beats, irregular heart rhythm, or other problems with your heart? [Probe further]
- What kind of treatment have you found helpful for your eating disorder in the past? [Probe further]
- What medications have you been on? Was this/were these effective? What dose were you on and for how long? What side effects did you have? [Probe further]
- What triggers have you noticed in the past that seemed to make your symptoms worse? [Probe further]

Case Examples

Note. The cases below are illustrative. They draw concepts (but not real case material) from the collective practice of the authors.

Adult Case

Mr. V was a forty-four-year-old divorced male who initially presented to the weight management clinic at a large academic medical center, in hopes of undergoing bariatric surgery. At 5'11" tall, he weighed 293 pounds, resulting in a BMI of 40.9 kg/m². Upon evaluation, his obesity medicine dietitian discovered that, on a typical day, Mr. V. drank only coffee for breakfast, ate a turkey sandwich and potato chips for lunch, and then consumed an entire pepperoni pizza or a dozen donuts upon returning home from work. He denied purging or any other attempts to compensate for the caloric intake after these episodes, which had been occurring up to four times per week since his recent divorce. He initially joked about his "manly appetite," but ultimately revealed that he felt deeply ashamed of his binge eating behavior and was worried it would preclude him from benefitting from weight-loss surgery. In consultation with the dietitian, Mr. V's bariatric surgeon recommended that Mr. V work to resolve his binge-eating disorder before considering surgical intervention. Upon referral to the hospital's eating disorder clinic, Mr. V received ten sessions of guided self-help based on cognitive-behavioral therapy (CBT-GSH). During the course of CBT-GSH, Mr. V's psychologist asked Mr. V to use his smartphone to keep a daily record of his food intake. Through this exercise, Mr. V learned that returning home from work feeling hungry and tired were his primary triggers for binge eating. In addition, he learned that by adding a healthy breakfast and afternoon snack, he could return home less hungry and make healthier dinner choices. He also realized that he was more likely to binge eat when he felt sad or lonely. Through CBT-GSH, he identified distraction tactics to help him manage these negative emotions, including going for a brisk walk, taking a hot shower, or inviting his friends over to play cards. Finally, he learned to incorporate moderate portions of his previous binge foods (e.g., two slices of pizza, one donut) into pre-planned meals and snacks. After completing CBT-GSH, Mr. V achieved abstinence from binge eating. Although his weight had remained relatively stable at 289 pounds, his surgeon invited him to return to the obesity medicine clinic in six months to consider potential weight-loss treatment options.

Child Case

Violet was a twelve-year-old female referred by the pediatric gastrointestinal program for the evaluation of a suspected eating disorder characterized by a lack of weight gain and restricted food intake. Violet's referral had come following a complete medical workup that had failed to identify a physical explanation of her symptoms. At the initial evaluation, her parents shared that while Violet had always been slender, she had grown along the twenty-fifth percentile curve for height and weight until her weight began faltering at her ten-year wellness visit; in the last year, she had grown in height but without any weight gain, resulting in a current weight that was at the seventh percentile for her age and gender. Concomitant with a transition to middle school in the last year, her parents noticed that Violet was eating less at meals; playing with her foods at dinner; reporting decreased appetite, early satiety, and nausea; and also seeming more anxious and withdrawing from friends. At the initial evaluation, Violet tearfully expressed confusion about her parents' concern and stated that she wanted to be "skinny and healthy"; her parents reported that in recent weeks they had observed her reading food labels, wrapping her fingers around her wrists, and pinching at her stomach and legs in ways that made them worried she may be preoccupied with thinness. On the basis of her low weight, restrictive eating behaviors, inability to appreciate the potentially serious health impacts of her low weight, and inferred body image disturbance, Violet was diagnosed with anorexia nervosa. She and her parents, and her nine-year-old brother, participated in a nine-month course of outpatient family-based treatment. The initial focus of treatment was on weight restoration, facilitated by parents taking control over meal preparation and food choices for Violet, and supervising her at all meals and snacks. Key strategies parents employed included remaining calm and united in their firm message to Violet that restricting her eating was not an option. Violet's parents began to gain confidence in their ability to refeed her, viewing food as her medicine, and she slowly began to make weight gains. While Violet was initially angry, tearful, and appeared scared by the changes, her parents expressed that they could sense her relief that they were making these difficult decisions (e.g., to choose to eat when her previous inclination at the onset of her anorexia nervosa was to do otherwise) for her. By the fourth month of treatment, when Violet's weight was increasing steadily and she was approaching her previous growth curve, parents began to transition control back to Violet as appropriate – for example, letting her return to unsupervised lunches at school with friends, and making choices about the components of her meals or snacks. The family described that it was starting to feel like "Violet was back!" As her eating normalized, the family moved into the final phase of treatment, focused on adolescent development and relapse prevention. At the close of treatment, Violet was spending more time with friends and engaging in activities she enjoyed (e.g., painting at home, joining the school chorus), and she began to show signs of puberty.

References and Selected Readings

- American Psychiatric Association Work Group on Eating Disorders (2006). Practice Guideline for the Treatment of Patients with Eating Disorders (3rd Edition). *American Journal of Psychiatry*, 163 (suppl.), 1–54.
- American Psychiatric Association (2013). *Diagnostic and Statistical Manual of Mental Disorders*, 5th ed. Washington, DC: American Psychiatric Publishing.
- Anderson, K. E., Byrne, C. E., Crosby, R. D., and Le Grange, D. (2017). Utilizing Tele-health to Deliver Family-Based Treatment for Adolescent Anorexia Nervosa. *International Journal of Eating Disorders*, 50 (10), 1235–1238.
- Arcelus, J., Mitchell, A J., Wales, J., and Nielsen, S. (2011). Mortality Rates in Patients with Anorexia Nervosa and Other Eating Disorders: A Meta-Analysis of 36 Studies *Archives of General Psychiatry*, 68, 724–731.
- Becker, A. E., Burwell, R. A., Gilman, S. E., Herzog, D. B., and Hamburg, P. (2002). Eating Behaviours and Attitudes Following Prolonged Television Exposure among Ethnic Fijian Adolescent Girls. *British Journal of Psychiatry*, 180, 509–514.
- Becker, A. E., Thomas, J. J., and Pike, K. (2009). Should Non-Fat-Phobic Anorexia Nervosa Be Included in DSM-V? *International Journal of Eating Disorders*, 42, 620–635.
- Brownley, K. A., Berkman, N. D., Peat, C. M., Lohr, K. N., and Bulik, C. M. (2017). Binge-Eating Disorder in Adults. *Annals of Internal Medicine*, 166 (3), 231.
- Couturier, J., Kimber, M., and Szatmari, P. (2013). Efficacy of Family-Based Treatment for Adolescents with Eating Disorders: A Systematic Review and Meta-Analysis. *International Journal of Eating Disorders*, 46, 3–11.
- Eddy, K. T., Dorer, D. J., Franko, D. L., Tahilani, K., Thompson-Brenner, H., and Herzog, D. B. (2008). Diagnostic Crossover in Anorexia Nervosa and Bulimia Nervosa: Implications for DSM-V. *American Journal of Psychiatry*, 165, 245–250.
- Eddy, K. T., Swanson, S. A., Crosby, R. D., Franko, D. L., Engel, S., and Herzog, D. B. (2010). How Should DSM-V Classify Eating Disorder Not Otherwise Specified (EDNOS) Presentations in Women with Lifetime Anorexia or Bulimia Nervosa? *Psychological Medicine*, 40, 1735–1744.
- Eddy, K. T., Tabri, N., Thomas, J. J., Murray, H. B., Keshaviah, A., Hastings, E., ... and Franko, D. L. (2017). Recovery from Anorexia Nervosa and Bulimia Nervosa at 22-Year Follow-Up. *Journal of Clinical Psychiatry*, 78 (2), 184–189.
- Fairburn, C. G. (2008). *Cognitive Behavior Therapy and Eating Disorders*. New York: Guilford Press.
- Fairburn, C. G., Cooper, Z., Doll, H. A., O'Connor, M. E., Bohn, K., Hawker, D. M., Wales, J. A., and Palmer, R. L. (2009). Transdiagnostic Cognitive-Behavioral Therapy for Patients with Eating Disorders: A Two-Site Trial with 60-Week Follow-Up. *American Journal of Psychiatry*, 166, 311–319.

- Fairburn, C. G., Cooper, Z., Doll, H. A., O'Connor, M. E., Palmer, R. L., and Dalle Grave, R. (2013). Enhanced Cognitive Behaviour Therapy for Adults with Anorexia Nervosa: A UK–Italy Study. *Behaviour Research and Therapy*, 51, R2–R8.
- Hay, P. J., and Claudino, A. M. (2012). Clinical Psychopharmacology of Eating Disorders: A Research Update. *International Journal of Neuropsychopharmacology*, 15, 209–222.
- Hill, L. S., Reid, F., Morgan, J. F., and Lacey, J. H. (2010). SCOFF, the Development of an Eating Disorder Screening Questionnaire. *International Journal of Eating Disorders*, 43, 344–351.
- Hudson, J. I., Hiripi, E., Pope, H. G., Jr., and Kessler, R. C. (2007). The Prevalence and Correlates of Eating Disorders in the National Comorbidity Survey Replication. *Biological Psychiatry*, 61, 348–358.
- Institute for Health Metrics and Evaluation (IHME). (2016). GBD Compare, University of Washington. Available from https://vizhub.healthdata.org/gbd-compare/. Accessed March 2018.
- Jimerson, D. C., Wolfe, B. E., Carroll, D. P., and Keel, P. K. (2010). Psychobiology of Purging Disorder: Reduction in Circulating Leptin Levels in Purging Disorder in Comparison with Controls. *International Journal of Eating Disorders*, 43, 584–588.
- Lebow, J., Sim, L. A., Erwin, P. J., and Murad, M. H. (2013). The Effect of Atypical Antipsychotic Medications in Individuals with Anorexia Nervosa: A Systematic Review and Meta-analysis. *International Journal of Eating Disorders*, 46, 332–339.
- Marques, L., Alegria, M., Becker, A. E., Chen, C.-N., Fang, A., Chosak, A., and Diniz, J. B. (2011). Comparative Prevalence, Correlates of Impairment, and Service Utilization for Eating Disorders across US Ethnic Groups: Implications for Reducing Ethnic Disparities in Health Care Access for Eating Disorders. *International Journal of Eating Disorder*, 44, 412–420.
- McElroy, S. L., Hudson, J., Ferreira-Cornwell, M. C., Radewonuk, J., Whitaker, T., and Gasior, M. (2016). Lisdexamfetamine Dimesylate for Adults with Moderate to Severe Binge Eating Disorder: Results of Two Pivotal Phase 3 Randomized Controlled Trials. *Neuropsychopharmacology*, 41 (5), 1251.
- Micali, N., Martini, M. G., Thomas, J. J., Eddy, K. T., Kothari, R., Russell, E., ... and Treasure, J. (2017). Lifetime and 12-Month Prevalence of Eating Disorders amongst Women in Mid-Life: A Population-Based Study of Diagnoses and Risk Factors. *BMC Medicine*, 15 (1), 12.
- Murray, H. B., and Thomas, J. J. (2017). Rumination Disorder in Adults: A Cognitive-Behavioral Formulation and Treatment. In Anderson, L., Murray, S., Kaye, W. (eds.), *Handbook of Complex and Atypical Eating Disorders*, pp. 253–269. New York: Oxford University Press.
- Preti, A., Rocchi, M. B., Sisti, D., Camboni, M. V., and Miotto, P. (2011). A Comprehensive Meta-Analysis of the Risk of Suicide in Eating Disorders. *Acta Psychiatrica Scandinavica*, 124, 6–17.
- Rome, E. S., Ammerman, S., Rosen, D. S., et al. (2003). Children and Adolescents with Eating Disorders: The State of the Art. *Pediatrics*, 111, e98–108.
- Steinhausen, H. C. (2009). Outcome of Eating Disorders. *Child Adolesc Psychiatr Clin N Am*, 18 (1), 225–242.
- Thomas, J. J., and Eddy, K. T (2019). *Cognitive-Behavioral Therapy for Avoidant/Restrictive Food Intake Disorder: Children, Adolescents, and Adults*. Cambridge: Cambridge University Press.

- Waller, G., Tatham, M., Turner, H., Mountford, V. A., Bennetts, A., Bramwell, K., ... and Ingram, L. (2018). A 10-Session Cognitive-Behavioral Therapy (CBT-T) for Eating Disorders: Outcomes from a Case Series of Nonunderweight Adult Patients. *International Journal of Eating Disorders*, 51 (3), 262–269.
- Wilson, G. T., and Zandberg, L. J. (2012). Cognitive-Behavioral Guided Self-Help for Eating Disorders: Effectiveness and Scalability. *Clinical Psychology Review*, 32 (4), 343–357.

Self-Assessment Questions

1. Which of the following disorders can be diagnosed concurrently with another feeding/eating disorder?
    A. Anorexia nervosa
    B. Binge-eating disorder
    C. Pica
    D. Bulimia nervosa
    E. Rumination disorder
2. Which of the following clinical findings is most useful in distinguishing anorexia nervosa from bulimia nervosa?
    A. Body image disturbance
    B. Purging behaviors such as vomiting and laxative use
    C. Low body weight
    D. Co-morbidity with anxiety and depressive symptoms
    E. Dietary restriction
3. Which of the following interventions has the strongest evidence base for the treatment of binge-eating disorder in adults?
    A. Repetitive transcranial magnetic stimulation
    B. Psychodynamic therapy
    C. Cognitive-behavioral therapy
    D. Atypical antipsychotics such as olanzapine
    E. Family-based treatment
4. Which of the following interventions has the strongest evidence base for the treatment of adolescent anorexia nervosa?
    A. Selective serotonin reuptake inhibitors such as fluoxetine
    B. Interpersonal therapy
    C. Cognitive-behavioral therapy
    D. Atypical antipsychotics such as olanzapine
    E. Family-based treatment
5. A sixteen-year-old adolescent girl is brought to the urgent evaluation center by her parents due to concern about their daughter's recent severe social

withdrawal and weight loss. The patient has a current BMI of 16. The patient does not believe she has an eating disorder, though she has been severely restricting food intake in spite of having an appetite over the past few months. Her mother has twice discovered her inducing vomiting. The patient feels her body looks "okay." On physical examination, the patient is found to be bradycardic; BP is 70/40. The best intervention for this patient is:

A. Routine referral to an outpatient clinic in the community
B. Urgent referral to a clinic with eating disorder specialization, next available appointment
C. Referral to a partial hospitalization program specializing in eating disorders
D. Elective admission to a psychiatric inpatient unit
E. Admission to a pediatric inpatient unit for stabilization

Answers to Self-Assessment Questions

1. (C)
2. (C)
3. (C)
4. (E)
5. (E)

13 | Child Psychiatry and Neurodevelopmental Disorders
SCOTT SHAFFER AND STEVEN C. SCHLOZMAN

Child and Adolescent Psychiatry

Given that children and adolescents can never be thought of simply as "little adults" but rather as patients with their own unique developmental, psychological, and biological characteristics, it is crucial that clinicians recognize how psychopathology presents differently in this population. Key differences between children, adolescents, and adults regarding epidemiology, diagnostic criteria, and treatment are described below for mood disorders, anxiety disorders, trauma and stressor-related disorders, and psychotic symptoms.

Depression

Prior to the 1960s, depression was rarely recognized in children. However, growing research and clinical experience has revealed that children can indeed experience depression although it sometimes presents differently than in adults (Shatkin, 2009). The criteria for major depressive disorder in the DSM-V differ for children and adolescents in two key ways. In children and adolescents, an irritable mood can substitute for a depressed mood. In order to meet these alternate criteria, the irritable mood must be present most of the day, nearly every day rather than simply during specific moments of frustration. Along with significant weight loss when not dieting, failure to make expected weight gain is an acceptable vegetative symptom of depression in children. In addition to these differences in DSM-V criteria, it has been observed that children and adolescents frequently demonstrate less impairment in sleep, energy, appetite, and concentration than depressed adults typically do (Birmaher, Brent, et al., 2007). In addition, depressed young children may report somatic symptoms such as stomach aches or headaches (Engle, Winiarski, et al., 2018).

Epidemiology

The Center for Disease Control and Prevention (CDC) estimates the incidence of depression in children 3–5 years old to be 0.5 percent, 2 percent for 6–11-year-olds, and up to 12 percent for 12–17-year-olds. The gender ratio is 1:1 for children, but becomes 2:1 female:male in adolescence (Perou, Winiarski, et al. 2013).

Treatment

The American Academy of Child and Adolescent Psychiatry (AACAP) practice parameter indicates that "it is reasonable, in a patient with a mild or brief depression, mild psychosocial impairment, and the absence of clinically significant suicidality or psychosis, to begin treatment with education, support, and case management related to environmental stressors in the family and school. It is expected to observe response after 4 to 6 weeks of supportive therapy" (Birmaher, Brent, et al., 2007). Cognitive-behavioral therapy (CBT) and interpersonal psychotherapy are both evidence based therapies for depression in adolescents. CBT provides the patient with skills and strategies to identify and connect their thoughts, feelings, and behaviors. Interpersonal psychotherapy targets the adolescent's interpersonal skills as a way to improve their relationships, which then improves depressive symptoms.

Selective serotonin reuptake inhibitors (SSRIs) are the first-line treatment in children and adolescents with moderate to severe major depressive disorder (Birmaher, Brent, et al., 2007). Fluoxetine is FDA approved for children eight years and older, and escitalopram is FDA approved for children twelve years and older. Other SSRIs, while off-label, are frequently used to treat depression in children and adolescents as well, though the evidence base is weaker. Following a review of all studies of antidepressants in children and adolescents, a pooled analysis demonstrated that about 4 percent of patients taking medication reported thoughts of suicide compared to 2 percent of patients taking placebo. As a result, in 2003 the FDA issued a black box warning stating that children and adolescents treated with antidepressants "should be observed closely for clinical worsening, suicidality, or unusual changes in behavior" (Noel, 2015). Since depression itself increases the likelihood of experiencing suicidal ideation, proving the link between SSRIs and increased suicidality has been challenging. While close monitoring when prescribing SSRIs to youth is important, SSRIs are considered safe medications that have the potential of providing improvement in symptoms when prescribed appropriately.

Bipolar Disorder

A significant current controversy in child and adolescent psychiatry is the approach to the diagnosis of bipolar disorder in children and adolescents. Symptoms associated with mania, such as aggression, impulsivity, irritability, and risk-taking behavior, can be seen in children diagnosed with behavioral disorders such as ADHD and Conduct Disorder (Parems & Johnston, 2010).

It is rare for children and young adolescents to demonstrate discrete episodes of depression and mania with clear change from baseline that is consistent with Bipolar I Disorder (Parems & Johnston, 2010). Bipolar disorder is thought of as a spectrum, and behavioral dysregulation and "mood swings" in youth have been used to justify a diagnosis of bipolar disorder. However, the DSM-V criteria for a manic episode are the same in children, adolescents, and adults.

The diagnostic criteria for cyclothymic disorder differ for children and adolescents compared with adults. Young patients require only one year rather than two years of numerous periods with hypomanic symptoms that do not meet criteria for a hypomanic episode and numerous periods with depressive symptoms that do not meet the criteria for a major depressive episode. It is crucial that children and adolescents receive a thorough and comprehensive psychiatric evaluation to determine whether their symptoms can best be explained by bipolar disorder.

Epidemiology

The prevalence of bipolar disorder in clinical populations in the United States has ranged from 0.6 percent to 15 percent and varies depending on the setting, referral source, and methodology in defining the diagnosis. Whether this increase is due to overdiagnosis or a heightened awareness on the part of clinicians is a current controversy in the field. Patients with bipolar disorder have a high rate of comorbid diagnoses, including disruptive behavior disorders (30 percent to 70 percent), ADHD (50 percent to 80 percent), and anxiety disorders (30 percent to 70 percent) (International Association for Child and Adolescent Psychiatry and Allied Professions [IACAPAP], 2015).

Treatment

Lithium was the first medication to be approved by the FDA for the treatment of mania in children ages twelve to seventeen years. Several atypical antipsychotics are FDA approved for the acute treatment of manic or mixed episodes in children and adolescents: risperidone for ten- to seventeen-year-olds, olanzapine for thirteen- to seventeen-year-olds, aripiprazole for ten- to seventeen-year-olds, and quetiapine for ten- to seventeen-year-olds. Lurasidone is the only medication that is FDA approved to treat bipolar depression in children and adolescents.

It is important that children and families receive psychotherapy in addition to psychopharmacologic treatments. Patients and families can benefit from recognizing triggers and early signs of mood changes, and to receive emotional support for coping with a chronic mental illness. Child and family focused cognitive-behavior therapy (CFF-CBT) was specifically designed for eight- to eighteen-year-olds with bipolar disorder. CFF-CBT consists of twelve 60-minute sessions that are delivered weekly over 3 months. The intervention is designed to be employed across multiple domains – individual, family, peers, and school – to address the impact of bipolar disorder on the child's psychosocial functioning (IACAPAP, 2015).

Disruptive Mood Dysregulation Disorder

Throughout the 1990s and early 2000s, researchers observed that children and adolescents who demonstrated severe nonepisodic irritability were frequently diagnosed with bipolar disorder. Ellen Liebenluft, MD, captured these patients with her description of severe mood dysregulation, which she defined as "severe, none-pisodic irritability and the hyperarousal symptoms characteristic of mania but who lack the well-demarcated periods of elevated or irritable mood characteristic of bipolar disorder." Children with severe mood dysregulation were compared to those with bipolar disorder in longitudinal course, family history, and pathophysiology. Longitudinal data in both clinical and community samples demonstrated that nonepisodic irritability in youth was common and was associated with an increased risk for anxiety and unipolar depressive disorders, but not bipolar disorder, in adults. Data also suggested that children with severe mood dysregulation had lower familial rates of bipolar disorder than did those with bipolar disorder (Liebenluft, 2011). These important findings led to a new diagnosis in the DSM-V called disruptive mood dysregulation disorder. The diagnostic criteria include severe recurrent temper outbursts manifested verbally and/or behaviorally that are grossly out of proportion in intensity or duration to the situation or provocation. The temper outbursts are inconsistent with developmental level, and they occur on average three or more times per week. The mood between temper outbursts is persistently irritable or angry most of the day, nearly every day, and is observable by others. Symptoms are present for twelve or more months, and throughout that time, the patient should not have a period lasting three or more consecutive months without all of the symptoms. The symptoms are also present in at least two of three settings. The diagnosis should not be made for the first time before age six years or after age eighteen years, and the age at onset is before ten years. In addition, the full symptom criteria for a manic or hypomanic episode have not been met, and the diagnosis cannot coexist with oppositional defiant disorder, intermittent explosive disorder, or bipolar disorder.

Since this is a new diagnosis, information regarding epidemiology and treatment is limited. Based on prevalence estimates of chronic and severe irritability, the prevalence likely falls in the 2 to 5 percent range. Rates are expected to be higher in males and school-age children than in females and adolescents (APA, 2013).

Anxiety Disorders

Anxiety disorders are of particular interest in child and adolescent psychiatry because of their early onset. About 5 percent of children and adolescents in Western countries meet the criteria for an anxiety disorder. As in adults, there is about a 1.5–2 times difference in the presence of anxiety disorders in females compared to males. Of all psychiatric disorders seen in children, they are often the most early to appear but often go untreated due to a cycle of avoidance on behalf of the patient and families. Similarly to adults, evidence-based treatment of anxiety disorders in children and adolescents consists of selective serotonin reuptake inhibitors (SSRIs) and cognitive-behavioral therapy (CBT). For patients experiencing mild anxiety that is causing minimal impairment, a trial of cognitive-behavioral therapy alone is recommended. For patients who are experiencing more moderate-severe symptoms and greater levels of impairment, and/or who have failed a trial of cognitive-behavioral therapy, combined treatment consisting of CBT and an SSRI is recommended (Connolly, Sucheta, et al., 2007).

Separation Anxiety Disorder

The diagnostic criteria for separation anxiety disorder are the same as adults with one exception: the fear, anxiety, or avoidance lasts at least four weeks in children and adolescents rather than six months in adults. In children, six- to twelve-month prevalence is around 4 percent, and in adolescents, the twelve-month prevalence is 1.6 percent. It is the most prevalent anxiety disorder in children younger than twelve years old (APA, 2013). School refusal is a frequent manifestation of separation anxiety disorder, which leads to significant academic and social impairment.

Selective Mutism

Selective mutism is a disorder most commonly seen in early childhood. Patients demonstrate a consistent failure to speak in specific social situations in which there is an expectation for speaking despite speaking in other situations. It must interfere with educational or occupational achievement or with social communication; last at least one month; not be limited to the first month of school; is not attributable to a lack of knowledge of, or comfort with, the spoken language required in the social situation; and is not better explained by a communication disorder or occur exclusively during the course of autism spectrum disorder, schizophrenia, or another psychotic disorder. While the known prevalence is rare (between 0.03 and 1 percent, depending on the setting), this may be an underestimate, as many children with anxiety disorders do not come to clinical attention. The onset is usually before age five years, although it sometimes does not become noticed until the start of school. Symptoms may spontaneously improve without treatment as the child gets older but often become more consistent with social anxiety disorder (APA, 2013).

Specific Phobia

Specific phobias are extremely common in children and adults. The diagnostic criteria are the same for children and adolescents, with the additional notation that in children, fear or anxiety may be expressed by crying, tantrums, freezing, or clinging. Prevalence is about 5 percent in children and about 16 percent in 13–17-year-olds. Females more commonly have this diagnosis compared to males by a rate of about 2:1. It is important to recognize that fear of the dark, ghosts, monsters, and the like are developmentally normal in young children and should not be considered psychopathology.

Social Anxiety Disorder

Social anxiety disorder has identical criteria for children and adolescents in the DSM-V with two important specifications. The anxiety in children must occur in peer settings and not just during interactions with adults. The anxiety can be expressed by crying, tantrums, freezing, clinging, shrinking, or failing to speak in social situations. The prevalence is 7 percent, which is equivalent to the prevalence in adults. There is a greater prevalence in females, and this difference is more prominent in adolescents and young adults (APA, 2013).

Trauma- and Stressor-Related Disorders

Reactive Attachment Disorder

Child and adolescent psychiatrists often work with children who have been profoundly neglected resulting in severe impairment in their ability to form attachments to others throughout life. Reactive attachment disorder is characterized by a consistent pattern of inhibited, emotionally withdrawn behavior toward adult caregivers manifested by the child rarely or minimally seeking comfort when distressed and the child rarely or minimally responding to comfort when distressed. These children demonstrate minimal social and emotional responsiveness to others, have limited positive affect, and can have episodes of unexplained irritability, sadness, or fearfulness that are evident even during nonthreatening interactions with adult caregivers. These symptoms are the direct result of experiencing a pattern of extremes of insufficient care. In order to meet the criteria for this diagnosis, children must have a developmental age of at least nine months, and symptoms must be evident before the age of five. The prevalence of this condition is unknown and thought to be uncommon, occurring in less than 10 percent of children in populations of severely neglected children (APA, 2013). Treatment consists of providing the child with a stable caregiver who can help provide a secure attachment.

Disinhibited Social Engagement Disorder

This condition describes children who similarly have experienced a pattern of extremes of insufficient care, but who have quite a different presentation as those with reactive attachment disorder. They demonstrate a pattern of behavior in which a child actively approaches and interacts with unfamiliar adults and has reduced or absent reticence in approaching and interacting with strangers, exhibit overly familiar verbal or physical behavior, demonstrate diminished or absent checking back with adult caregivers after venturing away, and/or have a willingness to go off with an unfamiliar adult with minimal or no hesitation. The patient must have a developmental age of at least nine months. Symptoms can start at any age. While the prevalence is unknown, it is thought to be present in about 20 percent of children in high-risk populations (APA, 2013). Treatment consists of providing the child with a stable caregiver who can help provide a secure attachment, as well as behavioral therapy reinforcing appropriate social behavior.

Posttraumatic Stress Disorder

It has long been recognized that children who have experienced trauma in their lives can experience significant symptoms that severely impair their social and emotional functioning, yet present differently than posttraumatic stress disorder does in adults. In order to account for this, there are unique criteria in the DSM-V that address this difference in children six-years-old and younger. The differences include the following:

- Spontaneous and intrusive memories may not necessarily appear distressing and may be expressed as play reenactment.
- It may not be possible to ascertain that the frightening content of dreams is related to the traumatic event.
- Trauma-specific reenactment may occur in play.
- Patients can have persistent avoidance of stimuli or negative alterations in cognitions. Older children, adolescents, and adults are required to demonstrate both of these symptoms.
- Irritable behavior and angry outbursts can manifest as extreme temper tantrums (APA, 2013).

While SSRIs are first-line medications to treat PTSD in adults, the evidence for their use in children and adolescents is not as strong. However, trauma-focused cognitive-behavioral therapy has been proven in children and adolescents to be an effective therapeutic modality and is considered first-line treatment (Cohen, 2010).

Psychotic Symptoms in Children

Psychotic symptoms in young children are extremely rare. When hallucinations are described by prepubertal children, they are often best understood as secondary to more common etiologies, including anxiety, trauma, or language impairment. Children with intrusive thoughts will sometimes experience these intense thoughts as "voices." Children who have been exposed to trauma can be both hypervigilant and have intrusive thoughts, which can result in perceptual abnormalities that are similar to hallucinations. Children who have expressive language difficulties have difficulty expressing their emotions and experiences, and can sometimes express thoughts as "voices." Consequently, it is crucial that clinicians consider a broad differential diagnosis for a young child who reports these symptoms, and conducts a developmentally appropriate interview to best characterize what best explains the patient's experience.

Although uncommon, schizophrenia can be present in young children. Childhood-onset schizophrenia is defined as symptoms starting prior to age thirteen, in contrast to early-onset schizophrenia, which is defined as the onset of symptoms prior to age eighteen. The worldwide prevalence is estimated to be less than 1 in 10,000. A study of childhood-onset schizophrenia study at the National Institute of Mental Health demonstrated that these patients tend to have more premorbid impairment than patients with later onset of symptoms, increased prevalence of developmental issues, premorbid social difficulties, motor issues, and family history of schizophrenia (IACAPAP, 2015). Symptoms typically have a slow and gradual onset. Diagnostic criteria are the same for children or adults with schizophrenia.

The prevalence of psychotic disorders increases in adolescence and is estimated to be about 1 in 500 for eighteen-year-olds. The majority of these patients had relatively normal premorbid functioning, and then experience a prodrome, which is significant for low mood, anxiety, and functional deterioration (IACAPAP, 2015).

When there is a suspicion for a psychotic disorder in children and adolescents, it is extremely important to ensure that the patient has received a complete medical and neurological evaluation to rule out any medical etiology. These patients often require very close monitoring, and their families require an extensive amount of psychoeducation and support.

It is extremely important to note that many seemingly psychotic symptoms in children do not necessarily indicate the presence of a psychosis. Taken in a developmental context, many behaviors that would be interpreted as psychotic if present in adults are in fact entirely normal in children. This includes the very common phenomena of an imaginary friend, or instances in which children describe hearing a voice that they will, upon further inquiry, describe as what adults would refer to as the voice that helps to know what is the correct course of action in a given circumstance. Some children will call this the voice of the conscience. Because these behaviors are very typical of toddlers and early school-aged children, most parents and caregivers do not worry about these instances, and pediatricians and related clinicians are quick to reassure when parents do happen to express concern.

Side effects to commonly prescribed medications also can cause psychosis in children. For example, the anticholinergic effects of diphenhydramine, taken orally or applied topically for allergic reactions, have been etiologic for psychotic disorders in children. Corticosteroids such as prednisone have also caused paranoia and even hallucinations in younger and older children. Finally, there is always the possibility that the accidental ingestion of certain plants, medications, or psychoactive recreational substances can cause psychotic presentations. In particular, the increasing presence of edible THC candies (i.e., marijuana gummies) has understandably proven enticing to children who think they have discovered a cache of candy and thus ingest large quantities of psychotropically active foods.

Finally, all children who present with psychotic symptoms should undergo a thorough neurological exam. Children with brain occupying lesions, central nervous system infections, or more systemic illnesses such as connective tissue diseases, multiple sclerosis, and a host of genetic syndromes can all experience psychosis. Because a primary psychotic disorder in children is by definition a diagnosis of exclusion, clinicians must carefully screen and consider all young patients with psychotic symptoms with a broad and inclusive differential diagnosis in mind. It is beyond the scope of this textbook to detail all of the possibilities – entire textbooks have in fact been written on this subject. Given the rarity of primary psychotic disorders in children and early adolescents, every attempt should be made to consult the most recent literature on the subject. We have listed below some key references, but it is important to note that the data in these references will change frequently and markedly as the medical and scientific community learn more about childhood psychotic presentations (Giannitelli, et al., 2017; Sikich, 2013).

References and Selected Readings

- American Psychiatric Association (2013). *Diagnostic and Statistical Manual of Mental Disorders*, 5th ed. Arlington, VA: American Psychiatric Publishing.
- Birmaher, B., Brent, D., et al., AACAP Work Group on Quality Issues (2007). Practice Parameter for the Assessment and Treatment of Children and Adolescents with Depressive Disorders. *Journal of the American Academy of Child and Adolescent Psychiatry*, 46 (11), 1503–1526.
- Cohen, J. A. (2010). Practice Parameter for the Assessment and Treatment of Children and Adolescents with Posttraumatic Stress Disorder. *Journal of the American Academy of Child and Adolescent Psychiatry*, 49 (4), 414–430.
- Connolly, S. D., Bernstein, G. A., The Work Group on Quality Issues (2007). Practice Parameter for the Assessment and Treatment of Children and Adolescents with Anxiety Disorders. *Journal of the American Academy of Child & Adolescent Psychiatry*, 46 (2), 267–283.
- Engel, M. L., Winiarski, D. A., Reidy, B. L., and Brennan, P. A. (2018). Early-Life Somatic Complaints: Longitudinal Associations with Maternal and Child Psychopathology. *Journal of Developmental and Behavioral Pediatrics*, 39 (7), 573–579.
- Giannitelli, M., Consoli, A., Raffin, M., Jardri, R., Levinson, D. F., Cohen, D., and Laurent-Levinson, C. (2017). An Overview of Medical Risk Factors for Childhood Psychosis: Implications for Research and Treatment. *Schizophrenia Research*, 192, 39–49.
- International Association for Child and Adolescent Psychiatry and Allied Professions (2015). *IACAPAP Textbook of Child and Adolescent Mental Health*. Geneva: Author.
- Liebenluft, E. (2011). Severe Mood Dysregulation, Irritability, and the Diagnostic Boundaries of Bipolar Disorder in Youths. *American Journal of Psychiatry*, 168 (2), 129–142.
- Noel, C. (2015). Antidepressants and Suicidality: History, the Black-Box Warning, Consequences, and Current Evidence. *Mental Health Clinician*, 5 (5), 202–211.

- Parens, E., and Johnston, J. (2010). Controversies Concerning the Diagnosis and Treatment of Bipolar Disorder in Children. *Child and Adolescent Psychiatry and Mental Health*, 4 (9), 1–14.
- Perou, R., Bitsko, R. H., Blumberg, S. J., Pastor, P., Ghandou, R. M., Gfroerer, C. M., et al. (2013). Mental Health Surveillance among Children – United States, 2005–2011. *MMWR Supplement*, 62 (2), 1–35.
- Shatkin, J. P. (2009). *Treating Child and Adolescent Mental Illness: A Practical, All-in-One Guide.* New York: W. W. Norton and Company.

Self-Assessment Questions

1. Evidence-based treatments for depression in adolescents include all of the following except:
   A. Cognitive-behavioral therapy
   B. Fluoxetine
   C. Interpersonal psychotherapy
   D. Methylphenidate
   E. Escitalopram

2. Children and adolescents who have severe mood dysregulation have been shown in studies to be at increased risk of developing which condition as adults?
   A. Bipolar disorder
   B. Anxiety disorders
   C. Schizophrenia
   D. Depressive disorders
   E. B and D

3. The most prevalent anxiety disorder in children less than twelve years old is:
   A. Panic disorder
   B. Generalized anxiety disorder
   C. Separation anxiety disorder
   D. Social anxiety disorder
   E. Selective mutism

4. The first-line treatment of posttraumatic stress disorder in children and adolescents is:
   A. Atypical antipsychotic
   B. Trauma focused cognitive-behavioral therapy
   C. SSRI
   D. Beta blocker
   E. Dialectic behavioral therapy

5. A three-year-old boy named James is brought to his pediatrician after his parents express concerns that he insists that his invisible friend accompany him to his first week of preschool. Their son further notes that because the invisible friend – in this case, a talking cow named William – refuses to accompany him, he does not plan on going to preschool. The parents are worried about their son's state of mind and note that his paternal uncle developed schizophrenia in college. The best course of action for the pediatrician involves:

    A. A thorough discussion of the risks and benefits of antipsychotic medications for young children and suggesting a trial of risperidone (a second-generation antipsychotic).

    B. Asking James and his parents why William refuses to go to school and reassuring the parents that young children often invoke imaginary friends as a means of expressing thoughts that they are less comfortable expressing themselves.

    C. Ordering EEG and brain imaging studies to rule out the presence of a lesion or a seizure.

    D. Referring the family to counseling so that James can learn and accept that William is not real.

Answers to Self-Assessment Questions

1. (D)
2. (E)
3. (C)
4. (B)
5. (B)

14 | Sleep Disorders

SUSAN CHANG AND JOHN WINKELMAN

Introduction to Sleep Disorders

Sleep disorders are prevalent, disabling, and deleterious to an array of physiologic systems. Given the intricate relationship between sleep, cognition, and emotional regulation, it is not surprising that complaints about sleep are especially frequent in the psychiatry clinic. It is incumbent on the clinician to identify potential sleep disorders, as treatment can have substantial benefits for both physical and mental health.

When approaching the patient with a sleep disorder, it is often helpful to categorize the problem: insomnia (difficulty sleeping), parasomnia (abnormal behaviors during sleep), or hypersomnia (excessive sleep or sleepiness). The last of these is often the most challenging to correctly identify, since it may easily be confused with common medical and psychiatric symptoms such as fatigue (lack of energy) or apathy (lack of interest or concern). This distinction can be made by careful history. One may ask, "If you sit down to read a book, do you begin to nod off?" or "Do you have difficulty staying awake on a long drive?" An affirmative answer suggests true sleepiness.

Several tools can be helpful additions to clinical history in the evaluation of the patient with a sleep disorder. The Epworth Sleepiness Scale (ESS) is a commonly used instrument for patients with hypersomnia. The ESS poses a series of scenarios and asks patients to rate their likelihood of dozing in each case. Scores can be used to quantify the degree of sleepiness and to track changes during treatment of the sleep disorder. On the other hand, progress during treatment of insomnia or a parasomnia is best monitored using sleep diaries. Patients are asked to document on a daily basis their sleep times and/or nocturnal behaviors. These "real-time" records often provide a more accurate picture of the sleep problem compared to the patient's recollection at the time of the visit. This may allow the identification of important patterns and external influences that may assist in treatment.

Insomnia

Difficulty sleeping is one of the most common concerns among psychiatric patients. According to the DSM-V, insomnia disorder encompasses difficulty initiating sleep, difficulty maintaining sleep, and/or chronically nonrestorative sleep that are present at least three times per week for a minimum of three months. Among US adults, the prevalence of insomnia disorder is approximately 10–20 percent, and roughly half of those follow a chronic course. Insomnia is more common in women, the elderly, and those who are widowed, divorced, or of lower socioeconomic status. Insomnia is also overrepresented in psychiatry clinics due to very high rates of comorbidity with mood, psychotic, substance abuse, and anxiety disorders.

Insomnia is often triggered by a stressful life event – the precipitant. This could be a social, medical, or psychological stressor that temporarily disrupts the normal sleep pattern. Acute insomnia is common in this setting and frequently resolves without treatment, though a short course of hypnotic medication may be warranted if the sleeplessness is severe or distressing. However, a subset of patients will go on to develop chronic insomnia disorder. In these individuals, a variety of unfavorable predisposing and perpetuating factors maintain the unsatisfactory sleep pattern despite the resolution of the precipitating circumstances. Predisposing conditions may include an anxious diathesis, older age, or medical illness. Perpetuating factors are often compensatory responses to the insomnia that eventually become counterproductive and/or inadvertent conditioned negative responses to the sleeping environment. For instance, she may go to bed earlier, nap during the daytime, worry excessively about sleep, and focus unduly on the effort to initiate sleep despite heightened alertness.

Evaluation of the patient with insomnia should focus on a careful understanding of sleep patterns (including any daytime napping), precipitating and perpetuating factors, and daytime consequences of the sleep disturbance. Every patient, whether in the psychiatry clinic or elsewhere, should be queried about symptoms of mood and anxiety disorders, since these are common causes of insomnia that often warrant independent treatment. It is also important to ask about symptoms of restless legs syndrome, circadian rhythm disorders, and obstructive sleep apnea, as well as symptoms such as pain, nocturnal dyspnea, and frequent urination that can interfere with sleep, and whose treatment can improve sleep (Table 14.1).

Treatment of insomnia incorporates two strategies: cognitive-behavioral therapy (CBT) and pharmacologic therapy. The selection of a treatment approach should be made in collaboration with the patient and in response to his or her needs. Some patients have a preference to avoid medications, while others are unable to make the time commitment required for CBT. In those who are willing and able, a combination of the two approaches is probably the most effective for long-term management.

Cognitive-behavioral therapy for insomnia (CBT-I) is a multimodal approach that teaches patients to modify unhelpful behaviors and cognitive patterns. In CBT-I, the patient keeps sleep diaries that are reviewed with the therapist. A variety of strategies are taught in CBT-I, including sleep hygiene, relaxation techniques,

Table 14.1 Differential diagnosis of insomnia

Differential diagnosis of insomnia

Psychiatric illness (e.g., depression, anxiety)

Stress

Irregular sleep schedule

Disruptive sleeping environment (e.g., noise, light)

Excess caffeine

Substance abuse (e.g., alcohol, cocaine)

Symptoms of medical problems, e.g.:

- Pain
- Nocturia
- Shortness of breath
- Cough
- Palpitations
- Tinnitus

Neurodegenerative disorders

Menopause

Medications

Circadian rhythm disorders

Restless legs syndrome

Obstructive sleep apnea

and cognitive restructuring, but the two components with proven efficacy are sleep restriction and stimulus control.

Stimulus control is based on the principles of classical conditioning. In this model, the bedroom and the process of attempting to sleep become stimuli that produce anxiety and physiological arousal, thereby interfering with sleep and perpetuating insomnia. Accordingly, in CBT-I the patient is directed to get out of bed when awake and unable to sleep in order to preserve the bed as a place for drowsiness/sleep. Sleep restriction, the other key intervention in CBT-I, involves limiting the total time in bed to the actual amount of time slept. Initially, total sleep time will decrease relative to baseline, but the increased sleep drive that ensues will over time facilitate faster sleep onset and better sleep maintenance, reducing anxiety regarding sleeplessness and leading to re-establishment of a pattern of regular sleep. Time in bed is then gradually increased as long as difficulties with sleep initiation or maintenance do not return.

Pharmacotherapy of insomnia is appropriate for short-term management in many patients and may be indicated for the long-term in a subset of individuals with chronic insomnia that does not resolve with behavioral techniques. The most

Table 14.2 Pharmacological agents for insomnia

Drug	Half-life (hours)	Dose range (mg)	Side effects
Benzodiazepines			Common to all: Residual sedation, complex sleep-related behaviors, anterograde amnesia, Falls (elderly)
• Lorazepam	8–12	0.5–2	
• **Temazepam**	8–12	15–30	
• Clonazepam	20–60	0.25–1	
• **Triazolam**	2–3	0.125–0.375	
Benzodiazepine receptor agonists			
• **Zaleplon**	1–2	5–10	
• **Eszopiclone**	5–6	1–3	
• **Zolpidem**	2–3	5–10	
• **Zolpidem ER**	2–3	6.25–12.5	
• **Zolpidem sublingual**	2–3	1.75–3.5	
Dual orexin receptor antagonists			Common to both: Residual sedation
• **Suvorexant**	12–15	10–20	
• **Lemborexant**	17–19	5–10	
Sedating antidepressants			
• Trazodone	7–15	25–150	Dry mouth, OH, priapism
• Mirtazapine	20–40	7.5–30	Weight gain, OH, dry mouth
• Amitriptyline	10–100	10–100	Weight gain, OH, dry mouth, urinary retention
• Doxepin	10–50	3–25	Weight gain, OH, dry mouth, urinary retention
Antipsychotics			Common to both: weight gain, metabolic syndrome, OH, dry mouth, akathisia
• Quetiapine	7	25–200	
• Olanzapine	20–54	2.5–20	
Anticonvulsants			
• Gabapentin	100–900	5–9	Dizziness, cognitive impairment, weight gain
Melatonin agonists			
• **Ramelteon**	8	0.8–2	Dizziness, fatigue
Antihistamines			Common to both: dry mouth, urinary retention, constipation, OH
• Diphenhydramine	25–50	5–11	
• Doxylamine	25–50	10–12	

Medications that are FDA approved for sleep are marked **in boldface**. OH, orthostatic hypotension; ER, extended-release well-studied sleeping medications bind to the benzodiazepine site on GABA(A) receptors in the CNS. These include both the benzodiazepines and the newer benzodiazepine receptor agonists. Although the newer agents are somewhat more selective for a subtype of GABA(A) receptor, practically this makes very little difference, and the choice of hypnotic should be made based on pharmacokinetic considerations and the patient's tolerance and preference. If benzodiazepine agonists are ineffective, poorly tolerated, or contraindicated, alternative treatment options include sedating antidepressants, melatonin agonists, atypical antipsychotics, and anti-epileptics (Table 14.2).

Restless Legs Syndrome

Restless legs syndrome (RLS) is a common sensorimotor sleep disorder, present in around 5 percent of the population. RLS is characterized by a strong urge to move the legs that is provoked by rest, relieved with movement, and worst in the evening or at night. The urge to move is often accompanied by an uncomfortable sensation. The patient may describe this as a creepy-crawly, tingly, or tight feeling deep within the legs. Women are affected more commonly than men, and the prevalence increases with advancing age. Other special groups in whom RLS is much more common include pregnant women, patients with end-stage renal disease, and those with iron deficiency.

Restless legs syndrome is a circadian disorder, and the peak intensity of symptoms is around bedtime and the first few hours of the night for most patients. Thus RLS is a common cause of difficulty initiating and maintaining sleep. The majority of RLS patients also experience periodic limb movements of sleep (PLMS). PLMS are repetitive (usually every 20–40 sec) stereotyped limb movements during sleep that may be associated with brief arousals from sleep. For all of these reasons, RLS patients very often complain of poor quality sleep.

Evaluation of the patient with RLS should begin with the identification of any underlying cause. Serum iron studies should be tested in all patients with RLS, and supplemental iron is indicated when ferritin is <50 µg/L. Medications are another frequent cause of RLS, particularly serotonergic or tricyclic antidepressants and dopamine antagonists. In this case, decreasing or stopping the offending medication may be helpful. If none of these approaches is applicable or helpful, pharmacologic treatment is often indicated. Dopamine agonists (e.g., pramipexole, ropinirole, rotigotine) are first-line in many cases. However, these medications tend to become less effective over years of treatment. Ligands at the $\alpha_2\delta$ calcium channel receptor, such as gabapentin and pregabalin, are also effective for many patients. In advanced or refractory cases, opioid medications can provide marked relief.

Parasomnias

Parasomnias are unwanted behaviors that occur during sleep. These can be divided into REM-related and NREM-related disorders, based on the stage of sleep from which they arise. NREM parasomnias are also known as disorders of arousal, since they are thought to stem from the inability to arouse fully from the deepest stages of NREM sleep. NREM parasomnias include somnambulism (sleep walking), somniloquy (sleep talking), confusional arousals, and sleep terrors. All of these are most common in children and tend to wane with age.

Confusional arousals occur in 10–20 percent of healthy children. Indistinct speech, relative unresponsiveness, and simple motor behaviors are characteristic. Sleep terrors are more dramatic episodes that often include screaming or distressed verbalization, inconsolable crying, and the appearance of intense fear. The lifetime prevalence is around 10 percent, and they are rare after the age of twelve. Sleep-walking occurs at least once in about 30 percent of children, and 1–5 percent have repeated episodes. The most important intervention for all parasomnias is precautionary measures to ensure safety. Regularizing the sleep-wake pattern and minimizing sleep deprivation can also be beneficial. If pharmacotherapy is necessary, short-acting benzodiazepines are usually first-line treatment.

Although parasomnias occasionally persist into adulthood, the new onset in an adult should prompt consideration of an alternative explanation. Complex sleep-related behaviors such as sleep-eating and sleep-driving can be associated with the use of hypnotic medications. In this case, stopping the medication usually eliminates the parasomnia. Other conditions in the differential diagnosis include nocturnal panic attacks, dissociative episodes, or frontal lobe epilepsy. Psychiatric or neurologic symptoms during the day are most helpful for making this distinction. Other features suggestive of seizures include multiple episodes per night and highly stereotyped motor activity. When nocturnal epilepsy is considered, overnight polysomnography with full EEG is indicated.

REM parasomnias include nightmares and REM behavioral disorder. Nightmares are repeated episodes of waking from sleep with intense memories of disturbing dream content. These are more frequent in children, in whom reassurance is often sufficient. In adults, nightmares are seen most often comorbid with psychiatric disorders, particularly PTSD, depression, and anxiety disorders. Cognitive therapies focused on rescripting and rehearsal of the dream with more positive content can be effective in both adults and children.

REM behavior disorder (RBD) stands in contrast to other parasomnias in that it tends to happen in older individuals and follows a progressive course. Normally, REM sleep is characterized by generalized muscle atonia that prevents the enactment of dreams. RBD involves loss of this motor inhibition, and affected patients act out dream content, often with aggressive or even violent behavior. RBD may be a manifestation of or a precursor to one of the neurologic disorders charac-terized by the accumulation of α-synuclein (Parkinson's disease, dementia with Lewy bodies, or multiple system atrophy). Up to two-thirds of patients initially diagnosed with "idiopathic" RBD will go on to develop a synucleinopathy within ten to fifteen years. A more benign and possibly more common cause of RBD is the use of serotonergic antidepressant medications. In such cases, reduction or discontinuation of the medication and substitution of another nonserotonergic agent is indicated.

When RBD is suspected, overnight polysomnography is indicated. Excessive muscle tone during REM sleep is supportive of the diagnosis. Treatment is twofold. First, protective measures should be instituted to ensure the safety of the patient and the bedpartner. This may involve moving the bedpartner out of the bed, at least until symptoms are controlled. Pharmacologic treatment is often indicated and can be remarkably helpful. Intermediate-acting benzodiazepines and high-dose melatonin have well-established efficacy and should be offered to most pa-tients.

Hypersomnias

According to the DSM-V, disorders of excessive daytime sleepiness can be divided into three groups: (1) narcolepsy caused by hypocretin (orexin) deficiency; (2) Kleine-Levin syndrome; and (3) other syndromes of hypersomnolence not explained by hypocretin deficiency (generally without cataplexy).

Narcolepsy with hypocretin deficiency is believed to be due to autoimmune destruction of hypocretin-producing neurons in the hypothalamus in genetically susceptible individuals. Hypocretin is a peptide involved in the regulation of vigi-lance and the organization of sleep. Its absence results in the abnormal propensity to transition between wake and REM sleep that is characteristic of narcolepsy. In addition to daytime sleepiness, several other features are often seen but are not required for the diagnosis. These are (1) cataplexy (a sudden loss of muscle tone lasting seconds to minutes, generally precipitated by an emotional stimulus); (2) hypnagogic hallucinations (visual or auditory apparitions at the transition be-tween sleep and wake); (3) sleep paralysis (a brief period of inability to move while drifting into or emerging from sleep); and (4) disrupted nocturnal sleep, often characterized by frequent awakenings. The first three of these phenomena can occur occasionally in normal individuals, but recurrent episodes are unusual outside of narcolepsy.

Hypersomnolence without hypocretin deficiency is a less well-understood disor-der that likely encompasses a heterogeneous group of pathophysiologic processes. Similar to narcolepsy, patients complain of difficulty staying awake, but this is not clearly related to REM sleep. Cataplexy and other ancillary symptoms are usually absent. The final disorder in this group – Kleine-Levin syndrome – is a rare condition characterized by recurrent episodes of hypersomnia, cognitive disturbance, hyperphagia, and/or hypersexuality. Adolescent males are most commonly affected.

Evaluation of the hypersomnolent patient should focus first on identifying any secondary cause of sleepiness (Figure 14.1). Sleep deprivation is much more common than disorders of increased sleep drive. This may be due to not allowing adequate time for sleep or due to another primary sleep disorder that interferes with sleep continuity. If these have been ruled out, hypersomnia should be evaluated using the Multiple Sleep Latency Test (MSLT). During an MSLT, the patient is given a series of five nap opportunities over the course of one day. A short latency to sleep (usually less than 5 minutes) and the onset of REM sleep during at least two of the five 15-minute naps is characteristic of narcolepsy, whereas short sleep latency without REM is suggestive of hypersomnolence without hypocretin deficiency.

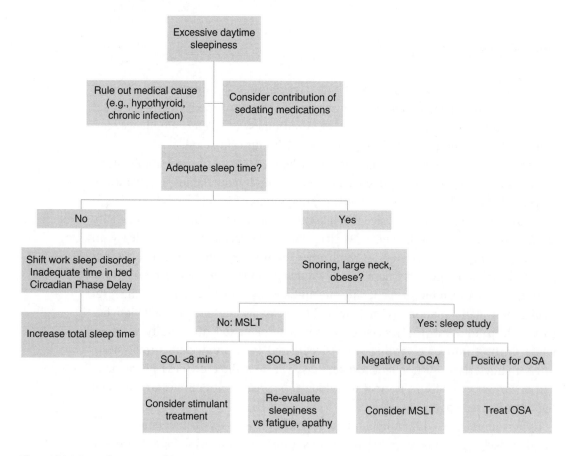

Figure 14.1 Secondary causes of insomnia

Narcolepsy typically requires pharmacologic treatment. Because daytime sleepiness is usually the most disabling symptom, the mainstay of treatment is a stimulant medication (e.g., modafinil, armodafinil, methylphenidate, amphetamine derivatives). In patients with frequent and bothersome cataplexy, REM suppression with the addition of an SSRI/SNRI is often effective. If daytime sleepiness and/or cataplexy persist despite these interventions (or if they are not well tolerated), sodium oxybate may be indicated. The mechanism of action of sodium oxybate in narcolepsy is poorly understood, but it can provide substantial relief for both daytime sleepiness and cataplexy in narcolepsy. Because of its short duration of action, sodium oxybate is usually administered twice per night. In the United States, it is distributed via a single central pharmacy and requires special registration to prescribe.

Circadian Rhythm Disorders

Circadian rhythm disorders arise from a mismatch between the endogenous circadian rhythm and the demands of the outside world. In some cases (e.g., advanced or delayed phase), the endogenous rhythm is "abnormal" compared to societal norms. In other cases, (e.g., jet lag or shift-work disorder), unusual demands are placed on an otherwise normally oscillating endogenous circadian rhythm. In both instances, the consequent misalignment of internal and external rhythms can result in adverse cognitive, physiologic, and emotional effects.

Delayed sleep phase disorder (DSPD) occurs in patients who are extreme "night-owls." They do not feel sleepy until 2:00–3:00 a.m., and if left to their own devices would sleep comfortably until 10:00–11:00 a.m. Often such individuals feel most productive in the late evening hours. The problem arises when they are required to adhere to a normal work or school schedule that requires them to be up by 6:00–8:00 a.m. Delayed circadian phase is common in young people and often becomes a problem when young adults finish college and join the workforce. On the opposite end of the spectrum, advanced sleep phase disorder (ASPD) generally occurs in older people who have difficulty remaining awake through the evening hours but wake up ready for the day at 3:00–4:00 a.m. Both advanced and delayed circadian phases are only considered disorders if the patient is dissatisfied with the pattern due to family or social demands or personal preference.

There are two main interventions that can shift endogenous circadian timing to help patients achieve their preferred schedule. Bright light is the most powerful treatment. The effect depends on when it is administered. Bright light in the morning shifts the endogenous rhythm earlier, while light in the evening pushes it later. Accordingly, patients with DSPD should be exposed to bright light in the morning and avoid light in the evening hours. The converse applies to ASPD patients in whom evening light is often the most effective therapy. Exogenous melatonin, although not as potent as light, can also be helpful when timed correctly. Melatonin is generally used to treat DSPD. When given approximately five hours before the natural bedtime, melatonin tends to shift the endogenous clock earlier.

Shift-work sleep disorder (SWSD) occurs when patients have insomnia or excessive daytime sleepiness that is temporally related to work scheduled during the usual sleep period. Although shift work universally produces circadian misalignment, a minority of individuals have extreme difficulty adapting (i.e., SWSD). Similarly, jet lag disorder occurs in those who have difficulty adjusting when traveling across time zones. There is no straightforward solution to either SWSD or jet lag. It is sometimes possible to strategize with the patient to adjust work or travel schedules to be less disruptive. For rotating shift workers, moving schedules in the clockwise direction is more likely to be tolerated; for overnight workers, it may be helpful to schedule a series of shifts in a row rather than shifting back-and-forth on a daily basis. Travelers trying to reduce jet lag should be advised to break up travel into multiple legs when possible or begin adjusting their bed and wake time toward appropriate times at their intended destination prior to travel. There are also more complex approaches utilizing strategically timed light, melatonin, and sleep scheduling.

Sleep-Related Breathing Disorder

Sleep-related breathing disorders include obstructive and central sleep apnea syndromes (OSA and CSA, respectively). Patients with OSA have repetitive partial or complete collapse of the upper airway during sleep, associated with oxygen desaturation and/or brief arousal from sleep. Common manifestations of OSA include loud snoring, witnessed apneas, dry mouth on awakening, difficulty with concentration, and/or excessive daytime sleepiness. The condition is more common in men, in overweight and obese patients, with advancing age, and in those with a small or posteriorly positioned mandible (micro/retrognathia). When untreated, OSA is associated with adverse cardiovascular (e.g., hypertension, atrial fibrillation), metabolic (e.g., insulin and leptin resistance), and neurocognitive (e.g., motor vehicle accidents, impaired work performance) consequences. Because OSA is a very common disorder with substantial repercussions and effective treatment, clinicians should have a low threshold to refer patients for testing (Figure 14.2).

Classically, evaluation of OSA involves overnight attended polysomnography in a sleep laboratory. Electroencephalogram, oro-nasal airflow, oxygen saturation, and abdominal respiratory effort are captured continuously throughout the night. Obstructive events are distinguished by absent or diminished airflow despite ongoing effort to breathe. The number of such events per hour of sleep is used to

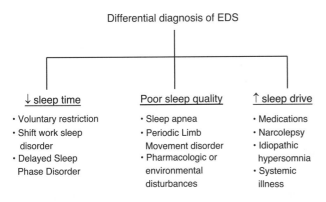

Differential diagnosis of EDS

↓ sleep time	Poor sleep quality	↑ sleep drive
• Voluntary restriction • Shift work sleep disorder • Delayed Sleep Phase Disorder	• Sleep apnea • Periodic Limb Movement disorder • Pharmacologic or environmental disturbances	• Medications • Narcolepsy • Idiopathic hypersomnia • Systemic illness

EDS, Excessive Daytime Sleepiness

Figure 14.2 Excessive daytime sleepiness

characterize the severity of OSA. In recent years, home sleep apnea testing (HSAT) using limited channels (usually airflow, oxygen saturation, and respiratory effort) has become more common for economic reasons. Although not as informative, HSTs are often sufficient to diagnose OSA. The treatment of choice for OSA is continuous positive airway pressure (CPAP), delivered by a bedside device that blows air in the upper airway through a mask placed over the nose and/or mouth. The air pressure stents open the upper airway to prevent collapse. For patients who decline or do not tolerate CPAP, an oral appliance for mandibular advancement or upper airway surgery can sometimes be beneficial. In addition, weight-loss counseling is appropriate for overweight or obese patients with sleep apnea.

Central sleep apnea involves the failure of neurons in the CNS to activate phrenic and intercostal muscles to generate a regular pattern of breathing. In contrast to obstructive events, central apneas are detected on polysomnography as absent airflow concomitant with an absent effort to breathe. Central sleep apnea may be an effect of medications (e.g., opioids) or may be associated with cardiac or neurologic disease. CSA should prompt a search for one of these causes, since primary CSA is rare. Treatment may involve CPAP or other advanced PAP devices.

References and Suggested Readings

* Aurora, R. N., Kristo, D. A., Bista, S. R., et al. (2012). The Treatment of Restless Legs Syndrome and Periodic Limb Movement Disorder in Adults – An Update for 2012: Practice Parameters with an Evidence-Based Systematic Review and Meta-Analyses: An American Academy of Sleep Medicine Clinical Practice Guideline. *Sleep*, 35 (8), 1039–1062.
* Buysse, D. J. (2013). Insomnia. *JAMA*, 309 (7), 706–716.

- Mignot, E. J. M. (2012). A Practical Guide to the Therapy of Narcolepsy and Hypersomnia Syndromes. *Neurotherapeutics*, 9(4):739–752.
- Rice, T. B., Strollo, P. J., and Morrell, M. J. (2011). Update in Sleep Medicine. *Am J Respir Crit Care Med*, 185 (12), 1271–1274.
- Winkelman, J. W., and Plante, D. T. (2010). *Foundations of Psychiatric Sleep Medicine*. Cambridge: Cambridge University Press.

Self-Assessment Questions

1. Which of the following sleep disorders typically has onset in childhood?
   A. Restless leg syndrome
   B. Sleep terror disorder
   C. REM behavior disorder
   D. Advanced sleep phase disorder

2. Which of the following is characterized as a parasomnia?
   A. Insomnia
   B. Obstructive sleep apnea
   C. Restless legs syndrome
   D. Narcolepsy
   E. Somnambulism

3. Which of the following is not indicated in the treatment of chronic insomnia?
   A. Cognitive-behavioral therapy (CBT)
   B. Zolpidem
   C. Trazodone
   D. Modafinil
   E. Ramelteon

4. Which of the following is not true of obstructive sleep apnea syndrome?
   A. Most common in older, overweight males
   B. Associated with an increased risk for hypertension and atrial fibrillation
   C. Rare disorder (<1 percent of the population)
   D. Best evaluation method is overnight polysomnography
   E. Treatment of choice is continuous positive airway pressure (CPAP)

5. Mr. C is a fifty-six-year-old divorced man who comes to his internist with complaints of poor concentration, daytime sleepiness, and increasing difficulty doing his job as an accountant. He finds himself making calculation errors and forgetting important tasks at work. His mood is generally good, though he sometimes finds himself irritable at work and down when he thinks about the difficulties he is having. The patient is 5 foot 10 inches with a weight of 260 pounds and a BMI of 37.3, placing him in the obese range. His medical history is significant for a 5-year history of hypertension well

controlled on medications. His alcohol intake is one to two glasses of beer or wine two to three days per week, most often on the weekends.

Which of the following is the most likely diagnosis in this patient?

A. Major depressive disorder
B. Restless leg syndrome
C. Obstructive sleep apnea
D. Shift-work sleep disorder
E. Alcohol abuse

Answers to Self-Assessment Questions

1. (B)
2. (E)
3. (D)
4. (C)
5. (C)

15 | Psychopharmacology and Neurotherapeutics

STEVEN SEINER, ROSS BALDESSARINI, JOAN CAMPRODON, DARIN
DOUGHERTY, LIOR GIVON, JEFFREY DEVIDO, AND JONATHAN E. ALPERT

Antidepressants

Background

Antidepressants are among the most widely prescribed medicines in the United States, particularly in psychiatry and primary care medicine. According to the US Centers for Disease Control, approximately 13 percent of the US population aged twelve years or older were prescribed an antidepressant in a recent year. Although antidepressants may be overprescribed in some patient populations and underprescribed in others, the overall high rate of antidepressant use is almost certainly related to the high prevalence of the conditions for which antidepressants are clinically indicated and approved by the US Food and Drug Administration (FDA). These conditions include major depressive disorder, generalized anxiety disorder, panic disorder, social anxiety disorder, obsessive-compulsive disorder, and posttraumatic stress disorder. In addition, certain antidepressants are used in the treatment of pain syndromes (e.g., fibromyalgia, migraine, or neuropathic pain), bulimia nervosa, binge eating disorder, premenstrual symptoms, somatic symptom disorders, irritable bowel syndrome, insomnia, and body dysmorphic disorder, as well as to help individuals quit smoking.

The first antidepressants of the modern era – tricyclic antidepressants and monoamine oxidase (MAO) inhibitors – were discovered by Serendipity in the 1950s. In the years that followed, it became apparent that all established antidepressants shared pharmacological activity on the monoamine neurotransmitter systems, particularly those mediated by serotonin and norepinephrine and, to a lesser extent, dopamine. This recognition largely drove subsequent drug development strategies until recently. Use of the older antidepressants has been limited by problematic adverse effects, drug interactions, and potential lethality in overdose. Research in the 1970s and 1980s yielded generally safer agents that represent current first-line medications for depression and anxiety. These pharmacotherapies are used either alone (monotherapy) or in conjunction with established forms of psychotherapy, including cognitive-behavioral, dialectical-behavioral, and psychodynamic approaches. For patients with relatively severe or otherwise treatment-resistant forms of depression, medication is sometimes coupled with neurostimulation approaches as well, particularly electroconvulsive therapy (ECT) or repetitive transcranial magnetic stimulation (rTMS).

Antidepressants can have dramatic and life-saving benefits for some patients, but meta-analyses of randomized, placebo-controlled antidepressant trials consistently show relatively small or moderate effect-sizes or drug-placebo differences. The small and variable effect-sizes of antidepressants probably reflects the considerable heterogeneity among patients diagnosed with major depressive disorder. Only about 1 in 3 patients respond to the first antidepressant they receive, even with increased doses. Some may respond to a different antidepressant, and multiple trials or even drug combinations are not uncommon.

Initial benefit from an antidepressant usually is not evident for two to four weeks after achieving an adequate dose, and full effects may require six to twelve weeks of sustained treatment. Owing to the frequent need to try more than one treatment, it often takes several months to determine whether antidepressant treatment works well for a particular patient. To deal with the heterogeneity of antidepressant responses, current research aims to identify clinically useful predictors. Some promising candidate predictors include pharmacogenomic data, neuroimaging patterns, or inflammatory markers, as well as clinical phenotypes. For the most part, such efforts have had limited success, though efforts to identify reliable predictors of response to antidepressants do and should continue.

Although all FDA-approved antidepressants interact with brain monoamine systems, many complex, secondary neurobiological effects of the drugs have been identified, and precise neurobiological mechanisms through which antidepressants alleviate depression or anxiety largely remain unknown. The observation that antidepressants have immediate effects on monoamine neurotransmission, including blockade of their inactivation by neuronal uptake or transport, but delayed effects on clinical symptoms suggest that the most relevant physiological mechanisms may be "downstream" from monoamine synapses and possibly slowly evolving. Some leading hypotheses concerning antidepressant mechanisms focus on neuroplasticity, inflammation, and brain energy metabolism. In addition, a number of promising investigational antidepressants appear to interact with the glutamate, GABA, and opioid systems rather than the monoamine systems, suggesting new avenues through which depression and anxiety conditions might be helped. Indeed, as noted later in this chapter, some of these agents, such as esketamine, have rapid effects on individuals who respond to them, with relief seen within hours to days rather than weeks.

Classification

Antidepressants have traditionally been classified according to their chemical structure (e.g., tricyclics [TCAs]) or mechanisms of action (e.g., monoamine oxidase inhibitors [MAOIs], selective serotonin reuptake inhibitors [SSRIs]).

The major classes of antidepressants in current use in the United States are as follows. The generic name of each medication is followed by the initial brand name in parentheses:

Selective Serotonin Reuptake Inhibitors (SSRIs)

- Citalopram (Celexa)
- Escitalopram (Lexapro)
- Fluoxetine (Prozac)
- Fluvoxamine (Luvox; FDA-approved for anxiety disorders but not depression)
- Paroxetine (Paxil)
- Sertraline (Zoloft)

All of these agents (except fluvoxamine) are FDA-approved for major depressive disorder; most are also approved for different forms of anxiety, including generalized and social anxiety disorders, and some for posttraumatic stress disorder (PTSD) and bulimia or binge eating disorder. Fluvoxamine is FDA-approved only for obsessive-compulsive disorder, though it is used to treat depression in other countries. No particular SSRI appears to be more effective than another for major depressive disorder (or anxiety conditions). Nevertheless, an individual patient may respond to or tolerate one SSRI better than another. For this reason, it is not uncommon to try a second SSRI even when a first has been unsuccessful.

Serotonin and Norepinephrine Reuptake Inhibitors

- Desvenlafaxine (Pristiq)
- Duloxetine (Cymbalta)
- Levomilnacipran (Fetzima)
- Venlafaxine (Effexor)

Like the SSRIs, the SNRIs are effective for major depressive disorder and for many anxiety disorders. In addition, agents that work on both serotonin and norepinephrine appear to be more effective for pain syndromes than are agents acting on serotonin only. These serotonin and norepinephrine reuptake inhibiting agents include both the newer SNRIs and the older tricyclic antidepressants (TCAs) such as amitriptyline (Elavil). For patients with depression or anxiety that is comorbid with pain syndromes such as fibromyalgia, SNRIs, or TCAs are considered the antidepressants of choice.

Norepinephrine and Dopamine Reuptake Inhibitor (NDRI)

- Bupropion (Wellbutrin, Zyban)

Among contemporary antidepressants, the only norepinephrine and dopamine reuptake inhibitor is the mild stimulant-anorexic agent bupropion. As the sole FDA-approved antidepressant devoid of serotoninergic activity bupropion is particularly well suited for individuals who have difficulty tolerating serotonin-related side effects, particularly sexual dysfunction. In addition, bupropion is the only antidepressant with demonstrated efficacy for smoking cessation. When used for this purpose, it is often prescribed in conjunction with nicotine replacement therapies and behavioral strategies. Bupropion also has some effectiveness for attention deficit hyperactivity disorder and is, therefore, one of the medication options for patients with ADHD who do not tolerate the more widely prescribed psychostimulants or whose risk for addiction may preclude the use of controlled substances. Unlike SSRIs or SNRIs, bupropion is not FDA indicated for the treatment of anxiety disorders; it is believed that serotonergic properties are required for an antidepressant to exert optimal anti-anxiety effects.

Miscellaneous Modern Antidepressants

- Mirtazapine (Remeron)
- Trazodone (Desyrel)
- Vilazodone (Viibryd)
- Vortioxetine (Trintellix)

Although these agents differ in molecular structure and pharmacological properties, they all share some effects on neurotransmission mediated by serotonin and norepinephrine. However, unlike the SSRIs and SNRIs, they have complex activities other than inhibition of neurotransmitter reuptake. At low doses, trazodone is also used as a non-addictive hypnotic agent. Another agent in this group, nefazodone (Serzone) is no longer used clinically, owing to high risk of liver toxicity.

Tricyclic Antidepressants (TCAs)

- Amitriptyline (Elavil)
- Clomipramine (Anafranil)
- Desipramine (Norpramin)
- Doxepin (Sinequan)
- Imipramine (Tofranil)
- Protriptyline (Vivactil)
- Nortriptyline (Pamelor)
- Trimipramine (Surmontil)

Prior to the introduction of the SSRIs in the late 1980s, the tricyclics, and particularly amitriptyline, were the most widely prescribed antidepressants. While the TCAs, like the SNRIs, block the neuronal reuptake of serotonin and norepinephrine, they also interact with other sites including adrenergic, histamine, and muscarinic receptors. These activities contribute to a variety of adverse effects, including drowsiness, dry mouth, blurred vision, constipation, weight gain, and hypotension. Notably, the TCAs also have quinidine-like depressant effects on cardiac conduction, and can induce potentially fatal arrhythmias, particularly in overdose or with preexisting cardiac conduction problems. Another unique aspect of the TCAs is that several commonly used TCAs have quite well established therapeutically optimal and safe serum concentrations that can be used for therapeutic monitoring.

Monoamine Oxidase Inhibitors (MAOIs)

- Isocarboxazid (Marplan)
- Phenelzine (Nardil)
- Selegiline (EMSAM)
- Tranylcypromine (Parnate)

MAOIs, like other antidepressants, enhance monoamine neurotransmission by interfering with monoamine metabolism, in this case by the enzyme MAO rather than blocking neuronal reuptake or by acting directly on monoamine receptors. MAO exists in two molecular forms, MAO-A and MAO-B. Type B is found in the liver and platelets, whereas MAO-A is typical of nerve terminals. At low doses, selegiline preferentially inhibits MAO-A, but at higher doses it inhibits both MAO-A and B. Blocking the catabolism of serotonin and norepinephrine appears to be relevant to its antidepressant efficacy. Other MAOIs block MAO-A and B at therapeutic doses and are more likely to induce potentially fatal hypertensive crises when taken with an indirect sympathomimetic amines such as tyramine (in cheese and other fermented foods) or neosynephrine. For this reason, MAOIs are used cautiously, with a diet that excludes tyramine and other sympathomimetic agents, and generally are reserved for individuals with severe depression unresponsive to other agents. Selegiline is available in transdermal (skin patch) form, whereas the other MAOIs are available for oral administration only.

MAOIs may be superior to TCAs for individuals with a type of depression known as "atypical depression," characterized by carbohydrate craving, oversleeping, temporary mood improvement after positive events ("mood reactivity"), and mood decline in the setting of perceived rejection or criticism ("rejection sensitivity"). These observations support a preference for MAOIs over TCAs for atypical depression, although SSRIs and SNRIs are more often used initially for their greater safety.

Adverse Effects of Antidepressants

Adverse effects associated with antidepressant treatment are summarized in Table 15.1. Despite the efficacy of most antidepressants in the treatment of anxiety disorders, paradoxically, transient "jitteriness" or increased anxiety is a common adverse effect during the first few days of treatment. Similarly, some patients experience insomnia or interrupted sleep as well as gastrointestinal symptoms, particularly mild nausea. These symptoms are also often, but not always, temporary and

Table 15.1 Adverse effects of antidepressants

Agents	Adverse effects
Tricyclic-type agents (TCAs)	
Amitriptyline, imipramine, doxepin	Anticholinergic-cognitive effects, hypotension, cardiac depressant, leukopenia
Amoxapine	Extrapyramidal symptoms, tardive dyskinesia, seizures (rare)
Clomipramine	Sedation, nausea, anticholinergic, cardiac depressant, hemolysis (rare)
Maprotiline	Seizures (high doses), rashes
Protriptyline	Agitation, photosensitivity
Monoamine-oxidase (MAO) inhibitors	
Phenelzine, tranylcypromine	Hypotension, mild hypertension, sexual dysfunction, hepatotoxicity (rare); severe hypertension with pressor amines, serotonin syndrome with serotonergic agents (SSRIs, meperidine, dextromethorphan)
Moclobemide	Less pressor risk, possible serotonin syndrome with other serotonergics
Selegiline	Less pressor risk at low doses, some risk of serotonin syndrome
St. John's wort	Possible serotonin syndrome with other serotonergics
Serotonin reuptake inhibitors (SSRIs) and serotonin-norepinephrine reuptake inhibitors (SNRIs)	
Citalopram, duloxetine, fluoxetine, sertraline, venlafaxine, and others	Nausea (especially early)
	Anorgasmia (men and women)
	Increased levels of other drugs
	Serotonin syndrome (with MAOIs)
	Withdrawal syndrome (high with paroxetine, venlafaxine; least with fluoxetine)
	Variable agitation/insomnia/lethargy
	Bleeding (platelet dysfunction, especially with NSAIDs or aspirin)
	QTc prolongation (mostly citalopram and fluoxetine)
	Neonatal distress (low Apgar, respiratory)
	Teratogenic risk low
Atypical antidepressants	
Bupropion	Seizures (high doses), stimulation, insomnia, anorexia, relatively low risk of manic-switching
Mirtazapine	Sedation, leukopenia (rare)
Trazodone	Sedation, hypotension, priapism

self-limiting. A more persistent increase in sweating, particularly night sweats, is not uncommon, particularly with the SNRIs.

Antidepressants also can be associated with mild hand tremor, which is particularly noticeable with arms outstretched or bringing a cup or spoon to one's mouth. This kind of tremor is distinct from the Parkinsonian resting (or "pill rolling") tremor associated with antipsychotic drugs or other antidopamine drugs. With the exception of bupropion and fluoxetine, many antidepressants are associated with modest to moderate weight gain, though with considerable variation across individual patients. Contemporary antidepressants particularly likely to cause weight gain include mirtazapine and paroxetine. TCAs and MAOIs also can cause weight gain. Drowsiness is common with some antidepressants, including mirtazapine, paroxetine, and trazodone, and most TCAs, particularly doxepin and amitriptyline.

All antidepressants with serotonergic activity can cause sexual dysfunction. Sexual side effects usually involve delayed ejaculation in men, diminished lubrication in women, and difficulty achieving orgasm. Decreased libido is also common. Since depression itself may reduce libido and sexual interest and performance, the net result of an antidepressant on sexual function may be positive as the depression lifts. The prevalence of sexual dysfunction during treatment with a serotonergic agent is as high as 30 to 60 percent. As a non-serotonergic agent, bupropion is especially unlikely to be associated with sexual dysfunction.

Anticholinergic (antimuscarinic) effects of antidepressants, particularly the TCAs, are associated with potential dry mouth, constipation, urinary retention, blurred vision, and memory impairment. These drugs should be dosed with care in older patients, particularly those with prostatic hypertrophy or mild cognitive impairment. In addition, TCAs can cause acute elevation of ocular pressure in patients with narrow-angle glaucoma.

Orthostatic hypotension can occur during treatment with trazodone or a TCA or MAOI. This is a particular concern in older patients vulnerable to falls. Clinicians often advise patients at risk to rise slowly after sitting and to dangle their feet at the edge of the bed for a few moments before standing.

When antidepressants are stopped abruptly, patients may experience discontinuation or withdrawal symptoms which, though not dangerous, can be highly distressing. Symptoms range from nausea, muscle aches, and tearfulness to unusual perceptual experiences such as sudden "zapping" sensations in one's scalp. The SSRIs, SNRIs, and especially paroxetine are particularly prone to cause these side effects, though they may occur upon sudden discontinuation of any antidepressant. Fluoxetine, by virtue of its very long half-life, is the least likely to cause discontinuation symptoms. The risk of discontinuation symptoms can be greatly reduced by slowly reducing the dose of antidepressants or switching to fluoxetine, although for some patients, discontinuing remains difficult. These withdrawal reactions are to be distinguished from high rates of early relapse into depression that follow abrupt or rapid discontinuation of antidepressant treatment.

Antidepressant-Related Emergencies
Although newer antidepressants have a high margin of safety, even in overdose, both newer and older antidepressants are associated with rare but life-threatening emergencies that all prescribers and users of antidepressants must be aware of. They include the following:

- *Mania*: While treating depression, antidepressants can activate manic or hypo-manic behavior in predisposed individuals. Such symptoms include decreased need for sleep, increased activity, racing thoughts, intense irritability, pressured speech, impulsive behavior, grandiose thinking, and even psychotic symptoms such as paranoia or hallucinations. Prior to prescribing an antidepressant to a depressed or anxious patient, inquiry about prior symptoms suggestive of bipolar disorder as well as relevant family history is crucial. Since antidepressants may precipitate manic symptoms in patients with no previous history suggestive of bipolar disorder, it is crucial to monitor all depressed patients closely for manic symptoms during the initial weeks of treatment, and to avoid antidepressants when *mixed* (hypomanic with depressive) features are present. Although antidepressants may precipitate mania and are not proved to be effective for bipolar depression, they are sometimes used in the treatment of depression in bipolar disorder. However, when doing so, the bipolar disorder is first treated with adequate doses of a mood-stabilizing agent or second-generation antipsychotic drug and patients must be monitored particularly closely for exacerbation manic symptoms or increased frequency of mood episodes (rapid cycling). The actual added risk of such mood-switching during antidepressant treatment is difficult to quantify, especially as risks of spontaneous emergence of mania among bipolar disorder patients are already quite high.
- *Suicidal ideation*: Although antidepressants generally reduce suicidal ideation along with other core depressive symptoms, a small number of patients appear to experience a paradoxical increase in suicidal thoughts, usually during the initial days or weeks of treatment. This reaction has been found most often among adolescents and young adults and may be associated with undiagnosed bipolar disorder in this age group. Since 2004, the FDA has required a so-called black box warning about this potential risk in pediatric patients and those below age twenty-five. This warning was followed by a temporary decrease in the diagnosis of major depression in juveniles and in prescribing of antidepressants, with concern about potentially increased risks of suicidal behavior due to inadequate treatment of depression. The possibility of an increase in suicidal thoughts early in antidepressant treatment warrants close monitoring, and the risk can be managed by reducing the dose of antidepressant or adding a mood stabilizer, antipsychotic, or sedative.
- *Cardiac arrhythmias*: Among their complex pharmacological effects, the TCAs have quinidine-like effects that slow cardiac conduction (QTc prolongation >500 msec) and increase the risk of life-threatening ventricular arrhythmias such as torsades de pointes, particularly in the setting of overdose. To a lesser extent, other antidepressants including trazodone, citalopram, and escitalopram may be associated with the risk of arrhythmia at high doses.
- *Seizures*: Most antidepressants lower the seizure threshold. This is particularly true of bupropion as well as clomipramine, which should be avoided or used

with expert consultation in patients at high risk for seizures such as those with brain lesions, head trauma, active eating disorders, or prior seizures.

- *Priapism*: Some antidepressants, most notably trazodone, have been associated with sustained, painful erection requiring emergency treatment to avoid penile damage. This uncommon adverse reaction has an incidence of approximately 1 in 6,000 men receiving trazodone.

- *Hypertensive crisis*: Use of MAOIs with sympathomimetic agents such as amphetamines, cocaine, or even over-the-counter decongestants such as pseudoephedrine or oxymetazoline can produce an abrupt, extreme elevation of blood pressure, often accompanied by notable symptoms such as severe headache, nausea, vomiting, confusion, or nosebleeds. Hypertensive crises are a potentially life-threatening emergency requiring immediate medical attention. In addition, because the MAO enzymes exist not only in the brain but in the gastrointestinal tract and liver, ingestion of foods that contain pressor amines, such as tyramine, typically inactivated in the gut and liver, also can produce hypertensive reactions in patients taking an MAOI. This effect is sometimes referred to as the "cheese reaction" as aged and fermented products are particularly likely to contain pressor amines. These include aged cheese, smoked, pickled or cured meats, draft beer, certain soy and yeast products, and overripened fruits, including bananas. For this reason, only patients who can reliably avoid such foods and drugs are candidates for treatment with MAOIs.

- *Serotonin syndrome*: High doses of serotonergic agents or, more commonly, combinations of highly serotonergic agents may lead to serotonin toxicity. Extreme toxicity can present clinically as "serotonin syndrome," which is characterized by clonus (involuntary rhythmic muscle contractions, such as at the ankle or arm), agitation, confusion, tremor, and potential fatality. The symptoms of serotonin syndrome overlap with those of neuroleptic malignant syndrome (NMS), which is related to the use of antipsychotic drugs. Both can be broadly considered forms of cerebral intoxication. However, muscle rigidity and fever traditionally have been more common with NMS than serotonin syndrome. Abnormal laboratory values are also more common with NMS than serotonin syndrome, including elevated white blood cell count and increased serum concentrations of the muscle enzyme, creatine kinase (CK). However, some of the classic features of NMS (marked muscle rigidity, elevation of creatine kinase and myoglobin) may not occur with intoxications associated with some modern antipsychotic drugs such as clozapine. As with NMS, there is no definitive treatment for serotonin syndrome other than immediate cessation of the offending drugs and supportive care, often requiring an intensive medical care setting. Although most serotonergic agents have been implicated in serotonin syndrome, the combination of MAOIs with highly serotonergic agents such as SSRIs or SNRIS, is particularly dangerous and should be considered absolutely contraindicated. Furthermore, certain opioid painkillers exert serotonin activity – in particular, meperidine (Demerol) and the antitussive agent dextromethorphan – should never be combined with an MAOI due to the significant risk of serotonin syndrome-like intoxication.

Selecting an Antidepressant

Given generally indistinguishable efficacy among antidepressants, the selection of a first antidepressant usually is based on side-effect profile, co-occurring conditions, prior responses to similar agents, and cost. For most uncomplicated depression or anxiety conditions for which antidepressants are approved, the SSRIs or SNRIs are reasonable initial agents. For comorbid pain conditions, the SNRIs (and tertiary-amine TCAs) appear to be more effective than the SSRIs. With co-occurring tobacco smoking or attention disorder (ADHD), bupropion as a mild stimulant may be advantageous, though less likely to benefit anxiety disorders. Bupropion may also be a good choice for patients who have experienced sexual dysfunction when taking a serotonergic agent. Because of the greater risk of adverse effects, drug interactions, and potentially fatal overdoses, the TCAs and MAOIs are usually reserved for patients whose conditions have not responded satisfactorily to one or more modern antidepressants.

Treatment Duration

For a first time, mild to moderate episode of major depressive disorder, antidepressant treatment usually is continued for six to nine months after depression has fully remitted, so as to get past the period of risk as indicated by the typical duration of an untreated depressive episode. As it often takes at least three months to achieve remission, the full course of antidepressant treatment is often a year or more. For individuals with more severe episodes of depression, such as those associated with significant work disability, suicide attempts, or psychotic symptoms, treatment is often extended for two to three years or longer. Long-term or "maintenance" antidepressant treatment is also used for patients with repeated episodes of depression in an effort to reduce the risk of recurrence and extend periods of wellness. For patients receiving maintenance treatment, its duration becomes an individualized decision in which the prescribing clinician and patient balance adverse effects and cost against the potential consequences of recurrences. Anxiety conditions treated with antidepressants, such as generalized anxiety disorder or social phobia, or with OCD, often are persistent, and several years of treatment may be warranted, particularly if treatment is helpful and well tolerated. As with depression, decisions about the duration of antidepressant treatment for anxiety are based on an individualized risk/benefit assessment, and should be reviewed regularly. Psychotherapy such as cognitive behavior therapy (CBT), when combined with an antidepressant, typically yields better outcomes than pharmacotherapy alone and probably reduces the risk of relapses and recurrences.

Treatment Resistance

As many as two out of three depressed patients do not respond to an initial antidepressant treatment, and as many as one in three remain symptomatic despite two or more antidepressant trials. Depression that has failed to respond to several adequate trials of treatment is referred to as "treatment-resistant depression" (TRD), though the precise definition varies. For such patients, it is very important to review basic information, including the diagnosis, the presence of other psychiatric, medical, or substance abuse disorders, adequacy of dosing, and the presence of other substances that may alter the clearance of an antidepressant, and to evaluate the patient's adherence to treatment. Repeated trials of similar medicines are unlikely to prove fruitful, but second and third trials with pharmacologically dissimilar agents may help, especially if doses are increased as tolerated. If that approach fails, it is not unusual to combine two antidepressants with complementary mechanisms, such as an SSRI with an NDRI (bupropion). Another strategy involves combining an antidepressant at an adequate dose with a potentiating agent. Some second-generation antipsychotics (notably, aripiprazole, quetiapine, and brexpiprazole) are the only agents specifically FDA-approved for antidepressant augmentation along with the combination of olanzapine and fluoxetine. However, other agents, including lithium, lamotrigine, thyroid hormone, dopamine agonists, and folic acid, have also been used as antidepressant boosters. For treatment-resistant anxiety disorders, other classes of medicines are sometimes considered, including benzodiazepines, some anticonvulsants (e.g., gabapentin, pregabalin, valproate), beta-adrenergic antagonists (e.g., propranolol), alpha-2 adrenergic agonists (e.g., clonidine), buspirone, and second-generation antipsychotics.

Rapid-Acting Antidepressants

An exciting recent development in the field of depression treatment has been the development of drugs that work through novel neural mechanisms not directly related to the potentiation of monoamine neurotransmitters; some exert remarkably rapid antidepressant effects. Two such agents were FDA-approved for depression in 2019: intranasal esketamine (Spravato) for adults with treatment-resistant depression, and brexanolone (Zulresso) for women with postpartum depression. Racemic ketamine, usually given intravenously in doses of about 0.5 mg/kg, had previously been found to have rapid antidepressant effects, and this widely used animal anesthetic agent, which acts as an antagonist of the N-methyl-D-aspartic acid (NMDA) type of excitatory glutamate receptor, has been used clinically to treat TRD on an off-label basis. An isomer of racemic R,S-ketamine, esketamine, is administered by nasal spray as it is not well absorbed through the GI tract. Racemic and esketamine can cause temporary dissociative reactions, agitation, elevated blood pressure, and, rarely, psychosis, especially at relatively high doses.

In addition, esketamine has the potential for misuse as a recreational agent. For these reasons, the FDA has required that esketamine be administered only in clinical settings rather than at home and that patients be monitored closely for several hours after dosing, as is also the standard practice with racemic ketamine. Esketamine is typically administered between twice a week to every two weeks, usually along with a standard oral antidepressant. The long-term risks of repeated administration of esketamine require further study, as do suggestions from studies of racemic ketamine that the agent may reduce suicidal thinking along with improving mood.

Brexanolone is a synthetic analogue of the naturally occurring neurosteroid, allopregnanolone. Brexanolone is a modulator of the inhibitory amino acid gamma-aminobutyric acid (GABA) receptor GABA-A. As with ketamine, the gastrointestinal absorption of brexanolone is poor, leading to its administration by intravenous infusion. A typical course of brexanolone involves a 60-hour infusion in a clinical setting with close monitoring. Adverse effects include drowsiness, dizziness, and occasional loss of consciousness. For individuals who experience benefit from esketamine or brexanolone, initial relief from depressive symptoms is often experienced within hours to days compared with weeks or longer with standard antidepressants. Though complicated by side effects, the need for parenteral administration, and high cost, the availability of these agents heralds a new era of antidepressant treatment, possibly of particular value for very severe depression and TRD.

Antipsychotic Drugs

Introduction

The era of effective pharmacological treatment for mania and psychotic disorders started with the discovery of antimanic and antipsychotic properties of the phenothiazine chlorpromazine in Paris in 1952. Its clinical effects included abnormalities of posture and movement, supporting the term "neuroleptic" to imply having broad effects on the nervous system. Many corporations responded to this important discovery by developing similar compounds. Older ("typical" or "first-generation") antipsychotics include phenothiazines (e.g., chlorpromazine, fluphenazine, perphenazine, thioridazine, trifluoperazine), thioxanthenes (e.g., thiothixene), phenylpiperidines (e.g., haloperidol, pimozide), and dibenzapines (e.g., loxapine). Most modern ("second-generation") antipsychotics (Figure 15.1) mimic the structure or actions of the highly effective dibenzapine clozapine, including potent antagonism of central serotonin $5HT_2$ receptors as well as some antagonism at central dopamine D_2 receptors.

Second-Generation

Clozapine

Olanzapine

Risperidone

Iloperidone

Aripiprazole

Paliperidone

Brexpiprazole

(A typical) Antipsychotics

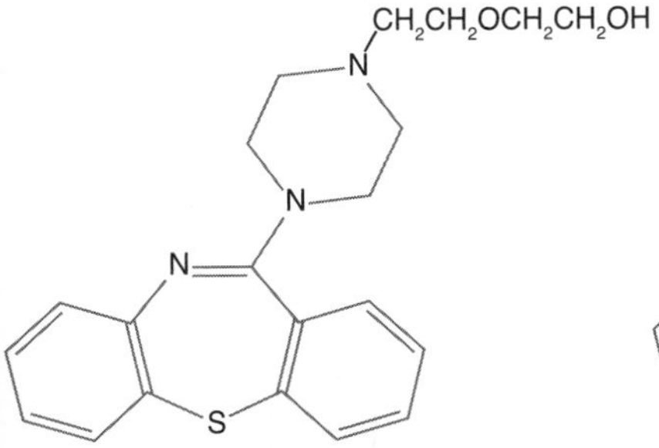

Quetiapine

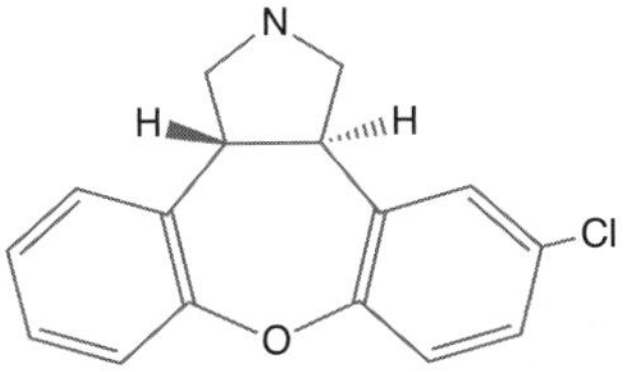

Asenapine

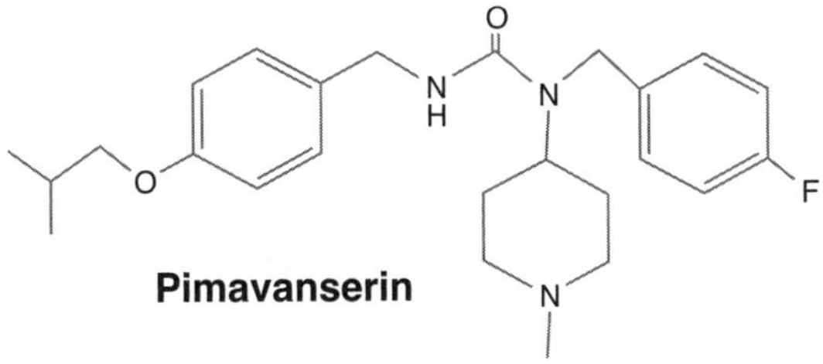

Pimavanserin

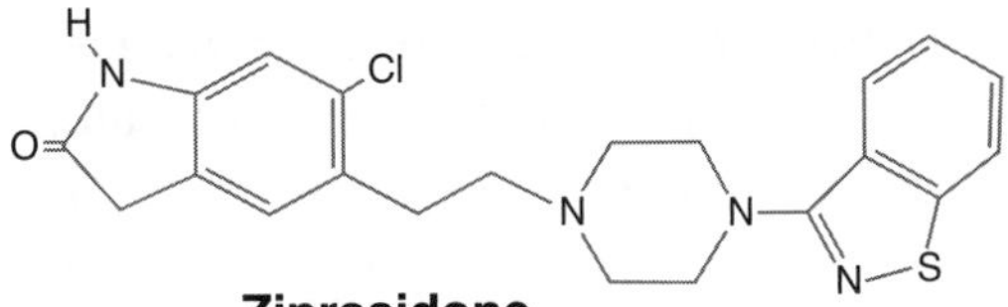

Ziprasidone

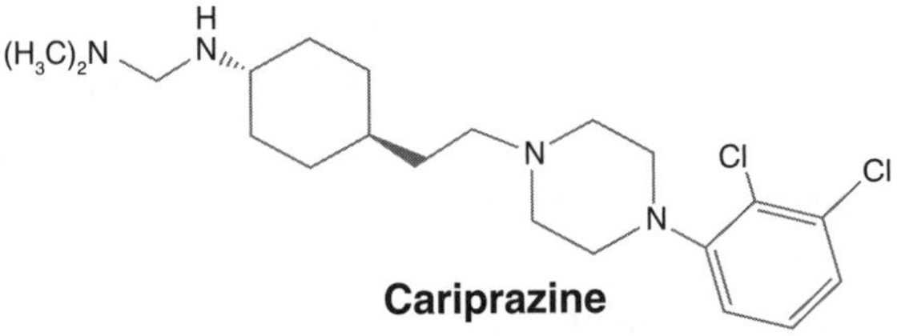

Cariprazine

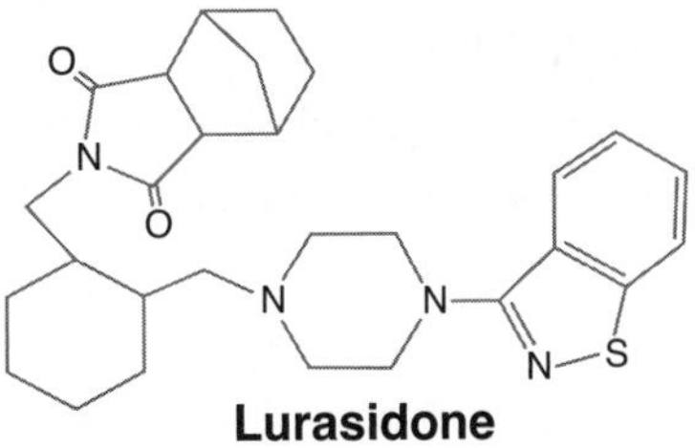

Lurasidone

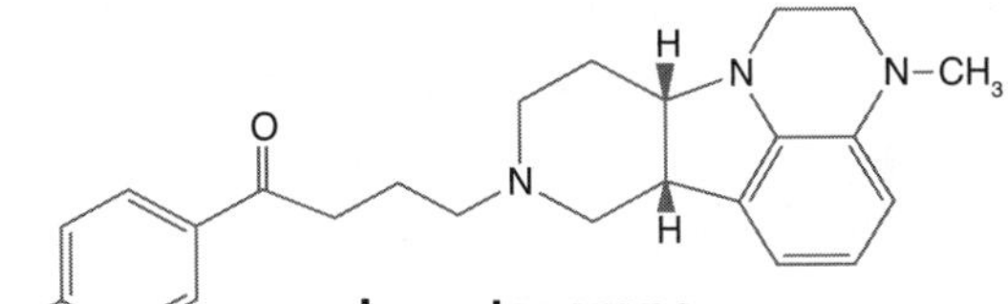

Lumateperone

Figure 15.1 Second-generation (atypical) antipsychotics

Antipsychotics are not specific for schizophrenia, and are particularly efficacious for acute psychotic disorders and mania, with some benefit in organic mental syndromes marked by agitation and psychotic features, as well as having adjunctive uses in severe depression. In addition, perhaps 60 percent or more of their usage is not FDA-approved ("off-label") for conditions other than psychoses, indicating broad clinical utility and diagnostic nonspecificity.

Antipsychotic drugs include rapidly orally dissolving preparations (for aripiprazole, clozapine, olanzapine, risperidone) that facilitate rapid responses for patients too confused to swallow pills reliably, and short-acting injectable forms (aripiprazole, olanzapine, risperidone, ziprasidone). Half-life averages approximately twenty-four hours, but butyrophenones have much slower tissue-elimination. Long-acting injected preparations are usually given every two to four weeks. They include slowly hydrolyzed decanoate esters of fluphenazine and haloperidol, risperidone in biodegradable carbohydrate microspheres, the palmitate ester of paliperidone, a pamoate complex of olanzapine, as well as a hydrate preparation and lauroxil ester of aripiprazole. Serum assays of most antipsychotics have not proved useful to guide dosing and safety in routine clinical practice.

Antipsychotics palliate acute psychotic symptoms, hasten remission, and limit risk of future exacerbations when continued in maintenance treatment of chronic or recurring psychoses. However, improvements in overall prognosis and functional outcomes in schizophrenia are limited and inconsistent. Controlled trials yield overlapping statistical confidence-intervals of pooled response rates for most antipsychotics, making secure ranking by efficacy difficult. Combinations of antipsychotics are unlikely to provide superior benefits or safety. Differences in adverse-effect risks (tolerability) and cost can usefully guide individual treatment-selection. Risks include neurological reactions with older, especially potent neuroleptics, whereas low-potency older neuroleptics as well as clozapine, olanzapine, and quetiapine are more likely to induce excessive sedative, hypotensive, and weight gain or metabolic effects (Table 15.2).

Short-Term Antipsychotic Treatment

Short-term applications are broad, and include neuromedical conditions as well as acute, primary psychotic illnesses, mania, exacerbations of chronic psychoses, and usually adjunctively in severe, psychotic, or bipolar depression. Research support for many short-term applications is remarkably limited. Basic questions pertaining to the process and time-course of recovery, optimal dosing, and the efficacy and tolerability of specific agents in specific subgroups of patients remain unanswered. Rapid, largely nonspecific sedating effects of antipsychotics occur early in the treatment of agitated, sleepless, anxious, and sometimes aggressive psychotic or manic patients; these can be enhanced with sedatives (e.g., clonazepam, lorazepam). Improvements in irrational thinking and abnormal sensations ("positive

Table 15.2 Properties of clinically employed antipsychotic drugs

Drug	Brand	Half-life (hrs)	Doses (mg/day)		Injectable	Preferred CYP	Adverse effect risks		
			Typical	Extreme			EPS	Sedation	Hypotension
Phenothiazines									
Chlorpromazine	Thorazine	24	200–600	30–1500	Yes	1A2, 2D6, 3A4	++	+++	++/+++
Fluphenazine	Prolixin	24	2–20	0.5–30	Yes+Depot	2D6	++++	+	+
Mesoridazine	Serentil	30	75–300	30–400	Yes	1A2, 2D6, 3A4	+	+++	++
Perphenazine	Trilafon	12	8–32	4–64	Yes	2D6	++	++	+
Thioridazine	Mellaril	22	150–600	20–750	No	1A2, 2D6	+	+++	+++
Trifluoperazine	Stelazine	20	5–20	2–30	Yes	1A2, 2D6	+++	+	+
Triflupromazine	Vesprin	– – –	50–100	10–150	Yes	– – –	++	+++	++/+++
Thioxanthene									
Thiothixene	Navane	18	5–30	2–30	Yes	1A2	+++	+/++	++
Phenylpiperidines									
Droperidol	Inapsine	2	2.5–5.0	1.25–10	Yes	– – –	++++	++++	+++
Haloperidol	Haldol	20	4–20	1–50	Yes+Depot	3A4	++++	+	+
Pimozide	Orap	55	2–6	1–10	No	3A4	++++	+	+
Benzepines									
Clozapine	Clozaril	12	150–450	12.5–900	No	1A2, 2D6, 3A4	+/-	+++	+++
Loxapine	Loxitane	16	60–100	20–250	Yes	– – –	++/+++	+	+
Olanzapine	Zyprexa	30	5–20	2.5–30	Yes+Depot	1A2	+	++	++
Quetiapine	Seroquel	6.5	300–600	50–800	No	3A4	+/-	+++	++

Table 15.2 (cont.)

Drug	Brand	Half-life (hrs)	Doses (mg/day) Typical	Doses (mg/day) Extreme	Injectable	Preferred CYP	EPS	Adverse effect risks Sedation	Adverse effect risks Hypotension
					Other heterocyclics				
Aripiprazole	Abilify	75	10–20	5–30	Yes	3A4, 2D6	+/–	+/–	+/–
Asenapine	Saphris	24	10–20	5–20	No*	1A2, 2D6	+/–	++	++
Iloperidone	Fanapt	26	12–24	2–32	Pending	2D6, 3A4	+/–	+/–	++
Lurasidone	Latuda	18	40–80	40–80	No	3A4	+	++	+
Molindone	Moban	2	50–200	15–225	No	2D6	+/++	++	+
Paliperidone	Invega	22	6–12	3–15	No	– – –	++	++	++
Risperidone	Risperdal	3+22	6–8	0.25–16	Yes+Depot	2D6, 3A4	++	++	++
Ziprasidone	Geodon	7.5	80–160	20–180	Yes	3A4	+/–	– – –	– – –

symptoms"), affective responsiveness, and self-care evolve over weeks; improvements in "negative symptoms" (impaired cognition, emotional and affective withdrawal) and functioning are more limited. Symptomatic improvement averages 50 to 60 percent within two months, with about two-thirds of eventual gains achieved within a month. Drug versus placebo rates of major clinical improvement typically differ as 40 to 50 percent versus 20 to 25 percent. Clinical remission is uncommon with antipsychotics (10–20 percent) but far less with placebo (1–2 percent). Nearly one-third of treated patients diagnosed with schizophrenia, though improved, remain substantially ill, and 5 to 10 percent show minimal improvement. Standard practice continues antipsychotic treatment at tolerated doses for many weeks following initial improvement in acute psychotic illnesses, and often for several months before considering gradual dose-reductions or cautious discontinuation – balancing current levels of recovery with critical assessments of individual strengths and vulnerabilities. For many chronically psychotic patients, it may never be feasible to discontinue or to rely on intermittent treatment.

Dosing with antipsychotics in acute psychotic illnesses typically involves the daily equivalent of up to 15–25 mg of haloperidol or fluphenazine, 300–500 of chlorpromazine, 2–6 mg of risperidone or paliperidone, or 10–25 mg of olanzapine. Daily dosing initially is divided to permit general adaptation, but moderate doses usually can soon be given once-daily. In acute psychotic episodes, there is little gain in efficacy with daily doses equivalent to several grams of chlorpromazine versus only about 300 mg, whereas risks of adverse effects are much greater with high doses. Most psychotic patients are managed safely with adequate medication plus skillful interpersonal and environmental management and support, ideally in a controlled clinical setting. Administratively shortened hospitalizations in the past, often with aggressive dosing, did not lead to more rapid improvement. Many psychotic patients leave the hospital substantially symptomatic and unstable, calling for the thoughtful planning of aftercare within limits of available resources, including the use of supervised partial-hospital or intensive outpatient settings.

Long-Term Antipsychotic Treatment

Many patients with chronic or frequently relapsing psychotic disorders are more stable when an antipsychotic is continued long-term. Major exacerbations of schizophrenia can be reduced by three- to fourfold by sustained antipsychotic treatment, but most other long-term applications are largely empirical, with little research support and variable regulatory approval. These indications include bipolar and schizoaffective disorders, and adjunctive treatment for major depression, particularly with psychotic features. Even in schizophrenia, many manifestations (particularly "negative" symptoms) are little-benefited by long-term antipsychotic treatment. As in short-term treatment, there is little evidence that particular antipsychotics, unusually high doses, or combinations consistently yield superior long-term benefits, with the notable exception of clozapine.

In long-term maintenance treatment, antipsychotic doses are individualized and adjusted to changes in levels of symptoms or stress. Typically, daily doses of 10–20 mg of aripiprazole, 100–300 mg of chlorpromazine or clozapine, 2.5–10 mg of fluphenazine or haloperidol, 5–15 mg of olanzapine, 300–600 mg of quetiapine, 2–4 mg of risperidone or paliperidone, or 80–120 mg of ziprasidone, or their equivalent, are adequate and tolerated. Far higher doses are unlikely to improve outcomes and increase adverse effects and expense. Treatment-nonadherence, a major contributor to poor long-term response, is increased by adverse effects that may not be obvious clinically, though troublesome to patients. Treatment adherence can be encouraged by conservative dosing and sensitivity to individual tolerability. Despite their theoretical advantages, the use of long-acting, injected preparations of antipsychotics has shown surprisingly limited average gains in clinical improvement (10–20 percent) over short-acting oral preparations in typical settings, and their acceptance by clinicians and patients varies greatly across cultures. Relapse-risk is markedly increased by the stressor of discontinuing antipsychotics rapidly; slow-gradual discontinuation of any prolonged psychotropic drug treatment is preferred.

Clinical management of chronically ill, psychotic-disorder patients requires long-term planning, considering the patient's symptoms, course and treatment response, as well as personal and family resources. Needed are support and efforts to minimize discouragement, abandonment, and social isolation, to encourage a tolerable quality of life, and to avoid depleting patient and family emotional and economic resources. Typical outcomes among schizophrenia patients include approximately 85 percent risk of appreciable clinical worsening within a year without specific treatment, 5–10 percent less with a placebo, about 25 percent less risk with psychosocial treatment only, perhaps 70 percent less with an antipsychotic drug alone, and perhaps 80 percent less with medicine plus cost-effective behavioral, educational, and family or group interventions with a supportive or rehabilitative orientation. Of note, the prevalence of long-term custodial hospitalization has decreased greatly, but re-hospitalization rates and incarcerations of the mentally ill in jails and prisons have increased several-fold as access to psychiatric services has declined.

Adverse Effects

Antipsychotic drugs carry substantial risks of adverse effects, ranging from uncomfortable symptoms to medically significant risks, and uncommon life-threatening effects. Common effects include a burden of excessive sedation, fatigue, decreased alertness, and decreased or slowed motility (Table 15.2). Some antipsychotics, especially those of relatively low potency, induce postural hypotension or fainting, particularly soon after starting a new drug. Nausea, altered appetite (increased or decreased), and dry mouth or blurred vision also are not uncommon. Importantly, antipsychotic drugs are associated with weight gain, with or without the metabolic syndrome of hypertension, hyperlipidemia, and type-2 diabetes mellitus. Such reactions are most closely associated with low-potency, older neuroleptics (e.g., chlorpromazine, thioridazine) and several modern agents (notably, clozapine, olanzapine, and quetiapine). Body-mass-index (BMI) values of 25–29 kg/m^2 (overweight) are found in about two-thirds of chronically psychotic and bipolar disorder patients, and ≥30 kg/m^2 (obese) in one-third, often at surprisingly young ages and brief exposures. Options include lower but adequate doses of antipsychotics, and selection of those less likely to increase weight, as well as encouraging exercise and dietary control, and possibly early introduction of hypoglycemic agents such as metformin.

Older neuroleptics were more likely to produce discrete neurological reactions that vary in timing, severity, pathophysiology, and treatment response. They include (a) *akathisia* (sustained restlessness), (b) acute dystonias, (c) gradually evolving and sustained *parkinsonism* (bradykinesia, variable tremor), and (d) late-emerging or *tardive dyskinesias and dystonias* (TD). In addition, a "neuroleptic malignant syndrome" (NMS) of cerebral intoxication can present in markedly dissimilar ways with older agents (fever, muscle rigidity, release of creatine kinase and myoglobin) versus modern antipsychotics (mainly delirium).

Cardiac arrythmias can arise with acute overdoses of some antipsychotics, notably thioridazine and mesoridazine. A more predictable risk, however, is prolongation of the repolarization phase of the electrocardiographic (ECG) cycle (QTc >500 msec). Such QTc-prolongation, altered size and shape of ECG T-waves, paroxysmal atrial tachycardia, hypokalemia, hypomagnesemia, hypertension, and advanced age increase risk for rare but potentially fatal ventricular arrhythmias, including torsades de pointes, and cardiac arrest. Sudden cardiac deaths, though uncommon, have been associated with long-term treatment with all types of antipsychotics. QTc-prolongation is especially likely with thioridazine or mesoridazine, may occur with chlorpromazine, haloperidol, and pimozide, and among modern agents, especially with ziprasidone, but also iloperidone and quetiapine. Risk increases with additional agents that inhibit cardiac repolarization, including tricyclic antidepressants and class Ia, sodium-channel blocking, antiarrhythmics such as quinidine, procainamide, and disopyramide. Antipsychotics of all types also are associated with increased mortality in the elderly, and particularly dementia patients, often in association with sudden death, strokes, and other cerebrovascular events.

Potent neuroleptics paliperidone and risperidone induce hyperprolactinemia (40–100 ng/mL) by blocking dopamine D$_2$ receptors in the anterior pituitary; serum prolactin levels >200 ng/mL suggest pituitary adenoma. Prolactin-elevation can be associated with breast-engorgement, sexual dysfunction, and osteopenia. It may promote the growth of prolactin-sensitive metastases of mammary carcinoma, but the risk of *causing* breast cancer appears to be low.

Clozapine presents particular risks, notably including uncommon agranulocytosis (neutrophil count $\leq 500/\text{mm}^3$), with risks of sepsis and death, within the first several months of treatment, leading to required, regular monitoring of white blood cell counts. Risk of agranulocytosis averages approximately 0.03 percent/month for 6 months and much less thereafter. Further use of clozapine following severe leukopenia is not recommended, and recurrences have been reported. Additional risks peculiar to clozapine include annoying sialorrhea that probably represents decreased ability to clear saliva by pharyngeal and esophageal mechanisms; it may increase the risk of aspiration pneumonia. Clozapine also can induce life-threatening ileus, dose-dependent epileptic seizures, and rare myocarditis and later cardiac myopathy.

Mood-Stabilizing Drugs

Introduction

The concept of "mood-stabilization" remains somewhat controversial as it applies to bipolar disorders (type I with manic as well as major depressive episodes, type II with depressive and hypomanic recurrences, and cyclothymic disorder). There are established antimanic effects of several types of drugs (antipsychotics, lithium, carbamazepine, valproate), and both lithium (greater effect versus mania than bipolar depression) and lamotrigine (not antimanic but reduces the risk of recurrences of bipolar depression) are accepted for long-term maintenance treatment. Several second-generation antipsychotics also have demonstrated efficacy in acute bipolar depression (cariprazine, lurasidone, olanzapine-with-fluoxetine, quetiapine), but their effectiveness and tolerability for long-term prophylactic treatment remains under investigation.

Acute episodes of adult bipolar I disorder are relatively stereotyped, but a high proportion of cases of apparently unipolar depression or other disorders of adults and juveniles often are unrecognized clinically as probable cases of bipolar disorder, sometimes for years. Available treatments are effective in acute mania but far less so (and far less well investigated) in bipolar depression, both acute and recurrent. No treatment has explicit regulatory approval for bipolar II disorder, although antidepressants are widely used, often with lithium or a putatively mood-stabilizing anticonvulsant. Lithium carbonate is the oldest and best-studied mood stabilizer, and remains a standard despite a lack of commercial interest in this unpatentable mineral. Most antipsychotics are rapidly antimanic. In addition, several anticonvulsants (particularly carbamazepine and divalproex) have antimanic effects (but remain unapproved for long-term treatment despite extensive off-label use with prophylactic intent), and lamotrigine has long-lasting mood-stabilizing effects selective for bipolar depression (Tables 15.3 and 15.4; Figure 15.2).

Table 15.3 Properties of FDA-approved mood-stabilizing anticonvulsants

Property	Carbamazepine	Divalproex	Lamotrigine
Brand names	Equetro®, Tegretol®	Depakote®	Lamictal®
Indication–approvals			
Mania/Mixed-state	2004	1994	no
Bipolar depression	no	no	2003
Maintenance		1994	
Doses (mg/day)			
Typical	400–1200	750–1500	200–400
Extreme	200–1600	250–4200	25–600
Serum concentrations (µg/mL)	6–12	50–120	5–10
Elimination half-life (hours)	18–65 (later 10–20)	9–16	14–34
Metabolism	CYP-3A4	Mitochondrial oxidation, glucuronidation	Glucuronidation
Actions	Blocks voltage-gated Na⁺ channels; can potentiate GABA	Potentiates GABA, inhibits GABA-transaminase; blocks voltage-gated Na⁺ channels & T-type Ca²⁺ channels; inhibits histone deacetylase to alter DNA function	Blocks voltage-gated Na⁺ channels, inhibits glutamate release
Adverse effects	Sedation, headache, leukopenia, SIADH, rashes (rare Stevens-Johnson), withdrawal seizures	Weight gain, hepatic toxicity (especially in children given other anticonvulsants), hyperammonemia, CNS intoxication, blood dyscrasias, withdrawal seizures, polycystic ovary, and masculinization	Common rashes; Rare dermonecrolysis (Stevens-Johnson), CNS intoxication, some leukopenia, withdrawal seizures
Teratogenicity	Multiple cardiac & other anomalies, spina bifida	Multiple cardiac & other anomalies, severe risk of spina bifida; cognitive effects (?), autism (?)	Midline clefts suspected but unlikely
Drug interactions	Induces metabolism of many drugs & itself; grapefruit inhibits 3A4	Increases lamotrigine, carbamazepine, tricyclic antidepressants; blocks folate absorption; salicylates can increase valproate concentrations	Valproate increases levels; estrogen increases
Other applications	Epilepsy, migraine, neuropathic pain, trigeminal neuralgia	Epilepsy, migraine, neuropathic pain; experimental in cancers and dementia–prevention	Epilepsy, migraine, neuropathic pain; adjunct for unipolar depression (?)

Table 15.4 Indication approval status for second-generation antipsychotics in bipolar disorder

Drugs			Indications		
Agent	Brand	Mania	Mixed	Depressed	Maintenance
Aripiprazole	Abilify®	2004	2004	no	2006
Asenapine	Saphris®	2009	2009	no	no
Cariprazine	Vraylar®	2015	2015	2019	no
Chlorpromazine	Thorazine®	1973	no	no	no
Iloperidone	Fanapt®	no	no	no	no
Lurasidone	Latuda®	no	no	2013	no
Olanzapine	Zyprexa®	2000	2000	2003 (+fluoxetine)	2009
Paliperidone	Invega®	off-label	no	no	no
Quetiapine	Seroquel®	2004	2004	2006	2008 (+ Li or VPA)
Risperidone	Risperdal®	2003	2003	no	2009 (LAI)
Ziprasidone	Geodon®	2004	2004	no	2009 (+ Li or VPA)

FDA-approved indications include acute mania, mixed-states, or bipolar depression.

Abbreviations: LAI: long-acting injectable; Li: lithium carbonate; VPA: valproate; plus (+) indicates FDA-approved for use adjunctive use only.

Lithium Salts

Description of antimanic effects of the putative anti-gout, salt-substitute, lithium carbonate by John Cade in Australia in 1949, followed by more extensive research led by Mogens Schou in the Netherlands opened the modern psychopharmacologic era. Most of its substantial intoxicating risks are avoided by use of moderate, controlled doses and regular monitoring of fluctuating serum [Li$^+$] concentrations at their daily nadir (8–12 hours post-dosing); concentrations of ≤1.00, and usually 0.60–0.75 mEq/L (at typical daily doses of 900–1500 mg of lithium carbonate [Li$_2$CO$_3$]) are safe, effective, and avoid potentially toxic, initial peak concentrations. Lithium has an unusually low therapeutic index (margin of safety, or ratio of toxic to effective doses or circulating levels of only 2–4). Once-daily dosing of lithium is convenient and may encourage adherence, but may not be well tolerated by some elderly or infirm patients, and has little beneficial effect on renal function. Complex actions of lithium include effects on production, storage, and release of cerebral neurotransmitter catecholamines and serotonin, and their intracellular molecular-effector mechanisms (reduced production of cyclic-adenosine monophosphate [cAMP] and activity of protein kinase-C [PKC]), some of which are shared with some antimanic anticonvulsants including valproate.

Lithium is available as generic tablets or capsules (with 8 mEq of lithium/300 mg of Li_2CO_3) and liquid (lithium citrate; 8 mEq Li^+/teaspoonful). Lithium is eliminated almost entirely renally; half-life averages 20–24 hours and slows moderately with advancing age. Cerebral concentrations of lithium are 20–40 percent lower than in plasma, based on nuclear magnetic resonance spectroscopy (MRS) to detect Li^+.

Mood-Altering Anticonvulsants

Several anticonvulsants are effective in bipolar disorder. Three are FDA-approved: carbamazepine for acute mania and mixed manic-depressive states, valproate (usually as sodium divalproex) for mania, and lamotrigine for long-term maintenance, mainly to limit depressive recurrences (Figure 15.2).

Carbamazepine is FDA-approved only to treat acute mania and mixed-states despite its empirical long-term, off-label use. Usual doses are 400–1200 mg/day (serum concentrations, 6–12 µg/mL). Carbamazepine induces the metabolic clearance of many other drugs and itself. Its own initial elimination half-life of 15–65 hours is shortened by induction of hepatic cytochrome-P450 (CYP) microsomal oxidases, including its preferred pathway (CYP-3A4). Adverse effects include excessive sedation, headache, leukopenia and thrombocytopenia, the syndrome of inappropriate secretion of antidiuretic hormone (SIADH) with hyponatremia, benign rashes as well as rare but potentially fatal Stevens-Johnson dermatomuconecrolysis, as well as major teratogenic effects.

Valproic acid was an industrial solvent synthesized in the 1880s and discovered serendipitously in France to have anticonvulsant and psychotropic properties in the 1960s. Typical oral doses of 750–1500 mg/day achieve serum concentrations of 50–120 µg/mL. Valproate is efficiently metabolized primarily by mitochondrial oxidation, followed by glucuronide conjugation and excretion; further oxidization can yield reactive, unsaturated derivatives that may contribute to hepatic toxicity, particularly when other anticonvulsants are given.

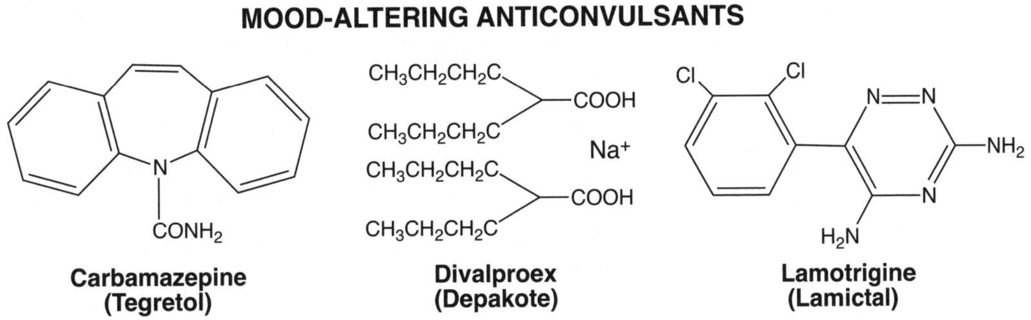

MOOD-ALTERING ANTICONVULSANTS

Carbamazepine (Tegretol)   **Divalproex (Depakote)**   **Lamotrigine (Lamictal)**

Figure 15.2 Mood-altering anticonvulsants

Lamotrigine was the first FDA-approved drug for long-term mood-stabilizing effects (in 2003) since lithium (in 1974, though initially mainly for recurrent mania). Unusual in lacking antimanic effects, it is a rare drug specifically approved for long-term treatment of bipolar depression. Its short-term applications are limited by the need to increase doses slowly (weeks) to limit the risk of dermatologic toxicity. It has been used off-label for a variety of depressive disorders.

Other anticonvulsants lack evidence of efficacy in bipolar disorder. Oxcarbazepine (carbamazepine analog, not a metabolite) has limited ability to induce drug-clearance or blood dyscrasias, making it simpler to use clinically, except for a relatively high risk of SIADH with hyponatremia. However, it lacks compelling evidence of having antimanic effects and remains inadequately studied and lacks regulatory approval for short or long-term use in bipolar disorder.

Antipsychotic-Antimanic Drugs

In addition to their effects in psychotic disorders, antipsychotics have powerful and rapid antimanic actions. Most modern agents (and chlorpromazine, but not lurasidone) are FDA-approved for acute mania. In addition, cariprazine, lurasidone, olanzapine combined with fluoxetine, and quetiapine are effective in acute bipolar depression and may also be beneficial long-term. In general, all mood-stabilizing medicines are more effective against recurrences of mania (and hypomania) than bipolar depression, long-term, whereas depressive and dysthymic phases of bipolar disorder are especially challenging to treat and carry a high risk of suicidal behavior and of disability.

Short-Term Treatment

Although lithium carbonate is effective and FDA-approved for acute mania, its therapeutic onset is relatively slow, and adverse-effect risks relatively high, especially if dosed aggressively. Since such slow action is incompatible with currently limited hospitalization, lithium is best used after initial control of mania by more rapid means. These include initial reliance on antipsychotic agents or antimanic anticonvulsants, such as divalproex (dosed to 10–20 mg/kg/day). Temporary adjunctive use of a sedative (e.g., lorazepam or clonazepam) also can be helpful.

Controlled trials indicate only modest differences (approximately 10 percent) in apparent efficacy among specific antimanic treatments, and a credible ranking of specific agents by efficacy remains elusive. However, antipsychotics are probably more rapidly acting than anticonvulsants, and this is clearly so for lithium. Placebo-associated response rates in mania, remarkably, are often ≥30 percent and have been rising. However, "placebo" responses involve many clinically important factors: quiet, orderly, non-provocative, protective and structured environments, use of sedative-hypnotics to restore sleep, and regular meals and schedules all can have major benefits. It is often possible to reduce mania symptom ratings substantially within several weeks (typical of controlled treatment trials), but full and sustained clinical remission requires many weeks or even months.

Treatment of bipolar depressive phases remains unsatisfactory and inadequately studied. Antidepressants are widely used without specific regulatory approval for bipolar depression. They are associated with some increased risk of pathologically excited states (mania, hypomania, mixed-states, psychosis, rapid cycling, or emotional instability), though probably only moderately more than occur spontaneously. Moreover, evidence concerning the relative efficacy of antidepressants in bipolar versus unipolar depression remains inconsistent. Encouraging findings have emerged concerning the treatment of acute bipolar depression with cariprazine, fluoxetine-plus-olanzapine, lurasidone, and quetiapine, whereas lamotrigine is less effective and requires impractically slow initial dosing. Experimentally, cautious administration of ketamine and the addition of the anti-narcolepsy stimulant armodafinil or omega-3 fatty acids to standard mood stabilizers also may benefit bipolar depression, but require further study.

Long-Term Prophylactic Treatment

Most bipolar disorder patients have multiple recurrences over many years, in highly variable numbers and timing, with acceleration of mood cycling over time only in a minority. However, the polarity of initial episodes is predictive of later predominant morbidity (mania: to mania or psychosis; depression or mixed-states: to more of the same). Since major illness-recurrences can be clinically dangerous, most bipolar disorder patients, especially of type I and after more than two recurrences, are candidates for long-term, often indefinite, treatment with mood stabilizers with long-term support and rehabilitation. Even after a first episode, medication and close clinical follow-up should continue for at least six to twelve months, aiming at full remission. Relapse risk is high within the months following acute episodes, and higher if medication is discontinued rapidly. After treatment for about a year, more prolonged maintenance can be considered, based on critical assessment of individual strengths and vulnerabilities, and patients' previous illness-experiences.

Many, especially young, patients are reluctant to accept prolonged treatment. Experience with relapses can encourage acceptance of prolonged treatment and clinical supervision. In addition to erratic treatment-adherence, unfavorable response to long-term treatment is predicted by rapid cycling (≥ 4 episodes/year), tendency to shift from depression into mania rather than the opposite, substance abuse, and multiple complex or mixed states. Prolonged delay of sustained mood-stabilizing treatment and higher recurrence-counts appear not to predict inferior treatment-response.

There is no ideal treatment for bipolar disorders, but medication alone is unlikely to be sufficient for comprehensive clinical care. Even with effective treatments, patients with bipolar disorder are unwell between 40 to 50 percent of the time according to naturalistic long-term follow-up studies. For most patients, depressive symptoms are even more prevalent than manic symptoms effects of and longer lasting. Multiple treatments are given in hopes of enhancing outcomes, though very few combinations have systematic, long-term assessments of added benefits/risks. Adding lithium to carbamazepine or valproate may be more effective than the anticonvulsants alone, though little more than lithium alone. Adding an antipsychotic to either lithium or valproate also may add long-term benefits, particularly versus manic recurrences. Olanzapine combined with fluoxetine, and adding lamotrigine to lithium may also enhance stability.

In recent quantitative, meta-analytic reviews of controlled trials of common long-term treatments for bipolar disorders, lithium, olanzapine, quetiapine, and risperidone showed evidence of protective effects against recurrences of mania. Against recurrences of bipolar depression, lamotrigine, lithium, olanzapine-fluoxetine, and quetiapine appeared to be effective. Evidence that antidepressants have a long-term ability to limit the risk of recurrences of bipolar depression is weak and largely negative, with some increased risk of new mania and a high risk of increased rapid cycling. Overall, benefits are clearest versus recurrent mania and protection against recurrences of bipolar depression requires further study.

Of particular concern are extraordinarily high risks of premature mortality from both violent and natural causes among bipolar disorder patients, including effects of co-occurring cardiovascular and other general medical disorders. Suicide rates in bipolar disorder are among the highest in any psychiatric disorder and are only slightly higher in type I than type II bipolar disorder. Lithium treatment may reduce the risk of suicides and attempts, perhaps more than other mood stabilizers, and long-term treatment generally may reduce mortality from all causes.

Adverse Effects

Mood-stabilizing agents have a range of adverse or toxic effects as well as interactions with other drugs; such effects contribute to treatment-discontinuation and poor outcomes (Table 15.5). They include the characteristic adverse effects of antipsychotics, with weight gain and metabolic syndrome as well as excessive sedation and variable or minimal extrapyramidal effects with lithium or anticonvulsants, high risks of teratogenic effects with divalproex and carbamazepine, and potentially life-threatening but rare dermatologic reactions to lamotrigine, divalproex, and carbamazepine. Retrospective analyses have raised questions about suicidal risk with anticonvulsants among patients with epilepsy, though evidence of such an effect in bipolar disorder is lacking. Although several second-generation antipsychotic drugs have beneficial effects and an emerging role in the treatment of bipolar disorder patients, they also carry risks characteristic of such agents, including excessive sedation, appreciable risks of akathisia, and low risks of tardive dyskinenesia.

Table 15.5 Adverse effects of mood-altering medicines used for bipolar disorder

Effects	Lithium	Anticonvulsants	Antipsychotics	Antidepressants
Poor short-term efficacy	no	LTG in mania	no	debated (avoid with mixed features)
Prophylaxis uncertain	no	CBZ, VPA (both off-label)	probably effective	yes
Sedation or lethargy	variable	variable	yes	uncommon
Neurological	mild cognitive, rare EPS	cognitive	variable EPS, akathisia	no
Headache	no	yes	no	rare
Gastrointestinal distress	early	variable	no	SRIs
Weight gain	yes	yes	especially CLZ, ONZ, QTP	variable
Hypertension	no	no	no	variable
Type II diabetes	no	no	especially CLZ, ONZ, QTP	no
Hypothyroidism	uncommon	no	no	no
Renal effects	predictable	no	no	no
SIADH/ Hyponatremia	rare	oxCBZ (not antimanic), CBZ	variable	SRIs
Dermatologic	yes	LTG (rare SJS), CBZ	rare	no
Hepatic damage	no	VPA, CBZ	rare	no
Pancreatitis	no	VPA	rare	no
Bone marrow dysfunction	no	CBZ, VPA	CLZ	rare
Masculinization (PCOS)	no	VPA	no	no
Drug-interactions	NSAIDs, diuretics, CCBs increase [Li]	CBZ decreases other drugs; VPA potentiates LTG	rare	SRIs
Teratogenic	uncommon (Ebstein's)	VPA>>CBZ	not proved	not certain

Abbreviations: CBZ (carbamazepine), CCBs (calcium-channel blockers), CLZ (clozapine), EPS (extrapyramidal neurological syndromes), LTG (lamotrigine), NSAIDs (non-steroidal anti-inflammatory drugs), ONZ (olanzapine) oxCBZ (oxcarbazepine), PCOS (polycystic ovary syndrome with increased testosterone secretion and masculinization), QTP (quetiapine), SIADH (syndrome of inappropriate secretion of antidiuretic hormone with water-retention and risk of hyponatremia), SJS (Stevens-Johnson dermatomucosal necrosis); SRIs (serotonin reuptake inhibitors), VPA (valproate). Among drug interactions, carbamazepine induces metabolism of itself and other agents; some SRIs block metabolism of other agents.

Anxiolytics and Hypnotics

Anxiolytics and hypnotics typically are used for the short-term treatment of anxiety and for insomnia. In the past, a series of classes of sedative or tranquilizing drugs have been employed to treat anxiety and insomnia. They include antihistamines (e.g., diphenhydramine), barbiturates, chloral hydrate, ethchlorvynol (Pacidyl), glutethimide (Doriden), meprobamate (Miltown, Equanil), methaqualone (Quaalude), paraldehyde, and others. These widely used drugs preceded the introduction of chlordiazepoxide (Librium) in 1960 and other benzodiazepines soon thereafter. In earlier decades, clinicians would even prescribe alcohol, usually as an elixir, including as a tincture of opium, in attempts to treat anxiety or insomnia. Most of the early sedatives were abandoned for the risk of pharmacodynamic tolerance, overuse, dependency, and as agents of suicide. Combining modern sedatives with alcohol is not uncommon, and increases the risk of adverse effects, intoxication, respiratory depression, coma, and even death.

The most widely employed anxiolytics are the benzodiazepines. Widely used benzodiazepines include alprazolam (Xanax), chlordiazepoxide (Librium), clonazepam (Klonopin), diazepam (Valium), estazolam (Prosom), flurazepam (Dalmane), hydroxyzine (Atarax), lorazepam (Ativan), oxazepam (Serax), quazepam (Doral), temazepam (Restoril), and triazolam (Halcion). These agents differ mainly in their speed of onset and duration of effect. As a class of agents, they facilitate central neurotransmission by the inhibitory neurotransmitter gamma-aminobutyric acid (GABA), interacting at a separate site from that for GABA itself on $GABA_A$ receptors to produce an allosteric effect leading to an increased influx of chloride ions (Cl^-), resulting in neuronal stabilization or hyperpolarization.

Benzodiazepines ideally are used for brief times as adjuncts to treatment of anxiety disorders with antidepressants and psychotherapy for episodes or recurrences of acute anxiety. Their beneficial effects are relatively short-lasting, and treatment with a benzodiazepine is best limited to a few days or weeks for several reasons. First, tolerance often develops, leading to the need for increasing doses to sustain a beneficial effect. In addition, abrupt cessation (versus gradual dose-reduction), especially of high doses, can result in withdrawal symptoms, potentially including epileptic seizures. In addition, some patients may become dependent on benzodiazepines and overuse them.

Buspirone is a selective $5\text{-}HT_{1A}$ mixed agonist-antagonist without effects at GABA receptors that has some anxiolytic activity. Unlike benzodiazepines, it is nonsedating and has little effect on motor performance. However, buspirone requires several days to begin to exert anxiolytic effects, is often ineffective, and many patients experienced with antianxiety agents may prefer the subjective effects of benzodiazepines. Other alternatives to benzodiazepines include the SSRI antidepressants, antihistamines, and possibly beta-adrenergic blockers. The group of highly sedating "z-drugs" employed as hypnotics has largely displaced benzodiazepines for the treatment of insomnia. They include the cyclopyrrolones eszopiclone (Lunesta) and zopiclone (Imovane), the pyrazolopyrimidine zaleplon (Sonata), and the imidazopyridine zolpidem (Ambien). These agents are chemically different from benzodiazepines, but their pharmacodynamic actions at the $GABA_A$ receptor are very similar. With prolonged use, they also can undergo tolerance or loss of effect, and insomnia can return or worsen, and can produce dependency. They also carry a considerable risk of inducing fugue-like dissociative states with loss of memory.

Medicines for Addiction

It is useful to think of medications for the treatment of substance dependency or addictive disorders in several categories: (1) those that replace an abused substance with a drug with similar pharmacologic actions (maintenance treatment), and (2) those that aim to modulate the experience of taking an abused substance by (a) blocking the effects of the substance, (b) reducing craving for it, (c) diminishing or altering the reinforcing effects of taking the abused substance, or (d) creating an aversive experience when the abused substance is taken.

There are three FDA-approved maintenance therapies: (1) nicotine replacement for tobacco users with nicotine dependence, and (2) methadone, or (3) buprenorphine for opioid dependence. Nicotine replacement is available in several forms: transdermal patches delivering 7, 14, or 21 mg of nicotine over 16 or 24 hours, lozenges and gum delivering 2 or 4 mg of nicotine, as well as nicotine inhalers, both used "as needed." Another treatment that can reduce the craving for nicotine is the mild stimulant-antidepressant, bupropion.

Methadone has been the mainstay maintenance treatment for patients with opioid dependence for more than fifty years. Unlike other full mu (μ)-opioid agonists, such as heroin or oxycodone, methadone has a long half-life that can prevent withdrawal symptoms and reduce craving up to twenty-four hours, if the dose is adjusted to the requirements of individual patient's requirements. However, like other opioid full-agonists, methadone carries a risk of overdose, especially if taken with another respiratory suppressant such as another opioid, alcohol, or benzodiazepines. Methadone also has many drug-drug interactions and adverse physical effects, including diaphoresis, constipation, weight gain, and cardiac QTc prolongation, which can limit its use. Moreover, methadone maintenance treatment of opioid dependence is available only through federally approved clinics and dispensaries, which generally also require comprehensive and intensive substance abuse treatment.

In contrast, buprenorphine, a high-affinity mu-opioid receptor partial-agonist used for maintenance treatment of opioid dependence, is less likely than methadone to produce dangerous overdose owing to being a partial-agonist, which provides a "ceiling effect" and limits the agonistic effects of abused opioids Buprenorphine, like methadone, also has a twenty-four-hour elimination half-life that allows for once-daily dosing. It is commonly manufactured with the opioid antagonist naloxone embedded in tablets or films (Suboxone) to prevent intravenous misuse since naloxone has poor oral bioavailability and is active only if taken parenterally. In further contrast to methadone, buprenorphine can be prescribed through a physician's office, making it attractive to those who do not have a convenient methadone clinic or are unwilling or unable to adhere to the strict regulations and rules associated with most methadone clinic programs.

One manner in which medicines can modulate the experience of using an abused substance is that they can block the effects of the abused agent altogether. For example, naltrexone, a potent μ-opioid receptor antagonist available as an oral tablet and a long-acting intramuscular injection, can effectively block the effects of opioids. Opioid-abuse patients who may be at risk of relapse after being treated with naltrexone should be warned that their tolerance for opioids may have plummeted during maintenance treatment, so that previously tolerated doses of opioids could now prove lethal.

For alcohol-dependent patients, naltrexone can modulate the experience of drinking by reducing craving for alcohol and reducing the pleasurable experiences of drinking, presumably by blocking the effects of small amounts of endogenous opioids released in the brain that positively reinforce the drinking experience. Through mechanisms that are not well understood, naltrexone may also decrease the craving for alcohol. Due to the rare occurrence of hepatitis associated with naltrexone use, liver function tests (LFTs) should be monitored regularly during such treatment.

Similarly, acamprosate (Campral) (N-acetylhomotaurine) is believed to decrease craving for alcohol through its purported stabilizing effect on dysregulated GABA and glutamate receptors, by acting as a positive allosteric modulator (like benzodiazepines) at inhibitory $GABA_A$ receptors and as an inhibitor of excitatory NMDA transmission. Acamprosate usually is dosed three times a day owing to its low oral bioavailability rather than a short half-life, which can be a helpful reminder of ongoing sobriety despite the inconvenience of repeated dosing.

Varenicline (Chantix), a nicotinic acetylcholine partial-agonist, can decrease nicotine craving and support abstinence from tobacco use. Controversy about possible cardiac side effects and a putative increase in suicidal thinking have dogged varenicline for years, but both concerns lack research support. Nonetheless, varenicline is typically reserved for patients for whom nicotine replacement and treatment with bupropion have been unsuccessful.

Through mechanisms not well understood, but possibly related to its dopamine and norepinephrine reuptake blockade, bupropion also modulates craving for nicotine. Bupropion may also derive some of its anti-nicotine effect from its antidepressant and anorexic effects, both of which can counteract some of the common complaints contributing to the use of nicotine: depressed mood and weight-gain.

Finally, some medicines can create an aversive experience when combined with a substance of abuse. *Disulfiram* (Antabuse), for example, has been a cornerstone of the treatment of alcohol dependence for more than fifty years. It works by irreversibly inhibiting the enzyme alcohol dehydrogenase, which allows the toxic metabolite of alcohol, acetaldehyde, to accumulate and cause a miserable combination of nausea, vomiting, flushing, and blood pressure fluctuations. Through this aversive experience, patients begin to psychologically disassociate alcohol with its pleasurable effects and to respect or fear the highly aversive effects of drinking alcohol while taking disulfiram. As with many of the medications described previously, disulfiram is only as effective as a patient's compliance with taking it. Many families or significant others develop supportive daily rituals around disulfiram dosing that can enhance medication compliance. Due to its rare association with fulminant hepatic failure, liver enzymes must be monitored regularly in patients taking disulfiram.

Medicines for Cognitive and Attentional Disorders

Treatment of Progressive Cognitive Deficits

With increased life expectancy and as the world population ages, heterogeneous and progressive neurodegenerative dementias are becoming more widespread. Alzheimer's disease (AD) is the most common dementia among the elderly (50–70 percent of dementias), and becomes more prevalent with age, rising from a prevalence of 1–2 percent at age of 65 to 35–50 percent by age 85. Cognitive deficits in AD range from mild cognitive impairment (MCI) to progressive and profound loss of mental capacities severe enough to interfere with activities of daily living and quality of life, that ultimately lead to death. In AD, motoric fluency and coordination are lost (apraxia), and language (aphasia), memory (amnesia), and executive functioning abilities become progressively impaired. While MCI is not necessarily a prodrome of dementia, progressive cognitive loss occurs in some cases of MCI. Effective pharmacotherapy and other interventions to prevent dementia or progression of MCI to dementia are not established. In the early stages of cognitive decline, periodic monitoring and healthy lifestyle choices are recommended as the search for effective treatments continues.

The pathophysiology of AD is characterized by loss of synaptic connectivity and loss of neurons in subcortical and cortical areas of the forebrain, resulting in atrophy and volume loss in the temporal and parietal lobes, frontal cortex, and cingulate gyrus. Beta-amyloid plaques and neurofibrillary tangles composed of hyperphosphorylated microtubule tau protein are distinct cytologic findings seen under the microscope, and such peptide markers as assayed in serum are being developed as diagnostic tests for AD. Decreased cerebral acetylcholine synthesis has been associated with memory decline and learning impairments, and anticholinergic agents are powerful inducers of delirium. Such findings have encouraged attention on the cerebral acetylcholine (ACh) system as a target for most of the medicines currently available to counter cognitive decline in AD.

Acetylcholinesterase Inhibitors

Several FDA-approved acetylcholinesterase inhibitor (AChEI) agents are available. They include donepezil (Aricept), galantamine (Reminyl), and rivastigmine (Exelon). Another such drug, tacrine (Cognex), is rarely used due to hepatotoxicity. AchEI agents inhibit the ACh-degrading enzyme acetylcholinesterase (AChE) and increase concentrations of ACh, with moderate beneficial effects on cognition and self-care. While they share similar mechanisms of action, these agents differ in their pharmacological properties. Donepezil (half-life 70 hours) is a reversible and highly selective AChEI, and galantamine is shorter-acting (half-life 6–8 hours) and both an AChEI and a nicotinic agonist. Both drugs are metabolized by CPY450 3A4 and 2D6 hepatic microsomal isoenzymes. Rivastigmine is an even shorter-acting (half-life 1–2 hours) AChEI. These three drugs are similarly, though moderately efficacious for mild to moderate AD.

Donepezil is widely used to treat mild to moderate AD and may be of some benefit for severe dementia. It is available in an oral formulation as immediate-release (5 or 10 mg), sustained-release (23 mg), and oral rapidly disintegrating (5–10 mg/day) preparations, and is FDA-approved for advanced dementia (at an average dose of 10 mg/day). It is generally well tolerated, with relatively low risk of liver toxicity. Its common adverse effects include indigestion, loss of appetite, nausea, vomiting, abdominal pain, diarrhea, muscle pain, dizziness rash, and pruritis. Donepezil has limited progression from MCI to dementia for the first 12 months of its use compared to placebo, but these gains were lost within 3 years. High doses of donepezil (averaging 23 mg/day) were FDA-approved in 2010 for the treatment of moderate-severe dementia after showing somewhat greater benefit than lower doses, though with greater risk of adverse events.

Galantamine is indicated for the treatment of mild to moderate AD and vascular dementia. It is available in 4, 8, and 12 mg tablets and 8, 16, and 24 mg capsules. Adverse effects associated with galantamine are similar to other AChEIs, and gastrointestinal symptoms are the most common complaint. Several clinical studies lasting 21–26 weeks found that 16 and 24 mg/day doses of galantamine were more effective than placebo.

Rivastigmine is indicated for the treatment of mild to moderate AD and dementia associated with Parkinson's disease. It is administered orally, starting at 1.5 mg twice a day, increased gradually to 6 mg twice daily, as tolerated. It is also available as a transdermal patch, given at an average dose of 9.5 mg/24 hours, which appears to reduce the risk of nausea and vomiting.

N-methyl-D-aspartate (NMDA) Receptor Antagonist

Glutamate is an excitatory neurotransmitter that is important in learning and memory functions, though excessive stimulation of glutamate receptors is excitotoxic, leading to cell death, which may occur in AD, Parkinson's disease, and multiple sclerosis. *Memantine* (Namenda; half-life 70 hours) is a non-competitive glutamate NMDA receptor antagonist and has moderate effectiveness in the treatment of moderate to severe AD, which may not be as great as with some AChEIs. Its adverse effects include confusion, dizziness, headache, and fatigue.

Combination Therapy AchEI and NMDA Receptor Antagonist

Combining an AchEI with memantine has yielded significant benefits for AD, as indicated by reducing decline in cognition and functioning over six months. Meta-analysis for such combination treatment showed small but statistically significant benefits in several clinical ratings of cognition and functioning.

Newer Treatments for Dementia

The search continues for disease-modifying treatments for dementia. Recent leads include immunological (monoclonal antibodies) and other treatments that may modulate deposition of amyloid and tau proteins in the brain that are characteristic of AD, alter their metabolism or their interactions with other molecules to reduce neuron-destroying effects, modify the production of neurofibrillary tangles, or reduce cerebral inflammatory responses.

Medicines for Attention Deficit Hyperactivity Disorder (ADHD)

ADHD affects children, adolescents, and adults, impairing academic progress, employment, and social interactions. Before starting treatment for ADHD, especially in children, a thorough clinical and diagnostic assessment should be undertaken. For pre-school children, individual and family therapy are recommended as a basic treatment, with a critically evaluated medication trial of several months to follow if needed. The main FDA-approved class of treatments for ADHD are psychostimulants, which include methylphenidate and amphetamines. Additional options include a selective norepinephrine reuptake inhibitor (NRI), and alpha-2 (α_2) adrenergic agonists, as well as some antidepressant drugs.

Psychostimulants

Psychostimulants are especially commonly employed to treat ADHD at all ages due to their rapid onset of action and established record of safety and efficacy. These drugs enhance cerebral dopamine and norepinephrine neurotransmission to improve executive functions including planning, working memory, attention, mental flexibility, concentration, and problem-solving, as well as to limit impulsivity and behavioral disinhibition.

Psychostimulants are controlled substances requiring a schedule II prescription. Because of the potential for improved alertness, attention, and staying awake, the psychostimulants have a high potential for misuse and diversion among primary and high school students (5–9 percent) and even more among college students (5–35 percent). Of those prescribed psychostimulants, 16–29 percent sell, give, or trade these drugs. The psychostimulants are contraindicated in symptomatic cardiovascular disease, moderate to severe hypertension, hyperthyroidism, motor tics or Tourette's syndrome, substance abuse, glaucoma, and current or recent (≤14 days) use of monoamine oxidase inhibitors (MAOIs).

Methylphenidate (d,l-racemate Ritalin, extended-release Concerta, and skin-patch Daytrana, as well as the *d*-enantiomer Focalin and Focalin-ER) is a short-acting dopamine and norepinephrine reuptake inhibitor, increasing their availability in the synaptic cleft, similar to the action of cocaine. Methylphenidate (half-life 4–12 hours) is taken orally with a duration of action 3–6 hours for immediate release, 3–8 hours for sustained release, and up to 12 hours for extended-release formulation (Concerta). Methylphenidate patch (Daytrana) delivers methylphenidate transdermally, with a duration of up to 12 hours, but can be removed early. Long-acting formulations are made available so that children will not have to take additional doses while at school. *Dexmethylphenidate* is the d-enantiomer of methylphenidate (Focalin) and is efficacious at approximately half the dose of methylphenidate. Common adverse effects of methylphenidate are dependence and tolerance, agitation, anxiety, irritability, insomnia, decreased appetite, headache, abdominal cramps, nausea, dizziness, heart palpitations, slowing of growth (height and weight) in children, seizures, blurred vision, hypertension, tachycardia, and visual hallucinations.

Amphetamines are available as dextroamphetamine (Dexedrine) or as a mixture of amphetamine enantiomers (Adderall), available in both immediate- and continuous-release preparations. Lisdexamfetamine (Vyvanse) is a prodrug that is metabolically converted to dextroamphetamine and acts for up to 10 hours. Common adverse effects associated with amphetamines include: delayed sleep onset, decreased appetite, weight loss, linear growth delay, headache, stomach upset, tachy-cardia and hypertension, jitteriness, emotional lability, and the development of tics.

Selective Norepinephrine Reuptake Inhibitor

Atomoxetine (Strattera) is the first FDA-approved nonstimulant for the treatment of ADHD in children (aged >6 years), adolescents, and adults. Its efficacy is probably not as great as with psychostimulants, but as a non-controlled substance, it is recommended for patients with a personal or family history of substance abuse, with tics, or with an intolerance for psychostimulants. Atomoxetine is provided as a capsule with 10–12 hours duration of action, taken once or twice daily. Efficacy may be better with morning dosing, but evening dosing may have lesser adverse effects. Dosing is weight dependent, not to exceed 1.4 mg/kg or 100 mg. Atomoxetine is metabolized through the hepatic microsomal cytochrome P450 (CYP) 2D26 isoenzyme pathway, which can be inhibited by other drugs including paroxetine and fluoxetine, with the need for dosage adjustments. Common adverse effects include weight-loss, abdominal pain, decreased appetite, vomiting, nausea, dyspepsia, headache, dizziness, somnolence, and irritability. Atomoxetine has a black box warning for possible increased risk of suicidal thinking in adolescents (reported incidence 0.4 percent). It has been associated with the emergence of motoric tics. Contraindications to treatment with atomoxetine include hypersensitivity, use of an MAOI within 14 days, glaucoma, current or past history of pheochromocytoma, and severe cardiovascular disorders.

Alpha-2 Adrenergic Agonists

The alpha-2-adrenergic agonists clonidine (Catapres) and immediate-release guanfacine (Tenex) are prescribed for children and adolescents who respond poorly to a trial of psychostimulants or atomoxetine, have intolerable adverse effects, or contraindication to psychostimulants or atomoxetine. Alpha-2-adrenergic agonists may take up to two weeks for clinical response (compared with minutes or a few hours for the psychostimulants), and there is less information regarding their efficacy.

Clonidine has been shown to reduce ADHD symptoms in patients suffering from tics, aggression, and conduct disorder. The immediate-release formulation requires multiple daily dosing. Extended-release clonidine (Kapvey) was approved in 2010 for the treatment of ADHD for patients ages 6–17 years old, both as monotherapy and as adjunct to psychostimulants, with a prescribed maximum dose of 0.4 mg/day in divided dosing, following slowly increased doses. A weekly clonidine transdermal patch is also available. While clonidine is effective in reducing symptoms of ADHD, it was not as effective as the psychostimulants. The combination of extended-release clonidine and psychostimulant medications is also effective in reducing symptoms in children with a partial response to psychostimulants. Clonidine may be useful in over-aroused, easily frustrated, highly active, or aggressive individuals. Side effects of clonidine include sedation, depression, bradycardia, headache, and possible hypotension. Discontinuation of clonidine requires gradual dose-reduction to prevent a rebound hypertension. Clonidine is not a controlled substance and has no known abuse potential.

Guanfacine has a higher selectivity as an alpha-2 adrenergic agonist. Its effectiveness and tolerability have been shown in treating hyperactivity and inattention in those suffering from ADHD with tic- and Tourette's disorders. Extended-release guanfacine (Intuniv) was FDA-approved in 2009 for the treatment of ADHD with once-a-day dosing (maximum 4 mg/day). Guanfacine has a longer half-life and less risk of side effects compared to clonidine. Most common adverse effects of guanfacine include somnolence, headache, fatigue, abdominal pain, and bradycardia.

Antidepressants

Tricyclic antidepressants (TCAs), particularly imipramine (Tofranil), desipramine (Norpramin), and nortriptyline (Pamelor), inhibit neuronal reuptake of norepinephrine and serotonin and have been used in the treatment of ADHD, especially for patients who have failed or not tolerated trials of other treatments. Adverse effects associated with the TCAs are dry mouth, constipation, and lowering of the threshold for seizures. In addition, concern arising from several cases of sudden death among children treated with desipramine led to disfavor of TCAs in the treatment of children. Prior to starting a TCA, patients should be evaluated for cardiac disease, palpitations, dizziness, and syncope, as well as family history of sudden death at age <40 years, long QT syndrome or arrhythmias, and cardiomyopathy. An electrocardiogram should be obtained at baseline and when the TCA dose has been optimized. TCAs not only have little risk of inducing tics, but may actually improve spontaneous tics or those induced by stimulant drugs.

The dopamine and norepinephrine reuptake inhibitor bupropion (Wellbutrin) also has been used in the treatment of ADHD. It has more stimulant properties than the TCAs and modest efficacy in decreasing hyperactivity and aggressive behaviors. Adverse effects include irritability, anorexia, insomnia, motor tics, and a decreased seizure threshold, especially at doses >450 mg/day.

Medication Adherence

A very common reason for relapse of most psychiatric illnesses involves nonadherence to treatment. Patients may discontinue treatment for a variety of reasons including stigma, cost, adverse effects, forgetfulness and complexity of treatment regimens, lack of efficacy, or impaired judgment due to psychiatric illness, among others. Occasionally due to problems of access to medical care, patients may be unable to obtain a prescription refill. Transitions in care, such as a change from inpatient care to residential or outpatient care, can be a particularly common place for these access issues to arise, as well as representing a time of unusually high suicide risk. It is important that prescribing clinicians remain alert to possible nonadherence and seek to understand its cause. When psychiatric drugs are stopped abruptly, several adverse outcomes can occur, ranging from the inconvenient and uncomfortable to the potentially fatal.

Relapse or Recurrence

One of the questions in every assessment of patients with recurring or worsening illness should be about adherence to prescribed treatment. Sudden or rapid discontinuation of most classes of psychotropic medicines can lead to rapid clinical worsening, as has been demonstrated repeatedly with antidepressant, antipsychotic, mood-stabilizing, and anxiolytic drugs. The risk involved is highly dependent on the rate of dose reduction, and the latency to recurrence can be much shorter than would be predicted by the natural history of the untreated illness. To some extent, discontinuation can reflect the psychology of the long-term treatment situation. If the treatment is helpful or effective, the patient's subjective experience is mainly the discomfort of adverse or "side" effects. Indeed, the concept that he may become ill again after discontinuing treatment may be hard to grasp, and may even require some experience to be appreciated and to motivate treatment adherence. Managing or overcoming such treatment reluctance requires direct and repeated discussion of the aims of long-term maintenance treatment and of the risks in interrupting it, supported by a solid patient-clinician alliance. Sometimes it may be appropriate to discontinue a maintenance treatment, such as in the presence of annoying or intolerable adverse symptoms, or to explore uncertainties about the value of treatment continued for very long times. In such circumstances, it is prudent to reduce the doses of all psychotropic agents as slowly as is feasible and the medical conditions may permit, so as to minimize the risk of worsening or recurrence of the disorder being treated.

Discontinuation or Withdrawal Syndromes

Physiological withdrawal syndromes occur with some psychotropic drugs. Classic examples include alcohol, opioids, and most sedatives, including benzodiazepines as well as barbiturates and other older agents. Usually the risk of withdrawal reactions rises with growing evidence of tolerance of the effects of a drug, and a state of dependency that is often associated with rising dose-taking to counter the loss of beneficial effects with prolonged treatment. Abrupt discontinuation, especially of high doses, can result in tremulousness, anxiety, irritability, and even seizures, delirium, coma, and death. Opiates, similarly have a markedly uncomfortable withdrawal, but it is usually not as physically dangerous.

A particular class of withdrawal syndromes are so-called discontinuation syndromes associated with the shorter-acting SSRIs including paroxetine, as well as some NSRIs, particularly venlafaxine. Common symptoms, again, include anxiety and restlessness, peculiar sensory experiences, dizziness, tremor, insomnia, gastrointestinal upset, flu-like symptoms, and a general sense of unease. Such reactions, especially when arising with ongoing psychiatric illness, can be highly distressing and very hard to tolerate, may increase suicidal risk, and need to be taken seriously.

Management of withdrawal or discontinuation syndromes associated with antidepressants sometimes proves to be quite difficult. As a first approach, very slow dose-reduction and discontinuation may be feasible. An alternative is to switch to very slowly eliminated fluoxetine and then reduce its doses slowly. If changing to another pharmacologically similar drug is tried, it is usual to increase its dose gradually as doses of the initial drug are slowly lowered. Such a "crossover" procedure requires caution about the risk of cerebral intoxication of the serotonin syndrome type when serotonergic agents are combined, particularly with rapid and aggressive dosing. Sound practice calls for a discussion with patients of the risks of discontinuing treatment, especially rapidly or from a relatively high dose, and of the need to discuss and plan any proposed discontinuation.

Neurotherapeutics

Despite the increasing number of psychopharmacologic agents, many psychiatric patients prove to be poorly responsive to several trials of dissimilar medicines or intolerant of them. For such patients, other physical or "neurotherapeutic" options can be considered. These include electroconvulsive therapy (ECT), as well as more recently developed techniques, such as repetitive transcranial magnetic stimulation (rTMS) and other forms of brain stimulation.

Electroconvulsive Therapy (ECT)

ECT was first used in Rome in 1930s, and since then has been modified to make it safer and better accepted, including by use of brief general anesthesia and muscle relaxants, as well as improved medical monitoring; in addition, research continues to clarify benefits and risks of particular characteristics of the applied electrical stimuli (wave-form, pulse-rate, amplitude). ECT involves inducing a generalized epileptic seizure using brief pulses of electrical stimulus. It can be applied to one side of the brain (unilateral) or to both (bilateral or bifrontal) with separate electrodes. For many years, ECT was considered a treatment of last resort, due to the adverse effects of unmodified treatment as well as its unfavorable representation in literature and films. Indeed, in some areas, access to ECT is limited by legal and regulatory restrictions. Nevertheless, modern, modified ECT is a valuable, safe, and effective treatment of a variety of mental disorders.

Primary Indications

1. *Depression.* ECT remains a highly effective option for the treatment of major depressive disorder, especially with very severe depression, with psy-

chotic features, and following failed trials of pharmacological treatments, as well as being an option for acutely and severely suicidal patients. No treatment has ever been shown to be more effective than ECT for short-term treatment of severe depression. Currently, too, a minority of depressed patients not adequately managed with antidepressants or other medicines, are maintained with occasionally repeated ECT on an outpatient basis.

2. *Catatonia.* This syndrome can be life-threatening. Currently, many cases arise in psychotic affective disorders more often than in schizophrenia. Though often responsive to high doses of potent benzodiazepines such as lorazepam or clonazepam, such pharmacological treatment may be unsatisfactory. ECT is a useful alternative, and is effective in 80–90 percent of cases of catatonia.

3. *Bipolar disorder.* Both bipolar depression and mania can be treated effectively and safely with ECT, including in pregnancy. The treatment can be complicated by a risk of acute cerebral intoxication in the presence of lithium, and with the use of anticonvulsants as mood stabilizers. Such circumstances require withholding lithium and adjusting stimulus parameters with anticonvulsants.

4. *Schizoaffective disorder or schizophrenia.* ECT can often be helpful both early in the illness-course and during periods of symptomatic exacerbation of chronic psychotic disorders, especially if pharmacological treatments are not adequately effective or tolerated.

5. *Severe agitation in dementia.* ECT is an option to be considered as the risks of stroke and fatalities associated with antipsychotic drugs have become more evident.

Safety and Adverse Effects
ECT has become quite safe as currently modified. Infrequently, direct stimulation of jaw muscles can result in dental damage, but bone fractures and other severe injuries are now rare, as are hypotension and cardiac arrhythmias. Patients with intracranial lesions, including tumors, aneurysms, or arteriovenous malformations, require careful assessment to minimize the risk of cerebral herniation or intracranial bleed. The risk of dying from ECT is approximately 1/25,000 treatments.

Cognition
A leading concern about ECT is the risk of adverse effects on memory and cognition. Extensive research indicates that adverse cognitive effects of ECT are not uncommon, but usually are mild and resolve within weeks, including rapid recovery of immediate and short-term memory, although infrequently some degree of retrograde memory loss can persist. Precise statistics about these risks are difficult to determine, owing to variation in the clinical condition of patients treated, including cognitive impairment associated with depression, and in details of the

technique employed. For example, relatively low-intensity, square-wave pulses, and unilateral placement of electrodes may be better tolerated. Most often, ECT-associated memory loss is spotty, and typically more annoying than significant, but some patients experience an upsetting amount of loss as retrograde amnesia. To minimize memory loss, the following steps can be taken:

1. Unilateral treatment (typically on the nondominant right hemisphere) is usually preferred when possible. Unilateral ECT probably causes less memory loss than bilateral, but may be less effective than bilateral stimulation; although with adequate stimulus strength, unilateral stimulation can yield benefits that approach those of bilateral treatment.
2. Specific electrical characteristics of ECT stimuli may also affect risk, severity, and duration of memory loss. Ultra-brief pulse ECT shortens the width of the electrical pulse so as to match the depolarization time of cerebral neurons. This technique seems to result in less retrograde amnesia and faster cognitive recovery.
3. Reduced frequency of treatments may limit cognitive effects, such as twice rather than three times a week.
4. Monitoring of cognitive effects throughout treatment with standard memory testing can be helpful.

Repetitive Transcranial Magnetic Stimulation (rTMS)

While ECT directly applies electrical stimuli to the brain, rTMS induces an electrical current within the brain using repetitive magnetic pulses applied superficially, usually over the dorsolateral prefrontal cortex. This readily tolerated, FDA-approved treatment takes about 10–40 minutes/session and can be done in a medical office without anesthesia. Typically simulation is applied to the left side, with high-frequency pulses. However, some experts prefer right-sided rTMS and low-frequency impulses. FDA approval of rTMS in 2008 was for a specific device (NeuroStar rTMS by Neuronetics Corp.) and for a relatively narrow indication: major depressive disorder in adults who have failed to achieve satisfactory improvement from at least one prior antidepressant trial at or above the minimal effective dose and duration in a current depressive episode.

Efficacy

At least two large multicenter, sham-controlled, randomized trials of rTMS have been reported. They suggested that at least four weeks (sometimes six) of five-times-a-week treatment was necessary to achieve an adequate antidepressant response. Remission rates in these controlled trials were only 14–17 percent, but responses to active treatment separated significantly from the sham control condition. Furthermore, in unblinded extensions of these trials, remission rates eventually reached 20–30 percent. A recent assessment has found response rates of 58 percent and remission rates of 37 percent. Some of these differences may reflect the continued use of antidepressants or not, illness severity, and differences in the techniques employed. These studies suggest that rTMS can be expected to yield about a 50 percent chance of a clinically significant response and perhaps a 30 percent chance of remission. The procedures used for rTMS continue to evolve and may improve, but the method appears to yield somewhat lesser results than with ECT, though patients often prefer rTMS.

Safety and Adverse Effects

One of the great appeals of rTMS is that it is very well tolerated and acceptable to patients. Unlike ECT, rTMS does not impair memory or cognition, and no anesthesia is required, making rTMS safer and more accessible. The most common adverse effects of rTMS are headache and scalp discomfort, which rarely lead to discontinuing treatment. There is a potential risk of seizure, but at currently recommended treatment parameters, these have been very rare.

Innovative methods of external brain stimulation are under development. These include transcranial direct current stimulation (tDCS) and the use of high-frequency magnetic stimuli to induce seizures (MST), possibly with a lower risk of memory impairment.

Deep TMS

A "Deep TMS" device (Brainsway Corp.) was recently FDA-approved for depressed patients who have not responded to antidepressant treatment, and for the treatment of obsessive-compulsive disorder (OCD). This device uses a coil design to allow deeper penetration of the magnetic pulses. It is typically given at five treatments per week for five weeks for depression and six weeks for OCD, followed by two per week for up to 12 weeks for depression and a seventh week at four per week for OCD. The clinical utility and availability of the treatment are currently evolving, and it is under investigation for other psychiatric indications.

Vagus Nerve Stimulation (VNS)

Vagus nerve stimulation (VNS) was FDA-approved for refractory epilepsy in 1997. Many patients with epilepsy have co-occurring depression, which also was found to improve during VNS treatment. Trials of VNS for treatment-resistant depression (TRD) led to FDA approval for this indication in 2005, with the requirement that a candidate has failed to respond in at least four antidepressant trials. The mechanism of action of VNS is not fully understood, but the vagus nerve projects to brain regions implicated in the pathophysiology of mood disorders.

The surgical procedure for implanting the VNS device involves a small incision in the left side of the neck to allow access to the carotid sheath, containing the carotid artery, internal jugular vein, and the vagus nerve, around which electrodes are placed. The left vagus nerve is used to avoid the parasympathetic branches to the heart in the right vagus. A second incision on the left chest allows for the implantation of an electrical pulse generator (IPG) connected to the vagal electrodes. An external device communicates with the IPG transcutaneously to control stimulus parameters (amplitude, pulse width, and frequency). Response typically requires 3–12 months of continuous stimulation. Adverse effects are usually well tolerated, and appear to arise from stimulation of branches of the vagus nerve (e.g., coughing or throat discomfort from stimulation of the laryngeal and pharyngeal branches). Clinical use of VNS has been limited for several reasons, including the high cost of establishing the implanted devices, widespread lack of insurance compensation in the US despite FDA approval, and a lack of adequately trained clinicians to apply it. Further advances in vagus nerve stimulation are arising with the use of transcutaneous VNS, which is less invasive than current methods of stimulation.

Deep Brain Stimulation (DBS)

Deep brain stimulation (DBS) has been used for more than a decade for the treatment of severe, treatment-refractory movement disorders such as Parkinson's disease, dystonia, and essential tremor. For treatment-resistant depression, electrodes are placed stereotactically and connected to a subcutaneous pacemaker surgically implanted in the chest wall. For movement disorders, preferred cerebral targets are the globus pallidus interna or subthalamic nucleus. The pacemaker can be programmed transcutaneously to deliver electrical stimuli at specific amplitudes and frequencies, for example, as guided by amelioration of abnormalities of movement.

DBS has been introduced more recently as an experimental treatment for severely unresponsive major depression or OCD. The most extensively studied target sites include the subgenual anterior cingulate cortex for depression, the anterior limb of the ventral internal capsule-ventral striatum for depression and OCD, and nucleus accumbens for depression. Several unblinded trials have yielded encouraging findings, especially for TRD (with response rates averaging 50 percent and remission rates of about 30 percent), though more recent, controlled trials have been less encouraging, as have trials for OCD and Gilles de la Tourette syndrome.

Current and Future Directions

Psychiatry and its related basic and clinical sciences have undergone rapid changes in recent years. A growing focus on translational neuroscience has catalyzed this process and is ongoing. Treatment discovery and improvement are primary goals for the field, and are advancing in different simultaneous pathways. The following discussion highlights some emerging trends and needs for biomedically based psychiatric therapeutics.

It is fair to state that the development of modern psychopharmacology and biological psychiatry since the 1950s has had a revolutionary impact on the theory and practice of psychiatry throughout the world. Yet remarkably little in the field of psychiatric therapeutics is fundamentally new since 1960, with many very similar drugs in each class, some of which are better tolerated, but almost none proved to be superior in efficacy. This circumstance highlights the need for therapeutic innovation, as well as the optimization of existing treatments. The development of novel treatments should be closely related to the understanding of pathophysiology. Recent decades have brought major advances in neuroscience and in the understanding of basic brain mechanisms, including their relationship to mood, thinking, and behavior. Nevertheless, there has been a remarkably limited impact of such advances on understanding the pathophysiology, let alone etiology, of most psychiatric disorders. Lack of such knowledge severely limits the impact of efforts at innovation aimed at improving treatment. Notably, these realities have led a growing number of pharmaceutical corporations – the major source of new drugs – to diminish or abandon their programs in psychopharmaceutical and other CNS drug development.

Pharmacological treatments are critically important in psychiatry, and they have come to dominate much of psychiatric therapeutics in recent decades. Currently, available medicines have been extensively characterized for their effects on one or more neurotransmitter systems. However, there has been a great deal of circularity in the process of developing novel, more effective, faster-acting, and safer treatments, based on mimicking partial knowledge of the pharmacodynamics of earlier drugs discovered largely by serendipity. This strategy has been employed with considerable success but has yielded many very similar drugs in each class, with some gains in safety and tolerability, but rarely improved efficacy.

A striking recent advance has been the discovery that NMDA glutamate receptor antagonists, notably ketamine and esketamine, have rapid antidepressant effects, even in otherwise treatment-resistant depressions. They can induce major improvements of symptoms within hours rather than weeks after administration. This strategy again arose from focusing on modulation of a specific neurotransmitter system, albeit glutamate rather than a monoamine. Clinical trials of ketamine for depression were encouraged by a series of findings of activity in animal behavioral models of depression dating back to the 1970s, as well as recognition of the drug's risk of abuse as a recreational agent in high doses, in addition to its activity as a dissociative anesthetic – but not clearly from a knowledge of the role of glutamate neurotransmission in a biology of depression. Other efforts at therapeutic innovation are moving further away from neurotransmitter biology, aiming for other targets such as second-messenger systems, gene-modulation, inflammatory pathways, cell-mediated immune responses, oxidative stress, mitochondrial processes, and neurodegeneration. Some of these approaches show promise, but it remains to be seen if they will lead to novel and better psychotropic medicines.

In recent years, a series of novel neurostimulatory treatment methods have appeared, including rTMS, deep TMS, VNS, and DBS, as reviewed above. All have limitations and risks and require technical refinement as well as additional research to optimize their clinical applications. An indirect benefit of these developments is renewed interest in improving understanding of the role of specific brain regions and neurophysiological mechanisms related to clinical manifestations of major mood, psychotic, and behavioral disorders.

It is important to point out that many basic questions remain with existing psychopharmacological and physical treatments, including the relative efficacy and risks of specific drugs or stimulation methods. Notably, it has been very hard to distinguish individual drugs by the averaging process represented by meta-analysis, but with very few head-to-head comparisons. Also inadequately tested are optimal drug dosing or stimulus parameters for particular groups of patients, including by age and clinical subtype. A major challenge is the need to specify which drug is a best first choice, or most likely to be effective and tolerated, for which patient or clinical circumstance.

Efforts also continue to define pathophysiological changes that are characteristic, if not diagnostic, of major psychiatric disorders, and which might contribute to more objective and precise diagnosis and to optimizing matches between individual patients and specific treatments. Nevertheless, as noted previously, current biomedical understanding of mechanisms and abnormalities underlying nearly all psychiatric disorders remains very limited, as might be expected with illnesses that lack a secure organ or tissue pathology. Some investigators propose that the very basis of contemporary psychiatric nosology, relying on clinical signs and symptoms, illness course, and treatment responses, itself, is a major limitation to therapeutic progress. To date, however, credible alternative diagnostic systems based on neuroimaging, genetics and molecular biology, metabolism, and pathophysiology have remained elusive.

A fundamental hope for a biomedical approach to psychiatric illness has been that a better understanding of putative pathophysiologic mechanisms, coupled with a sophisticated neurobiological understanding of the actions of psychiatric treatments, would lead to new "markers" or laboratory tests that would guide diagnosis and optimize and individualize treatment. This attractive and desirable perspective, too, has yet to be realized at the level of routine clinical practice, despite decades of efforts.

In conclusion, despite the frustrations involved, efforts to develop meaningful applications of emerging findings from neuroscience to psychiatric diagnosis and therapeutics continue and should be encouraged. Lest we abandon much of the progress from the past 150 years, it is also important to continue efforts to improve understanding of psychiatric disorders at the descriptive level, based on psychopathology, epidemiology, psychology, and sociology – ideally with ongoing reciprocal discussion of advances from both neuroscientific and clinical approaches.

References and Suggested Readings

- Baldessarini, R. J. (2013). *Chemotherapy in Psychiatry*, 3rd ed. New York: Springer.
- Bauer, M., Severus, E., Möller, H.-J., and Young, A. H., WFSBP Task Force on Unipolar Depressive Disorders (2017). Pharmacological Treatment of Unipolar Depressive Disorders: Summary of WFSBP Guidelines. *International Journal of Psychiatry in Clinical Practice*, 21 (3), 166–176.
- Cipriani, A., Furukawa, T. A., Salanti, G., Chaimani, A., Atkinson, L. Z., Ogawa, Y., Leucht, S., Ruhe, H. G., Turner, E. H., Higgins, J. P. T., Egger, M., Takeshima, N., Hayasaka, Y., Imai, H., Shinohara, K., Tajika, A., Ioannidis, J. P. A., and Geddes, J. R. (2018). Comparative Efficacy and Acceptability of 21 Antidepressant Drugs for the Acute Treatment of Adults with Major Depressive Disorder: Systematic Review and Network Meta-analysis. *Lancet*, 391 (10128), 1357–1366.
- Ionescu, D. F., and Papkostas, G. I. (2017). Experimental Medication Treatment Approaches for Depression. *Translational Psychiatry*, 7, e1068.
- Schatzberg, A. F., and Nemeroff, C. (2017). *The American Psychiatric Association Publishing Textbook of Psychopharmacology*, 5th ed. Washington, DC: American Psychiatric Publishing.
- Stahl, S., and Munter, N. (2013). *Stahl's Essential Psychopharmacology: Neuroscientific Basis and Practical Applications*, 4th ed. New York: Cambridge University Press.
- Stern, T. A., Fava, M., Wilens, T. A., and Rosenbaum, J. F. (2015). *Massachusetts General Hospital Psychopharmacology and Neurotherapeutics*. New York: Elsevier.

Self-Assessment Questions

1. Which of the following statements about antidepressant medications is *false*?
    A. 1 in 3 patients with major depressive disorder respond to the first antidepressant prescribed.
    B. Antidepressants that act on both serotonin and norepinephrine are more effective for pain syndrome than agents that affect serotonin alone.
    C. In comparing antidepressant medication to placebo, there is a large effect size.
    D. Sexual effects, including anorgasmia, and moderate weight gain are common adverse effects of antidepressants.
    E. Antidepressants can activate manic symptoms in predisposed individuals.

2. A paradoxical increase in suicidal ideation in depressed patients treated with antidepressants:
    A. Is common with this form of treatment.
    B. Is more common in the geriatric population than in children and adolescents.
    C. Is reportedly more likely at ages below twenty-five years versus older patients.
    D. Is unrelated to undiagnosed bipolar disorder in adolescents.
    E. Is a contraindication to the use of antidepressants in children and adolescents.

3. Which of the following medicines does not lower the seizure threshold?
    A. Clomipramine
    B. Bupropion
    C. Carbamazepine
    D. Clozapine

4. Which of the following is not indicated for acute mania?
    A. Carbamazepine
    B. Lithium Carbonate
    C. Oxcarbazepine
    D. Risperidone
    E. Cariprazine

5. For which of the following is there strong evidence for protective effectiveness against recurrent mania?
    A. Divalproex
    B. Lamotrigine
    C. Lithium carbonate
    D. Carbamazepine

Answers to Self-Assessment Questions

1. (C)
2. (C)
3. (C)
4. (C)
5. (C)

16 Psychosocial Interventions

MARSHALL FORSTEIN, ALFRED MARGUILES, ROBERT GOISMAN,
ELIZABETH SIMPSON, ELEANOR COUNSELMAN, MIRIAM TEPPER,
JENNIFER GREENWOLD, ZEV SCHUMAN-OLIVIER, AND DARSHAN MEHTA

What Is Psychotherapy?

Psychotherapy is an overarching term for any type of professional treatment for psychological and physical distress using verbal and nonverbal communication. Talking together, the patient and therapist engage collaboratively to understand the source of a dysfunction or suffering in order to reverse either maladaptive self-regulatory processes or to adapt and develop psychological strengths to cope with pathological conditions, developmental concerns, or trauma. Psychotherapy addresses multiple levels of functioning, including the neurobiology of the brain itself, the perception of the self to itself, the relationship of the self to others, the role of the individual in the social world, and the conceptual frameworks and beliefs that also may affect emotions and behavior.

Complex language is a unique characteristic of being human, and talking about thoughts, feelings, and behavior can help people feel connected to the world and make sense of the human condition. Listening to another human being is an active therapeutic intervention itself. In psychological or physical pain, the patient feels is seen and heard, thus validating the internal experience of the patient.

The following sections of this chapter explore some of the currently used forms of psychotherapy. What is common to all is the importance of the relationship between the patient and the therapist, establishing a trust (therapeutic alliance) that the process will lead to an improvement in feelings, thoughts, or behavior.

Psychotherapeutic interventions differ according to the "frame" of therapy. This "frame" varies in terms of parameters related to time (short visits, long visits), length of treatment (short term, long term, number of sessions, open-ended), and modality of treatment.

Sometimes referred to simply as "talk therapy," psychotherapy may be used alone or in conjunction with psychoactive medications to alleviate anxiety, depression, and many other psychiatric disorders. Other somatic interventions, such as ECT (electroconvulsive therapy), TMS (transcranial magnetic stimulations), or VNS (vagus nerve stimulation) may also be used concurrently. Many physiological changes in brain function have been documented as a result of psychotherapeutic treatments.

Therapists may work with individuals, couples, families, or groups of people of any age. Pre-verbal and young children may be engaged in "play therapy," while older children and adults talk with therapists about problems that help them become better at coping with difficult situations, relationships, or illness.

A useful concept corresponding to biological functioning is that of "mental homeostasis." As with biological homeostasis, mental functioning occurs within a "bandwidth" of "normal" function (i.e., ability to be resilient, flexible, and adaptive to the trials and tribulations of life or to the impact of biological processes on mental function and coping). The more severe the disruptions are in the "hard wiring" of the brain, the greater the possibility for mental dysfunction. Psychotherapy requires the ability to process information, to have a basically intact remote and working memory, and to tolerate emotions and bodily sensations that arise in the course of treatment. As within the immune system, there are multiple mechanisms for restoring homeostasis when affected by either internal changes in biological function, or external assaults on the integrity of the organism. Similarly, when the "mental homeostasis" is disrupted by changes in brain function or external events that impact the capacity of the person to manage, psychological defenses are employed to try to maintain or restore a sense of psychological well-being. These defenses, although sometimes maladaptive, are intended to keep the person functioning at the highest level of function possible.

"Dynamic" forms of psychotherapy rooted in the psychoanalytic tradition often explore psychological defenses, enhancing their usefulness or replacing them with more effective ways to diminish suffering and maladaptive behavior. Distinguishing what are "normal" anxieties and mood fluctuations from internal or external experiences that impinge on the ability to function in the day-to-day world can enhance coping skills. "Cognitive" therapies make use of understanding the role of negative thinking in creating ambivalence or fear about change may diminish dysfunction. Negative thoughts, for example, about the past, may predispose the individual to anticipate that the future may be much the same, even when there are opportunities for it to be different. "Psychosocial interventions" using principles of psycho-education, help patients understand their psychiatric disorders and symptoms, and include rehabilitation strategies and social supports for improving quality of life, symptom management, and connection with the world. Often psychotherapy of any modality helps people learn to grieve and live with what may appear to be insurmountable barriers to living with loss that is an inevitable part of the human experience.

Research is underway to better define what type of therapeutic process is most effective with particular disorders. There is a growing body of research providing evidence, for example, that talk therapy in addition to antidepressant medication is most effective in treating more moderate and severe depression. In the following sections, each author describes the form of therapy and its indication for use. References are provided for further exploration of the various modalities of treatment.

Psychoanalysis

Beneath our conscious awareness lie forces that powerfully shape our behavior and indeed consciousness itself – and this is the terrain of psychoanalysis. Not rational in the sense of linear goal directedness, these irrational forces have their own logic and structure that are revealed through how we operationalize our approaches. And so this terrain of irrational behavior, the not-fully conscious, overlaps with other disciplines, a hot area of research in neurobiology, medication compliance and noncompliance, placebo effect, nocebo effect, pain, dream states, addictions, and medical errors. Moreover, recent research into nonconscious behavior extends beyond medicine to areas as diverse as economics and market behavior, advertising, unconscious stereotyping and racism, voting patterns and political rhetoric, rapid decision-making by experts and novices, facial displays and lying, unconscious jury bias, and more. What we mean by the unconscious or *nonconscious* is then rapidly expanding, and we are still coming to understand how these processes saturate our clinical work and, indeed, our everyday existence. Here psychoanalysis takes up the clinical relevance of these forces.

Though we pride ourselves on our rationality, scratch the surface and we encounter complex fantasies of love, desire, lust and sexuality; self-esteem and envy; aggression and hatred; power, dominance and hierarchy; deep attachments and tangled relationships; unbearable grief and fear and, of course, high ideals and a demanding and troubled conscience side-by-side with intense belief and hope. Complex creatures in a complex world, no wonder that we keep a lot unsaid – and even more out of mind. No wonder, too, that when it comes to the varieties of human suffering, these unconscious forces are particularly complex and daunting, with some aspects of non-rational mind and behavior close to awareness and some more elusive.

For example, a patient in her late twenties presented with feelings of unshakeable depression, lack of energy and interest in life, poor sleep, and difficulty accessing her feelings. These symptoms seemed to come out of the blue and were in contrast with what she thought was the promise of her life and its opportunities. About to leave the state for what should be an exciting job, she felt deadened and confused. In taking a history, it emerged quickly that she was seeking treatment almost exactly coinciding with the first year anniversary of her father's death – and, up until the moment of her saying this, she had not been aware of the connection. Indeed, over the past year, she was aware of pushing aside her grief because she felt it would hamper her caring for her family. As the oldest child, she took charge of her siblings after her mother abandoned them all. In his despair, her father had relied on her. And despite her father's death – especially with his death! – she never had the space to deal with her own feelings: others, she felt, still need to come first. But, this made no sense to her: life had settled down over the past year, her siblings were launched in their own lives, she herself now had a serious boyfriend, and it seemed strange to her that still she felt numb, closed up, and shutdown. And here in her first interview and for the first time since her father had died, she wept deeply in telling her story. Immediately she felt relief, freer, and eager to continue before she left town. Given the space to talk freely, this young woman quickly identified what had precipitated her depressive shutdown, and in doing so, her depressive symptoms evaporated. In subsequent meetings, she grieved with a lively openness (grief is not depression!), and spontaneously brought in family albums, talked about beloved memories of her father, and, more difficult to acknowledge, ways he both loved and disappointed her. She had never felt comfortable being angry with him because he meant so much to her. In talking, her father emerged as a fuller person – and so did she.

The Psychoanalytic Process

Perhaps more difficult to describe is the experience of the psychoanalytic process itself. The self-recursive process of reflection inherent in the analytic approach continually boot-straps awareness with the participatory help of another. That is, rather than attempting to remain outside of the observational field, the analytic clinician brings into mutual awareness the complex interaction as a vehicle to further unfold awareness. Some basic processes of this force field we refer to as "transference" and "counter-transference," and their mutual interaction as "enactment." Not so mysterious, transference is at heart a translation of earlier experiences, patterns of expectations, into present ones. Particularly when these patterns of experience involve important others, they become reflexive and entrenched, sometimes highly repetitive and self-defeating, ways of both experiencing and shaping the world at the same time. And so these interactions (transference, countertransference, enactment) entangle the participants (analyst and patient), but – and here's the subtle psychoanalytic process – rather than attempting to step outside of the forces (an ultimate impossibility in a participant-observer field), the analyst and patient move into and through them as a way of becoming more aware of the reflexive and habitual impact on ways of being in a world that we also construct.

For example, with the patient above who was in a psychoanalytically oriented psychotherapy, imagine that she returns a few years later, now struggling in a marriage and with children of her own. And here she has a return of depressive symptoms – numbness and a disinterest in life – that she does not fully understand and that are spilling over into the lives of her husband and children, and this alarms her. Further, she suspects it is precisely in her new role as a mother that old concerns are being reawakened: Why am I afraid to attach and commit to another? What does it mean to love one's children? Why did mother leave – didn't she love me? Wasn't I good enough? Why am I withdrawing? Why do I avoid conflict? How about love and loss, and what to do about anger and ambivalence? She wants to better understand how she lives – and the stakes feel high for everyone she loves. She is ready to go deeper.

Psychoanalysis is designed to deepen this self-exploration of memory, affect, longing, meaning, and significance. By intensifying the therapy through frequency and duration, there is a loosening of resistance to painful emotion so that there might be an opening up of a free flow of feelings, memories, and associations that are ordinarily pushed away from awareness. The analyst and patient take special notice of how repetitive patterns emerge within the analytic relationship itself (transference, countertransference) and how they entangle one another within enactments. And here awareness opens further. The aim is toward the freedom to speak one's mind fully, letting it go where it will, in the presence and in conversation with another – with the goal of freeing up new possibilities of choosing how to live.

More than a hundred years after Freud launched his first investigations, this sketch belies the subtlety of the still-evolving field of psychoanalysis and its rich branches of theory and inquiry. The interested student might find the following resources ways to begin, though engaging these readings in conversation with a psychoanalytic supervisor in the context of clinical work will, of course, open a deeper awareness of the process itself.

Cognitive-Behavioral Therapy

Cognitive-behavioral therapy (CBT) is a highly operationalized form of psychotherapy with a strong evidence base justifying its use. In this section, we will briefly discuss the history and development of CBT, describe some of the basic principles believed to underlie the effectiveness of this method, discuss its indications and limitations, and provide resources with which the reader can further pursue areas of interest.

CBT is not an absolutely unified, monolithic body of doctrine; there are schools of thought within CBT that agree, disagree, and sometimes both agree and disagree with each other. Many clinicians and investigators separate the various streams of thought within CBT into "waves" (Kahl et al, 2012). The first wave is represented by classical behavior therapy or "behavior modification"; this is largely based on classical and operant conditioning models as described in the early 1900s by Pavlov, Skinner, and their intellectual descendants. Exposure treatment for anxiety disorders is a present-day "first wave" therapy (Barlow, 2007). The second wave is that of cognitive therapy, as pioneered by and exemplified by the work of Aaron Beck (Beck et al, 1979), Albert Ellis, and many others. Cognitive therapy of depression, perhaps the best-studied form of psychotherapy currently in existence, is one very commonly utilized second-wave treatment. The third wave of CBT is a rather heterogeneous group of treatments that have in common their use of mindfulness techniques, Eastern spirituality, meta-cognitive approaches, acceptance of dysphoric states, and so on; dialectical behavior therapy (DBT) and acceptance and commitment therapy (ACT) are currently popular versions of third-wave therapies (Kahl et al, 2012).

There are, however, certain characteristics that all of these "waves" share, which collectively distinguish CBT from other forms of psychosocial treatment. These are:

1. Delivery of psychotherapy in a structured and operationalized manner
2. Derivation from learning theory, cognitive psychology, information processing theory, and social learning theory
3. Selection of cognitions and behaviors as treatment targets in the expectation that changing these will lead to remission of symptoms
4. Relatively greater emphasis on current determinants of behavior and factors maintaining symptoms than on past hypothesized causes of symptoms
5. Treatment being relatively short-term and typically including formal agenda-setting and the assignment of homework in a collaborative manner

There are a number of treatment modalities within CBT that form the "building blocks" of treatment. These modalities are used in virtually all applications of CBT. These are:

1. Exposure
2. Cognitive restructuring
3. Skill deficit remediation
4. Contingency management
5. Stimulus control

Briefly, exposure methods involve getting into contact with ("exposed" to) a stimulus that evokes dysphoria and then staying in contact with it until the aversive emotion abates (Barlow, 2007); typically the dysphoria is that of anxiety, although Linehan (1993) and others have discussed exposure methods for guilt, shame, and other negative mood states. Cognitive restructuring involves the elicitation of thoughts which occur in given situations, usually those which are painful or otherwise problematic; these are then rated in intensity, categorized in terms of what type of cognitive distortion may be present, and discussed Socratically as to their truthfulness and usefulness, after which a less distorted thought is constructed and substituted (A. Beck et al., 1979). Skill deficit remediation involves conceptualizing psychopathology as a series of acquired or at times inborn skill deficits that can be corrected over time by didactic instruction, in vivo exercises including role-plays, and homework assignments; this has been shown to be particularly helpful in schizophrenia (Liberman, 2008) and borderline personality disorder (Linehan, 1993).

Contingency management, at its heart an operant conditioning intervention, describes a strategy of managing the consequences of a given behavior, so as to increase the frequency of desired behaviors and/or decrease the frequency of undesirable behaviors; token economies are examples of very elaborate contingency management systems, whereas the "pass" system used on many locked inpatient units, in which weekend passes are granted or not in part as a consequence of the frequency of desired behaviors such as group attendance during the week, is a simpler application of the same principle. Finally, stimulus control is a term used to describe efforts to alter the proximity of stimuli or "triggers" to a given behavior so as to increase their availability for desired behaviors and decrease their availability for those considered undesirable; an example of this would be to prescribe that a patient in early stages of recovery from alcoholism stay away from bars and liquor stores and go to Alcoholics Anonymous meetings instead, or to prescribe that a patient with pedophilia stay away from day care centers (Marlatt and Donovan, 2005). Psychoeducation is often mentioned as a sixth basic modality of CBT, but since clinicians from many schools of thought use psychoeducation, it is not listed here.

The earliest clinical work using principles of CBT (then known as "behavior modification") was in the 1940s and 1950s with outpatients suffering from specific phobias and with long-term inpatients suffering from schizophrenia. From those two quite disparate starting points the indications for CBT have increased exponentially, so that in contemporary psychiatry CBT has been used for most of the types of illness listed in the Diagnostic and Statistical Manual. A reasonable list of specific indications for CBT would include:

1. Anxiety disorders (including post-traumatic stress disorder)
2. Depression
3. Borderline personality disorder
4. Schizophrenia
5. Bipolar disorder
6. Substance abuse
7. Eating disorders
8. Child psychiatric disorders (e.g., autism spectrum disorders, childhood obsessive-compulsive disorder, etc.)

Treatment for anxiety disorders usually involves exposure to the external or internal anxiety-provoking or phobic stimulus, often combined with cognitive restructuring around the actual dangerousness of the stimulus and some type of anxiety management training. Cognitive restructuring and behavioral activation are the main modalities used in the CBT of depression, and dialectical behavior therapy is the primary cognitive-behavioral method used in the treatment of borderline personality disorder. As an augmentation strategy for antipsychotic medication, CBT can be used in the treatment of schizophrenia via skill deficit remediation and also by some fascinating newer work in the cognitive restructuring of hallucinations and delusions (Kingdon and Turkington, 2005). Similarly, CBT can be used as an adjunctive treatment for bipolar disorder through psychoeducation, early detection of signs of relapse, lifestyle management, and some cognitive restructuring (Basco and Rush, 2007). Protocols for the cognitive-behavioral treatment of eating disorders and substance abuse disorders are easily found (e.g., Barlow, 2007). And the literature on CBT for children and adolescents is expanding rapidly (e.g., Szigethy et al., 2012).

Thus contemporary cognitive-behavioral therapy has emerged as a versatile set of interventions that can be helpful in the treatment of many types of psychiatric illness. CBT has the additional value of having a strong research base to provide evidence of its effectiveness and of the stability of its results over time. In addition to the sources cited here, there are a number of basic textbooks to which the interested reader can refer in order to obtain more information or to help clinicians who are novices in this area to get started (e.g., J. Beck, 2011; Wright et al., 2006). Further, the two major organizations promoting CBT in the U. S., the Academy of Cognitive Therapy in Philadelphia and the Association for Behavioral and Cognitive Therapies in New York, each have websites containing "Find a Therapist" listings, educational materials about CBT and its indications, and other useful information (www.academyofct.org, www.abct.org). In an era in which the perceived value of the doctor-patient relationship cannot be taken for granted, CBT offers an evidence-based method by which physicians can justify spending time with patients to their benefit.

Dialectical Behavior Therapy

People suffering with borderline personality disorder (BPD) are often quite miserable and tend to consume a lot of treatment, not always to great benefit. In response, Dr. Marsha Linehan, a professor of psychology at the University of Washington in Seattle, developed dialectical behavior therapy (DBT) to provide a principle-based, manualized approach to the complex myriad of problems of chronically suicidal, self-injurious women. In a randomized control trial, the first in the literature for this diagnosis, women with BPD were assigned to DBT or to "treatment as usual" in the community. In the final comparison, those who received DBT were much less likely to drop out of treatment, had fewer and less serious episodes of suicidal behavior, were less frequently hospitalized, used drugs and alcohol less, enhanced their social functioning and anger control, and were more globally improved (Linehan, Armstrong, et al., 1991; Linehan, Tutek, et al., 1993).

DBT posits a primary role for emotional dysregulation in the patient's difficulties. People with BPD are hypothesized to be biologically vulnerable to overwhelming emotional experience. Exquisitely sensitive to emotional cues and intensely reactive and expressive, sudden surges of emotional arousal may overwhelm cognitive resources, having devastating consequences on good judgment, sound decision-making, mentalization, and self-control. It is vital, therefore, to have some regulatory sway over this passion, but people with BPD have not learned to let reason and reflection guide emotion. They may act impulsively to curtail the feeling (e.g., by cutting or suicide crisis) or resort to ineffective efforts to down-regulate it (e.g., rumination, disordered eating, depressive withdrawal), aiming to escape or avoid the experience of the emotion, rather than to solve the problem which elicited it.

Emotional dysregulation exerts its most ruinous consequences in relationships. Through interaction, all parties to any social exchange are vulnerable to unpredictable changes in their emotional state which may be potentially dysregulating (think of the crying baby on an airplane). The emotional arousal of one will influence that of the other, and vice versa, in a transaction of mutual effect, for good or for ill, in service of cooperation or conflict. People with BPD tend to experience the therapeutic context as the Marriott buffet of emotional cues, and their dysregulation creates an intense and potentially volatile context.

When things get hot, DBT activates acceptance and dialectics to keep the patient in the room. Dialectical philosophy guides the therapist to approach the patient with an open-minded curiosity, assuming that problem behavior makes sense from the patient's perspective or they would not be doing it. Letting go of efforts to change the patient, at least for the moment, the therapist focuses on understanding and accepting him as he is, and communicating that acceptance to him. Typically, validation lowers arousal and facilitates the cooperative relationship necessary for change. In early stages, validation can be used to facilitate acceptance of primary emotions, to cue adaptive emotions, to strengthen their capacity for self-reflection, and to highlight what matters to the patient.

In balance to acceptance, Stage I DBT provides a comprehensive array of change-oriented interventions. It is a highly structured, outpatient treatment, consisting of weekly individual therapy and group skills training sessions, with a renewable one-year treatment contract. A behavior therapy, DBT is focused on current determinants of behavior and is highly collaborative. It combines cognitive behavioral therapy (chain analysis, contingency management, exposure, skills training, stimulus control, and cognitive modification) with mindfulness (to train attentional control) and dialectical strategies (to develop and enhance flexibility of perspective and social cooperation).

Problems are organized into a hierarchy and are targeted directly. For example, suicidal urges and actions are monitored on a diary card, incidents are functionally analyzed to determine controlling variables, and alternative responses, taught in the skills group, are proposed and rehearsed in the individual session. The therapist is available for telephone coaching after hours to assist with the implementation of the new behaviors into the patient's life. The ultimate goal is to be able to engage in functional, life-enhancing behavior, even when strong emotions are present (Lynch, Chapman, et al., 2006).

In short, DBT therapy is a mindful dance between these fundamental truths: the wisdom in what is and the need for change. As a wise old analyst once said, "Meet the patient where they are and take them where they don't want to go."

Group Therapy

There are many kinds of group therapy: standard interpersonal or psychodynamic therapy groups, cognitive-behavioral (CBT), dialectic behavioral (DBT), psycho-drama, and psycho-educational to name a few. This section will describe general interpersonal/psychodynamic group therapy. Such groups can be time-limited or open-term. The overall efficacy of group psychotherapy has been discussed in a meta-analysis by Burlingame, Fuhriman, and Mosier, 2003. Group psychotherapy can be useful for patients with general interpersonal difficulties (Yalom & Leszcz, 2005; Rutan, Shay & Stone, 2007). Group therapy is effective for symptoms such as depression (McDermut, Miller, and Brown, 2001) and for specific populations: for example, people infected with HIV, (Himelhoch, Medoff, and Oyeniyi, 2007), people with PTSD (Sloan, Bovin, and Schnurr, 2013), and school-age children (Matta and Terjesen, 2012). (See "Group Works!" on the American Group Psychotherapy Association website for additional references on different populations: www.agpa .org/group/consumersguide2000.html.)

What is helpful about group therapy? There is considerable evidence linking specific therapeutic factors and mechanisms with patient improvement in groups. A number of therapeutic factors in group therapy have been identified: universality, altruism, installation of hope, imparting information, corrective recapitulation of primary family experience, development of socializing techniques, imitative behavior, cohesiveness, existential factors, catharsis, interpersonal learning – input, interpersonal learning – output, self-understanding (Yalom & Leszcz, 2005).

A major therapeutic advantage of group is that in individual sessions a patient can talk *about* interpersonal problems, but in a group session, the patient will actually *have* them. The therapist can facilitate constructive feedback for the patient and the group setting provides a safe and protected space for the patient to try out new, more effective ways of relating. Many patients are not aware of the ways that they protect themselves emotionally and the impact of their defenses on relationships; group therapy with its "hall of mirrors" helps patients learn and change. An example of such change was the pleasant young man from an extremely critical family. He had learned not to reveal anything about how he felt inside because it would be judged. Not surprisingly, his relationships stayed very superficial, and he did not know why. In group therapy, he was gently helped to see how much he feared judgment and therefore protected himself with platitudes that deprived others of any real connection with him. In the safety of the group, he gradually risked revealing more of his inner experience and was able to develop deeper connections first with other group members and subsequently in his outside life.

A common factor across all types of therapy groups is the basic human support that membership in a group can offer – the sense of belonging. Research supports the therapeutic relationship as the mechanism of action that functions across all types of therapies (Martin et al., 2000). Furthermore, that relationship appears more significant for client improvement than any specific mechanism of action in formal treatment protocols (Norcross, 2001; Wampold, 2001). For group therapy, the equivalent of a therapeutic relationship is group cohesion – that is, the multiple relationships between members, between members and leader, and between members and group as a whole. Group structure, verbal interaction, and emotional climate have been found to significantly increase group cohesion (Burlingame et al., 2002).

As in individual therapy, a group must feel safe for effective work to occur. The role of the leader is to create and maintain a group climate that facilitates the work. An effective group leader establishes a group agreement that each member must understand and commit to. This agreement includes the basics of time and place, attendance requirements, fee, purpose of the group, confidentiality, and rules about outside contact with other members. The leader serves as gatekeeper and is responsible for screening and preparing prospective group members. In the pre-group screening, which consists of one or more individual meetings, the group therapist establishes an initial alliance with the patient, gives information about the group including the group agreement, deals with expectable anxiety about entering the group, explores any resistance, and assesses whether the patient is appropriate for the group being considered.

The selection of members for a group is dependent on the nature of the group. General principles include the ability to uphold the group agreement, the capacity to benefit from the group, and some capability for empathy and/or wish for connection. Most interpersonal groups are composed of members at the same level of psychological functioning. Groups typically have eight to ten members and can be led by a single leader or a co-leader pair. Co-leadership is an excellent training model but does add the co-leader relationship as an additional dimension.

Some patients should be excluded from group therapy. A general rule is that individuals should not be placed in group therapy if due to logistical, intellectual, psychological, and/or interpersonal reasons they cannot engage in the activity of the group (Yalom & Leszcz, 2005). As premature dropouts are hard on groups as well as the member who drops out, great care should be taken with patient selection and preparation. The best question to consider is: Is this the right group for this patient at this time?

A number of models of group development exist in the literature (Bion, 1961; MacKenzie, 1994; Tuckman, 1965; Rutan, Stone & Shay, 2007). All describe various stages of group development: (1) early "forming" or dependency, (2) a "storming" or counterdependency, (3) "norming" or intimacy, (4) "performing" or mature working, and (5) separation (of individual members) or termination (of the whole group). These stages are epigenetic, developing gradually over time, although various group events such as the entrance of a new member or a leader vacation can cause a group to regress back into an earlier state. For example, a group may react to the leader's approaching vacation with greater reliance on the leader to facilitate (dependency) or may experience increased latenesses or absences (counterdependency). Also, groups with particular populations may tend to stay in a single stage; for example, a group for the chronically mentally ill may stay a dependency group and still offer considerable benefit to its members.

Group dynamics operate on a number of levels: individual, subgroup, group as a whole, and the larger system in which the group is embedded (e.g., hospital or clinic). At all times, the leader must attend to both content and process and needs to monitor the individual members, as well as the climate of the whole group.

Group therapy has risks as well as benefits. Possible risks include group pressures such as harsh confrontation or verbal abuse, inappropriate reassurance, isolation, and scapegoating (Corey & Corey, 1997). Poor member selection may result in inappropriate placement and a failed group therapy experience. Confidentiality cannot be guaranteed in group therapy in the same way as it can in individual treatment because clients are not bound (or protected) by the same restrictions as therapists.

In summary, with appropriate patient selection and preparation along with competent leadership, group therapy helps patients confront and change problematic interpersonal behavior, improve their social skills, decrease loneliness and isolation, deal with losses more effectively, diminish feelings of helplessness, enhance self-esteem, resolve feelings of shame, and develop hope. Notably, in an era of medical cost containment, it is economical because one therapist treats multiple patients at the same time. Thus group therapy is a cost-effective form of treatment worth considering for many psychiatric problems.

Community-Based Programs for Serious Mental Illness

Psychiatry has historically provided a bleak forecast to individuals with serious mental illnesses such as schizophrenia. However, in recent years there has been growing awareness that prognosis is in fact quite heterogeneous. A growing body of research has demonstrated that if provided supports, skills, opportunities, and early interventions, many people with schizophrenia do quite well (Harding et al, 1987). We have come to recognize that to treat a person like he or she will never improve is a self-fulfilling prophecy, since hope is a critical ingredient in clinical and functional improvement.

The recovery movement emerged in this context, originating from the increasing vocal perspectives of consumers, or persons with the lived experience of mental illness. (Frese et al, 2009). (In this section we will use the words "consumer," preferred by many in the recovery movement, and "patient," historically used in the medical context, interchangeably.) Recovery is understood as living a meaningful and nuanced life, as opposed to recovery from disease or the complete absence of symptoms (Deegan, 1993). Recovery is often described as a process emphasizing themes of hope, empowerment, and meaningful life activity, rather than long-term disability (Torrey, 2005). This approach is not inconsistent with the fact that for most people with serious mental illness, treatments do not "cure" the illness; indeed, clinical and functional problems remain for the majority.

Psychosocial interventions that address recovery are an area of intense interest and ongoing research (Lehman, A. F., 2004). Some evidence-based practices (EBPs) target residual symptoms, some help families, and some assist with daily living and employment. Others target the overall poor health status of persons with schizophrenia. However, despite a growing research base, only a minority of patients can access these EBPs, a disparity some have called the "science to service gap" (Drake, 2009). We discuss interventions that merit particular attention to a student of psychiatry as follows.

Many individuals with serious mental illness do not remain engaged with critical psychiatric services (Kreyenbuhl et al., 2009). Many people who are resistant to visiting clinics or hospitals benefit from having services and supports brought to them. Assertive community treatment (ACT) is an extensively studied, team-based method of delivering care to individuals with serious mental illness. An ACT team is a small, interdisciplinary group of clinicians who provide all of the service needs of a group of mental health consumers, twenty-four hours a day, seven days a week. The specific mix of services provided addresses any area of life in which support is needed from medication management to assistance with daily living and crisis management. Staff-to-consumer ratios are small, and typically consumers are familiar with all team members (Phillips SD et al., 2001). Studies have found that individuals with ACT teams report improved satisfaction with their care over traditional services and lower levels of substance abuse. ACT has also shown to be cost-effective for patients with previously high levels of hospitalization (Scott et al., 1995).

For people with serious mental illness work remains an important life domain. Employment is associated with a wide range of benefits including improved self-esteem. However, employment rates for the mentally ill are low (Marwaha et al., 2004). Sheltered workshops, long the traditional approach to vocational rehabilitation, have been proven generally unsuccessful at helping people obtain competitive jobs. Supported employment is a vocational intervention in which people are placed in jobs and then provided with ongoing support and training to maintain these jobs (Drake et al., 2000). Individuals determine what kind of work they would like to do, and also choose when and how to disclose their illness to their employer.

Interpersonal interaction is one of the most fundamental elements of life satisfaction. Social skills training (SST) programs have been designed to remediate crucial interpersonal skills. SST programs teach skills via role modeling, behavioral rehearsal, positive reinforcement, corrective feedback, and home assignments (Kern, 2009). A key feature of SST is bringing these skills from the clinic into real world scenarios (Kopelowicz, 2006).

Clubhouses are another means of helping individuals with serious mental illness have greater social interaction, as well as a sense of belonging. Developed after the closure of the state hospital system, clubhouses provide a consumer-driven community fostering participation, social connectedness, and employment. Clubhouses blend professional staffing with an egalitarian, client-driven philosophy. Clubhouses are organized along internationally validated standards to ensure quality outcomes (Mowbray, 2006).

Having a family member with a serious mental illness places tremendous burdens on families. Family psychoeducation is aimed at educating and supporting families around the illness. It can not only reduce caregiver burden but also improve outcomes for patients, including reducing rates of relapses and hospitalizations (Pharoah et al., 2010). Some interventions focus on individual families and others use a multi-family approach to teach stress reduction, problem-solving, and illness management (Meuser et al., 2013).

People with schizophrenia have an average life expectancy of twenty to thirty years less than that of the general population. Unhealthy lifestyles including poor diets, little exercise, and high rates of smoking and substance abuse contribute to this astonishing rate of early mortality (Laursen, 2011). The metabolic side effects of second-generation antipsychotics also contribute to obesity and high rates of diabetes and vascular disease in this population. Healthy living interventions such as smoking cessation initiatives, nutritional education, and exercise and weight management programs are being developed to address these concerns (Bradshaw et al., 2005).

There is a growing recognition that people with mental illness should be involved in all decisions that affect their lives, whether related to policy or clinical care. The statement "nothing about us, without us," is embodied in the peer movement, in which individuals with their own lived experiences of mental illness work as service providers. Peer providers might work in any role in a hospital, clinic, or rehabilitation agency. They may also staff "warm lines," consumer-operated businesses, and peer-run education and support/self-help groups. Evidence suggests that peer support interventions help service recipients have a greater sense of control, better satisfaction with their social lives, decreased psychotic symptoms, reduced hospitalizations, and decreased substance use (Davidson et al., 2012).

Contact with a person with lived experience can be important not only for individuals with mental illness themselves but also for their families. Many families have found support through the National Alliance on Mental Illness (NAMI), the largest advocacy group in the nation for people with mental illness. NAMI is primarily an organization to support and educate the families of affected individuals, as well as lobby for political/organizational change (www.NAMI.org).

A Brief Introduction to Motivational Interviewing

During medical training and practice, physicians have many opportunities to discuss behavioral change with their patients. Some conversations will be conducted in a familiar *directing style* – the physician tells the patient what to do and how to fix her illness. For many situations, this will work just fine (e.g., "Take this antibiotic for five days."). While a *directing style* can be effective for acute medical issues, it often falls short when addressing long-standing behavioral patterns underlying chronic illness, mental health, or addiction. Many behavioral patterns seem not only to endure physician interventions but also to survive despite mounting significant negative health consequences. Shouldn't having a heart attack be enough to persuade a patient to quit smoking, change his diet, and exercise more? Shouldn't the threat of kidney failure, blindness, and amputations from diabetes be enough to motivate weight loss and glycemic control? Unfortunately, even when initiated with the best of intentions, many conversations physicians have with people about changing behaviors occur in a dysfunctional way, potentially even limiting the power of transformative negative medical events to motivate behavioral change.

This section will provide a broad overview of an evolving clinical method called *motivational interviewing* (*MI*), which was first described by William Miller in 1983. There are currently more than 1,200 publications on this treatment method, including more than 200 randomized clinical trials, reflecting a wide array of behaviors, professions, practice settings, and nations (Miller, 2013). MI uses observations from natural language about change to help physicians have more effective conversations about behavioral modification with patients, finding a constructive way through the challenges that often arise in these encounters. Since patients' attitudes about change are actively shaped by their own speech (Bem, 1967), MI arranges conversations so patients talk themselves into change, based on their own values and interests. MI does this through the use of a collaborative *guiding style*, allowing patients to solve their own dilemmas for themselves.

Most people who need to make a change are *ambivalent* about doing so. They see both the reasons to change and the reasons not to change. They want to change and don't want to change at the same time. Ambivalence about change is a normal human experience. Being ambivalent is a state that holds within itself the possibility for change. Yet ambivalence can be uncomfortable and frustrating, and patients often get stuck there. During conversations about behavioral change, patients can provide *change talk*, their own self-motivational statements favoring change. They will also provide *sustain talk*, the patient's own arguments for not changing and sustaining the status quo. Once someone has contemplated making a change, an internal debate is unleashed inside. As physicians encountering this internal debate and seeing the future dangers of the behavior, we often instinctively follow our own *righting reflex* (the desire to fix what is wrong with someone and promptly put them back on the right course), and we fall back on our *directing style*. In many cases, well-meaning doctors provide uninvited advice or instruction about changing longstanding behavior. Despite our good intentions, the natural patient response is to take up the opposite side of the debate, hardening the patient's position for sustaining the behavior. Conversations can be overtaken by defensiveness, discounting advice, arguing, or outright explosive anger. Nonverbal responses such as avoidance, eagerness to leave, passivity, or feeling not understood can occur. For this reason, MI was developed as a collaborative conversation style that physicians can use for strengthening a person's own motivation and commitment to change.

The spirit of motivational interviewing is more essential than any set of technical linguistic skills or communication abilities. Four aspects are vital to the spirit of, M. I., including partnership, acceptance, compassion, and evocation. Acting with a guiding style, the physician is in a partnership with the patient, helping her activate her own motivation and resources for change. In order to do this, the physician must accept what the patient brings to the encounter. This does not mean that the physician necessarily approves of the person's actions or beliefs. Rather, the accepting physician honors each person's *absolute worth* and potential as a human being, recognizes and supports the patient's *autonomy* to choose and to have his own beliefs, seeks through *accurate empathy* to understand the world through the patient's eyes, and finally provides *affirmations* of the person's strengths and efforts already taken. When practicing *acceptance*, the physician has let go of the idea and the burdensome belief that physicians must (or can) make people change. This is a relinquishment of a power that we never had in the first place. Instead of taking on the role of a change maker who knows what is best for others, the MI-trained physician embraces *compassion*, which is a deliberate commitment to pursue the welfare and best interests of others. The final aspect of MI spirit is *evocation*, which derives from the premise that patients already have within them much of what is needed to make the change, and the physician's task is to evoke it and call it forth. The integration of these four principles represents *MI spirit*, and MI technical skills and communication tools have been developed to help physicians maintain this spirit during clinical encounters focused on change.

Four foundational *processes* underlie a motivational interview. First, the physician works on *engaging* the patient, forming a working relationship in which the patient feels understood. Engagement uses several skills adapted from client-centered therapy (Rogers, 1951), including *open-ended questions, affirmations, reflections*, and *summaries (OARS)*. Second, the physician engages in *focusing* the conversation about change by developing and maintaining a specific health-promoting direction. In traditional client-centered therapy, clinicians use a *following style* that lets the patient go in whatever direction they want to go. In contrast, MI keeps the direction of the conversation focused on strengthening motivation and confidence for a specific behavioral change (e.g., reducing alcohol use). Third, the physician engages in *evoking* the patient's own motivation for change. Patients *develop a discrepancy* between their current status and their beliefs, goals, values, and dreams. This allows them to develop their own *intrinsic motivation* for change, which is likely to be more enduring than their physician's external reasons for change. When evocation skills are used, physicians can observe patients expressing *preparatory change talk* and *mobilizing change talk*; then physicians can respond to these statements in ways that help the patient build the momentum toward a decision to change. Clinical studies of MI using a structured rating scale have demonstrated that the production of *change talk* and reduction of *sustain talk* during an interview predicts lower levels of alcohol use at follow-up (Moyers et al., 2007), and *MI-consistent* counselor responses result in a higher *change talk-to-sustain talk ratios* among patients (Glynn and Moyers, 2010; Gaume et al., 2010). Techniques have been developed to respond to *sustain talk* when it arises by circumventing discord and conflict, a process referred to as "rolling with resistance." Fourth, once a patient has significant motivation and confidence to change, then the physician collaborates with the patient in *planning*. During this process, a *change plan* is developed and the physician focuses on strengthening commitment and supporting persistence of the change.

So how do you give medical advice about behavioral change without increasing *sustain talk*? With an authentic acceptance of the patient's autonomy, you can request permission using *elicit-provide-elicit (E-P-E)*. First, ask for permission to give them advice about the topic. Then provide the information and advice in a non-judgmental manner, while stating your respect for their freedom to make their own choice. Finally, ask them how they understood or felt about hearing this information. In general, when advice about chronic behavioral issues is delivered in this way, people are willing to hear it and are able to process your suggestions without reactivity, allowing the flow of *change talk* to continue.

Motivational interviewing is an evolving clinical method with a strong evidence base supporting its use in behavioral change interventions. The process of *screening, brief intervention, and referral to treatment* (SBIRT) has recently been widely disseminated as a format allowing medical staff in various contexts to provide a brief motivational intervention to those who screen positive for substance use disorders or tobacco (McCance-Katz and Satterfield, 2012). Motivational interviewing can be learned in introductory and advanced workshops; however, studies suggest that reaching a state of proficiency in motivational interviewing requires ongoing practice and the support of feedback through ratings of sessions (Miller et al., 2004). Encouraging the development of healthy behaviors and helping people reduce unhealthy behaviors is important no matter what medical specialty one goes into. For this reason, motivational interviewing is a crucial method for all physicians who want to provide optimal care.

1. Advice Giving Using Elicit-Provide-Elicit:

MI-inconsistent (NOT MI):

DOCTOR: "You really need to stop eating fried foods and red meat and start eating more vegetables!"

Patient is thinking to himself, "But I can't afford to buy fresh vegetables on my weekly check, and my back hurts too much to carry groceries and then stand to cook. What does she know about my life?"

PATIENT: "Thanks Doc, I'll try." He leaves the office feeling discouraged and unable to even imagine how to change, thinking about how the doctor is wealthy and can shop wherever she wants and hire a cook.

MI-consistent:

DOCTOR (ELICIT):   "What do you already know about diet and its role in preventing another heart attack?"

PATIENT: "I should eat less red meat and fries. I should probably eat more fruit and eat my spinach."

DOCTOR (PROVIDE): "You're right. Eating more fruits and vegetables and avoiding fried food and red meat is important for your heart and could prevent a second more deadly heart attack."

DOCTOR: (ELICIT): "What are your reactions to this information?"

PATIENT: "It sounds important and I want to protect my heart, but I am honestly not sure how to do this on my weekly check and my back hurts too much to carry grocery bags and stand up cooking."

DOCTOR (DOUBLE-SIDED REFLECTION, ASKING FOR PERMISSION): "Figuring out how to make this change may take some thinking together, but you feel it is important to eat in a way that protects your heart. Can we take a few moments to think together about how you can solve the issues you brought up?"

2. Evocative Questions: A few examples for evoking types of *preparatory change talk (in parentheses)*

"Tell me what you don't like about how things are now." (*Desire*)

"If you did really decide you want to quit smoking, how would you do it?" (*Ability*)

"What might be the good things about exercising more frequently?" (*Reasons*)

"How important is it for you to lose weight?" (*Need*)

"On a scale of 0 to 10, where 0 means 'not at all important' and 10 means 'the most important thing for me right now', how important would you say it is for you to lose weight?"

Followed by: "and why are you at a _____ and not 0 (or a lower number)?" **Key point**: By asking the question this way, the doctor elicits change talk. If the doctor were to ask 'and why are you at ___ and not at 10', then the patient would respond with sustain talk.

3. Selective Responding and Rolling with Resistance:

PATIENT: "So what if I drank too much and blacked out? I am in college and everyone drinks. If I don't drink, then I will have no friends and be lonely."

Possible responses that will avoid *sustain talk* and possibly evoke *change talk:*

Double-sided reflection: "On the one hand, it feels like people are overreacting and, on the other, you know that you drank more than you would have liked to."

Agreement with twist: "You're right ... it is challenging to be sober in college ... and I get how important it is for you to have good friends who care about you ... and yet there may be better ways for you to find the friends you are looking for."

Figure 16.1 Motivational interviewing examples

Acknowledgment: Gratitude to Joji Suzuki, M. D., for his contributions to my motivational interviewing training and to this section.

Mind-Body Therapies

Mind-body therapies (MBT, also known as mind-body medicine) refer to a culturally diverse group of practices that have gained significant popularity over the past several decades. Data from the 2017 National Health Interview Survey found that 18.7 percent of the US adult population (more than 46 million people) had practiced a form of meditation during the previous 12 months (J Macinko & D Upchurch, 2017). According to the National Institutes of Health, MBT focuses "on the interactions among the brain, mind, body, and behavior, and on the powerful ways in which emotional, mental, social, spiritual, and behavioral factors can directly affect health. It regards as fundamental an approach that respects and enhances each person's capacity for self-knowledge and self-care, and it emphasizes techniques that are grounded in this approach." Examples of MBT include hypnosis, guided imagery, biofeedback, relaxation therapy, yoga, meditation, and tai chi, among others. These modalities have been found to have clinical effects in the management of common medical conditions including depression, insomnia, anxiety, acute and chronic pain, hypertension, congestive heart failure, as well as symptoms associated with chronic illnesses (such as coronary artery disease, HIV, and cancer) and their treatment.

Epidemiology

Nearly 1 in 5 adults in the United States used some MBT over the past year. Among complementary and alternative therapies, several MBT practices ranked among the top complementary health approaches used by adults. These included deep breathing, meditation, yoga, tai chi, progressive relaxation, and guided imagery. Individuals who suffer from common neurological conditions (regular headaches, migraines, back pain with sciatica, strokes, dementia, seizures, or memory loss), insomnia, anxiety, and depression use MBT more frequently than the general population. In several studies, individuals used MBT more often when conventional treatments were perceived ineffective. In addition, many users of MBT perceive its benefit to be helpful. There are also differences in the utilization patterns of MBT; for example, anxiety and depression are conditions most commonly treated with relaxation techniques, whereas low back pain was the condition most commonly treated with yoga/tai chi. Utilizers of MBT are found among all socio-demographic characteristics; however, a higher prevalence of MBT users are found among those with younger age, female sex, and higher educational and income levels, as compared with the general population (Bertisch, Wee, Phillips, & McCarthy, 2009).

Historical Perspective

Many MBTs have origins in multiple cultural and spiritual traditions throughout the world. For example, many yoga traditions have their origins in India from more than 2,000 years ago. Tai chi has its roots in Chinese traditions over the past millennium. Meditation practices are found through many religious traditions, including Hindu, Buddhist, Judaic, Christian, and Islamic traditions. In the United States, the popularity of MBT was heavily influenced by several meditation practices, including mindfulness-based stress reduction (MBSR) and transcendental meditation (TM). Both are examples of practices that have been extensively studied in the medical literature. In addition, there has been an explosion of yoga and tai chi programs throughout the United States as an alternate option to promote physical fitness and the maintenance of health and well-being.

TM was developed by Maharishi Mahesh Yogi in India and brought to the United States in the 1960s (V. A. Barnes & Orme-Johnson, 2012). Clinical studies of TM demonstrated changes in various physiologic and clinical parameters. In the 1970s, cardiologist Herbert Benson characterized this physiologic state as the relaxation response (RR; Benson, Beary, & Carol, 1974). The RR was described as a voluntary elicitation that was associated with decreases in oxygen consumption, respiratory rate, and blood pressure, along with an increased sense of well-being (Dusek & Benson, 2009). Moreover, the RR was described as the final common pathway among all MBT, as a state of decreased sympathetic nervous system arousal.

In the 1980s, mindfulness practices evolved as an adaptation of Buddhist techniques in a model entitled *mindfulness-based stress reduction* (*MBSR*). Mindfulness has been often defined as a non-judgmental present moment awareness. The MBSR model was developed by Jon Kabat-Zinn, and it introduced different MBT in the context of reducing suffering, enhancing positive emotions, and improving quality of life. It consists of various MBT including sitting meditation, body scan, and mindful movement. The MBSR model has been widely disseminated through the training of providers, with hundreds of programs in the United States. In addition, there have been many adaptations and variations of MBSR including mindfulness-based cognitive therapy (MBCT), mindfulness-based eating awareness therapy (MB-EAT), and mindfulness-based relapse prevention (MBRP). There are hundreds of clinical trials looking at MBSR interventions and their adaptations. The medical literature has been particularly favorable for MBSR, especially in depression, anxiety, and chronic pain (Grossman, Niemann, Schmidt, & Walach, 2004).

Biological Mechanisms in MBT

There are several psychoneuroimmunological mechanisms thought to be important in MBT (Taylor, Goehler, Galper, Innes, & Bourguignon, 2010). Initial models (e.g., Benson) generally focused on specific mechanisms – inhibition of the sympathetic nervous system via the sympatho-adreno-medullary and hypothalamic-pituitary axis and activation of the parasympathetic nervous system through the vagus nerve. In addition to these peripheral neural pathways, there are mechanisms at play in the central nervous system. Specifically, there have been changes found in the fronto-limbic system, including regions of the prefrontal cortex, insular cortex, and the anterior cingulate gyrus. MBTs have also been found to influence chemical mediators, including nitric oxide, NF-κB, and interleukin-6. Most recently, studies of MBT have found changes in genetic expression. For example, there are changes in telomerase activity; in addition, pathways involved with energy metabolism, particularly the function of mitochondria, have been found to be upregulated, whereas other pathways known to have a prominent role in inflammation, stress, trauma, and cancer have been found be downregulated among individuals practicing MBT.

Clinical Applications

Especially over the past twenty years, there has been a significant increase in research on MBT. For the majority of research in MBT, many conclusions that have been drawn are tentative simply because of methodological challenges. Most investigations of the effects of MBT lack a control, are poorly controlled and are not randomized, or lack descriptions on which to evaluate the adequacy of randomization. Despite these limitations, there has been a greater understanding of the ways in which MBT influences health.

The efficacy of biofeedback has been found to be positive in conditions including female urinary incontinence, anxiety, attention-deficit/hyperactivity disorder, chronic pain, constipation, epilepsy, headache, hypertension, motion sickness, Raynaud's disease, and temporo-mandibular joint disorder. Meditation interventions have been found to be clinically relevant in conditions such as hypertension, cardiovascular disease, substance abuse, anxiety, and depression. Guided imagery has been studied among patients preparing for surgery and procedures. While quite heterogeneous in application, yoga practices have been found to have beneficial effects in overall stress management, type 2 diabetes, arthritis, asthma, chronic pain, depression, chronic disease risk factors, and adverse effects of aging. Tai chi has been found to have positive effects in cardiovascular conditions (e.g., congestive heart failure) and fall prevention (Barrows & Jacobs, 2002).

Many clinicians are beginning to incorporate MBT into their practice, given its potential benefits. There is an increasing number of training programs geared toward health care providers as to the incorporation of MBT in clinical practice, especially as useful adjuncts to conventional care. MBTs have become popular among the lay public. Clinicians may be able to provide more culturally competent care through an understanding of patient preferences and beliefs. As rigorous scientific examination continues, MBT may have important roles in disease prevention and wellness promotion; in addition, MBT may provide important roles in helping to decrease burgeoning health care costs and excessive health care utilization.

References and Selected Readings

- Auchincloss, E., and Samberg, E. (2012). *Psychoanalytic Terms and Concepts*. New Haven: Yale University Press.
- Barlow, D. (ed.) (2007). *Clinical Handbook of Psychological Disorders*, 4th ed. New York: Guilford Press.
- Barnes, P. M., Bloom, B., and Nahin, R. L. (2008). Complementary and Alternative Medicine Use among Adults and Children: United States, 2007. *National Health Statistics Reports*, 12 (12), 1–23.
- Barnes, V. A., and Orme-Johnson, D. W. (2012). Prevention and Treatment of Cardiovascular Disease in Adolescents and Adults through the Transcendental Meditation Program: A Research Review Update. *Current Hypertension Reviews*, 8 (3), 227–242.

- Barrows, K. A., and Jacobs, B. P. (2002). Mind-Body Medicine: An Introduction and Review of the Literature. *Medical Clinics of North America*, 86 (1), 11–31.
- Beck, A. T., Rush, A. J., Shaw, B. F., and Emery G (1979). *Cognitive Therapy of Depression*. New York: Guilford Press.
- Bem, D. J. (1967). Self-Perception: An Alternative Interpretation of Cognitive Dissonance Phenomena. *Psychol Review*, 74 (3), 83–200.
- Benson, H., Beary, J. F., and Carol, M. P. (1974). The Relaxation Response. *Psychiatry*, 37 (1), 37–46.
- Bertisch, S. M., Wee, C. C., Phillips, R. S., and McCarthy, E. P. (2009). Alternative Mind-Body Therapies Used by Adults with Medical Conditions. *Journal of Psychosomatic Research*, 66 (6), 511–519.
- Bradshaw, T., et al. (2005). Healthy Living Interventions and Schizophrenia: A Systematic Review. *Journal of Advanced Nursing*, 49 (6), 635–654.
- Burlingame, G. M., Earnshaw, D., Hoag, M., Barlow, S. H., Richardson, E. J., and Donnell, I. (2002). A Systematic Program to Enhance Clinician Group Skills in an Inpatient Psychiatric Hospital. *International Journal of Group Psychotherapy*, 52, 555–587.
- Burlingame, G. M., Fuhriman, A., and Mosier, J. (2003). The Differential Effectiveness of Group Psychotherapy: A Meta-analytic Perspective. *Group Dynamics: Theory, Research, and Practice*, 7, 3–12.
- Corey, M. S., and Corey, G. (1997). *Groups: Process and Practice*, 5th ed. Pacific Grove, CA: Brooks/Cole.
- Davidson, L., et al. (2012). Peer Support among Persons with Severe Mental Illnesses: A Review of Evidence and Experience. *World Psychiatry*, 11, 123–128.
- Deegan, P. E. (1993). Recovering Our Sense of Value after Being Labeled Mentally Ill. *Journal of Psychosocial Mental Health Services*, 31 (4), 7–11.
- Drake, R. E., and Essock, S. M. (2009). The Science-to-Service Gap in Real-World Schizophrenia Treatment: The 95 Percent Problem. *Schizophrenia Bulletin*, 35 (4), 677–678.
- Drake, R. E., et al. (2000). Evidence-Based Treatment of Schizophrenia. *Current Psychiatry Reports*, 2 (5), 393–397.
- Dusek, J. A., and Benson, H. (2009). Mind-Body Medicine: A Model of the Comparative Clinical Impact of the Acute Stress and Relaxation Responses. *Minnesota Medicine*, 92 (5), 47–50.
- Frese, F., et al. (2009). Recovery from Schizophrenia: With Views of Psychiatrists, Psychologists, and Others Diagnosed with This Disorder. *Schizophrenia Bulletin*, 35 (2), 370–380.
- Freud, S. (1886–1939). *The Standard Edition of the Complete Psychological Works of Sigmund Freud*, Vol. 1–24 (Strachey, J., ed.). New York: Norton.
- Gabbard, G., Litowitz, B., and Williams, P. (2011). *Textbook of Psychoanalysis*. Arlington, VA: American Psychiatric Publishing.
- Gaume, J., et al. (2010). Counselor Motivational Interviewing Skills and Young Adult Change Talk Articulation during Brief Motivational Interventions. *Journal of Substance Abuse Treatment*, 39 (3), 272–281.
- Glynn, L. H., and Moyers, T. B. (2010). Chasing Change Talk: The Clinician's Role in Evoking Client Language about Change. *Journal of Substance Abuse Treatment*, 39 (1), 5–70.
- Grossman, P., Niemann, L., Schmidt, S., and Walach, H. (2004). Mindfulness-Based Stress Reduction and Health Benefits. A Meta-Analysis. *Journal of Psychosomatic Research*, 57 (1), 35–43.

- "Group Works!" www.agpa.org.
- Harding, C. M., et al. (1987). The Vermont Longitudinal Study of Persons with Severe Mental Illness, II: Long-Term Outcome of Subjects Who Retrospectively Met DSM-III Criteria for Schizophrenia. *American Journal of Psychiatry*, 144, 727–735.
- Himelhock, S., Medoff, D. R., and Oyeniyi, G. (2007). Efficacy of Group Psychotherapy to Reduce Depressive Symptoms among HIV-Infected Individuals: A Systematic Review and Meta-analysis. *AIDS Patient Care and STDs*, 21, 732–739.
- Kahl, K. G., Winter, L., and Schweiger U (2012). The Third Wave of Cognitive Behavioral Therapies: What Is New and What Is Effective? *Current Opinion in Psychiatry*, 25 (6), 522–528.
- Kern, R. S., et al. (2009). Psychosocial Treatments to Promote Functional Recovery in Schizophrenia. *Schizophrenia Bulletin*, 35 (2), 347–361.
- Kingdon, D. G., and Turkington, D. (2005). *Cognitive Therapy of Schizophrenia*. New York: Guilford Press.
- Kopelowicz, A., et al. (2006). Recent Advances in Social Skills Training for Schizophrenia. *Schizophrenia Bulletin*, suppl. 1, S12–S23.
- Kreyenbuhl, J., et al. (2009). Disengagement from Mental Health Treatment among Individuals with Schizophrenia and Strategies for Facilitating Connections to Care: A Review of the Literature. *Schizophrenia Bulletin*, 35 (4), 696–703.
- Laplanche, J., and Pontalis, J.-B. (1973). *The Language of Psycho-Analysis* (D. Nicholson-Smith, trans.). New York: W. W. Norton and Co.
- Laursen, T. M., et al. (2012). Life Expectancy and Cardiovascular Mortality in Persons with Schizophrenia. *Current Opinion in Psychiatry*, 25 (2), 83–88.
- Lehman, A. F., et al. (2004). The Schizophrenia Patient Outcomes Research Team (PORT), Updated Treatment Recommendations 2003. *Schizophrenia Bulletin*, 30, 193–192.
- Liberman, R. P. (2008). *Recovery from Disability: Manual of Psychiatric Rehabilitation*. Washington, DC: American Psychiatric Publishing.
- Linehan, M. M. (1993). *Cognitive-Behavioral Treatment of Borderline Personality Disorder*. New York, Guilford Press.
- Linehan, M. M., Armstrong, H. E., Suarez, A., Allmon, D., and Heard, H. L. (1991). Cognitive-Behavioral Treatment of Chronically Parasuicidal Borderline Patients. *Archives of General Psychiatry*, 48, 1060–1064.
- Linehan, M. M., Tutek, D. A., Heard, H. L., and Armstrong, H. E. (1993). Naturalistic Follow-Up of a Behavioral Treatment for Chronically Parasuicidal Borderline Patients. *Archives of General Psychiatry*, 50, 971–974.
- Lynch, T. R., Chapman, A. L., Rosenthal, M. Z., Kuo, J. R., and Linehan, M. M. (2006). Mechanisms of Change in Dialectical Behavior Therapy: Theoretical and Empirical Observations. *Journal of Clinical Psychology*, 62, 459–480.
- Macinko J, Upchurch DM. Factors Associated with the Use of Meditation, U.S. Adults 2017. J Altern Complement Med. 2019 Sep;25(9):920–927.
- MacKenzie, K. R. (1994). Group Development. In A. Fuhriman and G. Burlingame (eds.), *Handbook of Group Psychotherapy*. New York: Wiley, 223–268.
- Marlatt, G. A., and Donovan, D. M. (eds.) (2005). *Relapse Prevention: Maintenance Strategies in the Treatment of Addictive Behaviors*, 2nd ed. New York: Guilford Press.

- Marwaha, S., and Johnson, S. (2004). Schizophrenia and Employment – A Review. *Social Psychiatry and Psychiatric Epidemiology*, 39 (5), 337–349.
- Matta, A. R., and Terjesen, M. D. (2012). Efficacy of School-Based Group Therapy with Children and Adolescents: A Meta-analytic Review. APA 120th Annual Convention, Orlando, Florida, August 2–5, 2012.
- McCance-Katz, E. F., and Satterfield, J. (2012). SBIRT: A Key to Integrate Prevention and Treatment of Substance Abuse in Primary Care. *American Journal of Addiction*, 21 (2), 176–177.
- McDermut, W., Miller, I. W., and Brown, R. A. (2001). The Efficacy of Group Psychotherapy for Depression: A Meta-analysis and Review of the Empirical Research. *Clinical Psychology: Science and Practice*, 8, 98–116.
- Miller, W. R. (1983). Motivational Interviewing with Problem Drinkers. *Behavioural Psychotherapy*, 11, 147–172.
- Miller, W. R., et al. (2004). A Randomized Trial of Methods to Help Clinicians Learn Motivational Interviewing. *Journal of Consult Clin Psychol*, 72 (6), 1050–1062.
- Miller, W. R., and Rollnick, S. (2013). *Motivational Interviewing: Helping People Change*, 3rd ed. New York: Guilford Press.
- Mowbray, C. T., et al. (2006). The Clubhouse as an Empowering Setting. *Health Social Work*, 31 (3), 167–179.
- Moyers, T. B., et al. (2007). Client Language as a Mediator of Motivational Interviewing Efficacy: Where Is the Evidence? *Alcohol Clinical and Experimental Research*, 31 (10 suppl.), 40s–47s.
- Mueser, K. T., et al. (2013). Psychosocial Treatments for Schizophrenia. *Annual Review of Clinical Psychology*, 9, 465–497.
- Norcross, J., and Goldfried, M. (2001). *Handbook of Psychotherapy Integration.* New York: Oxford University Press.
- Pharoah, F., et al. (1999). Family Intervention for Schizophrenia. *Cochrane Database Systems Review* 4, CD000088.
- Phillips, S. D., et al. (2001). Moving Assertive Community Treatment into Standard Practice. *Psychiatric Services*, 52 (6), 771–779.
- Rogers, C. R. (1951). *Client-Centered Therapy: Its Current Practice, Implications, and Theory.* Boston: Houghton Mifflin.
- Rutan, J. S., Stone, W. N., and Shay, J. J. (2007). *Psychodynamic Group Psychotherapy*, 4th ed. New York: Guilford Press.
- Scott, J. E., and Dixon, L. B. (1995). Assertive Community Treatment and Case Management for Schizophrenia. *Schizophrenia Bulletin*, 21 (4), 657–688.
- Sloan, D. M., Bovin, M. J., and Schnurr, P. P. (2012). Review of Group Treatment for PTSD. *Journal of Rehabilitation Research and Development*, 49, 689–702.
- Taylor, A. G., Goehler, L. E., Galper, D. I., Innes, K. E., and Bourguignon, C. (2010). Top-Down and Bottom-Up Mechanisms in Mind-Body Medicine: Development of an Integrative Framework for Psychophysiological Research. *Explore*, 6 (1), 29–41.
- Torrey, W. C., et al. (2005). Recovery Principles and Evidence-Based Practice: Essential Ingredients of Service Improvement. *Community Mental Health Journal*, 41 (1), 91–100.

Self-Assessment Questions

1. Which of the following psychotherapeutic approaches is based on classical and operant conditioning?
    A. Psychoanalytic psychotherapy
    B. Motivational interviewing
    C. Cognitive behavioral therapy
    D. Mind-body therapies

2. What is meant by *dialectical philosophy* in psychotherapy?
    A. The process by which earlier experiences are unconsciously translated into present relationships
    B. A strategy of managing the consequences of a behavior so as to increase the frequency of desired behaviors and decrease the frequency of undesirable behaviors
    C. An approach to the patient which includes open-minded curiosity and assumes that problem behaviors being addressed make sense from the patient's perspective
    D. The use of a collaborative guiding approach by the clinician to allow the patient to solve their own problems

3. Which of the following modalities are not part of a cognitive-behavioral intervention?
    A. Exposure
    B. Skill deficit remediation
    C. Contingency management
    D. Transference and countertransference interpretation
    E. Cognitive restructuring

4. A twenty-four-year-old female with a past diagnosis of borderline personality disorder and alcohol abuse disorder is referred for evaluation and treatment recommendation due to depression following a series of relationship disappointments. Which of the following treatment approaches is likely to meet this patient's needs?
    A. Motivational interviewing
    B. Dialectical behavior therapy
    C. Mind-body therapy
    D. Behavior therapy

Answers to Self-Assessment Questions

1. (C)
2. (C)
3. (D)
4. (B)

17 Psychiatric Evaluation in the Medical Setting

FREMONTA MEYER, ORIANA VESGA LOPEZ, FELICIA SMITH, ROBERT
JOSEPH, TED AVI GERSTENBLITH, THEODORE STERN, JOHN PETEET,
DONNA GREENBERG, AND DAVID GITLIN

Emergency Psychiatry

One out of every twenty emergency department (ED) visits in the United States is due to a psychiatric issue. Providing a gateway between the community and the mental health system, psychiatry emergency clinicians are responsible for assessing and managing a wide array of clinical presentations and conditions. Among emergency mental health-related visits, substance-related disorders, mood disorders, anxiety disorders, psychosis, and suicide attempts are among the most prevalent presentations. Although urgent conditions are common, increasing numbers of patients who present to the emergency department seek treatment for routine or non-acute psychiatric symptoms. Some patients self-refer to the emergency department, while others may be referred by family, friends, outpatient treatment providers, public agencies, or representatives of the law enforcement system.

Most physicians will manage a number of psychiatric emergencies during the course of their medical careers, regardless of clinical specialty or practice setting. The overall scope of emergency psychiatry training includes the development of attitudes, skills, and knowledge necessary to perform a focused and efficient psychiatric assessment that guides acute interventions and treatment planning. The aim of this section is to provide a foundation for the clinical aspects of the psychiatric evaluation in the emergency setting. An approach to psychiatric interviewing in the emergency setting will be outlined, with a focus on the initial triage of patients presenting with psychiatric symptoms in the emergency department, the domains of the interview and the risk assessment, followed by a discussion of the focused medical assessment.

Triage

The psychiatric emergency evaluation should be focused and concise, with a primary goal of obtaining the necessary data to perform a diagnostic exam and risk assessment, to develop a brief psychosocial understanding of the patient, and to formulate a treatment plan. Just as in the general emergency department setting, the emergency psychiatric evaluation begins with a brief assessment of medical stability and safety (Table 17.1). The following questions should guide the process of triage: (1) Is the patient medically unstable? (2) Does the patient need to be

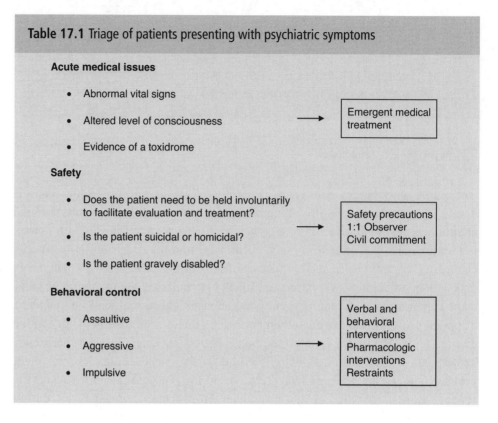

Table 17.1 Triage of patients presenting with psychiatric symptoms

Acute medical issues

- Abnormal vital signs
- Altered level of consciousness   ⟶   Emergent medical treatment
- Evidence of a toxidrome

Safety

- Does the patient need to be held involuntarily to facilitate evaluation and treatment?
- Is the patient suicidal or homicidal?   ⟶   Safety precautions 1:1 Observer Civil commitment
- Is the patient gravely disabled?

Behavioral control

- Assaultive   Verbal and behavioral interventions
- Aggressive   ⟶   Pharmacologic interventions
- Impulsive   Restraints

held involuntarily to facilitate evaluation and treatment? (3) Does the patient have adequate behavioral control? The information obtained from this initial clinical assessment will be used to select the best next step in management, to guide placement within the emergency department, and to attend to the patient's and the staff members' safety by minimizing endangering behaviors throughout the evaluation and treatment process.

Psychiatric Evaluation

Interview

The foundation of the initial psychiatric interview is a thorough history of present illness that focuses on the reason for the presentation and the temporal association between precipitating factors and the development of symptoms that have led to the emergency room visit. Emphasis should be placed on examining the events that triggered the emergency visit on that particular occasion, the quality of the presenting symptoms, and the associated likelihood of imminent harm to the person himself/herself or others. Ambulance run sheets, police reports, family members, outpatient providers, and records of prior medical and psychiatric treatment are frequently useful sources of collateral information. Table 17.2 describes the domains of the psychiatric interview.

Table 17.2 Domains of the emergency psychiatry evaluation

Purpose of the evaluation: the purpose of the evaluation influences the focus of the examination.

- History of present illness: Chronologically organized history of pertinent positive and pertinent negative features of the present illness, context for the symptoms, and safety evaluation.
- Past psychiatric history: Including lifetime diagnoses, previous psychiatric hospitalizations, suicide attempts, self-injurious behaviors, violence, homocidality, and current treatment modalities.
- Substance use and abuse history: Assess course and pattern (route, amount, frequency) of substance use; sequelae; history of sobriety; withdrawal syndromes; and previous treatment.
- Past medical history: Focus on active medical problems, particularly those which may be relevant to the current presentation.
- Current medications: Dosage, route of administration, and compliance.
- Allergies and adverse reaction to medications.
- Family history: Including diagnoses and history of attempted or completed suicides.
- Social history: Including an assessment of the patient's baseline level of function (e.g., living situation, day structure, and social support), life events that might contribute to the current visit (e.g., homelessness, loss of job), and insurance status.
- Legal history.
- Medical review of systems: emphasis on symptoms that may account for, or be associated with, the patient's presenting problems.
- Vital signs and physical examination.
- Mental status examination.
- Directed medical workup.
- Collateral information: Especially when patients are not able to cooperate with the assessment, or when their clinical presentation differs from the stated factors prompting assessment.
- Assessment: Summary statement, diagnostic assessment, psychosocial formulation, safety risk assessment.
- Plan: Documentation of any specific recommendations and significant interventions.

Mental Status Examination (MSE)

Performing a systematic and focused evaluation of the patient's mental and cognitive status then narrows the initial differential diagnosis. The MSE is a systematic collection of data based on observation of the patient during the interview and responses to specific questions. The primary goals of the MSE are to identify symptoms and signs of mental disorders, to determine the presence of neuropsychiatric illness, and to determine whether this illness is primary or secondary (to a general medical condition). A systematic approach to assessing mental status in the emergency setting is key to identifying alterations in mental status, especially when subtle, and to directing diagnostic testing and management. For example, after assessing basic levels of alertness and orientation, some patients require a formal assessment of attention and memory. Assessing attention and memory in a structured way allows the examiner to better differentiate delirium from dementia or from psychiatric illness, thus facilitating the diagnostic evaluation and disposition. There are several validated examinations (e.g., the Mini Mental State Examination [MMSE] and the Montreal Cognitive Assessment [MoCA]) available to assess a patient's cognition in the emergency setting.

Safety Risk Assessment

Regardless of the presenting complaint, the safety risk assessment is a mandatory component of a psychiatric emergency evaluation. The primary goal of the safety evaluation in the emergency setting is to estimate the risk of physical harm to self or others by virtue of a mental disorder, and whether this risk is imminent or not. It is important to note that although the objective of such evaluation varies according to the treatment setting, the overall end goal is to estimate the level of risk, through knowledgeable assessment of risk and protective factors, rather than to "predict" the likelihood of a potential outcome. In the emergency setting, it is critical to develop a treatment plan that addresses the safety of the patient, of staff, and of individuals in the community, and to use the evaluation to institute acute interventions and guide the selection of an appropriate setting for treatment.

The primary function of the safety evaluation is the assessment of ideation, plans, and intent of self-harm (i.e., suicidality) or harm to others (i.e., violence or homicidality). The clinician must initially focus on the presence, extent, and persistence of suicidal or homicidal ideation. If ideation is present, the clinician should elicit details about the presence or absence of specific plans, and availability of a method, focusing on lethality, and any steps taken to enact or prepare for those plans; followed by an assessment of the individual's level of intent to harming himself/herself or others.

The second component of the evaluation is the identification of specific factors and features that may increase or decrease the potential risk for self-harm or harm to others. In weighing risk factors for suicide in an individual patient, consideration should be given to (1) sociodemographic and psychosocial information (e.g., gender, age, ethnicity, and recent psychosocial stressors); (2) relevant clinical information (e.g., specific symptoms such as hopelessness, anxiety, impulsivity or psychosis); (3) historical information (e.g., history of psychiatric or medical illness, history of prior attempts, family history of suicide); and (4) individual psychological strengths and vulnerabilities. Finally, it is important to remember that asking about suicidal ideation does not ensure that accurate or complete information will be received. As such, the safety evaluation should generally include contact with members of the patient's support system and/or with professionals who are currently treating the patient.

The assessment of factors that increase or decrease the risk of violence and homicidality is similar to that of the assessment of suicidality. Specific factors that should be assessed in these cases include (1) sociodemographic information (e.g., gender, age, ethnicity); (2) relevant clinical information (e.g., specific symptoms, such as impulsiveness, agitation, substance use, or psychosis); (3) historical information (e.g., history of violence, access to weapons); and (4) legal issues that might or might not be related to violence. In addition, the specific target of violence or homicidality should be assessed. If there is evidence of directed violence toward an identified person, there will be a duty to protect this individual, either through admission to inpatient treatment setting or warning of the identified target.

The presentation of suicidal ideation or violence in the context of agitation or acute intoxication is common in emergency settings and may require interventions to address behavioral symptoms first before a full psychiatric evaluation can be performed. The clinician should seek collateral information early on, followed by reassessment of the individual once the mental status has cleared. Under such conditions, the goal of the evaluation is to use the information that is immediately available to make a clinical judgment, with steps being taken to enhance the patient's and the staff members' safety in the interim. A further discussion of assessing suicidality and violence, respectively, is provided later in this chapter.

Focused Medical Assessment

Studies have demonstrated prevalence rates of coexisting medical disease between 30–50 percent in patients who present with psychiatric emergencies. The initial medical evaluation, and subsequent medical workup, is often referred to as "medical clearance." However, because of the ambiguity and ongoing variability of the process and definition of "medical clearance," the American College of Emergency Physicians has recommended the label of "focused medical assessment" to describe the process in which a medical etiology for the patient's symptoms is excluded, and other illnesses and/or injuries are detected and treated. Timely identification and treatment of medical conditions are essential to prevent morbidity and mortality resulting from attributing somatic symptoms to psychiatric illness. It is important to remember that patients may have co-occurring medical and psychiatric illnesses and require care for both.

History and Physical Examination

When evaluating a patient with a psychiatric emergency, it is important to obtain a focused medical history and physical examination. In one retrospective study of patients presenting to an emergency department with psychiatric complaints, history, physical examination, vital signs, and laboratory testing, had sensitivities of 94 percent, 51 percent, 17 percent, and 20 percent, respectively, for identifying a medical etiology. It is important to obtain information from as many sources as possible, including the patient, EMS, family or friends, and witnesses. Relevant historical questions include the onset and course of the symptoms, and the presence of symptoms that are commonly associated with organic etiologies (e.g., visual hallucinations). Determining the patient's past medical and psychiatric history, as outlined in the previous section, is of particular importance since the absence of a past psychiatric history has been found to be an important factor associated with organic etiologies. It is important to not be overly biased by the information. For example, new-onset psychiatric symptoms are medical in etiology until proven otherwise, but the converse is not always true. A past history of psychiatric illness does not necessarily imply that the present complaint is psychiatric in origin. The review of systems may also help to guide the evaluation toward medical illness. For example, a patient who presents with new-onset anxiety in addition to symptoms of palpitations, tremor, weight loss, or heat intolerance may have a primary diagnosis of hyperthyroidism. In this case, management of the underlying endocrine disorder will be the initial treatment of choice. A detailed list of the patient's medications and allergies should be obtained in every case, especially in the elderly, since recent changes or new medications may suggest drug-related side effects or toxicity.

It is important to obtain vital signs in every patient, even those who are combative or agitated, as this may point to particular etiologies. Finally, the general examination should proceed in a head-to-toe manner, and place emphasis on the neurologic examination. Table 17.3 presents a list of findings that should raise concern for organic etiology.

Laboratory Studies

History and physical examination are the best method of determining medical stability in alert, cooperative patients presenting to the ED with psychiatric symptoms. History and physical examination alone have exhibited far greater specificity and sensitivity than laboratory analyses in detecting medical problems in

> **Table 17.3** Findings suggestive of an underlying medical basis for psychiatric symptoms
>
> - Sudden onset of changes in cognition
> - New-onset behavior change
> - Late age (over forty) of onset of a new behavioral symptom
> - No past history of psychiatric illness
> - Presence of a toxidrome
> - Visual hallucinations
> - Known systemic disease with recent changes to medications
> - Abnormal vital signs
> - Disorientation or impaired attention
> - Impaired level of consciousness

Table 17.4 Diagnostic evaluation of patients with psychiatric symptoms

- Complete blood count
- Basic metabolic panel
- Liver function tests
- Pregnancy test
- Urine toxicology
- Basic serum toxicology
- Medication levels

Consider in certain cases:
- EKG (if recent cocaine use or risk factors for prolonged QTc)
- Chest radiograph
- Computed tomography (if history suggests focal lesion or trauma)

patients presenting with psychiatric complaints. However, laboratory testing can often contribute to identifying the etiology for some psychiatric presentations. Routine urine toxicology screens for drugs of abuse should be performed as part of the ED assessment, as the results of those tests are frequently used to determine the cause of the patient's symptoms, and to aid in disposition and long-term care of a patient. Regarding patients with alcohol intoxication, consensus panels recommend that the patient's cognitive abilities (rather than a specific blood alcohol level) be the basis on which clinicians initiate a psychiatric assessment. Routine laboratory testing (Table 17.4) is justified in elderly patients, patients with no prior psychiatric history who present with a new-onset psychiatric complaint, and patients who present with altered mental status.

Imaging

Imaging studies should be guided by the history, vital signs, and physical exam. Chest radiographs are obtained based on the presence of positive pulmonary findings on historical or physical examination. A noncontrast head computed tomography (CT) should be reserved for patients with a focal neurologic exam or altered mental status or behavior of undetermined etiology. Head CT should also be considered for high-risk patients, such as those who are on anticoagulants or have a coagulopathy, the elderly, and the immunosuppressed.

In summary, the focused medical assessment of psychiatric patients is analogous to that of medical patients. Directed (as opposed to routine) testing based on a patient's presenting symptoms, together with the history, mental status evaluation, and physical examination is the best way to assess the patient. Finally, the diagnostic testing of patients during the initial emergency evaluation should accomplish one of the following goals: (1) to aid in disposition and determine the safety of potential treatments; (2) to detect the presence of medical conditions that require or affect management; or (3) to provide baseline medical information to assist in monitoring course or response to treatment.

Disposition

Patients seeking or requiring an emergency psychiatric evaluation should be treated in the setting that is least restrictive yet most likely to prove safe and effective. Treatment settings include a continuum of possible levels of care, from ambulatory settings, to partial hospital and intensive outpatient programs, to voluntary or involuntary hospitalizations. The estimate of suicide risk and potential for dangerousness to others both play an important role in the choice of the treatment setting. However, the choice of a specific treatment setting is not invariably dependent upon the estimate of risk, but rather will rely on the balance between several elements from the complete psychiatric and medical evaluation.

Consultation-Liaison Psychiatry

Definition and Background

Consultation-liaison psychiatry, also known as psychosomatic medicine, emerged in the early twentieth century on the medical floors in several large hospitals and since then has expanded into most general hospitals as well as specialized inpatient and outpatient treatment settings. Consultation-liaison psychiatrists play a key role in educating medical teams about psychiatric issues and supporting them in the intense work of caring for patients with complex medical illness and/or psychological distress.

In the medical setting, early recognition of emotional disturbances is critical because psychiatric comorbidity may contribute to patient, family, and team distress, negatively impact the course of medical illness, increase hospital length of stay and re-admissions, and increase the cost of care. More studies are required to determine whether prompt psychiatric consultation may decrease health care costs. In the meantime, patients who are seen by psychiatry often experience reduced emotional suffering and receive more accurate psychiatric diagnoses and treatments. Medical providers appreciate the added expertise of the psychiatric consultant, and profit from assistance with disruptive patients as well as education around common behavioral responses to illness.

Approach to Assessment

Flexibility is essential for psychiatric consultants given the chaotic aspects of the modern hospital environment, including lack of privacy due to shared rooms and frequent interruptions by staff and visitors. Patients may be quite physically ill, cognitively impaired, and/or in pain and therefore unable to participate in a

Table 17.5 Procedural aspects of psychiatric consultation

Speak to the requesting physician
    Clarify how we can help
    Ask whether the patient is aware that a psychiatrist will be seeing them
    If the patient has not been notified, see if it is possible for the team to do so
        before you see the patient
Review current medical record and pertinent old records
Talk to nursing staff if available
Interview the patient
    Don't forget detailed mental status and cognitive exam
    Get patient's permission to speak to family and/or outpatient treaters
Confirm medications – both home and hospital medications
Get collateral history
Write your note
    Include specific guidelines on the use of medications
Speak to the requesting physician to discuss your recommendations
Provide periodic follow-up

lengthy exploration of past developmental or psychiatric history. Still, the psychiatric consultation should ideally include all of the elements described below and summarized in Table 17.5. Practical considerations often dictate return visits to complete the evaluation.

Speak to the Requesting Physician

Often, written or verbal consultation questions are quite vague (e.g., "flat affect, rule out depression"). Speaking directly to the referring physician in order to clarify the question is important for several reasons. First, it provides additional information about the patient and his/her hospital course; and second, it can illuminate patient-team dynamics prompting the consultation. The patient with "flat affect, rule out depression" may be depressed or delirious. Many situations may challenge the team's ability to express the problem in a few words. For example, the patient could also be subtly hostile and frustrating to the team due to non-adherence with medical interventions, terminally ill and prompting feelings of helplessness in the team, or constantly attended by an angry family member who is dissatisfied with the hospital's care. Obtaining this background helps ensure that the consultation is maximally useful to the patient and the team. When possible, the team should also inform the patient in advance that a psychiatric consultation has been requested.

Review the Current Records and Pertinent Old Records; Talk to Nursing Staff If Available before the Consult

Particularly in patients who have had long hospitalizations, chart review is essential. Frequently overlooked areas which may contain valuable information include

Table 17.6 Personality disorders which present problems in the medical setting and associated management strategies

Personality disorder	Characteristics	Common behaviors	Possible countertransference responses provoked in clinician	Suggested therapeutic response	Illustrative management quote
Paranoid	– Suspicious – Misinterprets others' actions as malevolent	– Resists medications or invasive procedures – Mistrusts clinician – Threatens legal action	Impatience, anger, fear	Take empathic stance, rather than overtly challenging patient's paranoid thoughts	Patient: "You are trying to poison me with this medication." Clinician: "I can certainly see why you feel that way. Chemotherapy is tough. If I were having chemotherapy I'd be suspicious too. Let's see how we can address the side effects."
Antisocial	– Charming and ingratiating – Manipulative – Has history of prior incarceration and probation	– Tells compelling stories about life difficulties that induce the clinician to offer extra help or favors; stories later turn out to be lies – Brings weapons to the hospital or clinic	Sympathy followed by anger and fear	Acknowledge effects of patient's actions on you and others; set limits without unilaterally terminating or dismissing patient; protect safety of staff	"You are scaring me and my staff. We want to continue to treat you, but we need to think about our safety, and will call security to have you escorted out of the clinic if you again talk about having a knife."
Histrionic	– Flirtatious or sexually provocative – Highly emotional (which hinders rational discussion of treatment options)	– Provides vivid or exaggerated descriptions of physical symptoms – Has difficulty tolerating delay or ambiguity – Amplifies somatic complaints, prompting workups	Arousal Fatigue	Schedule regular follow-up visits regardless of symptom levels, acknowledge that treatment may not be entirely curative	"The pain may get better than it is now, but you will probably always have some flare-ups, because our medications are only 80 percent effective. I don't think we need to get another scan right now but I want to monitor you closely and would like to see you every 3 months to check on this."

Table 17.6 (cont.)

Personality disorder	Characteristics	Common behaviors	Possible countertransference responses provoked in clinician	Suggested therapeutic response	Illustrative management quote
Dependent	Intensely needy, anxious, seeks constant reassurance	– Calls and pages frequently between appointments – Has difficulty making independent decisions – Has trouble leaving office – Fails to ask appropriate questions – Feels a need for intensive care and support, including hospitalization, when faced with medical setbacks	Fatigue, guilt, aversion	Set appropriate expectations of doctor-patient relationship, acknowledge limits of knowledge/skill as well as time and stamina, educate patient about medical care	"I am committed to be with you for the long haul. When you call me about questions that could easily wait until your next appointment, I get stressed, and it makes it harder for me to be there in the way I want to be for you."
Narcissistic	– Entitled – Exquisitely sensitive to losses in function experienced as a result of medical treatment – Behaves well in medical settings when needs are being met	– Requests special consideration – Directs even minor concerns to the attending physician rather than ancillary staff – Talks at length to extend appointment times – Becomes extremely distressed by problems that affect sexual function, physical appearance, cognitive abilities	Anger; wish to counterattack	Do not challenge entitlement, but channel it into partnership in providing the best care; emphasize and align with patient strengths	"You certainly deserve the best medical care we can give, and that's why it is best if you arrive on time so that you get the most out of our visit." "You have been very successful in managing your company in difficult times; you are also the leader of your treatment team, and we will do our best to meet your goals."

Table 17.6 (cont.)

Personality disorder	Characteristics	Common behaviors	Possible countertransference responses provoked in clinician	Suggested therapeutic response	Illustrative management quote
Borderline	– Emotionally labile – Angry – Fears abandonment – Frequently changes residences, jobs and/or relationships	– Displays impulsive behaviors such as self-injury, substance abuse, binge eating, or sexual promiscuity – Non-adherent with medications – Misses appointments – Develops new symptoms during transition points in treatment (e.g., when medical visits become less frequent) due to feelings of abandonment	Depression, self-doubt, anger	Work empathically and diligently but lower expectations and adjust goals; set non-punitive limits; share care with other clinicians to reduce burnout; regular team meetings (including support staff, if appropriate) to coordinate plan of care	"Like you, I'm only human, so when you swear at me, I get upset-- and that interferes with my thinking clearly about what you need."
Obsessive-compulsive	– High need for control, orderliness, and perfectionism – Focuses on details as opposed to the larger medical picture	– Repeatedly questions clinicians regarding small details of care – Keeps meticulous logs of symptoms and medications – Has difficulty tolerating the imperfections of the process of receiving medical care	Irritation, anger	Give patient control when possible; acknowledge and empathize with vulnerability produced by medical illness	"It is really hard to feel so out of control. While you are in infusion, I'd like you to keep a careful log of everything that you experience with the new drug so you can report it to me."

nursing notes (e.g., level of orientation, awareness, and agitation), physical/occupational therapy notes (e.g., motivation, energy, cognition, functional abilities), and social work notes (e.g., emotional responses to illness, family issues, and financial stressors). Of course, if psychiatric consultations have occurred during prior admissions or in outpatient settings, it is important to review these carefully as well. Nursing staff is an additional important source of collateral regarding the patient's behavior and coping style.

Interview the Patient

Overall, the psychiatric examination in consultation-liaison psychiatry parallels the evaluation in the emergency psychiatry setting (Table 17.2). It is essential to perform a complete cognitive evaluation given the increased prevalence of delirium, dementia, and other cognitive disorders in medically ill patients. In many inpatient consultations, testing orientation and attention early in the interview will yield the correct diagnosis (delirium). Other elements of the cognitive exam include memory, language, and executive function. Many consultants perform a structured bedside evaluation such as the Mini-Mental State Exam or the Montreal Cognitive Assessment, which facilitates serial re-assessment during the hospitalization. At a minimum, the consultant should review physical examinations performed by other physicians, but will often also wish to perform a neurological examination and other selected parts of the physical exam that may assist with diagnosis and treatment.

Confirm Home and Hospital Medications

Many side effects (such as toxicity and withdrawal) may result from inadequate medication reconciliation. Examples include inadvertently discontinuing home medications, or starting full doses of medications with which the patient had been nonadherent. If uncertainty exists, it is helpful to ask family members to check pill bottles, and/or call the patient's home pharmacy. Consultants should also check medication administration records to see what doses have actually been received, particularly for as-needed medications.

Get Collateral History

Histories from hospitalized patients may be unreliable or even nonexistent (e.g., when the patient is delirious or somnolent). Collateral data from family members, outpatient health care providers, and other sources is crucial. It is important to weigh data according to the reliability of the source. Considerations include how well the source knows the patient, along with whether the source may be in denial or have a personal agenda to advance.

Write the Note

The note should include a condensed version of all the elements of a general psychiatric evaluation, with a few additions. In particular, the first few sentences of the HPI should summarize key elements of the past medical and psychiatric history, the reason for the current medical admission, and the consultation question. Afterward, the consultant should provide a brief summary of the present medical illness, pertinent diagnostic findings, and hospital course. Laboratory and imaging data and pertinent physical and neurological exam findings should be summarized as well. Recommendations should include specific ways to clarify the diagnosis and therapeutic suggestions (both medication and behavioral). It is important to anticipate future problems (for example, providing a medication recommendation for treatment of agitation in a delirious or psychotic patient who is currently calm). Include clear guidelines on the use of medications (providing indication, doses, intervals, side effects, and maximum doses to be given per day). End with a statement indicating that the consultant will provide follow-up and include contact information.

Speak with the Referring Clinician

For time-sensitive issues, personal contact is critical. Some information may be confidential and best conveyed verbally rather than in the written note. This is because hospital charts are read by a variety of individuals, including some who may not be closely involved in the patient's care, as well as by patients themselves at times.

Provide Periodic Follow-Up

After completing the consultation, determine the appropriate frequency and duration of follow-up visits. Patients who are suicidal, delirious, or otherwise agitated require brief daily visits, while other patients who are adjusting to medical illness may benefit from less frequent but longer duration visits for therapy. Follow-up visits should be documented in the medical record. Once a patient stabilizes, it may be appropriate to sign off on a case; notify the team, and indicate this clearly in the chart.

Common Emotional Responses to Illness

Patients display diverse emotional and behavioral responses to the stress of medical illness. The psychiatric consultant's task is to help the team understand and manage these responses. Patients with personality disorders may be at particularly high risk for adverse responses. In some cases, severe stress results in regression and unmasking of maladaptive personality traits that do not normally result in functional difficulties for the patient. A serious medical illness often leads to intensified feelings of vulnerability, which exacerbates the underlying fears of neglect and abandonment that are so common in patients with personality disorders. This may in turn result in behavioral regression and further illumination of personality vulnerabilities. Table 17.7 presents the specific personality disorders that tend to cause problems in the medical setting, along with management strategies.

Table 17.7 Emotional responses to medical illness

Emotion	Special notes	Therapeutic strategies
Anger	Common response to illness; most difficult for clinicians	Empathy and limit setting
	Commonly seen with paranoid, narcissistic, borderline, or antisocial personality styles	Redirect anger toward more productive targets (e.g., fighting the illness instead of refusing treatment)
Sadness	Illness results in multiple losses (e.g., ability to work; ability to pursue life goals; physical and cognitive capacity)	Provide patient with analogy to the process of grief/mourning
	Perhaps higher risk of depression in setting of premorbid mood disorders	Do not prescribe antidepressants for a normal grief reaction
Anxiety or fear	Nearly ubiquitous	Avoid superficial, blanket reassurance
		Instead figure out what the patient's specific fears are (e.g., death, pain, dyspnea, dependence on caregivers, disfigurement)
Guilt or shame	Illness seen as punishment for earlier health behaviors, real or imagined sins	Ask directly if the patient thinks they did something to cause their illness
	May be productive if it provides motivation for positive behavioral change	Be nonjudgmental, clarify that the illness is not the patient's fault
	May be maladaptive if leads to self-blame and thus depression	

Denial

Denial frequently factors into consultation requests. It is a complex concept, and the consultant's first task is to figure out what the referring physician means by "denial." Denial may refer to several different scenarios. The patient may actually reject the diagnosis outright. Some patients may accept the diagnosis but fail to appreciate its implications and may delay or avoid medical treatment. Other patients may display a disquieting lack of emotional response to the diagnosis. Denial can be adaptive in nature. For example, a patient may benefit from experiencing a period of denial immediately after a life-threatening diagnosis, as it allows time to catch up emotionally while beginning a demanding course of treatment. Some degree of denial may also be helpful in terminal illness so as to allow a patient to remain motivated and hopeful and to focus on quality of life. Denial becomes maladaptive when it prevents the patient from seeking medical attention for a new problem or interferes with treatment adherence. Interestingly, studies of the impact of denial on medical outcomes have found both beneficial and adverse effects. When maladaptive denial exists, clinicians should avoid directly confronting the denial and instead attempt to elicit a narrative of how the patient developed the illness. This will often bring to light underlying emotions driving the need for denial (e.g., anxiety, anger, or fear; Table 17.7). Diminishing the intensity of such emotions through psychotherapeutic or even psychopharmacologic interventions can help to reduce denial.

Other Common Differential Diagnoses and Issues in Psychiatric Consultation

Depression versus Delirium versus Dementia

Hospitalized patients with delirium do not always display agitation. At times, blunted, depressed, or anxious affect can be the principal manifestations of an underlying hypoactive delirium. Impaired attention is the cardinal feature of delirium. Other findings include impairments in orientation, short-term memory, and executive function. A comprehensive cognitive exam will usually provide evidence of delirium and should be supplemented by careful chart review, which will often reveal waxing/waning mental status with nocturnal worsening. By definition, delirium is the result of an underlying medical or neurologic condition, so delirious patients need to be worked up to determine the underlying cause. Whenever possible, the psychiatric consultant should assist the medical team by providing hypotheses in this regard. Efforts should then be directed toward reversing the identified medical cause(s), which will generally result in improved mental status.

Patients with dementia are at very high risk of overlying delirium in the setting of medical complications, even seemingly minor ones such as urinary tract infections. In order to diagnose an underlying dementia in a delirious patient, the consultant should obtain collateral history from family and/or outpatient treaters regarding the patient's cognitive and functional baseline.

Adjustment Disorder versus Depression

It can be difficult to distinguish depression from adjustment disorders in the medical setting. Specifically, several of the diagnostic criteria for major depressive disorder are confounded by symptoms resulting from medical illnesses, particularly fatigue, poor appetite, altered psychomotor activity, disordered sleep, and impaired concentration. In assessing for major depression in medically ill patients, criteria of particular interest include anhedonia, early morning awakening, guilt (Table 17.8), and suicidal ideation. Further, fatigue that is already present early in the morning, as opposed to fatigue that sets in gradually over the course of the day, may suggest depression as opposed to expected effects of medical treatments. Other non-DSM criteria may support a diagnosis of major depressive disorder (Table 17.9).

Table 17.8 Clinical findings suggesting major depression

Disability out of proportion to medical condition

Somatic preoccupation

Sustained irritability

Pervasively negative outlook, e.g., failure to see anything positive resulting from the medical diagnosis or treatment

Hopelessness

Wish for hastened death (+/−)

Requests for physician-assisted suicide (+/−)

Table 17.9 Questions that elicit guilt in medically ill patients

Do you blame yourself for getting this illness?

Do you feel that you deserved to get sick?

Do you feel like you are a burden on your family?

Do you feel worthless?

Capacity

Consultation-liaison psychiatrists may assist medical teams in determining whether a patient has capacity to make a particular treatment decision, such as refusing a diagnostic procedure or leaving the hospital against medical advice. Applebaum describes four key elements of decision-making capacity: choice (ability to express a consistent choice); understanding (ability to recognize the benefits and risks of the proposed treatment); appreciation (ability to appreciate the broader implications of treatment options on one's life); and rationality (ability to rationally manipulate information about treatment options). All of these elements should be assessed during a capacity evaluation.

It is important to remember that capacity assessments relate only to specific decisions, and levels of scrutiny will differ according to the specific issue at hand (Table 17.10). While the psychiatric consultant may offer important opinions regarding patient capacity, only a court of law can declare a patient globally incompetent to make health care decisions. At times, requests for capacity evaluation may reflect underlying ethical dilemmas that should be assessed with the assistance of ethics committees.

Table 17.10 Capacity evaluations: Level of scrutiny needed according to risk-benefit ratio of treatment

	High risk	Low risk
High benefit	Scrutinize capacity closely (e.g., face transplant)	Scrutinize refusers > accepters (e.g., intubation for pneumonia in healthy young adult)
Low benefit	Scrutinize accepters > refusers (e.g., 4th line chemotherapy for metastatic pancreatic cancer)	No need for close scrutiny (e.g., cholinesterase inhibitors in dementia)

Summary

Consultation-liaison psychiatrists perform a variety of important functions in the general hospital as described above. Historically, many of these functions have occurred in an inpatient setting, but there is increasing interest in integrating these services (and others) into outpatient medical clinics, which will be described below.

Behavioral Health Integration in Primary Care

Psychiatry, unlike other specialties, has historically functioned separately from the rest of medical health care delivery. Other than the practice of consultation-liaison psychiatry and the occasional psychiatric unit in a general hospital, mainstream psychiatric practice has taken place in private psychiatric hospitals, independent clinics, community mental health centers, and the private consulting room. The reasons for this are myriad and will only be mentioned here as a way to highlight and contrast this historical trend with the evolving concept of "integrated mental health care." Integrated mental health care is embedded in medical clinics and exists in many centers, including both specialty medical (and surgical) clinics and primary care clinics. Specialty sites include transplant programs, women's and obstetric clinics, oncology, HIV, and select other medical specialty clinics. This discussion will focus on integration in primary care clinics.

Integrated mental health care has increasingly become recognized as a valuable, innovative and distinct model of psychiatric health care delivery. The rationale for integrating mental health care into primary care practice has been firmly established in the research literature of the last few decades. The supporting evidence for an integration model includes epidemiologic surveys that demonstrate the high prevalence of psychiatric disorders in the community and general medical practices and that more patients with psychiatric disorders are seen by primary care providers than by mental health professionals. This fact was captured by Regier's 1978 observation that primary care could be considered the "de facto" mental health delivery system in this country. The reasons why more patients with mental illness are seen in general practice rather than by mental health professionals are complicated, but include the lack of access to traditional psychiatric care, the stigma associated with seeking mental health, and the fact that many patients express distress via somatic (physical) rather than psychological symptoms. Unfortunately, less than 50 percent of psychiatric disorders that present in primary care are identified and if identified, treatment outcomes are often poor. This problem is exacerbated by the fact that most of these patients, if referred, fail to engage effectively in traditional mental health care. This is partly due to the lack of reasonable access to mental health services, but also to patients' reluctance to accept the necessity for such care and/or the sense that traditional mental health services do not meet their needs.

In addition, increasing awareness of the cost and morbidity associated with psychiatric disorders, the high rates of co-morbidity among psychiatric and medical illnesses, and the bi-directional negative influence of medical and psychiatric disorders strengthens the case for integrated services. There is considerable evidence that integrating mental health care into primary care is practical and leads to improved outcomes compared to usual care. The promise of improved care and cost savings with integrated care has caught the attention of policy makers and payers who have recently begun to encourage integration. Integrated care is prioritized in the establishment of "medical homes" and in new payment models such as accountable care organizations.

Models of Care

Many models of integration have been developed and are currently in use. Model development has occurred in response to the evidence stated previously, the perspective of population health and in response to the needs of local health care systems. Integration takes place across a continuum of several parameters including leadership (unified versus separate), payers (same versus distinct), clinical and communication (letters, email, phone, joint meetings, common electronic health record), and space (co-located versus separate). There is no single model of integration, and each of these parameters results in its own barrier to effective integration. Barriers include the lack of space in many medical clinics to accommodate mental health clinicians, divided administrative incentives, separate funding streams, and confidentiality concerns about specially protected mental health data. Despite the existence of many models of integration, they all involve one or more of the following strategies.

Planned, Population-Based Care

This aspect of integration acknowledges that providers have responsibility to the population of patients in their community and not just the individual patient at hand. The prevalence of mental illness, the lack of access to traditional mental health providers, and the fact that many of these patients seek treatment in primary care require efficient and effective methods of care delivery and close collaboration among mental health and primary care providers.

Chronic Disease Management Strategies

The Institute of Medicine report of 2001 emphasized that American health care was oriented toward acute illness and was failing many patients with chronic illnesses, which account for the majority of health-related morbidity in this country. This report led to the development of new models for the care of chronic medical and mental illnesses. Typically called "chronic disease management," it calls for both routine and proactive care of patients. This is often accomplished using a patient registry, specified monitoring periods, and standardized monitoring tools. A central feature of these disease management programs is the structural redesign of the health care team, moving away from the traditional dyad of doctor-patient toward a team approach where all members of the care team have essential and specified roles in the care of each patient. A critical member of this model's team is the care manager. This role can be fulfilled by a nurse, social worker, medical assistant, or other paraprofessional. The care manager maintains registries and evaluation metrics and reaches out to patients at specified intervals. In the case of mental illnesses, the care manager also has routine supervision from a psychiatrist to maximize effectiveness and address issues with patients who are not improving. The primary care provider directs the team effort and focuses on patients who are not doing well. All team members are trained to understand how the illness fits into the patient's life and help address issues that inhibit optimal health care. In addition, all team members are explicitly tasked with educating the patient about their illness and encouraging self-management strategies as well as employing techniques such as behavioral activation and motivational interviewing. The emphasis is to inform, engage, and activate patients in the service of their own health care while addressing barriers to health that may exist beyond the disease process itself.

Algorithm Driven Care

This strategy usually entails a system of screening for mental disorders (improving detection), monitoring progress, and using evidence-based treatment strategies that can be followed by the primary care team, with adequate education, support, and backup from mental health. Algorithms can include medication recommendation, dosing strategies, and guidance on whether/when therapy or a psychiatric consultation might be necessary. Evidence-based algorithms help ensure quality care. In this context, electronic medical records provide for ease of communication among providers in busy practices, transparency of monitoring tools, and joint treatment planning.

Co-location of Mental Health Providers

The co-location of mental health providers in medical clinics has many advantages. Co-location allows for ease of verbal communication among providers and limits the stigma and inconvenience of services for patients referred to the mental health clinician. Co-location, to be effective, involves some important distinctions from traditional mental health care. These innovations include methods to improve access such as an "open door" policy, which allows the primary care clinician real-time access to mental health expertise. It also includes the notion of "warm handoffs," whereby the mental health clinician can be introduced to the primary care patient at the time of the referral to ease ambivalence about follow-through. The co-located mental health provider tends to use short-term, problem-solving psychotherapeutic techniques rather than traditional dynamic, insight-oriented treatment approaches. Short-term techniques include all the behavioral techniques mentioned in the chronic disease section above as well as more formal cognitive-behavioral therapies for specific conditions. Such therapeutic techniques seem to be particularly suited to the needs of primary care patients who often present with somatic symptoms and have chronic medical as well as mental illnesses. Co-located mental health specialists may also have an important role in "wellness" programs where lifestyle changes are often critical to improving health outcomes. Short-term treatment models also allow the mental health clinician to maintain availability and serve more patients over time.

Stepped Care

Stepped care describes an approach where the intensity of the care plan corresponds to the severity of the patient's illness. This approach has particular utility for the management of mental illness in primary care clinics. Less severe disorders tend to be managed by the primary care team alone (using monitoring systems and algorithms as appropriate). Moderately complicated disorders may require psychiatric consultation and/or brief therapies whereas more severe disorders may require intensive, specialty mental health care. An example might be mildly problematic alcohol use which can be successfully addressed by some counseling by PCP and a referral to community self-help programs. Moderate alcohol use disorders might require specialized mental health counseling. Severe alcohol use disorders might require a detoxification program and a residential rehabilitation program. Stepped care is predicated upon active care management and monitoring of the patient's course along with increasing the intensity of service if the patient is not progressing.

Psychiatric Consultation

Expert psychiatric backup is critical for integrated programs to be effective. The psychiatrist (and other mental health professionals) can help develop treatment algorithms and educate and support the primary care team. In addition, a psychiatrist is often used to supervise the care manager responsible for mental disorders and provide expert consultation to primary care providers and to patients not responding to usual care.

Conclusion

The evidence for the benefit of the integration of mental health in primary care is extensive and compelling. Integrative programs are becoming more common, and usually include one or more of the elements noted previously. The most crucial elements seem to be the routine use of monitoring tools, active care management, and effective psychiatric consultation.

Somatic Symptom Disorders

More than half of the population experiences one or more bodily symptoms in any given week. Some individuals who have somatic symptoms develop persistent distress regarding the symptom, and this can lead to an overvalued belief that one is ill. The tendency to experience and report bodily symptoms (whether due to a known medical or psychiatric etiology or not) can become a form of chronic illness behavior. In severe cases, it can become the focus of one's life and cause disruption in everyday functioning. When an individual develops excessive and dysfunctional feelings (e.g., anxiety), behaviors (e.g., devoting excessive time to the symptom or its control), and cognitions (e.g., persistent beliefs about the seriousness of the symptom) about somatic symptoms, that person should be assessed for a somatic symptom disorder. Examples of somatic symptom-related disorders proposed by the *Diagnostic and Statistical Manual of Mental Disorders*, 5th edition, include somatic symptom disorder, illness anxiety disorder, conversion disorder, and psychological factors affecting medical conditions.

The first step in evaluating a patient who presents with specific somatic symptoms involves determining whether there is a true medical or psychiatric condition that can appropriately explain the patient's symptoms and distress. Importantly, not all clinical presentations with somatic symptoms meet the criteria for a somatic symptom disorder. In a similar fashion, one can have a somatic symptom disorder in the context of a serious medical illness. Careful attention should be given to conditions that affect multiple organ systems or that can produce variable presentations (e.g., HIV infection, scleroderma, rheumatoid arthritis, systemic lupus erythematosus, multiple sclerosis). One should also consider whether the presentation can be fully explained by another primary psychiatric disorder (e.g., affective, anxiety, substance-related, and personality disorders).

The next diagnostic step involves differentiating whether the patient's symptoms are true or feigned (in which case one should consider factitious disorder or malingering). An individual who has a somatic symptom disorder actually experiences their symptoms as real and believes that these symptoms have a medical cause.

Patients with somatic symptom disorders often over-utilize medical care, frequently seeking care from multiple doctors for the same symptoms when the earlier providers are unable to identify a medical etiology. Not surprisingly, such individuals are frequently unresponsive to myriad medical interventions. They may pressure physicians to pursue tests and treatment which may not be indicated, and are thus at risk for iatrogenic harm associated with misdirected drug trials, unnecessary surgeries, and ill-advised diagnostic procedures. These interventions can potentially worsen a patient's symptoms. Left untreated, their course is commonly chronic (with occasional fluctuations). Therefore, early intervention is crucial. Effective treatment involves promoting a healthy lifestyle and avoiding maladaptive behaviors (such as validating overvalued beliefs about one's illness). An approach to treatment is best remembered by thinking of this disorder as a behavioral syndrome, not as a disease.

The optimal treatment for afflicted individuals requires building a long-term doctor-patient relationship (usually with a primary care physician) in which the patient's distress is accepted and viewed as real. Once this relationship is established, the treatments initiated (e.g., providing reassurance in the case of conversion disorder) are predicated upon the signs and symptoms of the actual diagnosis. The overall goals of treatment include maintaining or improving the individual's overall functioning, monitoring for concurrent physical or psychiatric disorders, and placing an emphasis on care rather than on cure. The role of stress, rather than the persistent symptoms, should become the focus. The primary care physician should oversee the ordering of all tests and consultations, especially when a patient seeks out care from multiple providers, so as to prevent unnecessary and potential harmful interventions.

Regular, brief (non-symptom contingent) follow-up visits are helpful, even when the patient is functioning well. Over time, the patient may then give up some of the symptoms, as they are no longer needed to gain the care of the provider. Such individuals should be monitored for the development of new illnesses. When new signs or symptoms develop, the clinician should perform specific procedures and initiate treatments based on objective evidence from a focused physical exam rather than on subjective symptoms. Referral for psychiatric consultation, if the patient agrees, can help to confirm the diagnosis as well to identify and treat any co-morbid psychiatric disorders. Cognitive-behavioral therapy can clarify and re-structure cognitive distortions, unrealistic beliefs, worry, and behaviors that might drive the disorder. Referral to a vocational counselor can help assure that a patient does not put important activities on hold until the resolution of any somatic symp-toms (as not working reinforces illness behavior).

Factitious Disorder and Malingering

In contrast to patients with somatic symptom disorders, individuals with factitious illness seek out medical attention after intentionally producing or feigning med-ical or psychiatric signs or symptoms, the cause of which they hide. Individuals may fake or exaggerate symptoms, intentionally worsen symptoms, fabricate histories, or deliberately induce injury. They often develop extensive medical knowledge, and then use that information to develop false stories of real dis-ease states. In reality, almost any symptom or condition can be feigned. Physical examples include factitious fever (by heating the thermometer), hypoglycemia (from exogenous insulin), sepsis (by self-injecting feces into body parts), and wounds (self-inflicted). Psychiatric examples include suicidal ideation, psychosis, depression, anxiety, bereavement, and posttraumatic stress. Incongruent findings on the physical exam (such as neurologic signs that do not conform to known anatomical pathways) and unexplainable laboratory results are often found, but with appropriate testing, the hoax can often be ascertained (e.g., testing for low levels of C-peptide when suspecting exogenous insulin ingestion, or testing for phenolphthalein in the stool in the case of laxative abuse as a cause for chronic diarrhea).

The characteristic feature of this disorder is deception. The attention of oth-ers (i.e., the reward) serves to sustain the hoax. The motivating factor for the deception, while often difficult to ascertain, separates factitious disorder from malingering. Those with factitious disorder are driven to deceive without obvi-ous secondary gain other than obtaining the benefits of achieving the sick role (e.g., protection, blamelessness, attention, support, and release from work). Those who malinger, in contrast, are externally motivated by a clear "second-ary" gain (e.g., legal or financial benefits, such as being placed on disability).

The factitious illness usually begins in early adulthood, frequently after a med-ical condition, mental disorder, or hospitalization. Individuals with the condition commonly have a history of abandonment and childhood abuse. Their behavior often becomes a lifelong pattern with recurrent episodes rather than with one sol-itary symptomatic period. In contrast, the malingerer's symptoms often improve once their objective has been obtained. The prevalence of malingering is unknown but it is often co-morbid with antisocial personality disorder.

Munchausen syndrome, a subset of factitious disorder, accounts for the approximately 10 percent of factitious disorder cases that are more severe, chronic, and refractory. Traveling from hospital to hospital (peregrination), being admitted to hospitals repeatedly, and *pseudologia fantastica* (a form of pathological lying involving the production of wildly exaggerated stories) are three characteristics of this syndrome.

Diagnosing factitious disorder is difficult and it requires diligent detective work either (if shrewd or lucky) by catching the patient intentionally self-inflicting signs of illness or through gathering extensive collateral information (from previous and current treaters, family, medical records) along with appropriate laboratory testing to confirm findings reported as facts. Using a systematic approach decreases the chances of overlooking a condition with a physiologic source. The diagnosis should remain provisional until there is considerable evidence gathered to confirm it.

Those with factitious disorder often share similar features that can be suggestive of the disorder: multiple hospital admissions, multiple forms of identification or hospital medical record numbers, use of medical jargon, awareness of what conditions will lead to hospitalization, ability to a provide convincing history, and a persistent demand for specific interventions (e.g., surgeries or administration of a particular medication). The person with this condition might arrive at the hospital during the night or on a weekend when staff is less likely to identify him or her.

As with most psychiatric disorders, the diagnosis hinges on ruling-out other mental disorders that could better explain the behavior and symptoms. It is important to remember that individuals with factitious disorder can also have a true co-morbid medical or psychiatric disorder.

Unfortunately, there is no specific and effective treatment for factitious disorder. However, one should attempt to make the diagnosis as early as possible to prevent iatrogenic complications that can develop through diagnostic workups and treatment. Clear communication among team members is essential. One should attempt to treat any true medical problems, to address complications of any self-injurious behavior, and to treat any co-existing psychiatric conditions. Direct confrontation of the patient over the diagnosis, while controversial, is generally ineffective, as few patients admit to their deceptive behavior. Confrontation can result in defensiveness, irritability, and elopement from the hospital. Providing a face-saving solution for the patient can sometimes diminish the aberrant behavior.

Finally, patients who deceive and lie can elicit intense emotional and behavioral responses from caregivers, or result in cognitive challenges for physicians (who are trained to be caring, trusting, and eager to help). These responses can serve as a distraction when applying diagnostic skills, further delaying an accurate diagnosis. These reactions can also lead physicians to act on their anger (e.g., through ordering unnecessary procedures, dispensing dangerous treatments, or making errors). Maintaining physician awareness about their hostility can prevent one from acting on it.

In summary, patients with somatic symptom disorders *believe* that they are ill, while those with factitious disorders *pretend* that they are ill. If they are pretending without an obvious external reward, then factitious disorder should be considered. If there is an external incentive, then malingering should be considered.

Palliative Care

The still young specialty of palliative medicine has both enhanced the perspective of psychiatrists working with seriously medically ill patients, and heightened the importance of knowing when to ask for the involvement of a palliative care team.

Dr. Cecily Saunders, founder of St. Christopher's Hospice in London, was among the first to demonstrate a coherent approach to patients' combined physical, social, psychological and spiritual distress, which she referred to as "total pain." The first hospital-based palliative care programs in the United States opened in the late 1980's. Since, their numbers have dramatically increased so that today they number over 1400; eighty percent of US hospitals with over 300 beds now have a program. Rather than only focusing on care at the end of life, palliative medicine offers a continuum of care, beginning with the diagnosis of a life-limiting illness and extending through bereavement.

In 2009, the National Consensus Project Clinical Practice Guidelines for Quality Palliative Care defined palliative medicine as "medical care provided by an interdisciplinary team, including the professions of medicine, nursing, social work, chaplaincy, counseling, nursing assistant, and other health care professions focused on the relief of suffering and support for the best possible quality of life (QOL) for patients facing serious life-threatening illness and their families. It aims to identify and address the physical, psychological, spiritual, and practical burdens of illness."

Put more simply, palliative medicine focuses on comfort, continuity and communication in the face of life-limiting illness. Comfort is the state of peace that results from the effective, coordinated management of distress in all of its dimensions. A clinician with this perspective will be alert to physical distress (for example, in the form of pain), the quality and extent of social supports, the experience of emotional suffering, existential or spiritual distress, and the relationship among all of these sources of distress. For example, unrelieved pain in a patient who witnessed his father's painful death may be a source of existential distress over leaving his own children, resulting in anxiety which could be worsening his experience of pain. Rather than focusing only on this anxiety, however, a clinician with a palliative medicine perspective will also focus on assertively treating the patient's pain, and/or requesting a consultation with a pain expert who is equipped and ready to do so. Since fears about future suffering are a major component of patient distress, appreciating the nature of these fears can allow the clinician to provide appropriate reassurance, and to tailor treatment plans with the patient that address these concerns.

Continuity refers to optimizing both (a) the connection across treatment episodes and sites with providers who understand the patient's needs, and (b) a coherent sense of self in the face of serious illness. Clinicians with this perspective will attend to the problems that primary oncologists may have in following their patients closely enough in the hospital, or when referred to hospice. They also listen for opportunities to both enhance that connection, and if necessary to supplement it with an interdisciplinary team of providers who can extend continuous care through the end of life. Keeping in mind Eric Cassell's (1991) definition of suffering as a threat to the integrity of the self, they will value the patient's narrative of what her life has been about, and how it is shaped by illness.

Palliative medicine recognizes communication as critically important in achieving comfort and continuity. This begins with a focus on helping the patient clarify his or her own goals. For example, clinicians can ask a patient to rank top life priorities, using a list of frequently chosen options (Table 17.11).

Understanding the patient's preferences for information and for involvement in decision-making is also important in shaping the approach of the team to meeting the patient's wishes. Does the patient want to have as much information as possible, or only what he asks to be told? Does she want to share the process of making decisions, prefer strong guidance from the physician, or want to be guided by her family's wishes? Since the patient's surrogate or health care proxy frequently makes end-of-life decisions, who does the patient prefer to serve in this role, and

Table 17.11 Possible end-of-life priorities for patients to rank in order of importance

- Live as long as possible, no matter what
- Be at home
- Be physically comfortable
- Be mentally aware
- Be independent
- Make sure my family is supported
- Be at peace emotionally and spiritually
- Achieve a particular life goal (patient to specify what)

how does he view that role? Given that patients view impairments in functions differently and make different choices based on these views, what do they consider unacceptable functional states, and why? Have they had the opportunity to think about tradeoffs that might be necessary to achieve the outcomes they want – for example, weighing time in the hospital, invasive procedures, or treatments against the value of time at home or feeling well?

Achieving clarity on a patient's goals and preferences often depends on good communication regarding prognosis. What does the patient understand about his prognosis? How much does the patient want to know? How much has he discussed prognosis with his family? What is the physician's understanding of the patient's prognosis? Although it may be difficult for the physician to predict, what does he answer to the question, "Would you be surprised if this patient died this year?" Given the importance of family members to most patients, what is their understanding of the patient's illness and prognosis? What do they fear, expect to happen and hope for? How much have they communicated their concerns with the patient and the clinical team? If they are keeping concerns secret from the patient or other family members, are they aware of the costs of doing so? Are they satisfied with their communication with the team? Have they begun the process of anticipatory grieving?

Finally, palliative medicine emphasizes the importance of self-care for clinicians. Intense feelings aroused by witnessing suffering can lead to "compassion fatigue," with the potential for withdrawal from patients and avoidance of difficult conversations. Clinicians alert to these risks will monitor their capacity for holding sadness and practice ways of remaining fresh to their work, in addition to cultivating the traditional psychiatric awareness of oneself as a therapeutic tool, and of the countertransference which the patient has evoked within them.

How does this perspective relate to psychiatric assessment considered more broadly? At first glance, the traditional psychiatric emphasis on helping patients to take responsibility for themselves and on maintaining therapeutic boundaries may seem at odds with the emphases of palliative medicine on advocacy and nearness to suffering. However, the emphasis of both specialties on the human dimension of serious illness make these tensions more theoretical than real. A palliative medicine perspective builds on the traditional biopsychosocial model of psychiatry by extending the clinical focus to the relief of suffering of the whole person within the context of his entire life, including its value and spiritual dimensions. Palliative-care oriented clinicians actively advocate for comfort, continuity, and communication, prioritizing the identification and relief of physical symptoms, and recognizing the value of a multidisciplinary approach to meeting the patient's and family's needs. Every clinician concerned with the whole patient should be able to assess the basic needs of the patient and family in these domains, but should also recognize when challenging symptoms or complex team dynamics call for palliative medicine consultation. For their part, palliative medicine clinicians call on psychiatric consultants to help them treat complex cases of delirium, major mental illness, and character disorders, complicating the care of the patient by the medical team. The perspectives of psychiatry and palliative medicine complement and enrich one another in the shared pursuit of relieving the suffering of individuals and families made vulnerable by serious illness.

Bereavement and Loss

Grief is a normal psychophysiologic response to the loss of a loved one. It is both mental and physical: a distinct syndrome and an important mark on a person's emotional memory and life course. Man is not the only mammal who shows the yearning and searching naturally mediated by the limbic system's anatomy for attachment, separation, and grief.

Symptoms of normal acute grief include sensations of somatic distress occurring in waves of 20 minutes to one hour, tightness in the throat, shortness of breath, an empty feeling in the abdomen, lack of muscular power, and sighing respiration. Panic attacks, which include similar symptoms, often occur as well. Grief is a mental pain accompanied by exhaustion and a slight sense of unreality.

Bereaved patients may be intensely preoccupied with the image of the deceased and feel emotionally distant from other people. It is common for patients to feel guilty about what they might have said or done prior to the loss. Could they have prevented the death? If they knew that the person would be gone forever, would they have acted differently? In the context of this internal preoccupation, patients may temporarily lose their ability to relate empathically to others: they may respond with irritability or anger, and not want to be bothered. Also common are symptoms of tearfulness, emotional numbing, and the feeling of unreality (i.e., that the death did not happen). It is common for patients to hear their loved one calling their name or to believe they recognize their loved one in a crowd. A bereaved patient, identifying with the lost person, may seek medical attention for symptoms that are similar to those previously experienced by the loved one.

Importantly, grief provides a window into what attachments and losses have been important to a patient. During a medical or psychiatric history in a bereaved patient, a physician records the date of family members' death and the cause of death, illuminating the landscape of the patient's relational history. Anniversaries of loss often cause recurrent grief symptoms. In addition, the memory of past loss resonates in the setting of new losses.

When attachments are straightforward, rituals of mourning bring people together to ease the person's pain and to guide them through this passage. People grieve in different ways, and each culture allows for a ritual that brings people together with respect for the bereaved. It is helpful to stand by those in acute grief to facilitate their search for the lost person, to express condolences, to take care of immediate needs, and then to facilitate life-sustaining activities. Self-care should be constantly encouraged for grieving patients. There are other times when the love lost is taboo and cannot be publicly acknowledged. In those cases, a physician may enable the patient to acknowledge and process such a loss.

Pathological grief describes a grief syndrome that persists in a painful way that limits function or deviates from what is expected. On the extremes, it can be abnormal that no overt grieving is occurring, or that severe distress persists with anxiety, depression, and loss of function. Complicated grief is the current terminology for syndromes that persist in relation to the loss and that include intense intrusive thoughts, pangs of severe emotion, distressing yearnings, feeling excessively alone and empty, excessively avoiding tasks reminiscent of the deceased, persistent insomnia, or loss of interest in usual activities.

Grief stands as a paradigm for emotional loss. The numbness, ambivalence, anger, and guilt, the timeline of gradual acknowledgment and adjustment to reality, is useful for understanding how people tolerate other important losses like amputation, loss of health status, or job loss.

One practical question relates to when grief merges into depression and when the clinician should consider antidepressants and psychotherapy. Antidepressants are used when the syndrome is associated with failure to thrive and suicidal thoughts, and when the syndrome blurs into the criteria of major depressive disorder. It is all the more likely for grief to provoke an episode of clinical depression in a patient who has had previous episodes of depression.

Bereaved patients often find peer support groups to be helpful. Individual psychotherapy begins with the patient talking about the lost relationship. In grief work, patients express the uncomfortable mixed emotions that are naturally part of an intense relationship. These often include guilt about what was not done and anger at the person who left. The lost loved one may be idealized and/or fixed in memory as he/she was at the time of death. Over time, in the months after loss, this can give way to a more nuanced understanding of who the person was. The preoccupation with the lost person gives way to more concentration on the present, adjustment to life without the loved one, and gradual engagement in the future.

Case Examples

A forty-four-year-old woman, with a remote history of trauma and anxiety disorder previously well controlled on paroxetine, and a more recent history of breast cancer, status post surgery, chemotherapy, and radiotherapy (completed two months previously), presented to the emergency department with depressed mood and new-onset panic attacks. Stressors included coming to terms with infertility and returning to her demanding job as an international flight attendant after a one-year leave. In addition, the patient was in the midst of transitioning her antidepressant from paroxetine to venlafaxine, given anticipated need for tamoxifen; paroxetine inhibits CYP2D6, which converts tamoxifen into its more active metabolite. Vital signs were normal except for sinus tachycardia to 110 (previously in the 90s during clinic visits). The consultant noted these stressors but also urged a full medical workup, including for pulmonary embolism (PE), given her cancer status. The PE workup was negative, but she was found to be notably hyperthyroid by TFTs. Ongoing management included endocrinology consultation, temporarily pausing the antidepressant transition and intensifying her outside psychotherapy to focus on grief over infertility and concrete strategies to support her gradual re-entry into work.

References and Suggested Readings

- Abrahm, J. (2005). *A Physician's Guide to Pain and Symptom Management in Cancer Patients*, 2nd ed. Baltimore: Johns Hopkins University Press.
- American Psychiatric Association (2013). *Diagnostic and Statistical Manual of Mental Disorders*, 5th ed. Washington, DC: American Psychiatric Publishing.
- Applebaum, P. S., and Grisso, T. (1997). Capacities of Hospitalized, Medically Ill Patients to Consent to Treatment. *Psychosomatics*, 38, 119–125.
- Braun, I. M., Greenberg, D. B., Smith, F. A., and Cassem, N. H. (2010). Functional Somatic Symptoms, Deception Syndromes, and Somatoform Disorders. In Stern, T. A., Fricchione, G. L., Cassem, N. H., Jellinek, M. S., and Rosenbau, J. F. (eds.), *Massachusetts General Hospital Handbook of General Hospital Psychiatry*, 6th ed. New York: Saunders/Elsevier, pp. 173–187.
- Cassell, E. J. (1991). *The Nature of Suffering and the Goals of Medicine*. New York: Oxford University Press.
- Institute of Medicine (2001). *Crossing the Quality Chasm: A New Health Care System for the 21st Century*. Washington, DC: Institute of Medicine.
- Karas, S. (2002). Behavioral Emergencies: Differentiating Medical from Psychiatric Disease. *Emergency Medicine Practice*, 4, 1–20.
- Katon, W. (2012). Collaborative Depression Care Models: From Development to Dissemination. *American Journal of Preventive Medicine*, 42, 550–552.
- Meyer, F., and Block, S. D. (2011). Personality Disorders in the Oncology Setting. *Journal of Support Oncology*, 9, 44–51.
- Oh, E. S., Fong, T. G., Hshieh, T. T., and Inouye, S. K. (2017). Delirium in Older Persons: Advances in Diagnosis and Treatment. *Journal of the American Medical Association*, 318 (12), 1161–1174.
- Regier, D. A., Goldberg, I. D., and Taube, C. A. (1978). The De Facto US Mental Health Services System: A Public Health Perspective. *Arch Gen Psychiatry*, 35, 685–693.

- Smith, F. A. (2008). Factitious Disorders and Malingering. In Stern, T. A., Rosenbaum, J. F., Fava, M., Biederman, J., and Rauch, S. L. (eds.), *Massachusetts General Hospital Comprehensive Clinical Psychiatry*. Philadelphia: Mosby/Elsevier, pp. 331–336.
- Smith, F. A., Querques, J., Levenson, J. L., and Stern, T. A. (2005). Psychiatric Assessment and Consultation. In Levenson, J. L. (ed.), *The American Psychiatric Publishing Textbook of Psychosomatic Medicine*, 1st ed. Arlington, VA: American Psychiatric Publishing, pp. 3–15.
- Viederman, M., and Perry, S. W. (1980). Use of a Psychodynamic Life Narrative in the Treatment of Depression in the Physically Ill. *Gen Hospital Psychiatry*, 2, 177–185.

Self-Assessment Questions

1. In patients who present with psychiatric emergencies to the emergency department:
    A. Vital signs and laboratory testing are the most sensitive tools to diagnose a medical etiology for the symptoms.
    B. 30–50 percent will have co-existing medical disease.
    C. A noncontrast CT scan should be performed on all patients presenting with new-onset psychiatric symptoms.
    D. Vital signs taken on a combative or agitated patient are contraindicated as they are likely to mislead clinicians regarding the etiology of the presenting symptoms.

2. The cardinal feature of delirium is:
    A. Hypoactivity
    B. Agitation
    C. Impaired attention
    D. Visual hallucinations

3. The model of "stepped care" refers to:
    A. A system of detection of mental disorders which utilizes screening, monitoring of progress, and the use of evidence-based treatments that can be followed by the primary care team.
    B. Routine and proactive care of patients using a patient registry and standardized monitoring tools.
    C. Providers have a responsibility to the population of patients in their community rather than individual patients alone.
    D. The intensity of the care plan corresponds to the severity of the patient's Illness.

4. Which of the following is a sign that a bereaved person may be suffering from pathological grief?

A. Patient has feelings of emotional numbing and feelings of unreality in the weeks following the loss.
B. Patient experiences loss of function over an extended period of time following the loss.
C. Patient is intensely preoccupied with the image of the deceased.
D. Patient experiences new-onset panic attacks in the weeks following the loss.

Answers to Self-Assessment Questions

1. (B)
2. (C)
3. (D)
4. (B)

18

Psychiatry of Gender and Sexuality

AARON S. BRESLOW

Overview of Gender Identity and Sexual Orientation

The current chapter focuses on the complex, socially informed, and constantly evolving concepts of gender identity and sexual orientation. Although these topics are often taboo, they will arise in almost every interaction with patients in the medical setting. Gender identity and sexual orientation are present in everyone's life and have implications for relationships, biology, and health. As such, this chapter will attempt to explain key concepts and terms in order to increase your ease discussing these issues with patients and colleagues. Although most people are raised to conceptualize gender identity and sexual orientation as inherent, biologically fixed aspects of our lives, the chapter will discuss these concepts as both biologically informed and socially constructed processes of human life. They will be explored in the context of their social, medical, and psychiatric implications in order to increase your comfort providing evidence-informed, affirming care for diverse and multifaceted patients.

First, the chapter explains key terms, keeping in mind that language is constantly shifting and informed by cultural and social contexts. Second, the chapter outlines psychiatric implications, discussing the impact of gender and sexual minority stress as well as the importance of (and debate around) psychiatric diagnoses. This is followed by evidence-informed guidelines for affirming evaluation and treatment. The chapter ends with a discussion of future directions as well as sample cases and questions.

It is important when working with patients to be mindful of any preconceptions and biases that may naturally arise. Discussions of gender identity and sexual orientation are often complicated by stigma-related discomfort and bias, which can impede our self-awareness and ability as clinicians to provide patients with competent care. As you begin your work as a medical professional, we encourage you to keep an open mind about these topics in order to offer a supportive experience for those seeking your care. In doing so, you may also learn things more about the full range of human experiences, identity, and health.

Overview of Gender Identity

This first section briefly outlines key terms related to *gender*. This term is culturally and emotionally laden; it may evoke images related to femininity and masculinity, pink and blue, different types of clothing, or a figure above a restroom door.

Gender is a complex and important term informed by biology, social structures, and identity. It is commonly conflated with biological sex and thought of as an inherent, fixed aspect of a person's life. Yet psychiatry's conceptualizations of gender have become more complex and affirming in recent years. In order to provide a more nuanced understanding of gender, we define relevant terms below.

Sex

Historically, the terms "sex" and "gender" have been used interchangeably. These concepts, however, are distinct. The term "sex" typically refers to one's biology: chromosomes, genitalia, hormones, and secondary sex characteristics such as breasts, distribution of body hair, or an Adam's apple. Such physiological traits typically lead to sex assignment by a doctor, even before a baby is born. Babies with two X chromosomes are called "female." Those with one X and one Y chromosome are called "male." Most often, of course, doctors assign an individual's sex prior to birth through a process of prenatal sex discernment: a process of testing to determine the sex of a fetus. Moments after an individual is born, their sex is codified on their birth certificate – as female or male – and a complex process of socialization is set into motion.

Because of this medical tradition of assigning a baby the label of "girl" or "boy," sex is typically thought of as a *binary* paradigm, with each person fitting the label of either "female" or "male." Sex, however, is not binary. Approximately 1.5 percent of babies are born with genitalia, hormones, or secondary sex characteristics that do not fit into either category. These babies are typically referred to as having *intersex* traits. This concept is discussed further throughout this chapter and highlights that sex is not exclusively biologically determined, but also socially and medically ascribed.

Gender

Gender is a term describing the behavioral, cultural, and psychological traits associated with masculinity and femininity. Whereas sex is primarily biological, gender is primarily social. Gender is mutable and culturally dependent; it varies across culture, ideology, race/ethnicity, and time. The World Health Organization defines gender as "the socially constructed characteristics of women and men, such as norms, roles, and relationships of and between groups of women and men. It varies from society to society and can be changed." Every person's gender is informed by a complex interplay between their body, identity, and expression and role. Multiple concepts are discussed below that may sound similar though describe discrete constructs. For example, gender identity, expression, and roles inform each other though are different processes. For clarity, it may be helpful to think of examples and/or consider how these concepts manifest differently in your life.

Gender identity is a person's inner sense of being a girl/woman, boy/man, something else in terms of gender, having multiple gender identities, or having no gender identity at all. Gender identity refers to a person's feelings about themselves in terms of how they relate to masculinity, femininity, and a blend of similar traits. Although studies demonstrate a wide spectrum of gender identities, society reinforces a notion that gender is a binary phenomenon consisting of only two genders, girl/woman or boy/man. Gender identity is often thought of as internal, whereas gender expression is considered more external.

Gender expression refers to the behavioral manifestations of one's gender. It is the way we show our gender identity to the world around us. This includes behaviors and rituals we may take for granted: wearing pants rather than a skirt, using the women's bathroom, speaking with a bass rather than falsetto voice, and responding to particular pronouns such as "he," "she," or "they." Gender expression is defined by clothing, mannerisms, vocal patterns, and behaviors. Feminist and queer theorists typically define gender expression as a "performance" rather than something biologically predestined (Butler, 1990). Gender expression is informed by one's personal preferences and cultural experiences. For example, men are socialized to be strong, unemotional, ambitious, and competitive. Women are socialized to be *softer*: to take care of others, support families, and to acquiesce to men. Yet many people defy or transcend these expectations of gender expression and express their gender in diverse ways.

Gender roles are the social demands deemed appropriate, legal, and productive based on each person's gender. They are specific, gendered behaviors and expectations. Think about the ways you assume men and women behave in society; the professions, relational expectations, and political positions you may imagine differently for men versus women are examples of gender roles. A demonstrative illustration is the competitive world of business and economics. When we envision the key players working on Wall Street to influence the global marketplace, we may imagine white men in powerful positions aggressively negotiating deals and asserting their dominance in sleek, often colorless board rooms. When we think about women in this world, we think of administrative assistants or wives. These gender roles are informed by sexist and often racial ideologies and political structures that have a real impact on access to political power. Many people defy gender roles, though there are often social consequences for doing so.

Gender roles assign predetermined tasks, behaviors, and social expectations for individuals based on their assigned sex. They also have profound social, economic, and psychological impacts. To put this in context, a 2017 study by *Fortune* magazine analyzing the leadership of the 1,000 American companies with the largest annual revenue found that only 54 companies were run by women; among these companies, only 5.4 percent had a female CEO. This disparity can be understood in the context of gender roles. Women are generally not socialized to run businesses or compete in the global marketplace. Certainly, this gender gap has social, economic, and political causes and effects. The predominance of men in business may seem like a "given," considering this patriarchal system has persisted in Western civilizations for generations. It is important to consider the impact of gender roles in creating and perpetuating such a disparity.

Transgender

Transgender (often abbreviated to "trans") is an umbrella term for people whose gender identity or expression does not align in a traditional way with the sex they were assigned at birth. A *transgender man* is a person who was assigned female sex at birth and identifies as a man. Other common terms include trans man, female-to-male, FtM, and man of trans experience. A *transgender woman* is a person who was assigned male at birth and identifies as a woman. Other common terms include trans woman, male-to-female, MtF, and woman of trans experience. Many, though not all, transgender people pursue psychotherapy, surgery, and other biomedical interventions to assure their gender presentation aligns with their gender identity.

The term *cisgender* (often abbreviated to "cis") refers to a person whose gender identity and expression aligns in a traditional way with the sex they were assigned at birth. For example, a cisgender man is a person who was assigned male sex at birth and continues to identify as a man. Some scholars prefer the term "non-transgender" or "non-trans" because this language is easier to understand and may intentionally normalize the transgender experience. The terms *cissexism* and *transphobia* refer to sociopolitical and personal systems of norms, behaviors, and laws that privilege cisgender people.

Resilience and oppression play a significant role in the lives of transgender people. According to recent studies by the Centers for Disease Control and numerous community samples, transgender people experience numerous adverse health outcomes in comparison to non-transgender people, including elevated HIV/STI risk, incidence, and prevalence (particularly among transgender women of color); and psychiatric disorders, such as depressive disorders, anxiety disorders, and substance use disorders, and increased incidence and prevalence of suicidal ideation and attempts. Transgender people also face numerous barriers to care, including high costs, lack of access, and discrimination in health care settings. There is a vicious cycle of anti-transgender discrimination, lack of access to culturally sensitive health care, and health disparities (Reback, Clark, Holloway, & Fletcher, 2018), exacerbating what scholars see as a crisis in transgender health. Transgender people have a critical need for culturally sensitive, gender-affirming health care.

Transgender people also demonstrate remarkable *resilience*: individual- and group-level factors that buffer against the deleterious effects of stigma and adversity. Particular strategies for resilience may include the cultivation of self-acceptance, gender and racial identity pride, personal mastery, self-esteem, and emotion regulation skills. Transgender people also engage in group-level factors such as social support and collective action for transgender rights, both of which have been shown to improve health outcomes and reduce levels of risk and pathology.

People Born with Intersex Traits

Intersex is an umbrella term used to describe a wide range of natural bodily variations. It is often used when referring to individuals born with some combination of sex characteristics (e.g., chromosomes, genitalia, internal reproductive organs, or hormones) that defy binary notions of female and male sex. Although this definition may make such an occurrence sound rare, somewhere between approximately 0.05 to 1.7 percent of the world population is born with intersex traits. To put that number into context, babies born with red hair make up less than 2 percent of the population, as do babies with green eyes. For some people, their intersex traits are visible to doctors and parents at birth; for others, these traits may not emerge until puberty, adolescence, or even adulthood. Intersex traits tend to carry stigma, and it is critical to be mindful of judgments or knee-jerk reactions to want to "fix" a person's body that may, in fact, simply be different than your own.

According to many vocal intersex communities, doctors and medical professionals have historically subjected intersex babies to unnecessary surgeries and other medical interventions (e.g., repeated genital examinations, genital surgery in the first days of life, forced dilation) in order to address bodily differences. Intersex advocates argue against such surgical and medical interventions, which have been shown in many studies to be associated with emotional and physical trauma, identity diffusion, and elevated rates of suicidal ideation and attempts in this population (for a review, see Davis, 2013). Few data exist supporting the claim that surgery is necessary to correct these differences in sex development.

Many intersex advocates argue the majority of medical interventions may pose significant harm and recommend instead that collaborative care practices be followed, including shared decision-making and psychoeducation. In 2015, an advocacy group named InterACT: Advocates for Intersex Youth released a brochure outlining "What We Wish Our Doctors Knew." Suggestions for intersex-affirming care include: providing emotional support, encouraging peer and community affiliation, communicating honestly, avoiding stigmatizing terms such as "normal" or "transvestite," not taking photos of patient's genitalia, and allowing patients and their families to make informed decisions about which medical interventions (if any) to pursue.

Nonbinary/Gender Expansive and Other Fluid Categories

Gender identities and expressions are rapidly evolving. Given the recent shifts in acceptance for gender variation and creativity in gendered expression, many people identify as *nonbinary*: neither girl/woman nor boy/man or possessing a combination of traits or behaviors that may be a hybrid, combination, or even frank rejection of femininity, masculinity, and androgyny. The term "nonbinary" emerged from transgender communities who were eager to dispel notions that even transgender people must adhere to a strictly binary gender paradigm. Other common terms include genderqueer, gender-diverse, and gender expansive, among others. People with nonbinary gender identities are receiving increased attention and care within psychiatry. In 2015, for example, the American Psychological Association's Division 44 (Society for the Psychology of Sexual and Gender Diversity) released a fact sheet on nonbinary identities (Webb, Matsuno, Budge, Krisnan, & Balsam, 2015), calling for increased scientific and clinical focus for this unique population. Recent studies have demonstrated that nonbinary people, in addition to facing issues common among binary transgender people, also report higher levels of physical violence, sexual abuse, and economic/employment discrimination than both their binary transgender and cisgender counterparts (Harrison et al., 2012; Richards et al., 2016).

There are also many fluid categories of gender that transcend primarily white, Western, binary notions. Many societies explicitly incorporate and celebrate people in more fluid gender categories. For example, many Indigenous American cultures have long revered people who identify as *two-spirit*: embodying both feminine and masculinity spirits within one person (Wilson, 1996). Many South Asian countries similarly celebrate *hijra*: a respected community including eunuchs, intersex people, and transgender people. The Supreme Court in India, for example, formally recognized a "third gender" in 2014. These nuances of gender identity and expression remind us that Western, binary myths of gender are exactly that. We have a responsibility as clinicians – often on the front lines serving race- and gender-diverse communities – to respect patients' identities and provide affirming advocacy and care.

Overview of Sexual Orientation

This section briefly outlines key terms related to sexuality and sexual orientation. Similar to gender, sexuality is a construct that has been recently understood to be fluid, mutable, and socially determined. Conceding that sexuality is a social construction, of course, does not deny that it is core to the human experience and thus has important psychiatric implications. Sexuality involves processes of pleasure, intimacy, reproduction, and health: elemental drives and aspects of the human experience. It is also impacted by legal, cultural, moral, and religious aspects of life. In order to provide sexuality-affirming care, this section briefly explores the key concepts and terms, followed by a discussion of the psychiatric implications of sexual orientation.

Sexual Orientation

Sexual orientation, behavior, and attraction are historically conflated constructs. However, it is important to tease them apart. A common taxonomy organizes sexual orientation into three intersecting components: (1) *sexual orientation identity,* or who I am; (2) *sexual behavior*, or what I do; and (3) *sexual attraction*, whom I desire. These distinctions are important because they do not always line up for many people. When patients explore each process, they may experience curiosity and confusion, dissonance and integration, and a critical process of identity development. Sexual orientation is typically determined by the gender(s) of the person or people someone is attracted to. Data suggest that people's sexual orientations are typically more fluid than we may think; attraction, behavior, and identity exist more on a continuum of identity and desire rather than in discrete and cleanly categorical ways (Vrangalova & Williams, 2012).

Sexual orientation identity – who I am – describes how a person self-identifies their emotional, romantic, and physical attractions and behaviors. Typical examples of terms and communities related to sexual orientation identity include straight/heterosexual, lesbian, gay, bisexual, queer, pansexual, and asexual. The term "sexual orientation" connotes that a person is *oriented* in a particular way, such as a man with a primary desire for men. People typically prefer this term over "sexual preference," which connotes that individuals prefer – or choose – their sexual, emotional, romantic, and physical attractions.

Sexual behavior – what I do – is the manner in which a person engages in sexual activities. People engage in a variety of sexual acts, ranging from acts performed alone (e.g., masturbation) to acts with others (e.g., oral sex, vaginal intercourse, and other behaviors). When working with patients, it is important to explore both the potential risks and benefits of specific sexual behaviors.

Sexual attraction – whom I desire – is a person's emotional, romantic, and physical attractions. Why tease these apart? For many individuals, these three processes may be in tension. Think, for example, about a hypothetical man who is married to a non-transgender woman, has sex with men, and is sexually attracted to transgender women. For this individual, his sexual orientation identity, sexual behavior, and sexual attraction may not fit cohesively within a restrictive social environment. He may experience identity diffusion, shame, and stigma, and he may benefit from nuanced resilience strategies to manage these complex components of self.

Diversity of Sexual Orientations

A person who is *heterosexual* (i.e., straight) feels primary emotional, romantic, and/or physical attractions to people of a different gender. Examples include men primarily attracted to women and women primarily attracted to men. The term *heteronormativity* refers to the social and political system in which heterosexuality is privileged and other identities are marginalized.

A person who is *lesbian*, *gay*, or *homosexual* feels primary emotional, romantic, and/or physical attractions to people of the same gender. *Lesbian* is a sexual orientation referring to women with a primary attraction to other women. *Gay* is a sexual orientation referring to primary attraction to people of the same gender; this term is used to describe people of all genders, whereas *lesbian* is typically reserved for women. The term *homosexual* was historically used as a psychiatric diagnosis, so people who identify as lesbian and gay typically do not use this term to describe themselves.

A person who is *bisexual* experiences primary emotional, romantic, and/or physical attractions to more than one gender. Psychiatric research into clinical issues faced by bisexual individuals reveals themes of exclusion (i.e., feeling excluded both from straight and gay or lesbian communities) as well as bicultural self-efficacy (i.e., being able to participate in gay/queer and straight cultural practices and spaces).

Queer is an umbrella term for gender and sexual minorities. Originally a pejorative term, "queer" has been reclaimed by sexual and gender minority people to describe a sexual orientation, gender identity, or similar identity or expression that does not conform to dominant social norms of gender and sexuality. Many young people have adopted the term queer as an identity term to defy binary notions of gender and sexuality.

Pansexual is a similar term referring to a person with emotional, romantic, and physical attractions to people regardless of (rather than because of) genders. A person who is *asexual* typically denies significant sexual attraction to others or reports minimal desire to engage in sexual activity.

Monogamy is the practice of engaging in an emotional, romantic, or physical relationship with only one partner. *Compulsory monogamy* refers to the cultural expectation that people marry one person and engage in an exclusive relationship with that one person. Conversely, *consensual non-monogamy* (CNM) describes the practice of engaging in emotional, romantic, or physical relationships with multiple partners. It is important to distinguish CNM from *cheating*, the practice of engaging in multiple relationships without the consent of one's spouse or partner. CNM is a separate practice in which one or more partners *consensually* engage in multiple relationships. People of all gender identities and sexual orientations may practice both monogamy and CNM. A recent meta-analysis revealed that people who engage in CNM report similar or higher rates of relational satisfaction and psychological well-being compared to people who engage in monogamy (Brewster et al., 2017). Many people engage in *kink* behaviors, an umbrella term describing a broad range of sexual behavior typically considered to be unconventional. Examples include spanking, dripping candle wax, cross-dressing (wearing clothing typically considered normative for a person of a different gender), and engaging in sexual role play. Again, despite carrying stigma, engaging in kink does not pose significant implications for psychiatric functioning or well-being and is often considered a normative expression of sexual and romantic desire.

Psychiatry of Gender Identity and Sexual Orientation

The second section will discuss psychiatric implications and concerns related to gender identity and sexual orientation. Particular topics include identity development, gender and sexual minority stress, and the history and contemporary guidelines for relevant psychiatric diagnoses.

Gender and Sexual Identity Development

Throughout the evolution of the field of psychiatry, multiple models have dominated thought about *how* and *why* people develop particular gender identities and sexual orientations. Psychiatry has long been curious about what drives and motivations lead to particular sexual attractions, behaviors, and identities. There has long been a discrepancy between those who believed gender and sexuality were produced by "nature," or a child's genetic and biological influences, versus those who argued that gender and sexuality are due to "nurture," or the environment in which a child is raised. For psychiatrists seeking to understand the reasons humans have particular experiences related to gender and sexuality, this has been a vital question. The current state of psychiatric science posits that both play a role, suggesting a dual nature-nurture understanding of how gender identity and sexual orientation develop.

There are several arguments within the field of psychiatry that sexuality and gender are determined by *nature*: one's chromosomes, genes, and natal development. Within these frameworks, sex is fundamentally biological in nature, determined by variations in a single chromosome: the 23rd pair of 23 along the cell nucleus. Human sex chromosomes, a typical pair of mammal allosomes, determine the sex of an individual. Most females have two X chromosomes in their 23rd pair and most males, rather, have an X chromosome and a Y chromosome. Knowledge about sex chromosomes dates back to 1905, when geneticist Nettie Stevens published a study on the chromosomal makeup of sperm and egg cells produced by mealworms.

These findings were applied and extended in research with human biology and psychiatry: the widespread understanding in medicine for decades to come was that sex and gender were determined by biology alone. Indeed, Charles Darwin and other early, eminent scholars, including Francis Galton and Edward L. Thorndike, wrote about gender-as-nature: arguing that women were naturally passive, intellectually inferior, and motivated by evolutionary instinct to nurture.

Discourse on the development of sexual identity emerged around this time as well, beginning largely with works by Sigmund Freud. In *Three Essays on the Theory of Sexuality*, Freud (1905) commented that young infants (0–5 years old) have, in analytic terms, *polymorphous perversity*: driven to seek pleasure from any object, person, or being, regardless of gender. Before children are educated in the social, legal, and political norms of their culture, Freud wrote, they simply turn to various bodily parts for sexual gratification. Throughout childhood development, however, their desires are circumscribed by education, social norms, and their parents or caregiving. This leads to repression: an amnesia or subjugation of primitive, polymorphous sexual desires. Freud wrote that heterosexual adults retain some homosexual desires, which are sublimated due to pressure from society. Although Freud lay a foundation of pathologizing theories about the development and persistence of queerness (i.e., positing it occurs due to arrests in sexual development), he later argued against an analytic "cure" or repudiation of people with same-sex desire. Indeed, the majority of contemporary psychoanalytic organizations (including the prominent American Psychoanalytic Association) have denounced early theories and may advocate for sexual and gender minority communities.

Throughout the mid-1900s, psychiatry and medical interventions were developed to "treat" gender and sexual diversity. These interventions were based on a belief that gender and sexual minority people had stunted or "inverted" identity development. They were often subjected to medically unnecessary and often harmful interventions, including electroconvulsive therapy, psychosurgery (e.g., lobotomy), supposedly reparative psychoanalysis, and chemical castration. It was due to early advocates within the field of psychiatry and sex research that marginalized communities were later de-pathologized and treated with more respect and care by the field. In contemporary practice, so-called "conversion therapy" (the pseudoscientific practice of attempting to change a patient's gender identity and/or sexual orientation) has been debunked and criminalized due to its harmful effects and lack of empirical validity.

More recent psychiatric conceptualizations of gender and sexuality are dominated by a belief that identity development is determined by an interaction of nature and nurture. According to a recent review (Eagly & Wood, 2013), psychiatry has shifted dramatically toward a less pathologizing, more integrated (nature *and* nurture) understanding of the roles of both biological factors and socialization. A prominent recent conceptualization of sexual identity development is the *multiple continua model* posited by Hammack (2005). Proponents of this model argue that sexuality is best understood as "a matrix of mental-emotional-behavioral experiences occurring across a wide range of contexts" (Moe, Reicherzer, & Dupuy, 2011, p. 230). This concept transcends the nature-nurture debate by integrating both sides of the date into its understanding of sexuality.

It has been well-documented in the literature that lesbian, gay, bisexual, transgender and queer (LGBTQ) people have unique developmental milestones in terms of how they may develop awareness, social expression, and integration of their sexual and/or gender minority status. Cass (1979), for example, posited a six-stage gay and lesbian identity development model, beginning at Stage 1 (Identity Confusion) and resolving in Stage 6 (Identity Synthesis). Similar models have been established among bisexual people, transgender people and gender nonbinary people, though models incorporating intersecting identities in their conceptualization (i.e., the influence of racial minority status on sexual orientation identity development) continue to be underresearched.

Gender and Sexual Minority Stress

Minority stress theory is the most prominent theoretical framework for understanding LGBTQ health disparities. This theory argues that high rates of psychiatric distress among LGBTQ communities are best explained by the high rates of prejudice, harassment, and discrimination experienced by LGBTQ people. Minority stress theory posits both direct and indirect links between discrimination (e.g., experiences of homophobia, or anti-gay prejudice and transphobia, or anti-transgender discrimination) and distress (e.g., symptoms of depression, substance use, high rates of psychosocial stressors). Numerous scientific studies have demonstrated that gender and sexual minorities experience a high degree of prejudice, harassment, and discrimination. According to this framework, these experiences have significant consequences for health and quality of life. LGBTQ people thus experience adverse health outcomes as a result of the stress involved in contending with discrimination. Experiences of anti-LGBTQ stigma and related victimization *predict* elevated rates of psychological distress: including symptoms of depression, anxiety, suicidal ideation, and decreased health-related quality of life (Meyer, 1995).

Despite shifts in perception, LGBTQ people often experience discrimination and disproportionate psychological distress. For many years, the field of psychiatry debated the reasons these disparities were so pronounced. Were LGBTQ people engaging in higher-risk health behaviors? Were they not taking care of their health? These myths have been challenged in recent decades with data demonstrating links between high levels of stigma-related discrimination and elevations in stress, which are in turn associated with adverse mental and physical health outcomes. Despite strides in the rights of LGBTQ people, these communities continue to face structural and interpersonal discrimination, manifesting in violence and harassment, economic/employment discrimination, non-affirming health care, police brutality, and microaggressions.

When working with LGBTQ communities, it is thus crucial to acknowledge that experiences of social stressors may lead to the development of psychological distress and adverse health outcomes. LGBTQ people also demonstrate resilience and group-specific coping strategies, including the development of stress-related growth, self-efficacy, and social support. With all patients, it is important to consider the impact of gender identity and sexual orientation in the context of their other identities. The *intersectionality model* suggests that identifying with multiple marginalized and privileged groups (e.g., race, social class, disability status, gender identity, sexual orientation, citizenship) leads individuals to have novel, complex experiences of both marginalization and resilience.

History of Gender- and Sexuality-Related Psychiatric Diagnoses

The DSM-V categorizes gender- and sexuality-related distress in three ways, as outlined in the following section. In order to diagnose and treat these disorders, and to provide affirming care with regard to issues of gender and sexuality, it is important to understand how psychiatry has addressed these issues historically. The field of psychiatry has a painful history of pathologizing gender and sexual diversity. It was not until 1973 that the American Psychiatric Association removed the diagnosis of "homosexuality" from its *Diagnostic and Statistical Manual*, after years of protest and resistance within the fields of psychiatry and psychology.

For centuries, sexual difference was criminalized in Western societies. The mid- to late-1800s saw a profound medical revolution, defined by a push for nationalized efforts to prevent disease and regulate public health. Health provision became regulated for the first time, and this reinforced a profound shift in societal perspectives on morality, wellness, and acceptable behavior. The late 1800s saw the first formal psychiatric response to gender and sexual diversity. Prominent scholars began to write about gender and sexual "deviance" as a threat to public health, a sign of pathology and disease. A prime example is Austro-German psychiatrist Dr. Richer Freiherr von Krafft-Ebing, who published *Psychopathia Sexualis* (translated to *Psychopathy of Sex*) in 1886. Krafft-Ebing wrote extensively about homosexuality, a behavior he ascribed to a mental disease caused by degenerate heredity.

In the 1970s, psychiatry underwent a tremendous cultural change in its conceptualizations of human sexuality. Scholars within the field, alongside community activists, had begun to formally challenge stigma within the field. Scholars such as Alfred Kinsey, Clellan Ford, Frank Beach, and others began to publish studies suggesting divergence from mainstream heterosexual behavior was more prevalent – and less disordered – than the field had assumed. In 1957, for example, psychologist Evelyn Hooker published *The Adjustment of the Male Overt Homosexual*. In this paper, Hooker conducted a study comparing the psychiatric health of thirty heterosexual and thirty homosexual men, finding no significant difference between the groups. Discussing the study's results, for example, Hooker wrote: "Homosexuality may be a deviation in sexual pattern which is within the normal range, psychologically." She presented these results in 1956 at the annual meeting of the American Psychological Association, contributing to a remarkable change in the field's understanding of and attitudes toward gay men.

Homosexuality, however, was still codified as a disease in the 1968 edition of the DSM. Throughout these years, community responses among gay men and lesbian women persisted, and activist groups often protested at psychiatric meetings and conventions. In the 1970s, community activists protested at conferences, demanding homosexuality and gender diversity be removed from the compendium of mental illnesses. In 1973, the American Psychiatric Association's Board of Directors voted to remove it from the *DSM-III*.

It is important to understand existent diagnostic categories while remaining critical of the impact of pathologizing gender identity and sexual orientation. The medicalization of gender and sexual diversity continues to have deleterious effects. During much of the twentieth century, psychiatry continued to define lesbian, gay, and bisexual desire, as well as gender diversity as psychiatric pathology. It is important to remember that this stigma and pathology does not only affect LGBTQ people. Any heterosexual/straight-identified people whose behaviors or desires may diverge from mainstream conceptualizations of "healthy" sexuality also face stigma and pathology.

Similar advocacy within the field has mitigated some of the psychiatric stigmas for transgender people. Throughout the field's history, various iterations of the *DSM* conceptualized gender "deviance" in changing ways. The *DSM-I* (1952) did not have any gender-specific diagnoses. The *DSM-II* (1968) diagnosed *transsexualism* under the parent category of sexual deviations. In the *DSM-III* (1980), *transsexualism* was retained but moved to the parent category of psychosexual disorders, then moved to the parent category of disorders usually first evident in infancy, childhood, or adolescence in the *DSM-III-R* (1987). The *DSM-IV* (1994) and *DSM-IV-TR* defined a diagnosis of gender identity disorder in the parent category of sexual and gender identity disorders. Most recently in the *DSM-V* (2013), the American Psychological Association renamed the diagnosis as *gender dysphoria* within its standalone parent category. This continues to be a controversial diagnosis for patients, providers, and community organizers. Indeed, carrying such a diagnosis may imply gender-diverse people are mentally ill simply due to their identities.

DSM-V Psychiatric Diagnoses Related to Gender Identity and Sexual Orientation

It is important to keep this history in mind when learning about the diagnostic categories that persist in the current, fifth edition of the DSM. Each of the following diagnoses is marked by the presentation of gender or sexual "difference" for a socially determined norm, as well as psychiatric symptoms (e.g., clinically significant distress or impairment in social, occupational, or other important areas of functioning) that subsequently affect one's life. There are three categories of gender- and sexuality-related diagnoses.

Gender Dysphoria

The first is *gender dysphoria*, defined by distress experienced by an individual whose gender identity does not match the sex they were assigned at birth. Gender dysphoria can be understood as a psychiatric conflict between one's physical/

legal/social sex and one's gender identity. Some people who meet the criteria for this diagnosis report significant distress and problems functioning due to this psychiatric conflict. Some people may socially transition, using a self-determined name, pronoun, and/or clothing to present to others in a specifically gendered way. Gender Dysphoria is not the same as *gender nonconformity*, which refers to engaging in behaviors that do not match socially sanctioned expressions and roles for girls/women and boys/men. Instead, gender dysphoria refers to distress or impacted functioning due to a discrepancy between one's gender identity and assigned sex at birth.

Diagnoses related to gender include (1) gender dysphoria in children, (2) gender dysphoria in adolescents and adults, (3) other specified gender dysphoria, and (4) unspecified gender dysphoria. Adolescents and adults may be diagnosed with gender dysphoria in the case that they report significant distress and impaired functioning due to a persistence of at least two of the following criteria (paraphrased for simplicity) for at least six months: (1) marked incongruence between one's experienced/expressed gender and primary and/or secondary sex characteristics; (2) strong desire to be rid of one's primary and/or secondary sex characteristics; (3) strong desire for the primary and/or secondary sex characteristics of the other gender; (4) strong desire to be of the other gender; (5) Strong desire to be treated as the other gender; and (6) strong conviction that one has the typical feelings and reactions of the other gender.

Children may be diagnosed with gender dysphoria in the case that they report significant distress and impaired functioning due to a persistence of at least six of the following criteria (paraphrased for simplicity) for at least six months: (1) strong desire to be of the other gender or an insistence that one is the other gender; (2) strong preference for wearing clothes typical of the opposite gender; (3) strong preference for cross-gender roles in make-believe play or fantasy play; (4) strong preference for the toys, games or activities stereotypically used or engaged in by the other gender; (5) strong preference for playmates of the other gender; (6) strong rejection of toys, games, and activities typical of one's assigned gender; (7) strong dislike of one's sexual anatomy; and (8) strong desire for the physical sex characteristics that match one's experienced gender.

For details, please consult the *DSM-V* as well as relevant discussions in the literature by transgender and nonbinary scholars concerning nuances of each diagnostic category and the utility of diagnostic categories more generally for gender-diverse communities.

Sexual Dysfunctions

The second category of gender/sexuality-related diagnoses in the *DSM-V* is *sexual dysfunctions*, defined by distress with sexual experiences and behaviors understood to be insufficiently intense in duration, magnitude, and/or frequency. Diagnoses include (1) delayed ejaculation; (2) erectile disorder; (3) female orgasmic disorder; (4) female sexual interest/arousal disorder; (5) genito-pelvic pain/penetration disorder; (6) male hypoactive sexual desire disorder; (7) premature (early) ejaculation; (8) substance/medication-induced sexual dysfunction; (9) other specified sexual dysfunction; and (10) unspecified sexual dysfunction.

Sexual dysfunctions are typically managed and/or treated by addressing underlying physiological and/or psychological processes affecting desire, performance, and/or role functions within relationships. Before medications and/or psychotherapy are utilized, it is typically recommended that patients assess for medical and physiological concerns. In the absence of such etiology, treatment may include mechanical aids, sex therapy, behavioral treatments, talk psychotherapy, and education and communication with partners. One common therapeutic practice within relationship therapy is *sensate focus*, developed by foundational sex researchers Masters and Johnson in the 1960s. Sensate focus therapy involves a series of behavioral exercises members of relationships can engage in to reduce relational pressure, enhance intimacy, and promote connection and communication.

Paraphilic Disorders

The third category of gender/sexuality-related diagnoses in the *DSM-V* is *paraphilic disorders*, defined by distress experiences related to sexual desire or behaviors understood to be illegitimate due to an unconventional sexual object choice. Diagnoses include (1) voyeuristic disorder; (2) exhibitionist disorder; (3) frotteuristic disorder; (4) sexual masochism disorder; (5) sexual sadism disorder; (6) pedophilic disorder; (7) fetishistic disorder; (8) transvestic disorder; (9) other unspecified paraphilic disorder; and (10) unspecified paraphilic disorder. Again, please consult the *DSM-V* for specific criteria and treatment recommendations, which typically include psychotropic medication (with significantly low effect sizes), individual and group psychotherapy, behavioral modification, and aversive classical conditioning (pairing a source of pleasure with aversive punishment). Etiology and treatment modalities for paraphilic disorders continue to be informed by stigma and criminal/forensic concerns and are disproportionately underdeveloped.

Psychiatric Evaluation and Treatment of Gender- and Sexuality-Related Issues

The evaluation of mental health concerns related to gender and sexuality has historically received relatively minimal attention. Traditionally, gender difference and sexual orientation diversity have been assessed through the use of psychological assessments measuring personality traits and capturing variations in femininity and masculinity. Perhaps the most frequently employed test is the Minnesota Multiphasic Personality Inventory (MMPI), a psychological assessment tool developed in the 1930s to capture variations in personality and mental health versus illness. Composed of 10 scales, the MMPI's scale 5 captures *masculinity-femininity*, assigning a score to the degree to which a subject identifies with social norms related to their gender. This scale was originally constructed to screen for homosexuality, demonstrating a historic conflation of gender diversity and sexual diversity within psychiatry. The field has come a tremendous way since then in its ability to evaluate and address diverse issues related to gender and sexuality.

In the last two decades, increased attention to sexual and gender minorities within psychiatry has led to more nuanced processes and mechanisms for evaluating gender- and sexuality-related concerns, stigma, and diagnostic questions. This has become increasingly crucial given the field's contemporary acceptance of *minority stress theory*, including awareness of the impact of heterosexism and transphobia on gender and sexual minorities. As such, current guidelines suggest any evaluation of issues related to gender and sexuality include questions about stigma, pleasure, community affiliation, and identity development and integration.

One example of such guidelines is *The Handbook of Gender and Sexuality in Psychological Assessment* (Brabender & Mihura, 2016), which makes the following practical suggestions when conducting affirming, comprehensive assessments related to these issues. Assessors are encouraged to (1) be attuned to the multifaceted aspects of patient's gender and sexual orientation identities and lives; (2) be aware of how gender- and sexuality-related biases may impact a provider's evaluation of the patient; (3) consider how stigma may influence a patient's responses during the evaluation process; (4) understand interactions between personality, intellectual strength, environmental stressors, and environmental support on the patient's identity development and expression; and (5) identify strategies to mitigate stressors impacting the patient's functioning with regard to gender and sexuality. These guidelines are relevant across all sexual orientations and gender identities. The following section will describe LGBTQ-specific guidelines for evaluation and care.

Psychiatric Evaluation with LGBTQ Patients

Recent calls for increased quality of evaluation and care among LGBTQ communities have led to robust guidelines for collecting patient data on gender identity and sexual orientation. In 2018, for example, the National LGBT Health Education Center at the Fenway Institute released guidelines and tips for providers to conduct comprehensive, affirming evaluations. These guidelines begin with the registration/intake form; medical sites are encouraged to integrate such questions in the demographics and social history sections of new/returning patient forms. Language is crucial with marginalized populations, and as such should model openness, flexibility, and an ever-changing, culturally syntonic lexicon utilized by LGBT communities. Recommended questions include: (1) What sexual orientation do you think of yourself as?; (2) What is your current gender identity?; and (3) What sex were you assigned at birth?

The rationale for asking both gender identity and sex assigned at birth is to capture the diverse medical and social needs of transgender people. These guidelines also recommend facilitating patient-centered communication with LGBTQ patients by asking for a patient's name in two ways *and* recording the patient's pronouns. For example, forms and providers may ask: (1) What name would you like us to use?; (2) What name is on your insurance records (if applicable)?; and (3) What are your pronouns? (e.g., he/him, she/her, they/them). After capturing these data, medical providers are encouraged to use a patient's chosen name and pronouns indicated on the initial evaluation materials. These guidelines also explicate strategies to effectively discuss gender identity and sexual orientation during the clinical encounter. Strategies include normalizing the conversation, avoiding assumptions, creating a welcoming and inclusive medical site, and building knowledge and resource lists related to LGBTQ issues and cultural humility.

Data on sexual orientation and gender identity (often referred to as "SOGI data") have only recently been collected with the rigor, cultural competence, and breadth necessary to properly measure the diversity and scope of such identities as they occur in patient populations (Cahill et al., 2014). To address the historically scant nature of SOGI data, prominent medical research institutions (e.g., The Institute of Medicine and the National Institutes of Health) have called for improved data collection procedures in clinical settings, academic research, and electronic health records. This push for increased collection of SOGI data is seen as a step to validate and support sexual and gender minority communities who have historically been excluded from national surveys and misrepresented in the electronic health record and insurance claims reports. For detailed steps to increase competency, please review guidelines put forth by the National LGBT Health Education Center at the Fenway Institute as well as the Center for Transgender Excellence at the University of California, San Francisco.

Psychological Evaluation with Transgender and Nonbinary Patients

There are particular, nuanced strategies to evaluate the psychiatric functioning and wellness of transgender and nonbinary patients, which are outlined in the *Standards of Care* published by the World Professional Association for Transgender Health (WPATH). Psychiatrists and other mental health professionals are often tasked with evaluating patients' gender dysphoria in the context of a psychosocial assessment. According to standards of care, this evaluation must include an assessment of gender identity and dysphoria, history and development of gender dysphoric feelings, impact of stigma, and availability of social and community support. Such an evaluation may or may not result in a gender dysphoria diagnosis per the *DSM-V* and may also reveal other psychiatric issues present in the patient's life. An important aspect of this evaluation is determining whether gender dysphoria is secondary to another psychiatric diagnosis. In the case that a patient presents with coexisting mental health concerns, it is critical that these concerns are treated with psychotherapy and psychotropic medications, as necessary, in order to increase the likelihood of a successful gender affirmation and/or quality of care.

The WPATH also outlines guidelines for providing information related to options for gender identity, gender expression, and gender-affirming interventions. The most important task is often to educate patients about the myriad pathways to alleviate dysphoria, which may include social affirmation, family systems interventions, increasing community support, psychotherapy, and medical interventions such as hormone therapy and surgical procedures. Although not all transgender patients desire medical intervention, some may, and psychiatrists are frequently tasked with assessing eligibility, preparing patients, and referring often complex cases for care. When referring a patient for a surgical procedure (e.g., breast/chest reductions or implants, genital surgeries), WPATH recommends including the following material in a letter: (1) patient's identifying characteristics; (2) results of patient's psychosocial assessment, including gender-related and coexisting diagnoses; (3) duration and quality of provider's contact with the patient; (4) explanation that criteria for hormone therapy are met, as well as clinical rationale; (5) statement of informed consent from patient; and (6) statement that referring psychiatrist is available for coordination of care.

Assessments should be conducted collaboratively with patients by using their chosen name and pronouns, communicating clearly about the limitations of the dysphoria framework for transgender communities, and collective data about psychosocial support and resilience. For patients seeking nonsurgical interventions (e.g., gender-affirming hormone therapy or social transition), a psychiatric assessment/letter is not required. Collaboration across disciplines is crucial when supported transgender patients. Often, a primary care provider may conduct an evaluation of the capacity to provide informed consent and mental health clinicians may not need to be involved especially when there are no significant concerns about psychiatric distress. Best practices recommend a primary care provider who is unsure of a patient's medical decision-making capacity to provide informed consent may collaborate with a mental health clinician to help with the capacity evaluation. For surgical intervention, however, a mental health clinician may need to provide a letter of referral to surgery. Patients undergoing medical interventions of any kind benefit from psychological preparation and practical readiness; this may be increasingly crucial for patients pursuing gender-related treatments that are complicated by stigma and gender minority stress.

Gender- and Sexuality-Affirming Psychiatric Treatment

Given these issues, how can we provide support for patients seeking treatment for psychiatric issues informed by gender and sexuality? We have discussed at length that LGBTQ people, in addition to contending with general psychological stressors, also must contend with systemic and interpersonal barriers to adequate, culturally affirming health care. Yet all people must contend with gender- and sexuality-related processes of exploration, development, and integration.

Current guidelines for gender- and sexuality-affirming psychiatric care tend to focus on providing culturally-sensitive, evidence-informed care for LGBTQ patients. Indeed, the need for such protocols has become increasingly salient, given the documented impact of discrimination on LGBTQ patient populations. Consequences include avoiding health care, poor retention in outpatient services, and decreased quality of care. Guidelines for addressing these issues (Tschurtz & Burke, 2014) include (1) collecting feedback from LGBTQ patients and community members; (2) ensuring communication with patients reflects a commitment to LGBT health; and (3) educating patients and staff about LGBTQ health issues. Providers are increasingly called upon to take an active role in shifting the culture of medicine and psychiatry toward being LGBTQ-affirming. Strategies to do so may include changing physical characteristics of a psychiatric clinic, such as increasing access to all-gender bathrooms and including images of people of diverse gender identities and sexual orientations on flyers and patient materials. For further information, please consult the *Guidelines for Psychological Practice with Lesbian, Gay, and Bisexual Clients* published by the American Psychological Association in 2012.

There are also numerous guidelines for micro-level interactions with patients when addressing issues related to gender and sexuality. Indeed, the goal of psychotherapy is to increase patients' overall psychological wellness, quality of life, and self-fulfillment (WPATH, 2012). For transgender, intersex, gender nonbinary, and gender-diverse people, this may include helping patients achieve long-term comfort in gender expression through social, psychiatric, and medical support. For patients in the midst of exploring gender identity or sexual orientation, clinicians can normalize the complexities of these experiences and encourage both introspection and social support.

A wide range of therapeutic modalities, including cognitive-behavioral, psychodynamic, and acceptance-commitment psychotherapies, have been adapted to buffer against minority stress and promote resilience among diverse sexual and gender communities. This includes empirically-informed individual and group techniques to reduce stigma and promote psychosocial functioning as well as promote community support and intrapsychic resources. When working with LGBTQ people of color, women, people with disabilities, and intersecting communities contending with multiple forms of marginalization, it is recommended that providers incorporate community strengths as well as ethics of transparency and humility into the therapeutic relationship. For further information, please consult the recommended readings at the end of the chapter.

Summary

Human sexuality and gender are complex phenomena informed by culture, biology, and psychiatric processes. In this chapter, key terms, constructs, and theories relevant to psychiatric assessment and treatment have been discussed. This has included an overview of gender identity and sexual orientation; psychiatric implications of gender identity and sexual orientation; evaluation and treatment; and specific guidelines for working with sexual and gender minority communities. When working with all patients, it is important to explore nuances in terminology and identity related to these concepts and to engage in self-reflection about your professional and personal biases, limitations, and assumptions. As the field's understanding of sexuality and gender continually evolves, you are in a powerful position as an emerging provider to advocate for and support marginalized and diverse communities.

Case of Transgender Identity Development

Identifying Information and Chief Complaint

Caleb is a twenty-five-year old, black, queer-identified transgender man living in a major city with no children and little family and social support. He presents to your adult outpatient psychiatry department seeking help for "feeling depressed and lonely but not knowing whom to turn to." Caleb is working-class and employed as a custodian for an office building. He denies remarkable medical history or past psychiatric hospitalizations. Caleb has been in outpatient psychotherapy twice before (last treatment was five years prior) and reports a diagnostic history of persistent depressive disorder as well as symptoms of anxiety in particular related to being harassed or "outed" as a transgender man. He denies a history of hypomanic/manic symptoms and reports his mood is significantly more depressed during times when he experiences rejection related to his transgender identity. He denies psychotic symptoms, though reports "Worrying I am crazy because I'm so anxious about people looking at me and knowing I'm transgender." Caleb uses marijuana one to two days per week to manage his mood.

In terms of his gender identity development, Caleb has identified as male since middle school and has recently begun to socially transition. For example, he has started to wear men's clothing, use masculine pronouns (i.e., "he," "him," "his"), and use the name Caleb rather than his name assigned at birth. Caleb has also begun to disclose his gender identity to select friends, though has isolated since beginning his social transition. He is concerned his family will reject him and thus has not been in contact with his parents or siblings. In terms of his sexual orientation identity, Alex identifies as "queer" and finds himself attracted to men, women, and gender nonbinary people.

In terms of transition-related concerns, Caleb reports desire to pursue masculinizing hormone therapy (i.e., use testosterone by patch) in order for his voice, distribution of hair, distribution of body fat, and overall muscle mass to feel more congruent with his internal gender identity. He does not desire surgical intervention. Caleb is excited to begin a more formal transition, though anxious about the potential reactions from coworkers and friends.

Case Conceptualization and Recommendations for Treatment

One way to conceptualize this case is to use the *biopsychosocial approach*: to consider Caleb's symptoms through the lens of his biological, psychological, and socio-environmental stressors and strengths. This interdisciplinary approach will help you consider the interconnectedness of Caleb's inner world and external world to develop a conceptualization and treatment plan. In doing so, we will also consider the role of gender minority stress and transgender community connectedness as key components of psychiatric distress and well-being.

Step 1: Identify biological stressors and strengths. The *biological* component of the biopsychosocial model entails identifying sources of stress and strength related to the patient's medical and/or genetic issues, age, developmental milestones, and physiological characteristics. Caleb's biological presentation is relatively unremarkable, as he denies a significant medical history. However, due to lack of access to affordable, transgender-affirming healthcare, it is important to consider referring Caleb to low-fee, transgender-affirming comprehensive health services for further screening and treatment as indicated. Caleb reports using marijuana multiple times per week, which serves a role of managing depression, though may also impair functioning and emotional processing and connectedness. His substance use is consistent with research identifying disproportionate rates of alcohol, marijuana, and cocaine use among community samples of transgender adults. As such, it is important to further assess the impact of marijuana use on Caleb's medical and psychiatric functioning and engage him in psychoeducation and harm reduction interventions. In terms of developmental milestones, Caleb denies remarkable concerns during early childhood with the exception of early rejection due to his more masculine gender presentation. It is important also to inquire about family psychiatric history.

Step 2: Identify psychological stressors and strengths. The *psychological* component of the biopsychosocial model entails identifying sources of stress and strengths related to the patient's mental status, thoughts, behaviors, feelings, history of trauma, and resilience. Caleb is reporting longstanding symptoms of depression as well as acute anxiety. Upon further interviewing, Caleb reports his symptoms of depression include loss of interest in daily activities, feeling empty and sad, feeling hopeless, experiencing irritability and excessive anger, weight loss and poor appetite, and trouble sleeping. His symptoms of anxiety are related to being in public and include excessive worrying about what other people think about him as well as agitation, muscle tension, and difficulty concentrating while in public spaces. In terms of a working hypothesis, we can determine that Caleb likely meets criteria for (1) persistent depressive disorder (dysthymia) and (2) social anxiety disorder. He also likely meets criteria for (3) gender dysphoria, given symptoms of distress due to wanting to be recognized socially in a way consistent with his gender identity.

Step 3: Identify socio-environmental stressors and strengths. The *socio-environmental* component of the biopsychosocial formulation entails identifying sources of stress and strengths related to the patient's social, cultural, and systemic factors. Caleb faces multiple minority stressors. For example, he may experience discrimination related to being working-class, black, and identifying as a transgender man as well as the intersection of these three marginalized social locations. Caleb's depression and anxiety can thus be conceptualized in terms of minority stress. Transgender people, especially transgender people of color, frequently face multiple manifestations of discrimination and social exclusion. These experiences often lead to compromised psychological functioning and well-being. One particular of how this affects Caleb is his anxiety about being "found out" as a black transgender man. This may be a manifestation of *hypervigilance*: an enhanced state of sensitivity and anxiety about what other people think, often leading to exhaustion and burnout and very common among transgender people. Another key component of minority stress is the critical need to connect with other transgender people and build social support. Thus treatment may include referring Caleb to a transgender community support group and mitigating the impact of isolation. This connectedness may encourage behavioral activation, reduction in internalized transphobia (i.e., negative feelings about himself as a transgender person), and an increase in self-efficacy, self-worth, and resilience.

References and Selected Readings

- Brabender, V., and Mihura, J. L. (2016). *Handbook of Gender and Sexuality in Psychological Assessment*. New York: Routledge.

- Brewster, M. E., Soderstrom, B., Esposito, J., Breslow, A., Sawyer, J., Geiger, E., ... Cheng, J. (2017). A Content Analysis of Scholarship on Consensual Nonmonogamies: Methodological Roadmaps, Current Themes, and Directions for Future Research. *Couple and Family Psychology: Research and Practice*, 6 (1), 32–47.
- Butler, J. (2006). *Gender Trouble: Feminism and the Subversion of Identity*, 1st ed. New York: Routledge.
- Cahill, S., and Makadon, H. (2014). Sexual Orientation and Gender Identity Data Collection in Clinical Settings and in Electronic Health Records: A Key to Ending LGBT Health Disparities. *LGBT Health*, 1 (1), 34–41.
- Cass, V. C. (1984). Homosexual Identity Formation: Testing a Theoretical Model. *Journal of Sex Research*, 20 (2), 143–167.
- Davis, G. (2014). The Power in a Name: Diagnostic Terminology and Diverse Experiences. *Psychology and Sexuality*, 5 (1), 15–27.
- Eagly, A. H., and Wood, W. (2013). The Nature–Nurture Debates: 25 Years of Challenges in Understanding the Psychology of Gender. *Perspectives on Psychological Science*, 8 (3), 340–357.
- Erickson-Schroth, L. (2014). *Trans Bodies, Trans Selves: A Resource for the Transgender Community*. New York: Oxford University Press.
- Freud, S. (1953). Three Essays on the Theory of Sexuality (1905). In *The Standard Edition of the Complete Psychological Works of Sigmund Freud, Volume VII (1901–1905): A Case of Hysteria, Three Essays on Sexuality and Other Works*. (pp. 123–246). London: Hogarth Press.
- Goldberg, A. E. (2016). *The SAGE Encyclopedia of LGBTQ Studies*. Thousand Oaks, CA: SAGE.
- Harrison, J., Grant, J., and Herman, J. L. (2012). A gender not listed here: Genderqueers, gender rebels, and otherwise in the National Transgender Discrimination Survey. *LGBTQ Public Policy Journal at the Harvard Kennedy School*, 2 (1), 13–24.
- Krafft-Ebing, R. (1998). *Psychopathia Sexualis: With Especial Reference to the Antipathic Sexual Instinct: A Medico-Forensic Study*. New York: Arcade.
- Matsuno, E. (2019). Nonbinary-affirming psychological interventions. *Cognitive and Behavioral Practice*, 26 (4), 617–628.
- Meyer, I. H. (1995). Minority Stress and Mental Health in Gay Men. *Journal of Health and Social Behavior*, 36 (1), 38–56.
- Moe, J. L., Reicherzer, S., and Dupuy, P. J. (2011). Models of Sexual and Relational Orientation: A Critical Review and Synthesis. *Journal of Counseling and Development*, 89 (2), 227–233.
- Nadal, K. L. (2017). *The SAGE Encyclopedia of Psychology and Gender*. Thousand Oaks, CA: SAGE.
- Patterson, C. J., and D'Augelli, A. R. (2013). *Handbook of Psychology and Sexual Orientation*. Oxford: Oxford University Press.
- Reback, C. J., Clark, K., Holloway, I. W., and Fletcher, J. B. (2018). Health Disparities, Risk Behaviors and Healthcare Utilization among Transgender Women in Los Angeles County: A Comparison from 1998–1999 to 2015–2016. *AIDS and Behavior*, 22 (8), 2524–2533.

- Richards, C., Bouman, W. P., Seal, L., Barker, M. J., Nieder, T. O., and T'Sjoen, G. (2016). Non-binary or Genderqueer Genders. *International Review of Psychiatry*, 28 (1), 95–102.
- Singh, A. A. (2018). *The Queer and Transgender Resilience Workbook: Skills for Navigating Sexual Orientation and Gender Expression*. Oakland: New Harbinger.
- Tschurtz, B., and Burke, A. (2011). *Advancing Effective Communication, Cultural Competence, and Patient- and Family-Centered Care for the Lesbian, Gay, Bisexual, and Transgender (LGBT) Community: A Field Guide*. Retrieved from www.jointcommission.org/assets/1/18/LGBTFieldGuide_WEB_LINKED_VER.pdf.
- Vrangalova, Z., and Savin-Williams, R. C. (2012). Mostly Heterosexual and Mostly Gay/Lesbian: Evidence for New Sexual Orientation Identities. *Archives of Sexual Behavior*, 41 (1), 85–101.

Recommended Online Resources

Center of Excellence for Transgender Health, Department of Medicine, University of California, San Francisco. URL: https://prevention.ucsf.edu/transhealth

National LGBT Health Education Center, Fenway Institute, Fenway Health. URL: https://fenwayhealth.org/the-fenway-institute/education/the-national-lgbt-health-education-center/

Providing Ethical and Compassionate Health Care to Intersex Patients: Intersex-Affirming Hospital Policies. Published by interACT Advocates for Intersex Youth and Lambda Legal. URL: https://interactadvocates.org/wp-content/uploads/2018/09/interACT-Lambda-Legal-intersex-hospital-policies.pdf

Standards of Care for the Health of Transsexual, Transgender, and Gender Nonconforming People. Published by the WPATH World Professional Association for Transgender Health. URL: www.wpath.org/

Self-Assessment Questions

1. According to minority stress theory, high rates of psychiatric distress experienced by lesbian, gay, bisexual, transgender, and queer people are best explained by high rates of which of the following?
    A. Arrested sexual development in early childhood
    B. Medical and physiological disorders
    C. Paraphilic disorders
    D. Prejudice, harassment, and discrimination
2. The way a person self-identifies in terms of emotional, romantic, and physical attractions and behaviors is best defined by which of the following terms?

    A. Sexual orientation identity

    B. Gender roles

    C. Gender non-conformity

    D. Consensual non-monogamy

3. In 1973, for the first time since its first edition, the American Psychiatric Association did not include the diagnosis of "homosexuality" in its compendium of mental illness, the *Diagnostic and Statistical Manual of Mental Disorders* (*DSM*). Which edition of the *DSM* was this?

    A. DSM-II

    B. DSM-III

    C. DSM-IV

    D. DSM-V

4. The *DSM-V* distinguishes between sexual dysfunctions and paraphilic disorders. Which of the following is an example of a sexual dysfunction?

    A. Voyeuristic disorder

    B. Male hypoactive sexual desire disorder

    C. Exhibitionist disorder

    D. Sexual masochism disorder

5. Which of the following is an umbrella term for people whose gender identities or expressions do not align in a traditional way with the sex they were assigned at birth?

    A. Cisgender

    B. Transgender

    C. Gender binary

    D. Polymorphous perversity

Answers to Self-Assessment Questions

1. (D)
2. (A)
3. (B)
4. (B)
5. (B)

19

Health Policy and Population Health in Behavioral Health Care in the United States

KIRSTIN BEACH AND BRUCE SCHWARTZ

Introduction

The treatment of behavioral health disorders is impacted by the many complexities and challenges inherent in the United States health care system. Patients and their families struggle with limited access, availability and affordability of treatment, inadequate insurance coverage, and a fragmented system of care. To better understand these issues, this chapter provides an overview of the US health care system, with a focus on coverage and financing of behavioral health care; describes current challenges within the system; and highlights emerging solutions to improve behavioral health delivery and outcomes.

Health Care in the United States

The US Health Care System in the International Context

The US health care system has a mixed model of insurance coverage and of service delivery, with public and private sources of insurance and public and private health care providers. Unlike many countries in the Organization for Economic Cooperation and Development (OECD), the US does not have universal health care coverage.

While it lacks universal health insurance coverage, the United States spends far more on health care than any other nation. In 2017, total health spending per capita in the United States was $10,209, in comparison to $4,826 in Canada and $8,009 in Switzerland. When including social services and health care spending, the United States is much closer to the OECD average, highlighting the relative underpayment in the social services sector in the United States; 28.8 percent of US GDP is spent on social services and health care, compared to the OECD average of 21.4 percent of GDP (OECD, 2017). While the root cause of high health care spending is the subject of debate, it is clear that the United States is deriving less value for these expenditures than other OECD countries. Utilization of medical and hospital services is not the main driver of high health care spending, as patients in the United States do not use these services at a notably higher rate than patients in other nations. For example, Americans have an average of four physician visits annually compared to the OECD median of 6.5 visits (Squires, 2015). Lack of price control is likely a key driver of US spending compared to other nations (Anderson et al., 2003).

Sources of Coverage in the United States

The US health care insurance system is a patchwork of group health plans that are most often offered through employment arrangements, government-sponsored health insurance for defined populations, and non-group markets from which individuals to purchase coverage. In total, these insurance sources cover 91 percent of Americans, leaving more than 27 million individuals uninsured (OECD, 2017). Further, there is significant variability in benefits across insurance products, making it difficult for patients and providers to understand and obtain needed medical services, especially for behavioral health care. The largest sources of coverage are employer-sponsored health insurance (ESI), Medicare, and Medicaid.

Employer–Sponsored Health Insurance

In the United States, unlike many high-income countries, employment plays a major role in health care insurance coverage. More than 150 million Americans are covered by ESI, making it the largest source of coverage in the United States (Collins, Gunja, & Doty, 2017). This form of insurance was enabled by the Employee Retirement Income Security Act (ERISA) of 1974, which established minimum standards for retirement, health, and other welfare benefit plans. Employer-sponsored insurance receives preferred tax treatment, which encourages private businesses to provide it to employees. Employer and employee contributions for employer-sponsored insurance are excluded from income and payroll taxes, costing an estimated loss of approximately $250 billion in federal tax revenue annually (Congress of the United States Congressional Budget Office, 2013).

The cost of ESI has steadily grown faster than wages, concerning employers and employees alike. The growing ESI costs have led many employers to increase the amount employees must contribute for coverage through larger contributions to the premium and insurance plan designs that result in larger out-of-pocket costs and high deductibles for employees. For example, those enrolled in high-deductible plans must pay a substantial amount on their health care bills before insurance coverage is triggered. The share of people covered by ESI with deductibles of more than 5 percent of household income grew from 2 to 13 percent between 2003 and 2016 (Collins, Gunja, & and Doty, 2017). As a result, many individuals cannot afford to use their health insurance coverage – a phenomenon referred to as *underinsurance* – and forgo and delay necessary treatment.

It is also worth noting the variability in the regulation of ESI, depending on the size of the employer and the way the plan is administered. Some ESI plans are subject to state regulation and mandates, while others are subject to lesser federal oversight. This leads to significant variability in what ESI plans are required to cover.

Medicare

Medicare is a federal health insurance program for individuals aged sixty-five and older, as well as individuals under sixty-five with end-stage renal disease (ESRD), and with some disabilities. Medicare covers sixty million people. Traditional, or fee-for-service, Medicare is administered directly by the federal government and offers hospital insurance (Part A); physician services, outpatient services, and other medical services (Part B); and outpatient prescription drug coverage (Part D). Under Medicare Part C, also known as Medicare Advantage, private insurance companies administer the Medicare benefit through managed care programs. There are many notable gaps in Medicare, including long-term care, vision, hearing, and dental coverage, leading many beneficiaries to elect for supplemental insurance coverage (Cubanski et al., 2015).

Medicare is financed through federal taxes and beneficiary premium contributions. In 2016 Medicare accounted for 15 percent of total federal spending, and 20 percent of total public and private health spending in 2015 (US Centers for Medicare & Medicaid Services, 2018). Given the rising costs of health care and expected increases in enrollment due to the aging population, there is increasing concern about the future costs of Medicare.

Medicaid

Medicaid, which currently covers more than 67 million people, provides health insurance for people with low-income. Each state administers its own Medicaid program, which is jointly financed and overseen by the federal government. (US Centers for Medicare & Medicaid Services, 2018). To qualify for Medicaid, individuals must fall below income thresholds and meet categorical eligibility, such as being a child, a parent of an eligible child, or an aged adult. Although states must adhere to some federally mandated categories for eligibility, there is much discretion in designing Medicaid programs, leading to great variability in benefits from state to state.

The Affordable Care Act of 2010 (ACA) intended to expand Medicaid eligibility to all individuals under the age of 65 in households with income up to 138 percent of the federal poverty level. However, a 2012 Supreme Court ruling made the eligibility expansion optional for each state (Klees, Wolfe, & Curtis, 2017). As a result, many states chose not to expand their Medicaid programs. This has significantly hampered the ability of the ACA to reduce the uninsured and has resulted in even greater variability across state Medicaid programs.

Medicaid plays an especially important role in covering patients with serious mental illness. While only 14 percent of the adult population is covered by Medicaid, the program covers 21 percent of adults with diagnosed mental illness and 17 percent of adults with substance use disorders. In most states, individuals are automatically eligible for Medicaid if they qualify to receive Supplemental Security Income, the federal cash assistance program for the aged with low-income, blind, or disabled. Mental illness is a qualifying disability for program eligibility.

There are major differences between the states in Medicaid's behavioral health coverage and funding for psychiatric and substance abuse services. This especially affects the provision of mental health services as many states do not adequately reimburse the cost of care provided by community mental health clinics or hospital providers. The variability is particularly stark in terms of substance use disorders, where many Medicaid programs do not cover medication-assisted treatment. Further, federal Medicaid funding is prohibited for "institutions for mental disease," limiting access to residential and inpatient treatment settings (Social Security Act).

Population Health and Mental Health Indicators in the US

Despite high spending, the US generally has poorer outcomes on almost any health measure than other OECD countries. The US life expectancy at birth in 2015 was 78.8, compared to the OECD average of 80.6 (OECD, 2017). This difference may be driven in part by high rates of obesity and poorly managed chronic disease. The obesity rate in the US is 38.2 percent, nearly 20 percentage points higher than the OECD average of 19.4 percent (OECD, 2017).

Mental and behavioral disorders are among the leading causes of disability in the US and the most costly health conditions for adults under sixty-five, along with cancer and trauma-related disorders. Of the top twenty-five leading causes of disability and injury between 1990 and 2016, nine are mental, neurological, or substance use disorders (US Burden of Disease Collaborators, 2018). In 2016, deaths from overdose and suicide in the US exceeded deaths from diabetes (29 per 100,000 population versus 25 per 100,000 respectively) (Rockett et al., 2018).

The prevalence of psychiatric disorders in the US of adults ages 18 or older in 2016 was estimated at 44.7 million (18.3 percent), with a higher rate of occurrence among women (21.7 percent) than men (14.5 percent; SAMHSA 2017). In 2014, it was estimated that 20.2 million adults in the US aged 18 or older (8.4 percent) had a substance use disorder (SUD) and 39.1 percent had a co-occurring mental disorder and SUD. For adolescents aged 12 to 17 years, who had a past year SUD, 28.4 percent had a co-occurring major depressive episode (Park-Lee et al., 2017).

Challenges in Behavioral Health and Service Delivery

Inadequate Behavioral Health Coverage and the Search for Parity
Historically, health insurance, regardless of the source, has covered behavioral health differently than physical health. This lack of *parity* has meant that patients were often subject to higher cost-sharing for behavioral health services, limits on the number of inpatient and/or outpatient services covered, strict prior

authorization requirements, and annual and/or lifetime limits on behavioral health services.

Over time, policymakers attempted to achieve parity for behavioral health care. These efforts for parity began within states. However, state efforts were piecemeal and, because states generally cannot regulate ESI, which is regulated under federal law, the impact was limited (US Department of Health and Human Services Assistant Secretary for Public Affairs [ASPA], 2016).

The first major federal attempt at parity was achieved in 1996 when the US Congress passed the Mental Health Parity Act. This legislation required that any annual or lifetime limits on behavioral health benefits set by large employers be comparable to the limits set on physical health benefits. While this effort was largely effective in addressing lack of parity in annual and lifetime limits on behavioral health, health insurance companies continued to discriminate against psychiatric patients in their benefit design. Notably, four years after the passage of the legislation, among plans that were compliant with the law, 87 percent restricted mental health benefits more than physical health outpatient visits and hospital days (Schwartz, Stein, & Wetzler, 2017).

The Mental Health Parity and Addiction Equity Act (MHPAEA) of 2008 was passed with bipartisan support to address the shortcomings of the Mental Health Parity Act of 1996 and required that, if mental illness and substance use disorder benefits were offered by ESI plans, then coverage could be no more restrictive than that for physical health benefits. Notably, this law did not require that plans offer behavioral health benefits, nor did this requirement apply to Medicaid or Medicare. In 2009, of individuals insured through ESI, 2 percent had no behavioral health benefits whatsoever and 7 percent had no substance use benefits. Individuals covered by other types of plans had even lower coverage of behavioral health benefits (Frank, Beronio, & Glied, 2014). The Affordable Care Act extended parity protections to additional types of insurance coverage. However, implementation and enforcement of parity protection have been slow, and parity has still not yet been fully achieved.

Inadequate Access to Psychiatric Care

There are insufficient resources in almost all communities to provide access to specialized behavioral care given the prevalence of psychiatric and substance use disorders. The National Survey on Drug Use and Health from 2016 indicated that among the estimated 44.7 million adults with any mental illness, only 43.1 percent received mental health services in the past year (Park-Lee et al., 2017). For the 10.4 million adults with serious mental illness, 64.8 percent received mental health services, and more than 17.7 million adults who needed substance use treatment did not receive specialty treatment (Park-Lee et al., 2017). This data demonstrates the serious shortfall in the availability of behavioral health treatment resources across the United States.

This shortfall in treatment is driven in part by an inadequate supply of psychiatrists. The US Department of Health and Human Services estimates there are approximately 46,000 psychiatrists in the United States with a current shortage of over 6,000 to meet current demand; this shortage is expected to grow to between 14,000 and 31,000 psychiatrists by 2024 (Satiani et al., 2018).

The psychiatrist shortage is compounded by inadequate insurance reimbursement and, therefore, insufficient numbers of psychiatrists participating within insurance networks. The acceptance rate of private insurance and Medicare is significantly lower for psychiatrists (55 percent) than for other physicians (86 to 88 percent; Bishop et al., 2014). As a result, patients access out-of-network behavioral services at a rate of 4.8 to 5.1 times higher than for primary care. (Melek, Norris, & Paulus, 2014). This means that patients who are treated by psychiatrists are subject to higher out-of-pocket costs, even if they have insurance offering behavioral health benefits.

Primary care physicians and pediatricians necessarily become the front-line behavioral health providers for the majority of patients when they present for medical care (Norquist, Regier, 1996; Regier, Goldberg, & Taube, 1978). Depression is one of the most prevalent disorders, and it should be of no surprise that more than 70 percent of antidepressants are prescribed in primary care and are among the most frequently prescribed medications. Although treatment for behavioral disorders most likely occurs in a primary care setting, research demonstrates that enhanced treatment is most likely to occur in a specialty mental health setting as psychiatrists use higher doses of medications, and patients were more likely to continue medication for 90 days or longer (Mojtabai, Olfson, 2008).

The problem of accessing needed behavioral health services extends as well to inpatient psychiatric services. Many communities have seen the loss of inpatient psychiatric capacity driven by inadequate reimbursement, including the impact of overly stringent utilization review from behavioral managed care companies. The US now averages about 11 psychiatric beds per 100,000 population. This is 25 to 30 percent of other OECD countries and below the consensus of 50 beds needed per 100,000 population (Green, Griffiths, 2014; Treatment Advocacy Center, 2016).

Siloed Behavioral and Physical Health Systems Creates Fragmented Care

Inadequate reimbursement, limits on coverage, and stigma around psychiatric illness has led to and reinforced a system wherein psychiatric services are most often provided outside of the general system of medical care. Further contributing to the siloed treatment of behavioral health care is the confidentiality often accorded mental health care. Federal law requires unique, stringent privacy protections of substance use data in the patient's medical record. These protections often result in non-psychiatrist medical care providers being unaware of patients' mental health and substance abuse problems and the medications being prescribed for treatment. This is especially dangerous in emergency situations where the physicians evaluating a patient are potentially unaware of critical information.

The growing emphasis on quality and cost embodied in outcomes-based payment models is leading to a re-examination of the siloed system, especially in regard to the impact of behavioral disorders on co-morbid medical disorders, such as diabetes and hypertension. Many medical illnesses have etiologies with behavioral contributions such as diet, exercise, substance use, and social stressors. Depression is often co-morbid with chronic medical disorders and can interfere with medication compliance, dietary recommendations, or adherence to outpatient appointments. Individuals with comorbid behavioral health problems are 2.5 to 3.5 times more expensive to treat than those who do not have these problems (Malek, Norris, & Paulus, 2014). The fragmentation of care that is so prevalent and characteristic of the US health care system is now recognized as a potential driver of costs, which needs to be addressed.

Emerging Solutions and Innovations

The Integration of Medical and Behavioral Health Care Reduces Fragmentation

As discussed earlier, untreated psychiatric disorders can increase the severity and costs of medical disorders. Integrating behavioral health services into primary care, therefore, presents an opportunity to address unmet behavioral health needs, improve quality of life, and improve outcomes, which is increasingly tied to reimbursement.

While psychiatrists and other mental health providers can simply be collocated into primary care settings, the large unmet need for mental health services in this setting is better suited for a population-based approach that efficiently deploys the limited supply of psychiatrists. This imperative led to the creation of the IMPACT Model (Improving Mood: Promoting Access to Collaborative Treatment) by Dr. Jürgen Unützer and colleagues at the University of Washington. The IMPACT Model tries to provide efficient and effective use of resources by only intensifying treatment as clinically required.

The IMPACT Model involves a collaborative team approach in which care managers and psychiatrists work with primary care physicians to treat effectively patients who are identified as suffering from depression. Using a stepped-care model, patients with varying severity of depression begin with lower-intensity treatment. Treatment response is closely monitored and measured, and care is intensified for patients who are not responding.

The care manager tracks and documents, in a patient registry, the population of patients in the practice who are identified as suffering from depression. The care manager also maintains contact with the patient to assist with treatment engagement and medication compliance, and provide education and brief psychotherapy for depression, as needed. The psychiatrist in this model provides decision support to the primary care physician and care manager on treatment options, and moves, as needed, from indirect consultation to direct face-to-face consultation, especially for patients who are on the more severe spectrum of illness, such as those at risk for suicide or who are not responding to treatment. When possible, the model maintains care within the primary care setting. If the patient requires specialty mental health care, then the patient will be referred for needed services.

The IMPACT Model has demonstrated the substantial benefits of collaborative care. A study of 1,801 older adults with major depression and dysthymic disorder showed a 50 percent or greater reduction in depressive symptoms in 45 percent of intervention patients as compared to 19 percent of patients undergoing usual care. Intervention patients also experienced improved satisfaction with depression treatment, less functional impairment, and greater improvements in quality of life (Unützer et al., 2002). Evidence is building that intervention will reduce five-year mean total medical costs, especially for patients with depression and the most severe medical comorbidities (Katon et al., 2008). There is the potential that collaborative care not only for depression but also for substance use disorders can affect overall medical costs and improve medical outcomes and quality of life when implemented in medical care settings. The Medicare program now recognizes the importance and utility of collaborative care and allows primary care practices to bill for the services of behavioral health care managers.

In contrast to the IMPACT Model, which collocates behavioral health services within primary care, the "reverse-integrated" model of care, which offers primary care within clinics and practices providing mental health care, is also increasingly prevalent. It is estimated that patients with mental illness die ten years earlier than age-matched cohorts, and worldwide, approximately eight million deaths each year are attributable to mental disorders (Walker, McGee, & Druss, 2015). Many of the premature deaths among the mentally ill may be attributable to how difficult it is for this group of patients to access primary care services, which demonstrates how this reverse-integrated model has the potential to achieve significant gains in avoidable deaths.

Telehealth Presents an Opportunity to Improve Access

Technology is beginning to transform the practice of medicine, and telehealth presents one of the most promising opportunities to markedly improve access amid growing physician shortages and across remote geographies. Telehealth can be deployed directly to the consumer or used by providers to gain access to off-site psychiatrists for consultations and evaluations.

In telepsychiatry and telepsychotherapy models directed to consumers, the consumers use computers, tablets, and smartphones to connect with psychiatrists and nurse practitioners who can provide assessments, medication management, and psychotherapy services. These models have already gained a foothold and are rapidly gaining users. The ready, and at times instant, availability of services contributes to its popularity. Many companies that offer these services provide HIPAA compliant and secure videoconferencing and messaging platforms. Some products offer the ability to integrate with major electronic medical record systems, which can share files and medical records with other providers or systems. Multilingual services are also readily available and are offered by these platforms.

In provider-to-provider models, providers work with off-site psychiatrists for consultations and evaluations. For example, providers in remote emergency departments can videoconference with psychiatrists who can provide timely emergency evaluations of patients. The consulting psychiatrist can then determine whether the patient requires transfer to a psychiatric facility or referral for treatment. For less urgent cases, staff can obtain e-consults for patients using asynchronous store and forward technology. Telehealth also supports integrated care initiatives, such as the IMPACT model, as a consulting psychiatrist can remotely advise and provide decision support to the primary care provider.

As these services constitute the "practice of medicine," which is governed by the individual states, participating physicians or nurse practitioners usually must be licensed by the state in which the patient resides. Some psychiatrists provide services to an international patient base where psychiatric expertise is relatively unavailable or inaccessible.

Telemedicine and telepsychiatry companies currently offer their services on a subscription basis and/or with per-use fees. The major government payers, Medicaid and Medicare, are beginning to reimburse for these services, as are health plans and some large employers. While Medicare historically only reimbursed telemedicine services in rural areas, geographic restrictions are being progressively and gradually eased as there is increasing recognition of the utility and importance of these services, especially when specialized services would otherwise be unavailable, regardless of geography.

Among the advantages of telehealth are increased access and reduced costs. Providers can increase their caseloads as geographic limitations are not as relevant. Patients save on travel costs and are usually able to schedule visits at more convenient times. For patients who are home-bound or disabled, telepsychiatry may be the only option to receive services.

Another developing area is the provision of internet-based computerized psychotherapy. Several of these programs, especially those based on cognitive-behavioral principles have demonstrated efficacy for the treatment of depression, insomnia, and anxiety disorders (Spek et al., 2007). These iCBT (internet-based cognitive-behavioral therapy) programs are both efficacious and cost-effective. Many of these programs offer access to consultations from "live" clinicians when needed.

The landscape for telepsychiatry and technology-based interventions is rapidly evolving. Integration of these services with EHRs will further fuel their adoption by health care systems and providers. These technologies make it more efficient to monitor patient progress and outcomes with self-report measures that can improve quality of care and promote electronic monitoring of patients' symptoms. As our health care system focuses more on outcomes, quality, and efficiency, technology and telehealth services will become much more prevalent and useful to the practicing clinician.

Conclusion

Clinicians practicing in the United States are challenged daily with the complexities of the nation's health care system. This is particularly true for mental health providers and primary care providers who so often serve as de facto mental health providers. Patients struggle with high costs, fragmented care, and poor access. However, efforts to integrate behavioral health care into the physical health system are gaining ground, and these new models, especially when supported by telehealth, hold great promise to improve the delivery of behavioral health care.

References and Suggested Readings

- Anderson, G. F., Reinhardt, U. E., Hussey, P. S., and Petrosyan, V. (2003). It's the Prices, Stupid: Why the United States Is So Different from Other Countries. *Health Affairs*, 22 (3), 89–105.
- Bishop, T. F., Press, M. J., Keyhani, S., and Pincus, H. A. (2014). Acceptance of Insurance by Psychiatrists and the Implications for Access to Mental Health Care. *JAMA Psychiatry*, 71 (2), 176–181.
- Collins, S., Gunja, M., and Doty, M. (2017). *How Well Does Insurance Coverage Protect Consumers from Health Care Costs? – Findings from the Commonwealth Fund Biennial Health Insurance Survey, (2016).* New York: The Commonwealth Fund.
- Congress of the United States Congressional Budget Office (2013). *Options for Reducing the Deficit: 2014 to 2023.* Washington, DC: Government Printing Office.
- Cubanski, J., and Neuman, T. (2018). *The Facts on Medicare Spending and Financing.* San Francisco: Henry J. Kaiser Family Foundation.
- Cubanski, J., Swoope, C., Boccuti, C., Jacobson, G., Casillas, G., Griffin, S., and Neuman, T. (2015). *A Primer on Medicare: Key Facts about The Medicare Program and the People It Covers.* San Francisco: Henry J. Kaiser Family Foundation.

- Frank, R. G., Beronio, K., and Glied, S. A. (2014). Behavioral Health Parity and the Affordable Care Act. *Journal of Social Work in Disability and Rehabilitation*, 13 (1–2), 31–43.
- Green, B., and Griffiths, E. (2014). Hospital Admission and Community Treatment of Mental Disorders in England from 1998 to 2012. *General Hospital Psychiatry*, 36, (4), 442–448.
- Katon, W. J., Russo, J. E., Von Korff, M., Lin, H. B. E., Ludman, E., and Ciechanowski, P. S. (2008). Long-Term Effects on Medical Costs of Improving Depression Outcomes in Patients with Depression and Diabetes. *Diabetes Care*, 31 (6),1155–1159.
- Klees, B., Wolfe, C., and Curtis, C. (2017). *Brief Summaries of Medicare and Medicaid: Title XVIII and Title XIX of the Social Security Act.* Washington, DC: US Centers for Medicare and Medicaid Services.
- Melek, S. P., Norris, D. T., and Paulus, J. (2014). *Economic Impact of Integrated Medical-Behavioral Health Care: Milliman Report for the American Psychiatry Association.* Arlington, VA: American Psychiatric Publishing.
- Mojtabai, R., and Olfson, M. (2008). National Patterns in Antidepressant Treatment by Psychiatrists and General Medical Providers: Results from the National Comorbidity Survey Replication. *Journal of Clinical Psychiatry*, 69 (7), 1064.
- Norquist, G., and Regier, D. (1996). The Epidemiology Of Psychiatric Disorders and the De Facto Mental Health Care System 1. *Annual Review of Medicine*, 47 (1), 473–479.
- OECD (2017). *Health at a Glance 2017: OECD Indicators.* Paris: OECD Publishing.
- Park-Lee, E., Lipari, R., Hedden, S., Kroutil, L., and Porter, J. (2017). *NSDUH Data Review: Receipt of Services for Substance Use and Mental Health Issues among Adults: Results from the 2016 National Survey on Drug Use and Health.* Washington, DC: Substance Abuse and Mental Health Services Administration.
- Regier, D. A., Goldberg, I. D., and Taube, C. A. (1978). The De Facto US Mental Health Services System: A Public Health Perspective. *Archives of General Psychiatry*, 35 (6), 685–693.
- Rockett, I., Caine, E., Connery, H., and Greenfield, S. (2018). Mortality in the United States from Self-Injury Surpasses Diabetes: A Prevention Imperative. *Injury Prevention*, 25 (4), 331–333.
- Satiani, B., Satiani, A., Niedermier, J., and Svendsen, D. P. (2018). Projected Workforce of Psychiatrists in the United States: A Population Analysis. *Psychiatric Services*, 69 (6), 710–713.
- Schwartz, B., Stein, G., and Wetzler, S. (2017). Financing Integrated Care Models. In *Integrating Behavioral Health and Primary Care*. New York: Oxford University Press, p. 78.
- Social Security Act 42 USC. §§ 1905 (a) (B).
- Spek, V., Cuijpers, P., Nyklícek, I., Riper, H., Keyzer, J., and Pop, V. (2007). Internet-Based Cognitive Behaviour Therapy for Symptoms of Depression and Anxiety: A Meta-Analysis. *Psychological Medicine*, 37 (3), 319–328.
- Squires, D. (2015). *US Health Care from a Global Perspective Spending: Use of Services, Prices, and Health in 13 Countries.* New York: The Commonwealth Fund.
- Substance Abuse and Mental Health Services Administration (2017). *Key Substance Use and Mental Health Indicators in the United States: Results from the 2016 National*

Survey on Drug Use and Health (HHS Publication No. SMA 17–5044, NSDUH Series H-52). Rockville, MD: HHS.

- Treatment Advocacy Center (2016). *Going, Going, Gone; Trends and Consequences of Eliminating State Psychiatric Beds, 2016*. www.treatmentadvocacycenter.org/storage/documents/going-going-gone.pdf.
- Unützer, J., Katon, W., Callahan, C. M., Williams, J., John W, Hunkeler, E., Harpole, L., Hoffing, M., Della Penna, R. D., Noël, P. H., Lin, E. H. B., Areán, P. A., Hegel, M. T., Tang, L., Belin, T. R., Oishi, S., Langston, C., and for the IMPACT Investigators (2002). Collaborative Care Management of Late-Life Depression in the Primary Care Setting: A Randomized Controlled Trial. *JAMA*, 288 (22), 2836–2845.
- US Burden of Disease Collaborators (2018a). Burden of Diseases, Injuries, and Risk Factors among US States. *JAMA*, 319 (14), 1444–1472.
- US Burden of Disease Collaborators (2018b). The State of US Health, 1990–2016. *JAMA*, 319 (14), 1444–1472.
- US Centers for Medicare and Medicaid Services (2018a). *May 2018 Medicaid and CHIP Enrollment Data Highlights*. www.medicaid.gov/medicaid/program-information/medicaid-and-chip-enrollment-data/report-highlights/index.html.
- US Centers for Medicare and Medicaid Services (2018b). *NHE Fact Sheet*. www.cms.gov/research-statistics-data-and-systems/statistics-trends-and-reports/national-healthexpenddata/nhe-fact-sheet.html.
- US Department of Health and Human Services Assistant Secretary for Public Affairs (ASPA) (2016). *Parity Policy and Implementation*. www.hhs.gov/about/agencies/advisory-committees/mental-health-parity/task-force/resources/index.html.
- Walker, E. R., McGee, R. E., and Druss, B. G. (2015). Mortality in Mental Disorders and Global Disease Burden Implications: A Systematic Review and Meta-analysis. *JAMA Psychiatry*, 72 (4), 334–341.

Self-Assessment Questions

1. Which of the following is the largest source of health care coverage in the United States?
    A. Medicaid
    B. Employer-sponsored health insurance (ESI)
    C. The Affordable Care Act
    D. Medicare
2. The term *underinsurance* refers to:
    A. 9 percent of the US population is without health insurance.
    B. Insurance deductibles are prohibitively high in many plans, leading to many insured individuals being unable to use their health insurance.
    C. In the United States, individuals have an average of 4 physician visits annually compared to 6.5 visits in the Organization for Cooperative Development Countries (OECD).

D. Employment plays a major role in health care coverage in the United States.

3. Which of the following is true of Medicare?
   A. Covers long-term care for all enrolled individuals
   B. A state-funded health insurance program for low-income people
   C. A federal health insurance program for individuals aged sixty-five or older
   D. Each state administers its own Medicare program with federal oversight

4. With regard to psychiatric disorders in US adults in 2016, which of the following is false?
   A. The prevalence of psychiatric disorders is 8 percent.
   B. There is a higher prevalence of psychiatric disorders in women compared with men.
   C. 8 percent of US adults are diagnosed with a substance use disorder (SUD).
   D. Individuals with medical illnesses and comorbid mental health problems are 2.5–3.5 times more expensive to treat than those without mental health comorbidity.

5. Which of the following is true of health outcomes in the US compared with OECD countries?
   A. The US life expectancy is two years longer than OECD life expectancy.
   B. The US has poorer health outcomes on all measures compared with the OECD.
   C. Rates of obesity and chronic illness are similar in the US and OECD.
   D. OECD countries spend more on health care than the US

Answers to Self-Assessment Questions

1. (B)
2. (B)
3. (C)
4. (A)
5. (B)

20 Global Health and Mental Health Care Delivery in Low-Resource Settings

GIUSEPPE RAVIOLA

Introduction

Mental and neurological disorders present a significant burden of illness globally, with profound shortages of trained human resources, inadequate financing for mental health care delivery systems, and a lack of robust social and legal protections for people living with mental disorders. In low- and middle-income countries, the gap between the burden of illness and available treatments is especially acute, with a significant proportion of the world's population having little to no access to formal mental health and neurological services. This chapter provides an overview of challenges and opportunities for global health and mental health care delivery, with a focus on innovative care delivery solutions.

Global Health Challenges

Global Health and Mental Health

Global health has been described as a field that places a priority on improving health and achieving equity in health for all people worldwide (Koplan 2009). Broadly, low- and middle-income countries have made extraordinary progress over the past two decades in health care delivery and population health through global and national programming targeting diseases such as HIV/AIDS, tuberculosis, and malaria, and through basic interventions such as immunization. Mental health, however, remains overwhelmingly unaddressed, and represents an opportunity for the global health community given the significant burden of illness, the glaring treatment gap, the common co-morbidity of mental disorders with other conditions, and the proven effectiveness of treatments for mental disorders.

The World Health Organization (WHO) has defined "mental health" as "more than the mere lack of mental disorder," but rather as "a state of well-being" (WHO Fact File 2018). Mental health therefore encompasses a broad conception of health that includes wellness, ameliorating poverty and social determinants of mental illness, addressing early childhood development and preventive approaches to care, and providing clinical treatments that encompass psychological, pharmacologic and other approaches, for a broad range of mental and neurological disorders. *Severe mental disorders*, including schizophrenia and other psychotic illnesses; *common mental disorders*, encompassing major depression, anxiety, and stress-related conditions and post-traumatic experiences; and *epilepsy* together compose a significant proportion of the untreated global burden of mental disorders that current global health efforts are seeking to creatively address.

The focus of an emergent field of *global mental health* over the past several decades has been on reducing mental health disparities between and within nations, and seeking innovative community-based and systemic solutions to increasing access to care (Patel and Prince, 2010). The field of global mental health has primarily reflected significant research efforts showing evidence that mental health treatments originally developed in higher-income settings can be adapted and delivered in low- and middle-income countries. Overcoming the significant challenges that relate to bridging the treatment gap, and developing functional, sustained mental health systems, remains a significant challenge in global health. It requires a deep appreciation of the ways in which local culture and belief systems inform understandings of health and illness in communities; knowledge of the burden of illness; awareness of the effectiveness of various mental health treatments; familiarity with best practices in community health, including the engagement of nonspecialist providers such as community health workers; and skills in effective advocacy to also transform health systems and policy responses that can help lay the groundwork for interventions to be successfully embedded within local community, cultural, and biomedical contexts.

The Global Burden of Illness

Mental disorders represent the greatest collective cause of disability globally today. Over the past two decades, new methodologies and information on the prevalence of mental disorders have highlighted the global burden of illness. Recent estimates suggest that the disease burden of mental disorders accounts for 32.4 percent of years lived with disability (YLDs) and 13.0 percent of disability-adjusted life-years (DALYs) (Vigo et al., 2016). Mental disorders account for almost one in three years lived with disability globally. Depression, the most common mental disorder, affects an estimated 350 million people globally and represents the leading cause of disability (as measured by DALYs) around the world. Severe mental disorders, including schizophrenia, affect approximately 1 in 100 people globally, across cultures, with significant severity of illness, morbidity, low life expectancy, and economic impact on families. Mental disorders significantly impact people in low- and middle-income countries, with 80 percent of the world's population living in these regions; however, most formal, health system-based mental health resources are spent inhigh-income countries.

The Mental Health Treatment Gap

Resources that do get spent on mental health services, particularly in low- and middle-income countries, are often highly centralized and tend to be funneled toward national-level institutional facilities instead of being "decentralized" to create services at primary care clinics and in communities. In high-income countries socioeconomic disparities also limit the availability of mental health services within and across communities, particularly in rural areas, leading to similar challenges across low resource settings. Furthermore, the "treatment gap" for people with mental disorders exceeds 50 percent in all countries worldwide, approaching rates as high as 90 percent in the least resourced countries (Patel, Maj, et al. 2010). Epilepsy, for example, the most common serious neurologic disorder, could be treated in 70 percent of people if treatments were available; however, 76 percent of epilepsy remains untreated globally in all areas, with upwards of 90 percent in rural areas in low-income countries (Meyer et al. 2012). Neurological and neurodevelopmental services are also so limited in many contexts that within government ministries of health in low-income countries neurological care falls under the aegis of "mental health," with even greater gaps in the availability of neurologists.

With regard to child and adolescent mental health, more than 50 percent of mental disorders start before the age of 14, and 75 percent start before the age of 24 (Kessler 2005). One quarter of DALYs for mental disorders and substance abuse is borne by those 24 years old or younger, the age group that accounts for more than 40 percent of the world population (Mundi 2017, GBD 2017). Most children and young people in low-income countries do not have access to mental health care, with child mental health considered the "orphan's orphan" of health care across low-, middle-, and high-income countries (Lu et al. 2018, Mind Your Mind 2018). Even in high-income countries, there exists a crisis in child mental health service delivery and access. In Canada, for example, often cited as having a highly evolved health care delivery system, only one in five children who need mental health services receive them (CAMH 2018, *Huffington Post* 2018).

Reasons for the mental health treatment gap are numerous and include inadequate government budgets to fund adequate human resource, facility, and medication costs; the deleterious effects of locked hospitals in promoting stigma and fear and poor quality of care; limited access to care for a significant proportion of the population due to geographical distance for those living in rural or remote areas; the significant emotional costs of seeking care for people living with illness and their families; a general lack of sustained community-based care models that exist in context; lack of families' ability to pay for medications and exclusion of psychiatric medications from insurance payment plans if they exist; general lack of specialists trained in the provision of quality care practices; and community-wide stigma and fear of people living with mental disorders.

Human Rights and Institutional Care

An ongoing challenge for global health has remained a poor standard of clinical care delivered in resource-constrained, public institutional psychiatric facilities, combined with a lack of human rights protections for people living with mental disorders. This generally has reflected the limited resources allocated for mental health services by governments, which have tended to spend less than one percent of their budgets on mental health care despite the high disease burden, spending the limited funding on maintaining dilapidated facilities with inadequate human resources, and over-reliance on powerful neuroleptic medications. In higher-income countries, while more mental health services may be available in communities than in lower-income countries, people living with mental disorders can also find themselves incarcerated or homeless without social protections.

Of grave concern, in many low- and middle-income countries, asylums, mental and psychiatric hospitals continue to be the primary form of mental health care, a dire situation. Such facilities continue to be the sites of human rights abuses, also perpetuating economies of ineffective alternative healers in communities (Cohen and Minas, 2017). While traditional healing systems, and religious and spiritual practices, should ideally be integrated with more formal biomedical interventions for truly holistic, patient-centered care, in many instances local community providers drain the financial resources of families desperate to heal a family member living with a severe mental illness (often attributed to a culturally specific or spiritual cause). The promise of healing, and no other alternative, draws families to seek care at the psychiatric facility. Solutions to such facilities include the development of community-based services, the gradual opening of small acute psychiatric units in general hospitals, which can reduce admissions to centralized notional facilities, and legislation protecting the rights of people living with mental disorders. Greater investments need to be made in integrating care within primary care, and engaging additional cadres of providers in the health care system in various aspects of care, while not allowing centralized facilities to degrade and serve as monuments to fear and stigma related to mental illness in contexts where safe, effective and evidence-based clinical mental health services have not previously existed.

Global Mental Health Care Delivery

"Task Sharing" and Nonspecialist Care Delivery

Increasingly, and in response to the complete lack of formal, decentralized mental health services across most of the globe, over the past decade, a research evidence base has been developed for the effectiveness of provision of nonspecialist-delivered, community-based care for mental disorders in low-resource settings. Nonspecialists include community leaders, community health workers, nurses, physicians, and other members of the community and providers who can support the provision of certain mental health care tasks. Growing evidence about effective "task sharing" of psychosocial and psychological interventions – care delivered by nonspecialist providers – may be the most important advance made by an emergent field of *Global Mental Health* over the past decade (Whitley 2015). This was supported by a landmark *Lancet* series in 2007 (Chisholm 2007, Patel Araya 2007, Patel Flischer 2007, Prince Patel 2007), launching "a new movement for mental health" (Horton 2007), and subsequently followed with a 2011 *Lancet* series (Kakuma 2011, Lund 2011, Patel Boyce 2011), a 2011 *Nature* publication (Collins 2011), and a 2013 *PLOS* series on Grand Challenges in Global Mental Health (Kaaya 2013, Ngo 2013, Patel 2013, Rahman 2013, Whitley 2015). New funders also came onto the scene – the Wellcome Trust (UK), Grand Challenges Canada, and in 2011 a new US National Institutes of Mental Health (NIMH) Office for Research on Disparities and Global Mental Health (a title implying the relevance of solving disparities in mental health care provision in high-income countries as well, and the possibility of "reverse innovation" from low- to high-income settings such as in the United States). This movement itself, with its own history, has had as its stated aim "to improve services for people living with mental health problems and psychosocial disabilities worldwide, especially in low- and middle-income countries where effective services are often scarce" (GMHM website 2018). This aim distinguishes the global mental health movement from the decades of work within cultural psychiatry and medical anthropology that sought to understand local conceptions of mental distress and healing (Kirmayer and Pedersen 2014). The development of the field of global mental health reflected the historical neglect of mental health as a component of the global health agenda, what Arthur Kleinman called "a failure of humanity," as well as a historical overemphasis on the practices of the field of psychiatry as the main solution to the perceived problem: the aforementioned treatment gap (Kleinman 2009).

Since the early twenty-first century, significant work has been done to evaluate interventions and systems to address the treatment gap, and to build momentum toward identifying cost-effective, evidence-supported practices and services that could feasibly be made more widely available in low-income countries, leading to a "scale-up" of services. The World Health Organization (WHO) has taken an important role in this process through its Mental Health Gap Programme, which in 2011 published an Intervention Guide (IG) for "mental, neurological and substance use disorders in nonspecialized health settings" based on extensive literature review – emerging international consensus on best practices that can potentially be adapted to context, and acknowledgment of certain "universal" aspects to the way mental disorders present regardless of cultural context (WHO 2011). The WHO mhGAP-IG materials provide guidance for the treatment of depression, psycho-sis, bipolar disorder, and other conditions, suggesting social, psychosocial, psy-chological, and pharmacological interventions, and have been most relevant to the training and support of generalist physicians in delivering basic components of mental health care. A subsequent second edition was unveiled in 2016, and an additional version was developed for use in humanitarian emergencies (WHO 2016, WHO 2015). These guidelines to support the development of services for the long-term have intersected with the concurrent development of guidance for health sector agencies in providing support to populations during humanitarian crises, embodied by the 2007 Interagency Standing Committee Guidelines (IASC) on Mental Health and Psychosocial Support in Emergency Settings (IASC 2007). Taken together, these documents seek to ensure that the most appropriate actions are taken and resources expended at the right time and in the right way in the pro-cess of moving from acute emergencies to longer-term responses so that sustaina-ble mental health systems can be "built back better" (WHO 2013). At a policy level, the WHO has been deeply involved in supporting governments in strengthening mental health care, including with a WHO Comprehensive Mental Health Action Plan 2013–2020 (DeSilva et al. 2013, WHO MHAP 2013).

Strengthening Health Systems through "Decentralization" of Mental Health Services and Development of "Platforms"

Task sharing with nonspecialist providers cannot be the only component of func-tional, sustained, and decentralized models of mental health care. Health system strengthening efforts that engage nonspecialists in mental health care must con-sider strengthening the health system as a whole, from community to tertiary care levels. The improvement of primary care health systems through the delivery of services for HIV/AIDS and tuberculosis in various low-resource settings at the turn of the millennium led to a fundamental shift in global health toward the *strength-ening of health systems* through the building of more effective models of primary care. Given that mental health systems greatly benefit from strong primary care, the progress made in global health through the development of systems for other conditions lays a foundation for improvements in mental health care delivery sys-tems. Mental health services of various kinds can be developed and delivered at various levels in society, called *platforms*. Platforms can exist at the levels of the population (i.e., legislation and regulation, information and awareness), commu-nity (i.e., workplace, schools, neighborhood and community groups), and health care (i.e., self-care and informal care, primary health care, and specialist health care) (Patel et al. DCP 2015).

While *global health*, broadly, has concerned itself with the health of populations in the global context with a focus on achieving health equity, *global health deliv-ery* is a newer field focusing on the actual planning, service implementation, and sustained supply of modern, comprehensive, integrated medical and integrated preventive care to people living in resource-limited settings. In global health delivery, the mere existence of functional, sustained services that are decentralized can itself be an innovation, and this is certainly the case for mental health; however, while research has increasingly shown that mental disorders can be treated effectively not only in high-income settings, but also in settings where there are few specialists, the actual implementation and subsequent scaling up of sustained mental health services within existing public health systems has been slow. Research related to "collaborative care" delivery models in higher resourced settings has shown the importance of key system components: population-based care for specific disorders that prioritizes screening, treatment and tracking of outcomes; self-care support, including family and patient education about illness and treatments, self-monitoring, and adherence support skills; care management and measurement-based care using patient-reported outcomes focused on adherence, side effects, change in symptoms and course of care following evidence-based guidelines; treatment to target and systematic monitoring of severity, with treatment intensification for patients not improving, according to evidence-based guidelines; case registry to track clinical outcomes (e.g., depression severity scores) and key process steps, to facilitate transparent shared management across nonspecialist workers, primary care providers and consulting specialists; psychiatric consultation for more complex presentations; and the use of proven intervention strategies, including brief psychological treatments in addition to medications, consistent with mhGAP-IG (Kroenke and Unützer 2016). More broadly, additional general macro components that require attention as systems building blocks for mental health include governance and financing, information systems including electronic medical records as well as digital technologies, psychotropic medication supply chain, attention to the mental health workforce, and development of user and family associations to ensure that care systems are truly person-centered and driven by consumer needs and preferences (WHO-AIMS 2009). These all relate to catalyzing important actions for advancing the decentralization of integrated community-based services, including: empowering people living with mental disorders; building a diverse mental health workforce; developing collaborative and multidisciplinary mental health teams; using technology to increase access to mental health care; identifying and treating mental health problems early; and reducing premature mortality in people living with mental health problems (DeSilva et al. 2014).

Conclusion

Significant challenges remain to increasing the delivery of mental health care in low-resource settings globally. Innovative care delivery solutions such as task sharing of care with the support of nonspecialist providers, including community health workers, and increased use of digital technologies in supporting nonspecialist-delivered care, will advance the decentralization of mental health services to primary care and community-based platforms in the decades to come. The COVID-19 pandemic crisis has accelerated these processes. Psychiatrists will play an essential role not only as clinical experts but as team leaders and systems and technology experts in the creation of new care delivery models that will advance mental health service expansion in areas of need across low-, middle-, and high-income countries.

References and Suggested Readings

- CAMH website, https://cmha.ca/about-cmha/fast-facts-about-mental-illness (accessed August 8, 2018).
- Chisholm, D., Flisher, A. J., Lund, C., Patel, V., Saxena, S., Thornicroft, G., and Tomlinson, M. (2007). Scale Up Services for Mental Disorders: A Call for Action. *Lancet*, 370, 1241–1252.
- Cohen, A., and Minas, H. (2017). Global Mental Health and Psychiatric Institutions in the 21st Century. *Epidemiology and Psychiatric Sciences*, 26, 4–9.
- Collins, P.Y., Patel, V., Joestl, S. et al. (2011). Grand Challenges in Global Mental Health. *Nature*, 475, 27–30.
- Collins, P. Y., Insel, T. R., Chockalingam, A., Daar, A., and Maddox, Y. T. (2013). Grand Challenges in Global Mental Health: Integration in Research, Policy, and Practice. *PLOS Medicine*, 10 (4), e1001434.
- DeSilva, M., Samele, C., Saxena, S., Patel, V., and Darzi, A. (2014). Policy Actions to Achieve Integrated Community-Based Mental Health Services. *Health Affairs*, 33(9), 1595–1602.
- Horton, R. (2007). Launching a New Movement for Mental Health. *Lancet*, 370, 806.
- *Huffington Post* website, www.huffingtonpost.ca/2016/02/17/kids-mental-health-canada_n_9212872.html (accessed August 8, 2018).
- Inter-Agency Standing Committee (IASC) (2007). IASC Guidelines on Mental Health and Psychosocial Support in Emergency Settings. Geneva: IASC.
- Kaaya, S., Eustache, E., Lapidos-Salaiz, I., Musisi, S., Psaros, C., and Wissow, L. (2013). Grand Challenges: Improving HIV Treatment Outcomes by Integrating Interventions for Co-morbid Mental Illness. *PLOS Medicine*, 10 (5), 1001447.
- Kakuma, R., Minas, H., van Ginneken, N., Dal Poz, M. R., Desiraju, K., Morris, J. E., Saxena, S., and Scheffler, R. M. (2011). Human Resources for Mental Health Care: Current Situation and Strategies for Action. *Lancet*, 378, 1654–1663.
- Kessler, R. C., Berglund, P., Demler, O., Jin, R., Merikangas, K. R., and Walters, E. E. (2005). Lifetime Prevalence and Age-of-Onset Distributions of DSM-IV Disorders in the National Comorbidity Survey Replication. *Archives of General Psychiatry*, 62 (6), 593–602.
- Kirmayer, L. J., and Pedersen, D. (2014). Toward a New Architecture for Global Mental Health. *Transcultural Psychiatry*, 51, 759–776.

- Kleinman, A. (2009). Global Mental Health: A Failure of Humanity. *Lancet*, 374, 603–604.
- Koplan, J. P., Bond, T. C., Merson, M. H., Reddy, K. S., Rodriguez, M. H., Sewankambo, N. K., et al. (2009). Towards a Common Definition of Global Health. *Lancet*, 373, 1993–1995.
- Kroenke, K., and Unützer, J. (2016). Closing the False Divide: Sustainable Approaches to Integrating Mental Health Services into Primary Care. *Journal of General Internal Medicine*, 32 (4), 404–410.
- Lu, C., Li, Z., and Patel, V. (2018). Global Child and Adolescent Mental Health: The Orphan of Development Assistance for Health. *PLOS Medicine*, 15 (3), e1002524.
- Lund, C., De Silva, M., Plagerson, S., Cooper, S., Chisholm, D., Das, J., Knapp, M., and Patel, V. (2011). Poverty and Mental Disorders: Breaking the Cycle in Low-Income and Middle-Income Countries. *Lancet*, 378, 1502–1514.
- Meyer, A. C., Dua, T., Boscardin, W. J., Escarce, J. J., Saxena, S., and Birbeck, G. L. (2012). Critical Determinants of the Epilepsy Treatment Gap: A Cross-National Analysis in Resource-Limited Settings. *Epilepsia*, 53(12), 2178–2185.
- Mind Your Mind website, https://mindyourmind.ca/blog/youth-mental-health-care-canada-orphans-orphan (accessed November 5, 2020).
- Ngo, V. K., Rubinstein, A., Ganju, V., Kanellis, P., Loza, N., Rabadan-Diehl, C., and Daar, A. S. (2013). Grand Challenges: Integrating Mental Health Care into the Non-communicable Disease Agenda. *PLOS Medicine*, 10 (5), e1001443.
- Patel, V., Araya, R., Chatterjee, S., Chisholm, D., Cohen, A., DeSilva, M., Hosman, C., McGuire, H., Rojas, G., and van Ommeren, M. (2007a). Treatment and Prevention of Mental Disorders in Low-Income and Middle-Income Countries. *Lancet*, 370, 991–1005.
- Patel, V., Belkin, G. S., Chockalingam, A., Cooper, J., Saxena, S., and Unutzer, J. (2013). Grand Challenges: Integrating Mental Health Services into Priority Health Care Platforms. *PLOS Medicine*, 10 (5), e1001448.
- Patel, V., Boyce, N., Collins, P. Y., Saxena, S., and Horton, R. (2011). A Renewed Agenda for Global Mental Health. *Lancet*, 378, 1441–1442.
- Patel, V., Flisher, A. J., Hetrick, S., and McGorry, P. (2007b). Mental Health of Young People: A Global Public-Health Challenge. *Lancet*, 369, 1302–1313.
- Patel, V., Maj, M., Flisher, A. J., De Silva, M., Koschorke, M., and Prince, M. (2010). Reducing the Treatment Gap for Mental Disorders: A WPA Survey. *World Psychiatry*, 9 (3), 169–176.
- Patel, V., and Prince, M. (2010). Global Mental Health: A New Global Health Field Comes of Age. *JAMA*, 303, 1976–1977.
- Patel, V., Chisholm., D., Dua, T., Laxminarayan, R., and Medina-Mora, M. E. (eds.) (2015). *Mental, Neurological, and Substance Use Disorders. Disease Control Priorities*, 3rd ed., vol. 4. Washington, DC: World Bank.
- Prince, M., Patel, V., Saxena, S., Maj, M., Maselko, J., Phillips, M. R., and Rahman, A. (2007). No Health without Mental Health. *Lancet*, 370, 859–877.
- Rahman, A., Surkan, P. J., Cayetano, C. E., Rwagatare, P., and Dickson, K. E. (2013). Grand Challenges: Integrating Maternal Mental Health into Maternal and Child Health Programmes. *PLOS Medicine*, 10 (5).
- Vigo, D., Thornicroft, G., and Atun, R. (2016). Estimating the True Global Burden of Mental Illness. *Lancet Psychiatry*, 3 (2), 171–178.

- Whitley, R. (2015). Global Mental Health: Concepts, Conflicts and Controversies. *Epidemiology and Psychiatric Sciences*, 24, 285–291.
- World Health Organization (2011). *mhGAP Intervention Guide for Mental, Neurological and Substance Use Disorders in Non-Specialized Health Settings*. Geneva, Switzerland: WHO.
- World Health Organization (WHO) (2013a). *Building Back Better: Sustainable Mental Health Care after Emergencies*. Geneva, Switzerland: WHO.
- World Health Organization (WHO) (2013b). *WHO Comprehensive Mental Health Action Plan 2013–2020*. www.who.int/mental_health/action_plan_2013/en/.
- World Health Organization (2015). *mhGAP Humanitarian Intervention Guide (mhGAP-HIG): Clinical Management of Mental, Neurological and Substance Use Conditions in Humanitarian Emergencies*. Geneva, Switzerland: WHO.
- World Health Organization (2016). *mhGAP Intervention Guide for Mental, Neurological and Substance Use Disorders in Non-Specialized Health Settings: Mental Health Gap Action Programme (mhGAP) – version 2.0*. Geneva, Switzerland: WHO.

Self-Assessment Questions

1. Which of the following statements about mental disorders globally is false?
   A. Mental disorders represent the greatest collective cause of disability globally.
   B. Schizophrenia is the most common mental disorder globally.
   C. The majority of mental health resources are spent in high-income countries.
   D. Most of the world's population live in low- and middle-income countries, where mental illness burden is the highest.

2. With regard to the mental health treatment gap in child and adolescent disorders, which statement is false?
   A. 50 percent of mental health disorders have their onset before the age of fourteen.
   B. Most children and adolescents in low-income countries do not have access to mental health care.
   C. The treatment gap for children and adolescents with mental health disorders in high-income countries is minimal.
   D. Reasons for the mental health treatment gap for children and adolescents globally include stigma and fear, inadequate government funding, lack of specialists, and poor quality of care.

3. Challenges to global mental health care include:
   A. Overuse of powerful neuroleptic drugs
   B. Lack of human rights protection for people with mental illness

      C. Overabundance of locked psychiatric facilities in resource-constrained low-income countries

      D. Lack of local, community-based services for people with mental illness

      E. All of the above

4. Which of the following interventions have been found to effectively address the mental health treatment gap in low-income countries?

      A. Decentralization of mental health care

      B. Task-sharing with nonspecialists

      C. Improvement of primary health care systems in low-resource communities

      D. Strengthening of information systems, including electronic medical records

      E. All of the above

Answers to Self-Assessment Questions

    1. (B)
    2. (C)
    3. (E)
    4. (E)

Index

The page numbers in "**bold**" are tables and those in "*italics*" are figures.

5-HT₃ serotonergic, 179

absolute risk
  calculating, 12
  first-degree relative and, 12
  of schizophrenia, 14
abstinence syndromes,
    190–191
  babies and treatment for
    opioid, 192
  physical examination and, 191
Academy of Cognitive Therapy,
    396
acamprosate, 209–210, 372
acceptance and commitment
    therapy (ACT), 156
acetylation, histone, 18
acetylcholinesterase inhibitors
    (ACHEIs), 277, 374–375
  NMDA combination therapy,
    375
acute and transient psychotic
    disorder (ATPD), 107
acute grief, 443, 444
acute intoxication, 190, 191, 419
acute opioid intoxication, 196
acute stress disorder (ASD),
    153, 166, 167, 168, 169
  case, 176
  etiological insights into, 174
  future directions for
    treatment of, 175
  sample interview questions,
    175
  treatment of, 171–172
acute syndromes, substance
    use disorders and,
    195–197
addiction
  behavioral change and, 403
  medication for, 371–373
  risk for, 345
adjustment disorders, 166–167,
    168, 169

acute stress disorder (ASD),
    168
  anxious mood and, 134
  diagnosis of, 170
  treatment of, 174
  vs. depression, 430–431
  with depressed mood, 84
adolescents
  evidenced-based prevention
    programs and, 228
  psychiatric disorders and, 2
  psychiatry, 318
  psychotic symptoms and, 30
  substance use disorders and,
    227
  substance use disorders
    screening tools, 227
adoption studies, 186
adrenocorticotropin hormone
    (ACTH), 27
advanced sleep phase disorder
    (ASPD), 337, *See also*
    sleep disorders
Affordable Care Act (ACA)
    2010, 475
  and parity protections, 477
agonist therapy
  buprenorphine for treatment
    of opioid use disorders, 212
  methadone for treatment
    of opioid use disorders,
    211–212
agoraphobia, 129, 132, 133
  case example, 142–143
  phobic neurosis diagnosis,
    129
alcohol dehydrogenase, 187
alcohol use disorders, 52, 179,
    191, 200
  acamprosate for treatment
    of, 209–210
  Alcohol Use Disorders
    Identification Test
    (AUDIT), 199

consumption patterns, 179
dependence, 219
depressive symptoms and, 83
detoxification from alcohol
    use, 206–207
disulfiram for treatment of,
    210, 213
early intervention and
    prevention, 179
family history of, 185–187
FDA approved medications
    for, 210
known history of, 198
naltrexone for treatment of,
    208–209
psychoactive properties of,
    179
specialized mental health
    counseling, 435
statistics and, 184
suicides and, 184
treatment of, 203, 208–211,
    218, 229
withdrawal seizures and,
    179
Alcohol Use Disorders
    Identification Test
    (AUDIT), 199
Alcoholics Anonymous (AA),
    204, 210, 216, 395
aldehyde dehydrogenase, 187
algorithm-driven care, 434
allostasis, 191
alpha-2 adrenergic agonists,
    377
Alzheimer's Association, 266
Alzheimer's disease (AD), 124,
    267, 373
  Anti-Amyloid Treatment, 283
  cause of dementia, 265
  interventions for, 283
  major or mild NCD, 263
  medications for, **279**
  Memantine and, 279

Alzheimer's disease (AD) (*cont.*)
  neurocognitive disorders due
    to, 268–269
  stages of, **266**
American Academy of Child
    and Adolescent Psychiatry
    (AACAP), 319
American Academy of
    Neurology, 275
American Board of Psychiatry
    & Neurology (ABPN), 2
American Psychiatric
    Association (APA), 43,
    303, 459, 460
American Psychological
    Association (APA), 453,
    459, 460, 466
anabolic-androgenic steroids,
    183
aneuploidy, 13
anhedonia. *See* depressive
    disorders
anorexia nervosa (AN), 289,
    See also eating disorders
  crossover to bulimia nervosa
    and, 294
  mortality and, 293–294, 300
  recovery and relapse,
    292–293
  treatment options for,
    304–305
  weight loss and, 297
antagonist therapy
  naltrexone for treatment of
    opioid use disorders, 213
anticonvulsants
  mood-altering, *365*, 365–366
  mood-stabilizing, **363**
antidepressant medication. *See*
    antidepressants
antidepressants, 10, 76, 88, 306,
    335, 342–343, 378, 390
  adverse effects, 346–347
  adverse effects of, **347**
  antidepressant-related
    emergencies and, 348–351
  choosing, 351
  classification of, 343–346
  discovery of, 19
  rapid-acting, 352–353
  self-assessment questions,
    387–388
  treatment duration, 351
  treatment of bulimia nervosa
    with, 305

tricyclic antidepressants,
    137, 279, 281, 333, 342,
    344, 345, 361, 378
  use for anxiety disorders,
    136–137
anti-NMDA-receptor
    encephalitis, 25
antipsychotic drugs, 10,
    353–358
  adverse effects of, 360–362
  atypical antipsychotics, 278
  long-term treatment, 359
  short-term treatment,
    356–359
  use for anxiety disorders,
    137
antipsychotic-antimanic drugs,
    366
antisocial personality disorders
    (ASPD), 64, 246–247
  cluster B disorders, 245–246
  malingering and, 439
  treatment, 246–247
  violent behavior and, 64
anxiety disorders
  and children, 321
  Anxiety Disorders Interview
    Schedule (ADIS), 135
  case examples, 141–142
  changes to classification
    of, 140
  classification of, 128–129
  clinical features and course
    of, 130–131
  diagnosis, 133–134
  epidemiology, 129
  etiological formulations, 139
  evaluation, 134–135
  FDA approved SSRIs and
    SNRIs, **137**
  genetic risks of, 12–13
  medical comorbidities and,
    129–130
  sample interview questions,
    140–141
  self-assessment questions,
    144–145
  social and economic burden
    of, 130
  suicidal ideation and
    behaviors, 130
  treatment, 135–138
anxiolytics and hypnotics,
    370–371
anxious distress, 74

Applebaum, P. S., 67, 431
appreciation, 68, 431
arousal/regulatory systems, 6
Asian population, alcohol
    consumption among, 187
Asperger's syndrome, 243
assertive community treatment
    (ACT), 401
associated management
    strategies, **424–426**
Association of American
    Medical Colleges (AAMC),
    2
Atomoxetine (Strattera), 377
attention deficit hyperactivity
    disorder (ADHD), 345
  hereditability and, 4
  medicines for, 375
attenuated psychosis
    syndrome, 107
atypical anorexia nervosa, 291
AUDIT-Consumption
    (AUDIT-C), 200
autism spectrum disorders
    (ASD), 153
  ADHD genetic overlap and,
    18
  communication and, 322
  food-related anxiety and, 296
  hereditability and, 4
  heritability and, 13
  high functioning variants
    of, 243
  paternal age and, 110
  risks for developing, 14
avoidant personality disorders
    (AVPD), 242, 243,
    255–256
  treatment, 255–256
avoidant/restrictive food intake
    disorder (ARFID), 290,
    294, 295

Babinsky, Joseph, 9
bath salts, 181, 193, 196
BDD-Symptom Scale, 155
Beach, Frank, 459
Beck, Aaron, 393
behavioral and physical health
    systems, siloed, 478–479
behavioral couples therapy
    (BCT), 218
behavioral health
  behavioral health provider
    (BHP), 3

billing for services of health care managers, 480
inadequate insurance coverage for, 476–477
integrated care, 220–221
integrated with primary care and, 3–4, 432–433
integration of with physical health care, 482
treatment of disorders and, 473
behavioral learning theory interventions, 216–217
behavioral therapies, 219
    pharmacotherapy use with, 219–220
    substance use disorders and, 214–215
Benson, Herbert, 409
benzodiazepines, 135–136
bereavement, 85–86, 443–444
beta-blockers, 135
    used for anxiety disorders, 137
binge-eating disorder (BED), 290, 295, See also eating disorders
    episode of, 291
    recovery and relapse, 293
    treatment options for, 306
biofeedback, 408, 410
bipolar disorders
    anticonvulsants in treatment of, 365–366
    children and adolescents and, 319–320
    classification of, 89–90
    clinical course, 90
    duration of treatment for, 98
    effect of on other medical illness, 91
    electroconvulsive therapy (ECT) treatment for, 381
    epidemiology of, 320
    evaluation of patient, 96–97
    full remissions, 94
    genetics and, 12
    hereditability and, 4
    hypomanic episode phase, 93–94
    incidence of, 12
    long-term prophylactic treatment for, 367–368
    major depressive disorder (MDD) and, 91, 95

manic episode, 91–93
medication-induced, 90, 95
mood-stabilizing drugs for, 362–365
morbidity and mortality, 90
other mental conditions and, 95
prevalence of, 90, 320
psychotic symptoms and, 92
recurrent episodes of, 94
risk assessment and, 97
second-generation antipsychotics in, **364**
substance-induced, 95
suicide and, 94
treatment options for, 97–98
blood alcohol content (BAC), 195
Blood Oxygen Level Dependent (BOLD) signal, 30
body dysmorphic disorder (BDD), 146, 147
    case example, 159
borderline personality disorder (BPD), 76, 234, 245, 247–251, 396
    cognitive-behavioral treatment and, 396
    skill deficit remediation and, 394
    treatment of, 249–251
borderline schizophrenia, 240
boundaries, between clinicians and patients, 41–42
brain function, 26, 28, 125
    biological basis of, 20
    circuit-based understanding of, 9
    connection between immune molecules and, 24, 26
    emotional phenomena, 9
    mental homeostasis and, 390
    psychotherapeutic treatments and, 389
brain imaging techniques, 10
Brain on Fire, 25
brain pathology
    history and clinical syndromes, 9–10
brain signaling molecules, 19–22
brexanolone, 353
brief psychotic disorder, 106–107
    psychotic symptoms, 106

brief reactive psychosis, 107
Broca, Paul, 9
building blocks
    for mental health, treatment modalities and, 394
bulimia nervosa (BN), 289, 291, See also eating disorders
    crossover to anorexia nervosa, 294
    mortality and, 300
    recovery and relapse, 293
    treatment options for, 305–306
buprenorphine, 204, 212
    for opioid dependence, 372
    opioid use disorders treatment, 212
    treatment of opioid withdrawal, 208
bupropion, 348

Cade, John, 364
cancer
    depression and, 72
    heritability of ovarian, 13
cannabinoids, 181, 192
cannabis use disorders, 208, 214
    adolescents and young adults, 188
    cannabis intoxication, 192
    psychotic disorder and, 228
    schizophrenia and, 110
    treatment for, 181
capacity
    assessment, 66–68
    decision-making, 431
    evaluations, **432**
    self-assessment questions, 69
Carlsson, Arvid, 19
catatonia, 94
    electroconvulsive therapy (ECT) treatment for, 381
    major depression and, 76
Center for Transgender Excellence, 464
Centers for Disease Control and Prevention (CDC), 180, 318, 342, 451
central sigma receptors, 182
central sleep apnea syndromes, 338, 339, See also sleep disorders

cerebrovascular health and cognitive functioning, 282
characterologic dysphoria, 84
Charcot, Jean-Martin, 9
chief complaint, 44
child and adolescent psychiatry, 318, 323
shortage of child psychiatrists, 3
child- and family-focused cognitive behavior therapy (CFF-CBT), 320
child/children
anxiety disorders and, 321
depression and, 318
depressive disorders in, 320–321
disinhibited social engagement disorder and, 323–324
post-traumatic stress disorder PTSD) and, 324
psychiatric disorders and, 2
psychotic symptoms in, 324–326
selective mutism and, 322
separation anxiety disorder and, 322
specific phobia and, 322
substance use disorders and, 227
treatment for depression in children, 320
Chisholm, Brock, 1
chlorpromazine, 19
chronic disease management strategies, 434
cigarette smoking, decline of, 180
circadian rhythm disorders, 337–338
circuits
and brain signaling molecules, 19–22
converging, 28–32
classification systems, 5
Client-Centered Therapy, 405
mind-body therapies,
Clinical Institute Withdrawal Assessment for Alcohol (CIWA-Ar), 198
clinical interview, patients with MDD and, 86–87

clinical neurosciences, 7, 9, 33, 34, 35
self-assessment questions, 36
Clinical Opiate Withdrawal Scale (COWS), 198
clinical psychiatry, 6, 9, 26, 38
and symptom-based diagnoses, 6
clinician-rated instruments, 153
club drugs, 193
clubhouses, 402
cluster disorders
cluster A disorders, 240–241
cluster B disorders, 245–246
cluster C disorders, 254–255
cocaine, 23, 95, 181, 184, 188, 193, 196, 214, 350, 376, 468
administration in mice, 18
dependence, 219
intravenous, 187
withdrawal phases of, 83
cognitive and attentional disorders
medications for, 373–375
cognitive behavior therapy (CBT), 138, 171, 175, 217–218, 312, 321, 324, 351, 393–396, 397
obsessive-compulsive disorders (OCD) and, 155
therapy for depression in children, 319
treatment for insomnia, 330
treatment option for eating disorders, 301–302
cognitive impairment
differential diagnosis and, 272–273
evaluation, 273
cognitive processing therapy (CPT), 172
cognitive reserve model, 277, 282
cognitive systems, 6
cognitive therapy (CT), treatment for OCD, 155
collateral history, 423, 430
collateral history', 427
common variants, searching for, 14–16
compassion fatigue, 442

compassion, patient interview process and, 40–41
complex disorders, polygenic, 4
confusional arousals, 334
consultation-liaison psychiatry/psychiatrists, 422, 431, 432
contingency management (CM), 216–217
copy number variants (CNVs), 4, 15
corticotropin-releasing hormone (CRH), 27
Cotard's syndrome, 75
COVID-19, 7
neuropsychiatric manifestations of, 24
CRAFFT screen, 201–203
cue exposure, 216
cyclothymic disorder, 362
diagnostic criteria for children, 320
cytochrome p450 system, 15

deacetylation, 18
deep brain stimulation (DBS), 384
deep TMS device, 383
Delay, Jean, 19
delayed sleep phase disorder (DSPD), 337
deletion syndrome, 14
delirium, 263–279, 280
clinical features and onset, 264–265
evaluation of, 274
precipitating factors and, 280
predisposing factors for, 280
treatment of, 275–276
delusional disorder, 105–106
diagnostic criteria, 105
specify types of, 105–106
delusions
psychotic depression and, 75
dementia
age and, 265
associated neuropsychiatric syndromes treatment, 278
behavioral and psychological symptoms of, 277–280

cases, 285
cognitive symptoms of, 277
dementia electroconvulsive
 therapy, 280
electroconvulsive therapy
 (ECT) for, 381
factors for delirium, 281
future research and,
 283–284
neurodegenerative, 270, 373
new treatments for, 375
prevalence rates for, 283
progressive, 266
progressive
 neurodegenerative, 263
sample interview questions,
 284
self-assessment questions,
 286–287
treatments for
 neuropsychiatric
 symptoms, 278–280
dementia praecox, 102, 115, 125
demoralization, 85, 132
denial
 of a problem, 205
 response to illness, 195,
 429–430
Deniker, Pierre, 19
dependent personality disorder
 (DPD), 255–256
dependent personality disorder
 (DPD), 256–257
depressive disorders, 79, 81,
 86, 94, 346
 adjustment disorders and, 84
 alcohol use disorders and,
 83
 anxiety and, 74
 bereavement and, 85–86
 bipolar disorders and, 94
 children and, 318
 classification of, 70
 depressed mood or
 anhedonia, 73, 79
 depression,
 disruptive mood
 dysregulation disorder,
 320–321
 disruptive mood regulation
 disorder and, 82
 electroconvulsive therapy
 (ECT) treatment for, 380

epidemiology of and
 children, 318
episode specifiers, 94
following medical illness, 72
medication-induced, 83
mild depression and, 79
mixed mood features and,
 75
morbidity and mortality
 and, 72
neurovegetative symptoms
 of, 86
persistent, 79–81
rapid-acting antidepressants
 and, 353
related to another medical
 condition, 82–83
remission from, 79
seasonal variation pattern
 of, 77
self-assessment questions for
 children and adolescents,
 327–328
severe depression and, 64,
 79, 89
severe depression and
 electroconvulsive therapy,
 98, 280
short-term treatment for,
 366–367
statistics, 80
substance-induced, 83
treatment of, in children, 319
treatment options for, 87–89
treatment-resistant
 depression (TRD), 352
unipolar depression in
 children, 321
detoxification
 alcohol use disorders,
 206–207
 from other drugs, 208
 medically-supervised, 179
 opioids, 207–208
 program for severe alcohol
 use disorders, 435
 sedative-hypnotics, 206–207
diagnosable mental disorder, 1
Diagnostic and Statistical
 Manual of Mental
 Disorders, Fifth Edition
 (DSM-5), 5, 70, 128, 146,
 189, 436

(DSM-IV-TR), 166
diagnoses, 50
Diagnostic and Statistical
 Manual (DSM), 10
 psychiatric diagnoses
 of gender and sexual
 orientation and, 460
 system of categorization, 5
dialectical behavior therapy
 (DBT), 156, 250, 394, 395,
 396–398
diffusion tensor imaging (DTI),
 30
discontinuation (withdrawal
 syndromes), 379–380
disinhibited social engagement
 disorder, 323–324
dissociative drugs, 182, 193,
 196
disulfiram, 210, 213
dizygotic twins, 12, 308
domestic violence, 56
 assessing the risk, 59–60
 care with mental illness
 diagnosis, 60–61
 clinical documentation in,
 60–61
 clinical presentations of, 57
 definition of, 56–57
 interventions and, 61
 outcomes and, 61
 prevalence and impact of, 57
 referring victims to help, 60
 screening and assessment,
 58–59
Dominantly Inherited
 Alzheimer's Network
 (DIAN), 283
dopamine D2 receptor (DRD2),
 16
dopamine system, 21, 22, 124
dopamine transporter (DAT),
 23
Down's syndrome, 272
drug allergies, 47
Drug Assessment Screening
 Tool (DAST-10), 200
drug overdose, 2
drug reinforcement, 187
drug use disorders, 214
 statistics and, 184
Durable Power of Attorney for
 Health Care, 68

dysphoria, 24, 52, 86, 182, 278, 290, 394
  and personality disorders, 84
  gender, 460–461, 464–465, 469
dysphoric mania, 92

eating disorders
  adult case example, 312–313
  anorexia nervosa (AN), 31, 289, 291
  bulimia nervosa (BN), 291
  child cases of, 313–314
  classification of, 289–291
  course and outcome for, 292
  diagnostic crossover and, 294
  differencing from normative behaviors, 297
  differential diagnosis and, 295–296
  differentiating from a medical disorder, 296–297
  directions for research, **310**
  epidemiology and impact of, 291–292
  etiological factors and, 291–292
  evaluation of, 298–299
  family-based treatments (FBT) for, 302–303
  future research and, 309
  management team for treatment of, 307
  mortality and, 293–294
  neurobiological risk factors for, 308
  not otherwise specified (EDNOS), 291
  pharmacologic management of, 304
  recovery and relapse, 292–294
  residential and inpatient treatment for, 303–304
  sample interview questions, 311
  self-assessment questions, 316–317
  supplemental questions, 311–312
  suspected, 299–301
  treatment approaches for, 301–307
  types of, 289–290

electroconvulsive therapy (ECT), 76, 342, 380–381, 389
  cognition and, 381–382
  safety and adverse effects of, 381
Ellis, Albert, 393
emergency psychiatry, 415–416
empathy, 64, 76, 204, 253, 399, 404
  and the patient interview process, 40–41
Employee Retirement Income Security Act (ERISA) (1974), 474
employer-sponsored health insurance (ESI), 474
endocrine system
  endocrinologic disorders, 82
  link to psychiatric illness, 27–28
end-of-life priorities, **441**
end-stage renal disease (ESRD), 475
enzymatic attachment, 18
Epidemiologic Catchment Area (ECA) study, 184
epigenetics, 18
erotomania, 113
ethyl alcohol, 179
evidence-based psychotherapy, 88
evidenced-based prevention programs
  adolescents and, 228
evidence-based screening assessments, 221
exome sequencing, 14
exposure and response prevention (ERP) component, 155

factitious disorder, 438–440
factual understanding criteria, 67
Fagerstrom Test for Nicotine Dependence, 199
failure of humanity, a, 490
familial relative risk, 12
family and couples therapy, 218–219, *See also* family-based treatments (FBT)
family history, patients', 48
family psychoeducation, 402

family-based treatments (FBT), 218–219, 228
  eating disorders and, 302–303
Farmer, Paul, 1
feeding disorders, 290–291, 294–295
fluoxetine, 304, 305, 319, 348, 352
Ford, Clellan, 459
FRAMES model, 204–205
Freud, Sigmund, 10, 174, 393
  Three Essays on the Theory of Sexuality (Freud), 456
frontotemporal neurocognitive disorder (FTNCD), 270
functional brain imaging techniques, 10
functional neural connectivity field, 7

Galton, Francis, 456
gender and sexuality, 456–458
  affirming treatment, 466–467
  and non-binary/gender-expansive categories, 452–453
  Diagnostic and Statistical Manual (DSM-5) diagnosis of, 460
  history of psychiatric diagnoses of, 459–460
  minority stress and, 458–459
  psychiatric evaluation and treatment of issues with, 462–463
  sexual identity development and, 456–458
gender dysphoria, 460–461, 464–465, 469
gender expression, 450, 465, 466
gender identity, 448–449
  gender and, 449–451
  gender identity disorder, 460
  gender roles and, 450
  psychiatry of sexual orientation, 456–458
  sex and, 449
  sexual orientation and, 448
gene, 13
  DNA methylation, 18
gene expression, 18

generalized anxiety disorder (GAD), 6, 132, 234
  7-item Scale (GAD-7), 135
  case examples, 141–142
genetic heritability, 186, 308
genetic mutations, age and, 110
genetic risks, 18, 24, 308
  alcohol use and, 186
  Alzheimer's disease (AD), 282
  psychiatric disorders and, 4, 12
  schizophrenia and, 25
  vascular disease risk factors and, 282
genetics, psychiatric, 4–5
Genome-Wide Association Studies (GWAS), 16–18
  use of data from, 17
genotype, 13
Global Burden of Disease study, 108
global disease burden, 184
global health, 486–487, 491
  agenda, 490
  burden of illness, 486
  delivery, 491
  global health equity, 1
  standard of clinical care, 489
global mental health care delivery
  self-assessment questions, 495–496
global population, growth of, 2
global treatment gaps
  and integrated health care, 3
glutamate and gamma-aminobutyric acid (GABA), 20
G-protein inwardly-rectifying potassium (GIRK) ion channels, 179
grief, 392, 443–444, 445
  acute, 444
  unbearable, 391
Griesinger, Wilhelm, 9
Grisso, T., 67
group therapy, 398–400
Guidelines for Psychological Practice with Lesbian, Gay, and Bisexual Clients, 466

hair pulling disorder (HPD), 146, 148
  case example, 160
hallucinogens, 182, 193, 197
haplotypes, 16
head imaging (CT or MRI), and patient with delirium and, 274
health care coverage
  self-assessment questions, 484–485
  United States and, 473
health care proxies, 68
health care system, 433, 482, 489
  United States, 283, 473–474, 479, 482
health insurance
  behavioral health coverage and, 476
  employer-sponsored, 474
  federal, 475
  Medicaid, 475
  Medicare, 475
  sources of coverage, 474
  universal, 473
healthy living interventions, 402
heritability
  anorexia nervosa (AN) and, 308
  antisocial personality disorders (ASPD), 246
  avoidant personality disorder (AVPD) and, 255
  borderline personality disorder (BPD) and, 248
  dependent personality disorder (DPD) and, 256
  for a disorder, 13
  genetic, 186
  histrionic personality disorder and, 251
  mental illness and, 12
  missing, 15
  narcissistic personality disorder (NPD) and, 253
  obsessive-compulsive personality disorder (OCPD) and, 257
  paranoid personality disorder (PPD) and, 241, 243
  schizoid personality disorder (SzPD) and, 243

schizophrenia and, 16
  schizotypal personality disorder and, 244
Hispanics
  prevalence and treatment outcomes of mental disorders, 2
histocompatibility complex (MHC) locus, 17
histone acetylation, 18
histrionic personality disorder (HPD), 251
  treatment of, 252–253
HIV. See human immunodeficiency virus (HIV)
hoarding disorder (HD), 146, 147–148
  case example, 160
homosexuality, 459, 460
  codified as a disease, 459
hormones, 19, 28
  and mental illnesses, 26–28
  masculinizing therapy, 468
Human Connectome Project (HCP), 30
human genome, 4, 13, 16
human immunodeficiency virus (HIV)
  depression and, 72
  global health programs and, 486
  group therapy for people diagnosed with, 398
  injecting drug use and, 180, 185
  low testosterone and depressive symptoms in men with, 83
  neurocognitive disorders and, 263
  neurocognitive disorders resulting from, 271
  primary health care and, 491
  secondary mania and, 95
  stimulant use and risky behaviors and, 182
  transgender people's increased risk for, 451
human rights, and institutional care, 489
human sexuality and gender, 467
Huntington's disease, 271

hydroponically-engineered hemp plants, 181
hypersomnias, 335–337
hyperthymic temperament, 96
hypnotics and anxiolytics, 370–371
hypothalamic-pituitary-gonadal (HPG) axis, 28

illness
  medical, 428
imaging studies, 421–422
immune cell dysfunction psychiatric symptoms and, 25
immune system, 24–26
IMPACT Model (Improving Mood Promoting Access to Collaborative Treatment), 479–480, 481
informed consent, 66
inhalants, 183
injection drug use, 180, 185
Insel, Thomas, 10
insomnia, 329–333
  cognitive, 330
  differential diagnosis of, 331
  induced, 182
  initial, 86
  middle, 87
  suicide risk and, 53
  symptomatic treatment of, 174
  terminal, 87
institutional care, and human rights, 489
integrated behavioral health care, 220–221
integrated mental health care, 3
integrative health care programs, 436
Interagency Standing Committee Guidelines (IASC), 491
International Classifications of Disease (ICD-10) system, 104
International Genomics Consortium (PGC), 4
International Statistical Classification of Diseases and Related Health Problems-10, 5

interpersonal psychotherapy (IPT), for treating depression in children, 319
intersex traits, 452
intoxication syndromes, 183
intrauterine opioid exposure, 192

Kinsey, Alfred, 459
Kleinman, Arthur, 490
Kraepelin, Emil, 102

laboratory studies
  psychiatric symptoms and, 420–421
Lewy bodies, 263, 265, 335
  neurocognitive disorder due to, 269–270
LGBTQ people, 457, 458–459, 460, 463
  affirming treatment and, 466–467
  health disparities and, 458
  psychiatric evaluation of, 463–464
Liebenluft, Ellen, 320
Liebowitz Social Anxiety Scale (LSAS), 135
life expectancy
  of people with mental illnesses, 2
  United States, 476
lifestyle
  behavioral therapies and modification of, 215
  changes for improved health, 435
  cognitive behavior therapy (CBT), 396
  eating disorders and healthy, 298
  of people with schizophrenia, 402
  patients', 47
  sedentary, 308
  somatic symptom disorders and a healthy, 437
  substance use disorders and, 194
ligands, 180
Lindqvist, Maria, 19
linkage disequilibrium, 16
Lisdexamfetamine dimesylate (LDX), 306

lithium salts, 364–365
locus, 13
long term depression (LTD), 20
long-term antipsychotic treatment, 359–360
lower socioeconomic groups and schizophrenia, 110

maintenance therapies, 371–373
major depression. *See* major depressive disorders
major depressive disorder (MDD), 6, 73–74, 234
  atypical features of, 76, 91
  bipolar disorder and, 95
  catatonia and, 76
  clinical course and, 71–72
  clinical findings and, **431**
  clinical interview of patients, 86–87
  DSM criteria for children, 318
  DSM-5 diagnostic criteria, 73, **73–74**
  laboratory evaluation of patient with MDD, 87
  melancholic features of, 75–76
  morbidity and mortality and, 72
  norepinephrine depletion, 19
  onset of, 71–72
  peripartum onset and, 77
  persistent depressive disorder and, 79–81
  physical exam of patient, 87
  prevalence of, 71
  risk assessment of, 87
  self-assessment questions, 100–101
  serotonin depletion and, 19
  suicide and, 77–79
  treatment duration of, 351
  unipolar major depressive disorder, 89
  with psychotic features, 75
major depressive disorders (MDDD)
  psychotic symptoms and, 75
major psychiatric disorders
  discovery of pharmacological treatments for, 10

malingering, 438–440

Manhattan plot, 16

mania and psychotic disorders
pharmacological treatment,
353

MAPS TO diagnosis, 45

marijuana. *See* cannabinoids

masculinizing hormone
therapy, 468

Massachusetts General Hospital
Hairpulling Scale, 155

mediated neurotransmission,
179

Medicaid, 266, 475–476

medical and behavioral health
care, integration of,
479–480

medical detoxification, 206

medical history, 47

medical illnesses/problems, 7,
24, 82, 95, 251, 277, 417,
420, 428, 439
anxiety disorders and, 130
behavioral factors and, 479
bipolar disorders impact on,
91
emotional responses to,
428–430, **429**
impact of mental illness
on, 72
mental illness and, 2
psychiatric, 1
psychotic disorders and, 105
untreated psychiatric illness
and, 123

Medicare, 266, 475, 478, 480,
481
Medicare Advantage, 475

medications
adhering to treatment, 378
confirming using, 427
current, 47
for attention deficit
hyperactivity disorder
(ADHD), 375
mood-altering, **369**

meiosis, 16

memantine, 277, 278, 375

menopause, 71

mental disorders
classification of, 5–6
diagnosable, 1
future diagnostic system
and, 5–6

treating when comorbid
with an eating disorder,
306–307
worldwide prevalence of, in
children and adolescents, 2

mental health
clinicians, 4, 62, 433, 465
co-co-location of providers,
479
co-location of providers, 435
global challenges in care
delivery, 492
increase need for treatment, 2
integrated care, 3
integration of treatment, 3
models of care, 433
neglected healthcare, 7
providers, 482
providers, 434
shortage of clinicians, 3
treatment gap, 488
treatment settings, 247
treatments, 487
workforce shortage and, 2–3

mental health care delivery
global, 489–491
nonspecialist, 489–491
task sharing and, 489–491

Mental Health Gap program,
490

Mental Health Parity Act, 477

Mental Health Parity and
Addiction Equity Act
(MHPAEA), 477

mental health services
decentralization of, 491–492

mental homeostasis, 390

mental illnesses
assessing risks posed to
others, 62
cultural factors and, 72
global impact of, 487
heritability, 14
human suffering and, 1
life expectancy and, 6
patients and risk factors for
violence, 62–63
relapse or recurrence of, 379
serious and community-
based programs for,
400–403
statistics, 1
substance use disorders and,
184

suicide and, 2

mental status examination
(MSE), 48–49, 60, 87, 117,
171, 273, 298, 417–418
electronic medical record
system (EMR) and, 43, 481
electronic medical record
system (EMR) checklist, 48
laboratory evaluation and, 49
mini, 284
neurocognitive disorders
and, **273**
psychotic symptoms and, 118
substance intoxication and,
190

mentalization-based treatment
(MBT), 250, 254

mesocortical pathway, 21

mesolimbic system, 23

methadone, 196, 204, 217, 229
maintenance treatment
facilities usage in, 217
opioid use disorders and,
208, 371–372
opioid use disorders
treatment, 211–212
pharmacogenomics and, 221

methamphetamine, 181, 184

Miller, William, 403

mind-body therapies, 407–408
biological mechanisms and,
409
historical perspective,
408–409

mindfulness-based cognitive
therapy (MBCT), 409

mindfulness-based eating
awareness therapy
(MB-EAT), 409

mindfulness-based relapse
prevention (MBRP), 409

mindfulness-based stress
reduction (MBSR), 408

Minnesota Multiphasic
Personality Inventory
(MMPI), 463

minority stress theory, 458

missing heritability, 15

mixed mood episode, 75

monoamine oxidase (MAO)
inhibitors, 137, 256, 342,
376

monoamine receptors
blockade of, 19

monozygotic twins, 12, 19
and psychiatric disease, 13
mood disorders, 27, 52, 64,
96, 104, 105, 117, 134,
136, 306, 318, 383,
415, *See also* depressive
disorders, post-traumatic
stress disorders (PTSD)
and neuroimaging, 99
DSM-5 Classification of, **70**
mood-stabilizing agents
adverse effects of, 368
motivational enhancement
therapies, 215–216
motivational interviewing
approach, 194, 215, 216,
228, 403–407, 434
examples, 407

naltrexone, 208–209, 221, 372
opioid use disorders
treatment, 213
narcissistic personality disorder
(NPD), 253–254
treatment of, 253–254
Narcotics Anonymous (NA),
216
meetings of, 230
National Alliance on Mental
Illness (NAMI), 403
National Alzheimer's Plan
(2011), 283
National Center for
Complementary and
Alternative Medicine
(NCCAM). *See* National
Center for Complementary
and Integrative Health
(NCCIH)
National Center for
Complementary and
Integrative Health
(NCCIH),
National Comorbidity Survey
Replication (NCS-R), 129
National Consensus Project
Clinical Practice
Guidelines for Quality
Palliative Care, 440
National Health Interview
Survey, 407
National Institute of Aging,
266

National Institute of Mental
Health (NIMH), 6, 10, 108,
157, 325
National Institute on Drug
Abuse, 227
National LGBT Health
Education Center, 463
National Survey on Drug Use
and Health (NSDUH), 184,
194, 477
negative valence systems, 6
negativism, 76
neural circuits, 12, 28–30
identification of, 5
neurobehavioral disorder, 186
neurocognitive disorders
classification of, 263–264
criteria for, **264**
due to Alzheimer's disease
(AD), 268–269
due to other medical
illnesses, 272
evaluation of, **273**
HIV infection and, 271
Lewy bodies (NCDLB) and,
269–270
major, 268
major or mild, 265–266
medication/drug-induced,
272
mild, 266–267, **268**
neurodegenerative dementias,
270
neurohormone systems,
functioning of, 249
neuroimaging, 5
neurologic conditions
laboratory evaluation and,
97
neurological disorders/illnesses
(NCD), 82, 281–282, 486,
490
evaluation of patients with,
275
treatment of, 276
neuromodulation approaches
to mental health care, 7
neuropharmacology, 221
neurotherapeutics, 380
neurotransmitters, 19–22
technologies for studying,
23–24
nicotine dependence, 192, 371

pharmacotherapy for,
213–214
nicotine withdrawal, 180
nicotinic acetylcholine
receptors, 214
nicotinic cholinergic signaling,
179
nigrostriatal pathway, 21
NIMH RDoC system, 7
NMDA receptor antagonism,
182
NMDA-mediated
glutamatergic excitatory
neurotransmission, 179
N-methyl-D-aspartate (NMDA)
receptor antagonist, 375
non-binary patients
psychological evaluation of,
464–465
non-binary/gender-expansive
identities, 452–453
normative sadness, 86
nosology, 10–12
nucleosomes, 18
nucleotides, 13

obsessive-compulsive
personality disorder
(OCPD), 150, 234, 254,
257–258
hoarding and, 147
treatment for, 257
obsessive-compulsive and
related disorders (OCRDs),
146, 151, 153
case examples, 159–161
clinical features, 149–151
criteria of, 146
diagnosis of, 151
epidemiology and impact,
148–149
etiological insights, 151
future directions, 156–158
sample interview questions,
158
semi-structured diagnostic
interviews for, 153
obsessive-compulsive disorders
(OCD), 129, 146, 147
case example, 159
Obsessive-Compulsive
Inventory-Revised
measure, 154

treatment, 155–156
olanzapine, 352
one gene-one syndrome, 23
opioid use disorders, 192
    buprenorphine as treatment
        for, 212
    detoxification from opioids,
        207–208
    methadone as treatment of,
        211–212
    naltrexone as treatment for,
        213
    opioid withdrawal, 180, 192,
        198, 207–208, 209, 212
    opioids, 180
    overdoses and, 180
    treatment of, 229–230
opium poppy plant, 180
optogenetics, 7
Organization for Economic
    Cooperation and
    Development (OECD)
    universal health coverage,
        473–474
oxycodone, 204

palliative care
    case examples, 444–445
    medicine, 440–443
panic disorder, 131–132
    without agoraphobia, 142–143
Panic Disorder Severity Scale
    (PDSS), 135
paranoid personality disorder
    (PPD), 241–242
    prevalence of, 241
    treatment options and, 242
paraphilic disorders, 462
parasomnias, 334–335
Parkinson's disease, 271
paternal age, schizophrenia
    and, 110
patient interview, 38, 427
    confidentiality and, 40
    developing interviewing
        skills, 43
    directioning, 42–43
    importance of safety and
        respect, 42
    importance of therapeutic
        alliance to, 39–40
    purpose of, 39–40
    setting boundaries, 38

setting up (structure of),
    42–43
showing empathy and
    compassion, 40–41
patients
    and capacity to make
        decisions, 66–68
    collateral history of, 423,
        427
    diagnostic evaluation of,
        421
    interviewing the, 427
pedophilia, 395
peer movement, 402
peripartum onset, 94
    major depression and, 77
persecutory delusions, 113
persistent depressive disorder,
    79–81
personality disorders, 233–238,
    424–426
    antisocial personality
        disorders (ASPD), 64,
        246–247
    avoidant personality
        disorders (AVPD), 255–256
    borderline personality
        disorder (BPD), 76, 234,
        247–251, 394, 396
    case examples, 259–260
    cluster B disorders, 245–246
    cluster C disorders, 254–255
    dependent personality
        disorders (DPD), 256–257
    dependent personality
        disorders (DPD) treatment,
        255–256
    differential diagnosis and
        comorbidities, 236–238
    dysphoria in, 84
    future research and, 258
    histrionic personality
        disorder (HPD), 251
    histronic personality
        disorder (HPD) treatment,
        252–253
    narcissistic personality
        disorder (NPD), 253–254
    narcissistic personality
        disorder (NPD) treatment,
        253–254
    obsessive-compulsive
        personality disorder

(OCPD), 147, 150, 234,
    257–258
    obsessive-compulsive
        personality disorder
        (OCPD) treatment, 257
    paranoid personality
        disorder (PPD), 241–242
    paranoid personality
        disorder (PPD) treatment,
        242, 243
    pharmacologic treatments
        for, 238
    prevalence of, 234
    psychotherapy treatment
        for, 238
    sample interview questions
        and, 259
    schizoid personality disorder
        (SzPD), 242–243
    schizotypal, 102, 240
    schizotypal personality
        disorder (StPD), 244–245
    treatment of, 239–240
personality type, hyperthymic
    personality, 96
PET studies, 5
pharmacodynamics, 15
pharmacogenomics, 221
    genetic variation and, 15
pharmacological treatments
    discovery of, 10
    personality disorders and,
        235
pharmacotherapy, 87, 277
    behavioral therapy use with,
        219–220
    treatment for substance use
        disorders, 206
phobia, specific, 132
phobic neurosis, 129
physical exam
    patient with MDD, 87
physioneurosis, 174
pica, 294
pleiotropy, phenomenon of, 4
pluripotent stem cells (iPSCs),
    12
polygenic complex disorders, 4
polygenic risk score (PRS), 17
polysubstance use, 197
population-based care
    and mental illness, 434
population growth, US, 2

positive valence systems, 6
positron emission tomography (PET), 23
post-traumatic stress disorder (PTSD), 129, 167, 168–169, 174, 175
children and, 324
course of, 169
evaluation of patient with, 170–171
prevention of, 171–172
self-assessment questions and, 177–178
treatment of, 172–174
victims of domestic violence and, 57
potentiation of glycine, 179
potentiation of inhibitory GABA$_A$, 179
pre-menstrual dysphoric disorder (PMDD), 81
psychotic symptoms and, 82
prescription amphetamines, 181
prescription opioid, 192
prescription stimulant, 184
present illness
history of, 45, 117, 298, 416, 417
primary care
and integration with behavioral health care, 3–4
behavioral health integration and, 432–433
primary care provider (PCP) and, 3
Prion diseases, 271
progressive cognitive deficits treatment of, 373–374
Prolonged Exposure Therapy (PE), 172
prophylactic treatment long-term, 367–368
protein-coding sequence of DNA (exons), 14
psychiatric assessment
goals of a write-up, 43–44
outline of, 44–50
writing up the, 43–44
psychiatric care
inadequate access to, 477–478
psychiatric conditions

and stigma associated with, 7
psychiatric consultation, **423**, 436
and diagnoses, 430–431
approach to assessment, 422–423
periodic follow-up, 428
psychiatric disorders
early onset of, 2
genetics and, 4, 12–13
hereditability/heritability and, 4, 12–13
prevalence of, 1–2
prevalence of, in the United States, 140
psychiatric diagnosis and suicide, 52
psychotic symptoms and, 115
recategorizing, 10
spectrum disorders and, 5
transdiagnostic approach and, 6
understanding pathophysiology of, 9
psychiatric emergencies
self-assessment questions, 446–447
psychiatric evaluation
interview process, 416–417
note of, 427
psychiatric genetics, 4–5, 18–19
and rare variants, 13–14
research, 4
Psychiatric Genomics Consortium, 16
psychiatric illness
past history of, 45–46
pathophysiology of, 25
present, 45
psychiatric interview. *See* patient interview
psychiatric symptoms and disorders
scientific understanding of, 6
psychiatrists, practicing decreasing numbers of, 2
psychiatry
clinical, 9
consultation liaison, 422
current and future directions of, 384–387

emergency, 415–416
emergency and focused medical assessment and, 419
emergency safety risk assessment and, 418–419
emergency valuation domains, **417**
emergency, patient history and physical examination, 419–420
ethical issues and, 32–35
gender identity and sexual orientation and, 456–458
neuroscience and, 9
psychiatric examination, 427
psychiatric symptoms, **420**, **421**
scientific basis of, 4–5
psychoanalysis, 10, 391–392
process, 392–393
psychoeducation, 395
psychoeducational and counseling therapies, 216
psychoneuroendocrinology, 26
psychoneuroimmunogical mechanisms, 409
psychopharmacologic treatments, 320
psychosis
acute, 121–122
clinical examination and, 117–118
initial medial work-up, **119**
laboratory investigation and, 118
medical conditions associated with, **116**
post-psychotic phase of, 121–122
psychotic symptoms and, 117
psychosis diagnosis, 115–117
psychosomatic medicine, 422
psychostimulants, 376–377
psychotherapy, 87
and anxiety disorders, 138–139
discussion about, 389–390
evidence-based, 88
treatment for personality disorders, 238

psychotic disorders
  psychotic mood episodes, 95
  psychotic symptoms and, 52,
    64, 75
  psychotic symptoms in
    adolescents, 30
  schizophrenia and, 153
psychotic symptoms, in
  children, 324–326
psychosis
  phase-specific treatment
    goals and challenges, **120**
psychiatric emergency
  treatment settings, 422

rapid-acting antidepressants,
  352–353
reactive attachment disorder, 323
rebound syndromes, 191
recombination, 16
referring clinician, 428
reinforcement, 187
relapse prevention therapies,
  206
relaxation response (RR), 409
religious delusions, 113
repetition compulsion, 174
repetitive transcranial
  magnetic stimulation
  (rTMS), 157, 342, 380, 382
  efficacy of, 382–383
  safety and adverse effects
    of, 383
representative assessment
  outline of, 44–50
requesting physician
  speaking to, 423–427
Research Domain Criteria
  (RDoC) project, 6, 18, 33
  framework, 10–12
residential and inpatient
  treatment
    eating disorders and, 303–304
restless legs syndrome (RLS),
  333
restraining orders, 60
reuptake transporter, 22
rumination disorder, 290, 294
Rush, Benjamin, 9
Rx for Survival, Global Health
  Champions, 1

safety and respect, importance
  of, 42

Saunders, Cecily, 440
Saving Inventory-Revised
  measure, 155
schema-focused therapy (SFT),
  250
schizoaffective disorder, 96,
  104–105
  diagnostic criteria, **105**
schizoid personality disorder
  (SzPD), 242–243
schizophrenia, 95, 102–103
  advanced paternal age and,
    110
  burden of the illness, 108
  cannabis use and, 110
  classification of all spectrum
    disorders classification,
    102
  clinical features and course
    of, 111–113
  cognitive impairment and,
    272
  diagnosis of, 115–117
  diagnostic criteria, **103**
  early brain development,
    109–110
  electroconvulsive therapy
    (ECT) treatment for, 381
  etiological and
    pathophysiologic Insights,
    123–125
  evaluation of, 117–120
  excess dopamine and, 19
  family history and, 109
  future directions, 125–126
  hereditability/heritability
    and, 4
  life expectancy and, 402
  maintenance phase, 122–123
  neurocognitive testing, 119
  prevalence of, 108
  prodromal phase of, 121
  psychotic disorders and,
    153
  psychotic symptoms and, 95,
    111, 113
  risk factors for, 109–110
  self-assessment questions,
    126–127
  sex ratio, 110
  skill deficit remediation and,
    394
  socioeconomic status and,
    110

suicide risks and, 109
symptoms of, 113–115
treatment options and, 120
schizophreniform disorder, 106
schizotypal personality
  disorder, 102, 240,
    244–245
Schneider, Kurt, 113
school-based prevention
  programs, 228
Schou, Mogens, 364
SCOFF, 299
Screen, Assess and Refer (SAR)
  patients, 56
screening and assessment
  screening questions for
    domestic violence and,
      58–59
screening questions, 49, 199,
  299
  anxiety disorders and, 140
  substance use abuse and
    adolescents, 201
  violence risks and, 65
screening tools
  for adolescents at risk of
    substance use disorders,
      227
*Screening, Brief Intervention,
  and Referral to Treatment*
  (SBIRT), 406
seasonal pattern, 82, 94
  depression and, 77
secondary mood disorder, 95
secretion of antidiuretic
  hormone (SIADH), 365
sedative-hypnotics, 183
  detoxification from
    substance use, 206–207
selective mutism, 322
selective norepinephrine
  reuptake inhibitor (SNRIs),
    377
selective serotonin reuptake
  inhibitors (SSRIs), 19, 22,
    136, 305, 344
  and treating depression in
    children, 319
  antidepressants, 173
self-assessment questions
  clinical neurosciences, 36
  psychiatric emergencies and,
    446–447
  schizophrenia, 126–127

self-harm, 46, 57, 260
  in depressed patients, **78**
  intentional, 51, 52
  risk, 245
  risk of, 97
  safety evaluation, 418
self-report instruments
  OCRD assessment and,
    154–155
separation anxiety disorders
  and children, 322
serious mental illness,
    community-based
    programs for, 400–403
serotonin reuptake inhibitors
  (SRIs), 155
serotonin system, 22
serotonin-norepinephrine
    reuptake inhibitors
    (SNRIs), 19, 136, 173, 342,
    344, 346
sex assignment, 449
sexual dysfunctions, 136, 361,
    461–462
  alcohol use and, 179
  antidepressants and, 345,
    348, 351
  opioid use and, 180, 213
sexual orientation, 448,
    453–454
  diversity of, 454
shared psychotic disorder, 107
shift work sleep disorder
    (SWSD), 338
short-term antipsychotic
    treatment, 356–359
shut-in personality, 240
sickness behavior, 24
SIGECAPS, 74
siloed behavioral and physical
    health systems, 478–479
single nucleotide
    polymorphisms (SNPs), 4,
    15, 16, 123
singleton siblings, 12
skill deficit remediation, 394
skin picking disorder (SPD),
    146, 148, 155
  case example, 160
  Skin Picking Scale, 155
sleep apnea. *See* sleep
    disorders
sleep disorders, 329–338
  central sleep apnea, 338, 339

delayed sleep phase disorder
    (DSPD), 337
excessive daytime sleepiness,
    336
obstructive sleep apnea, 330
onset latency, *336*
self-assessment questions,
    340–341
sleep disturbances, 86
sleep-related breathing
    issues and, 338–339
SMART Recovery, 204, 216
smoking cessation, medication
    for, 181
social and developmental
    history, patients', 48
social anxiety disorder (SAD),
    133
  case examples, 143
  children and, 323
social phobia, 76, 133
social processes, systems for, 6
social rhythm therapy (IPSRT),
    98
SOCRATES (Stages of Change
    Readiness and Treatment
    Eagerness Scale), 205
somatic delusions, 113, 296
somatic symptom disorders,
    436–438
specific phobia, 132
  and children, 322
specified feeding or eating
    disorder (OSFED), 291
sperm, 183, 456
  copy number variations and,
    110
St. Christopher's Hospice, 440
stepped care, 435–436
steroids, anabolic-androgenic,
    183
Stevens, Nettie, 456
Stevens-Johnson Syndrome,
    365
stimulants/stimulant use,
    181–182, 193
stimulus control techniques,
    156, 331, 395, 397
stress and trauma-related
    disorders, 166–168
structural and functional MRI, 5
Structured Clinical Interview
    for DSM Axis I Disorders
    (SCID), 134

Substance Abuse and Mental
    Health Services Agency
    (SAMHSA), 199
substance abuse disorders. *See*
    substance use disorders
substance intoxication, 195
substance use disorders, 2,
    179, 352, 396
  abstinence syndromes and,
    190
  abuse history of, 46–47
  acute intoxication and, 190
  acute opioid intoxication,
    196
  acute syndromes and, 195–197
  agent, 187
  alcohol use and, 191
  assessment of substance use
    patterns and, 222
  cannabis use and, 192
  clinical evaluation and, 194
  clinical features of, 189–190
  cocaine and, 193
  consequences of substance
    use and, 222
  controllability, 222–223
  core features of, 190
  course of illness, 193–194
  CRAFFT screening of
    adolescents, 201–203
  diagnosis and, 194
  environmental factors and,
    188–189
  epidemiology of, 184–185
  epigenetic factors and, 194
  etiology of, 185
  hallucinogens, 193
  hereditary and, 185–187
  history of, 222
  host, 185–187
  individual protective factors
    and, 194
  individual risk factors and,
    194
  medical advice and, 204–205
  office-based detection
    screening, 198–201
  opioid use and, 192
  other mental illnesses and,
    184
  patient readiness to change,
    205–206
  pharmacotherapy treatment
    options for, 206

physical examination and biomarkers and, 191
polysubstance use, 197
prevention and early intervention in children, 227
reinforcement and, 187
safety issues and, 189
schizotypal personality disorder and, 244
screening of adolescents, 201
screening of pregnant women, 201
statistics for, 184–185
stimulant use and, 193
synthetic drug use and, 193
tobacco use and, 191
treatment options, 193, 206–207
substance use screening process
biomarkers and immunoassay, 203–204
suicide/suicidality
aborted/interrupted attempts, 51
alcohol use disorders and, 184
assessment of suicidality/ suicidal thoughts, 50, 53–54, 55
avoidant personality disorder (AVPD) and risk of, 255
bipolar disorder and, 94
historical risk factors for, 52
interview elements, 55–56
major depression and, 77–79
mental illnesses and, 2
mitigating factors for suicidality/suicidal thoughts, 54
risk factors, 51–53
schizophrenia and, 109
suicidal thoughts, 53, 349
suicidal thoughts and, 46, 87
young adults and, 2
supported employment, 402
synaptic cleft, 19, 20, 21, 23, 376
synaptic plasticity, 20
synthetic cathinones, 181
synthetic drug use, 193

systemic illnesses, 95
systems for social processes, 6
Systems Training for Emotional Predictability and Problem Solving (STEPPS), 250

tai chi, 408, 410
task sharing, and mental health care, 489–491
telehealth, 480
telepsychiatry, 3
therapeutic alliance
and the patient interview process, 39–40
Thorndike, Edward L., 456
tic disorders, 152
tobacco/tobacco use, 180–181, 191
long-term effects of, 180
short-term effects of, 180
topiramate, 305, 306
treatment for alcohol use disorders, 210
transcendental meditation (TM), 408
transcranial direct current stimulation (tDCS), 383
transcranial magnetic stimulations (TMS), 156, 389
transdiagnostic approach and psychiatric disorders, 6
transference focused psychotherapy (TFP), 250, 254
transgender, 451–452, 453, 458, 461, See also LGBTQ
identity case conceptualization and recommendations for treatment, 468–469
identity development and, 467–468
in the DSM-III, 460
psychiatric stigma for, 460
psychological evaluation of, 464–465
self-assessment questions, 471–472
social needs of, 464
transsexualism as a disorder, 460
women, 454

Transtheoretical Stages-of-Change Model, 205
trauma, 166
definition of reactions to, 166
definition of traumatic events, 166
epidemiology and impact of traumatic events, 167
exposure to traumatic events, 166
history of, 47
stress-related disorders and, 166–168
trauma and stressor-related disorders, children and, 323–326
Trauma History Questionnaire, 171
traumatic brain injury, 263, 270
traumatic events and, 47
traumatic events and hair pulling, 150
traumatic neurosis, 174
treatment
Alzheimer's disease (AD), 283
bipolar disorders, 97–98, 367
borderline personality disorder (BPD), 249–251
histrionic personality disorder (HPD), 252–253
major or mild NCD and, 276
narcissistic personality disorder (NPD), 253–254
new treatments for dementia, 375
obsessive-compulsive disorders, 155–156
obsessive-compulsive personality disorder (OCPD), 257
of mania in children, 320
paranoid personality disorder (PPD), 243
schizotypal personality disorder, 244–245
treatment plan, patients', 50
triage
emergency psychiatry and, 415
patients with psychiatric symptoms, **416**
trinucleotide repeats, 14

twin studies/twins, 12–13, 19,
  186
  monozygotic and dizygotic,
    12–13

unipolar depression, 98, 99
  antidepressants use and,
    367
  children and, 321
  differentiating from bipolar
    depression, 95
  genetics and, 97
  major depressive disorder
    and, 89
  neuroimaging and, 99
  suicide and, 52
United States
  cigarette smoking in, 180
  employer-sponsored health
    insurance in, 474
  health care system, 283,
    473–474, 479, 482
  population and mental
    health indicators, 476
  sources of health insurance
    coverage, 474
  universal health care
    coverage and, 473
United States Census Bureau, 2
United States military, heroin
  use and, 188

universal health insurance
    coverage
  in the United States, 473
Unützer, Jürgen, 479
urine toxicology, 193, 196
  cannabinoids users and, 192
  cocaine use and, 196
  drug abuse screening and,
    421
  opioid use and, 192
US Department of Health and
    Human Services, 478
US Food and Drug
    Administration (FDA), 342

vagus nerve stimulation (VNS),
    383–384, 389
valproic acid, 98, 365
varenicline, 372–373
vascular neurocognitive
    disorders (VNCD), 269
Vietnam War, 188
violence
  clinical risk factors and,
    63–64
  mental illness patients and,
    62–63
  neurologic impairment and
    the risk for violence, 64
  risk factors for, 63
  sample questions, 65–66

  treatments and
    interventions, 66
  violence risk assessment,
    64–65, 66

Wernicke, Karl, 9
withdrawal seizures, and
    alcohol, 179
withdrawal syndromes, 190,
    206, 379–380, 417
  stabilization of, 197–198
World Health Organization
    (WHO), 109, 184, 486
  and the Mental Health Gap
    program, 490
World Professional Association
    for Transgender Health
    (WPATH), 464

Yale-Brown Obsessive-
    Compulsive Scale, 154
Yogi, Maharishi Mahesh, 409
young adults
  anorexia nervosa (AN) and,
    303
  delayed circadian phase and,
    337
  social anxiety disorder
    (SAD) and, 323
  suicide and, 2, 136, 173,
    349